Lecture Notes in Statistics 179

Edited by P. Bickel, P. Diggle, S. Fienberg, U. Gather, I. Olkin, and S. Zeger

D.Y. Lin   P.J. Heagerty

Editors

Proceedings of the Second Seattle Symposium in Biostatistics

Analysis of Correlated Data

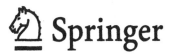 Springer

D.Y. Lin
School of Public Health
Department of Biostatistics, CB #7420
University of North Carolina
Chapel Hill, NC 27599-7420
USA
lin@bios.unc.edu

P.J. Heagerty
School of Public Health and Community
Medicine
Department of Biostatistics, Box 357232
University of Washington
Seattle, WA 98195
heagerty@biostat.washington.edu

Library of Congress Cataloging-in-Publication Data
Seattle Symposium in Biostatistics: Analysis of Correlated Data (2nd :
2000 : Seattle, Wash.)
    Proceeding of the second Seattle Symposium in Biostatistics : analysis
of correlated data / edited by D.Y. Lin, P.J. Heagerty.
        p. cm. — (Lecture notes in statistics, (Springer-Verlag) ; v.
179)
    Includes bibliographical references (p.   ).
    1. Biometry—Congresses.   I. Lin, D. Y. (Danyu Y.)   II. Heagerty, P. J.
III. Title.   IV. Series.
    QH323.5.S425   2000
    570′.1′5195—dc22   2004052209

ISBN 0-387-20862-3   Printed on acid-free paper.

Printed in the United States of America.   (SBA)

9 8 7 6 5 4 3 2 1   SPIN 10963296

springeronline.com

Contents

Preface

Preface

The First Seattle Symposium in Biostatistics: Survival Analysis was held on November 20 and 21, 1995 in honor of the twenty-fifth anniversary of the University of Washington (UW) School of Public Health and Community Medicine. The event was a big success. Exactly 5 years later, the *Second Seattle Symposium in Biostatistics: Analysis of Correlated Data* was held on November 20 and 21, 2000, and it was also very successful. The event was sponsored by Pfizer and co-sponsored by the UW School of Public Health and Community Medicine and the Division of Public Health Sciences, the Fred Hutchinson Cancer Research Center (FHCRC). The symposium featured keynote lectures by Norman Breslow, David Cox and Ross Prentice, as well as invited talks by Raymond Carroll, Peter Diggle, Susan Ellenberg, Ziding Fan, Mitchell Gail, Stephen Lagakos, Nan Laird, Kung-Yee Liang, Roderick Little, Thoms Louis, David Oakes, Robert O'Neill, James Robins, Bruce Turnbull, Mei-Cheng Wang and Jon Wellner. There were 336 attendees. In addition, 100 people attended the short course *Analysis of Longitudinal Data* taught by Patrick Heagerty and Scott Zeger on November 18, and 96 attended the short course *Analysis of Multivariate Failure Time Data* taught by Danyu Lin, Lee-Jen Wei and Zhiliang Ying on November 19.

When the UW School of Public Health and Community Medicine was formed in 1970, biostatistics as a discipline was only a few years old. In the subsequent thirty years, both the field and the UW Department of Biostatistics have evolved in many exciting ways. The Department had only seven faculty when it moved from the School of Medicine to the new School of Public Health and Community Medicine in 1970. The faculty roster currently lists 43 regular and research faculty and 34 adjunct and affiliate faculty. Ed Perrin was the Department Chair in 1970, succeeded by Donovan Thompson, Norman Breslow and presently Thomas Fleming. The faculty have been actively involved in methodological and collaborative research in addition to graduate teaching. The choice of *Analysis of Correlated Data* as the theme for the *Second Seattle Symposium in Biostatistics* was a tribute to the significant contributions made by the UW and FHCRC faculty to this important area of statistical science.

The Symposium Organizing Committee consisted of Thomas Fleming, Patrick Heagerty, Gordon Lan, Danyu Lin (Chair), Art Peterson and Lianng Yuh. The staff of the Biostatistics Department, including Diane Ames, David Fetrow, Michael Heroux, Barbara Jensen, Cynthia Marks, Alexandra MacKenzie, Jamie Miller, Rachel Rodke, Elaine Riot, Lian Schmidt and Eleanor Schweihs, provided great administrative support to the symposium. The UW President Richard McCormick, the School Dean Patricia Wahl, and the Department Chair Thomas Fleming delivered the opening remarks. The scientific sessions were chaired by Norman Breslow, Patrick Heagerty, Gordon Lan, Danyu Lin, Yasuo Ohashi, Masahiro Takeuchi and Elizabeth Thompson. We are grateful to the aforementioned people as well as all the speakers and participants for making the symposium a great success.

This volume contains most of the papers presented at the symposium. These papers encompass recent methodological advances on several important topics, such as longitudinal data, multivariate failure time data and genetic data, as well as innovative applications of the existing theory and methods. This collection serves as a reference for those working in the area of correlated data analysis.

Each of the 11 papers in this volume was refereed by two peer reviewers, and their comments were incorporated by the authors into the final versions of the papers. The referees are listed at the end of this book. We are indebted to them for their time and efforts. We also appreciate the guidance and assistance by John Kimmel of Springer-Verlag as well as the secretarial support by April Smyth and Pete Mesling during the preparation of this volume.

Finally, we would like to acknowledge the scientific and financial contributions by Pfizer. Without their generous support, it would have been impossible to hold this symposium.

D. Y. Lin
P. J. Heagerty

Whither PQL?

Norman Breslow

Department of Biostatistics, University of Washington

ABSTRACT Generalized linear mixed models (GLMM) are generalized linear models with normally distributed random effects in the linear predictor. Penalized quasi-likelihood (PQL), an approximate method of inference in GLMMs, involves repeated fitting of linear mixed models with "working" dependent variables and iterative weights that depend on parameter estimates from the previous cycle of iteration. The generality of PQL, and its implementation in commercially available software, has encouraged the application of GLMMs in many scientific fields. Caution is needed, however, since PQL may sometimes yield badly biased estimates of variance components, especially with binary outcomes.

Recent developments in numerical integration, including adaptive Gaussian quadrature, higher order Laplace expansions, stochastic integration and Markov chain Monte Carlo (MCMC) algorithms, provide attractive alternatives to PQL for approximate likelihood inference in GLMMs. Analyses of some well known datasets, and simulations based on these analyses, suggest that PQL still performs remarkably well in comparison with more elaborate procedures in many practical situations. Adaptive Gaussian quadrature is a viable alternative for nested designs where the numerical integration is limited to a small number of dimensions. Higher order Laplace approximations hold the promise of accurate inference more generally. MCMC is likely the method of choice for the most complex problems that involve high dimensional integrals

1 Introduction

Penalized Quasi-Likelihood is a technique for approximate inference in GLMMs and is not a rigorous statistical method in its own right.[33, p. 390, emphasis added]

The generalized linear model or GLM [35] is a prime tool of the applied statistician. It brings the power and flexibility of linear regression modeling to the analysis of data with outcomes, particularly discrete outcomes, that do not satisfy the conventional assumptions of least squares. The linear mixed model or LMM, with its multiple levels of random variation and best linear unbiased prediction of random effects [19], dominates statistical theory and applications in diverse fields including animal breeding and education. During the past decade these two models have been fused into a hybrid body of statistical theory and methodology known as the generalized linear mixed model or GLMM.[46, 40, 5, 49, 12, 31, 16, 29, 30] An even more general formulation, known as the hierarchical generalized linear model or HGLM, encompasses both normal and non-normal probability distributions for the random effects.[22, 23]

GLM and LMM parameter estimates are obtained from estimating equations that are unbiased under simple moment conditions and that may be solved by iterative solution of systems of linear equations. For the GLMM, by contrast, the specification of normally distributed random effects intrinsically defines the marginal likelihood and its logarithmic derivatives. The fact that the integrals in the GLMM estimating equations cannot be evaluated in closed form has seriously limited GLMM applications. Until recently the only available commercial software was the EGRET program [9] that implemented the logistic-normal model for clustered binary outcomes, unit level covariates and a cluster level random intercept. Thus substantial interest was generated by the work of Schall [40], Breslow and Clayton [5], Wolfinger [48] and others who developed a general approach to approximate inference. Their "penalized quasi-likelihood" or PQL procedure involved repeated fitting of the LMM using a working outcome variable and iterative weights that mimicked the standard iterative least squares algorithm used to fit the GLM.[28, §2.5] It was disseminated in macros written for several commercially distributed LMM programs: the GLIMMIX macro for PROC MIXED in SAS [26]; the PQL option for MLwiN [37]; and the HLM series distributed by SSI [38]. The IR-REML macro in GENSTAT [32] facilitated fitting of both GLMMs and HGLMs. This stimulated increasing use of these procedures in old disciplines such as sociology, where hierarchical models were already familiar, and in new ones like epidemiology [17], where they were just being discovered.

As usual when software for complicated statistical inference procedures is broadly disseminated, there is potential for abuse and misinterpretation. In spite of the fact that PQL was initially advertised as a procedure for *approximate* inference in GLMMs, and its tendency to give seriously biased estimates of variance components and *a fortiori* regression parameters with binary outcome data was emphasized in multiple publications [5, 6, 24], some statisticians seemed to ignore these warnings and to think of PQL as synonymous with GLMM.[7] In an apparent reaction to these developments, and to the algorithm's acknowledged shortcomings for binary outcome data, the authors of one recent textbook have recommended that PQL "not be used in practice".[30, p.234]

The purpose of this review is to take stock of PQL as a tool of the applied statistician now that some years have passed since it was first implemented in commercial software. In the interim, substantial advances have taken place in statistical computing. "True" maximum likelihood (ML) estimation is now available for a much wider range of problems by using numerical integration to calculate marginal likelihoods and solve score equations. In particular, the adaptive Gaussian quadrature methods [27, 36] implemented in SAS PROC NLMIXED [45] apply to clustered data problems where the dimensionality of the required integrations is in the low single digits. Higher order Laplace approximations [39], implemented for the logistic-normal model in the latest HLM program [38], may prove to be just as accurate as quadrature and more widely applicable.

Recent Monte Carlo approaches to numerical integration include Monte Carlo relative likelihood [13], Monte Carlo EM [29, 3] and Monte Carlo Newton-Raphson [20]. Kuk and Cheng [21] provide an excellent, comprehensive review of these stochastic procedures. Their use in practice to date has been limited by their longer computing times and the fact that none have yet been implemented in standard software packages. Booth and Hobert [3] argue that their "automated" Monte Carlo EM algorithm is an improvement on the Markov chain Monte Carlo (MCMC) version. It facilitates assessment of convergence and thus removes one of the main impediments to commercial implementation. Hierarchical Bayes procedures, which also depend on MCMC to evaluate posterior distributions, have been implemented in available, supported software and are increasingly used in applications. [8, 44, 34] These Monte Carlo methods will undoubtedly see much greater use with continuing improvements in computing technology. In view of their greater complexity, however, and the desire to keep this review focussed on the most immediate competitors to PQL, further discussion of Monte Carlo methods is left to investigators who are more familiar with their properties. Comparisons with the "h-likelihood" methodology of Lee and Nelder [22, 23] for inference in HGLMs also have been left for others.

2 GLMMs and PQL

The GLMM is a model for the hierarchical regression analysis of a series of n univariate response measurements y_i on p-dimensional covariates x_i associated with fixed effects and q-dimensional covariates z_i associated with random effects of interest $(i = 1, \ldots, n)$. Conditional on the unobserved values of a q-vector b of random effects, and on all the covariates, the y_i are assumed to be independent observations with means and variances specified by a GLM.[28] Specifically we suppose

$$E(y_i|b) = \mu_i^b = h(\eta_i^b) = h(x_i^T \alpha + z_i^T b)$$

$$\mathrm{Var}(y_i|b) = \frac{\phi}{a_i} v(\mu_i^b)$$

where $g = h^{-1}$ is the link function that relates the conditional means μ_i^b to the linear predictors η_i^b; $v(\cdot)$ is the variance function that relates the conditional means and variances to each another; ϕ is a scale factor assumed equal to one for the standard binomial and Poisson models; and a_i is a prior weight such as a binomial denominator. Specification of the model is completed by the assumption that b follows a q-dimensional normal distribution with mean 0 and variance matrix $D(\theta)$ depending on a vector of dispersion parameters θ. Examples of typical GLMM applications are considered in Sections 4 and 5.

The objective function for estimation of the GLMM parameters is the integrated quasi-likelihood $L(\alpha, \theta)$ given by

$$L = \frac{1}{\sqrt{(2\pi)^q |D(\theta)|}} \int_{R^q} \exp\left[-\frac{1}{2\phi}\sum_{i=1}^n d_i(y_i, \mu_i^b) - \frac{1}{2}b^T D^{-1}(\theta)b\right] db \quad (1)$$

where

$$d_i(y, \mu) = -2a_i \int_y^\mu \frac{y - u}{v(u)} du$$

denotes the weighted deviance.[28] If Y is Gaussian and $g(\cdot)$ the identity, the integral in (1) is normal and may be evaluated in closed form. Otherwise, maximization of this expression is intrinsically complicated by the integrations that must be performed numerically at each cycle of iteration. One approach to the integration, which eventually leads to the PQL algorithm, is to make a Laplace approximation. The term in square brackets in (1), the logarithm of the "penalized quasi-likelihood", is replaced by its quadratic expansion in b about the value $\tilde{b}$ at which it is maximized. Components of $\tilde{b}$ serve as predictors of the random effects. After some adjustments to the resulting normal integral, application of Fisher scoring to determine $(\hat{\alpha}, \tilde{b})$ as a function of θ leads to the familiar mixed model equations for joint estimation of fixed and random effects, as originally derived by Henderson [19], but now involving a working vector Y^* and iterative weights w_i. Further approximations lead to the standard REML equations for θ. Specifically, with $\hat{\mu}_i^b = h(x_i^T \hat{\alpha} + z_i^T \tilde{b})$,

$$Y_i^* = x_i^T \hat{\alpha} + z_i^T \tilde{b} + (y_i - \hat{\mu}_i^b)g'(\hat{\mu}_i^b)$$

and

$$w_i = \phi a_i [g'(\hat{\mu}_i^b)]^2 v(\hat{\mu}_i^b)^{-1},$$

the algorithm repeatedly applies mixed model REML estimation to the normal theory problem

$$Y^* = X\alpha + Zb + \varepsilon, \ b \sim \mathcal{N}(0, D(\theta)), \ \varepsilon \sim \mathcal{N}(0, W^{-1})$$

where $W=\text{diag}(w_i)$. See Breslow and Clayton [5] for details.

Although PQL yields REML estimates of variance components and regression coefficients in the Gaussian linear case, in general it only provides an approximation to these quantities. For the simplest GLMM involving clustered data with a single dispersion component θ, Breslow and Lin [6] expanded both the efficient score based on the true profile log-likelihood function, and the PQL variance estimating equation, in Taylor series about $\theta = 0$. They thereby showed that the asymptotic bias in the PQL estimator $\hat{\theta}_{\text{p}}$ was a nearly linear function of θ in a neighborhood of the origin. By determining the slope of this linear relationship, which is estimable from the standard GLM fit assuming $\theta = 0$, they derived a correction factor for $\hat{\theta}_{\text{p}}$ that removed the asymptotic bias for small θ at the cost of some increase in variability. Lin and Breslow [24] extended this work for models with multiple variance components, deriving a matrix correction factor, and termed the resulting procedure corrected PQL or CPQL.

An alternative derivation of the PQL algorithm developed by Schall [40] and others uses a linearization of the conditional mean as a function of fixed and random effects. Consider, for example, the two-level model with I clusters having n_i observations per cluster, $i = 1, \ldots, I$, and random effects b_i assumed independent between clusters. The jth observation in cluster i may be written

$$y_{ij} = \mu_{ij}^b + \varepsilon_{ij} = h(x_{ij}^T\alpha + z_{ij}^T b_i) + \varepsilon_{ij}$$

with $\text{var}(\varepsilon_{ij}) = \phi v(\mu_{ij}^b)/a_i$, $j = 1, \ldots, n_i$. Expanding h about the current estimates $(\hat{\alpha}, \bar{b})$ based on the current $\hat{\theta}$ gives

$$y_{ij} \approx \hat{\mu}_{ij}^b + h'(\hat{\eta}_{ij}^b)[x_{ij}^T(\alpha - \hat{\alpha}) + z_{ij}^T(b_i - \bar{b}_i)] + \varepsilon_{ij} \qquad (2)$$

which implies that the "working" observation $Y_{ij}^* = \hat{\eta}_{ij}^b + g'(\hat{\mu}_{ij}^b)(y_{ij} - \hat{\mu}_{ij}^b)$ satisfies

$$Y_{ij}^* = x_{ij}^T\alpha + z_{ij}^T b_i + \varepsilon_{ij}^* \qquad (3)$$

where, at least to an approximation for the ε_{ij}^*,

$$b_i \sim \mathcal{N}(0, D(\theta)) \quad \text{and} \quad \varepsilon_{ij}^* \sim \mathcal{N}\left(0, \phi[g'(\hat{\mu}_{ij}^b)]^2 v(\hat{\mu}_{ij}^b)/a_i\right). \qquad (4)$$

Updated estimates of (α, b, θ) are obtained by solving for them in the LMM defined by (3) and (4), i.e., by using the PQL algorithm.

A further expansion of the conditional mean in terms involving b_i alone adds $\frac{1}{2}h''(\hat{\eta}_{ij}^b)z_{ij}^T(b_i - \hat{b}_i)(b_i - \hat{b}_i)^T z_{ij}$ to the right hand side of (2). Goldstein and Rasbash [14, 16, 15] suggested that one ignore the cross-products involving different components of b_i, add the mean values of the resulting quadratic terms as offsets to the regression model and treat their residuals as additional random error terms with known variance. This modified procedure, implemented as PQL2 in MLwiN [37], is also intended to improve the estimates of variance components.

3 Adaptive Gauss-Hermite Quadrature

Consider the two-level GLMM with I independent clusters of observations $\{y_{ij}, \; j = 1, \ldots, n_i\}, \; i = 1, \ldots, I$ and a random intercept so that

$$\mu_{ij}^b = E(y_{ij}|b_i) = h(x_{ij}^T \alpha + b_i), \quad b_i \overset{i.i.d}{\sim} \mathcal{N}(0, \theta).$$

To simplify matters , suppose $g = h^{-1}$ is the canonical link function so that $v(\mu) = [g'(\mu)]^{-1}$ and furthermore that the scale factor and prior weights are all unity. This setup applies, for example, to two-level log-linear modeling of Poisson data and to logistic regression for clustered binary outcome data. The contribution to the marginal likelihood (integrated quasi-likelihood) for the ith cluster is

$$L_i = \frac{1}{\sqrt{2\pi\theta}} \int L_i^c(b) e^{-\frac{b^2}{2\theta}} db$$
$$= E_{\mathcal{N}(0,\theta)} L_i^c(b) \tag{5}$$

where $E_{\mathcal{N}(\mu,\theta)}$ denotes expectation with respect to the $\mathcal{N}(\mu, \theta)$ distribution and L_i^c is the conditional quasi-likelihood contribution

$$L_i^c(b) = \exp\{-\frac{1}{2} \sum_{j=1}^{n_i} d_{ij}(y_{ij}, \mu_{ij}^b)\}.$$

Ordinary Gauss-Hermite quadrature approximates the integral in (5) with the sum

$$L_i \simeq \frac{1}{\sqrt{\pi}} \sum_{r=1}^{R} w_r L_i^c(\sqrt{2\theta} t_r)$$

where the t_r are the R quadrature points, roots of the R-degree Hermite polynomial, and the w_r denote the associated weights.[11, p. 924] The problem with this approach is that the same quadrature points are used for each cluster, irrespective of the cluster outcomes. Thus, for some i, the conditional quasi-likelihoods $L_i^c(b)$ may take large values for b well outside the range covered by the points $\{\sqrt{2\theta} t_r, \; r = 1, \ldots, R\}$.

Let $\phi(b; \mu, \sigma^2)$ denote the density of the normal distribution with mean μ and variance σ^2. The basic idea behind adaptive quadrature as introduced by Liu and Pierce [27] is the same one that underlies the Laplace integral approximation, namely, to determine the normal density $\phi(b; \bar{b}_i, \bar{\sigma}_i^2)$ that best approximates the entire integrand $L_i^c(b)\phi(b; 0, \theta)$ in (5). The value that maximizes the integrand, $\bar{b}_i$, is obtained as the solution (in b) to $\sum_j(y_{ij} - \mu_{ij}^b) + b/\theta = 0$. The curvature in the log integrand at its maximum is the inverse of $\bar{\sigma}_i^2 = [\sum_j v(\mu_{ij}^{\bar{b}_i}) + \theta^{-1}]^{-1}$ [5, §2.1]. Once these are computed, the marginal likelihood contribution is approximated via

$$L_i = E_{\mathcal{N}(\bar{b}_i, \bar{\sigma}_i^2)} \left[\frac{L_i^c(b)\phi(b; 0, \theta)}{\phi(b; \bar{b}_i, \bar{\sigma}_i^2)} \right]$$

$$\simeq \frac{1}{\sqrt{\pi}} \sum_{r=1}^R \omega_r \frac{L_i^c(\bar{b}_i + \sqrt{2}\bar{\sigma}_i t_r)\phi(\bar{b}_i + \sqrt{2}\bar{\sigma}_i t_r; 0, \theta)}{\phi(\bar{b}_i + \sqrt{2}\bar{\sigma}_i t_r; \bar{b}_i, \bar{\sigma}_i^2)}$$

$$= \sqrt{2}\bar{\sigma}_i \sum_{r=1}^R \omega_r e^{t_r^2} L_i^c(\bar{b}_i + \sqrt{2}\bar{\sigma}_i t_r)\phi(\bar{b}_i + \sqrt{2}\bar{\sigma}_i t_r; 0, \theta). \quad (6)$$

The Laplace approximation is given by (6) for $R = 1$, $\omega_1 = 1$ and $t_1 = 0$.

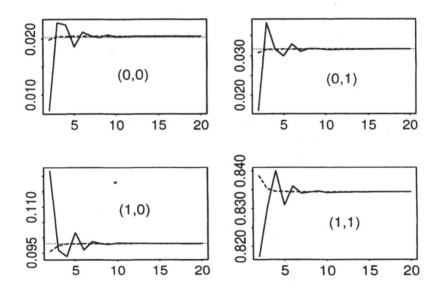

FIGURE 1. Marginal probabilities (ordinates) of each of four possible outcomes with matched pairs of binary outcome data estimated using standard (solid line) and adaptive (dashed line) Gauss-Hermite quadrature. The outcome vector is shown in the center of each panel. The abscissae show the number of quadrature points.

Use of standard and adaptive Gauss-Hermite quadrature to approximate the integrated likelihood is illustrated in Figure 1 for the special case of matched pairs of binary outcome data with a single binary covariate that varies within clusters. Defining $\text{expit}(x) = [1 + e^{-x}]^{-1}$, this model has $\mu_{i1}^b = \text{expit}(\alpha_0 + b_i)$, $\mu_{i2}^b = \text{expit}(\alpha_0 + \alpha_1 + b_i)$ and $v(\mu) = \mu(1 - \mu)$. The parameter values used were $\alpha_0 = 4$, $\alpha_1 = -2$ and $\theta = 4$. The four panels of the figure show plots of the approximated marginal probabilities of the four possible outcomes for (y_{i1}, y_{i2}), namely (0,0), (0,1), (1,0), and (1,1), as functions of the number R of quadrature points. Using the adaptive procedure, the integral approximations converged to the fourth decimal place with $R = 5$. By contrast, with the standard procedure, they continued to oscillate for R well beyond 5 .

Pinheiro and Bates [36] adapted this methodology for multidimensional integrals and their methods have been incorporated into PROC NLMIXED in SAS.[45] In the sequel we compare results using NLMIXED and GLIM-MIX, *i.e.*, using ML and PQL, with two well studied sets of data.

4 Meta Analysis of Clinical Trials Data

Our first example involves a series of 2×2 tables of counts of "successes" and "failures" among 293 patients distributed in treatment and control groups in eight clinical centers (Table 1). Introduced to statisticians by Beitler and

TABLE 1. Clinical trial of topical cream for infection

Center	Treatment	Response Success	Failure	Total patients	Success Rate (%)
1	Drug	11	25	36	30.6
	Control	10	27	37	27.0
2	Drug	16	4	20	80.0
	Control	22	10	32	68.8
3	Drug	14	5	19	73.7
	Control	7	12	19	36.8
4	Drug	2	14	16	12.5
	Control	1	16	17	5.9
5	Drug	6	11	17	35.3
	Control	0	12	12	0.0
6	Drug	1	10	11	9.1
	Control	0	10	10	0.0
7	Drug	1	4	5	20.0
	Control	1	8	9	11.1
8	Drug	4	2	6	66.7
	Control	6	1	7	85.7
Total	Drug	55	75	130	42.3
	Control	47	96	143	32.9

Source: Beitler and Landis [26]

Landis [2], these data have been widely used to illustrate different methods for mixed effects modeling of categorical data. The developers of GLIM-MIX, for example, noted that their macro converged more consistently if one first converted the table of counts to a series of binary outcome variables and covariates.[26, p. 440] The data also featured prominently in a recent review by Agresti and Hartzel [1] of methods for meta analysis of binary outcome data. The object of many of these analyses has been to estimate the clinic specific treatment effect, expressed as an odds ratio and assumed constant over clinics, while adjusting for clinic to clinic variation in baseline success rates via random effects modeling. There has also been interest in deciding whether there is evidence for treatment by center interaction.

Let y_{ij} denote the binary outcome (1 for success, 0 for failure) for the jth subject in the ith clinic. Suppose the covariate x_{ij} takes values $-\frac{1}{2}$ for control and $+\frac{1}{2}$ for treatment. This coding helps to orthogonalize the design matrix and render more plausible the implicit assumption of independence between random intercept and random slope (interaction) terms in what follows. Two models of interest are I: logit $\mathrm{E}(y_{ij}|b_i) = \alpha_0 + \alpha_1 x_{ij} + b_i^0$; and II: logit $\mathrm{E}(y_{ij}|b_i) = \alpha_0 + \alpha_1 x_{ij} + b_i^0 + b_i^1 x_{ij}$, the first corresponding to the hypothesis of constant odds ratio. The parameter of interest α_1 represents the *within clinic* log odds ratio comparing treatment and control groups. This is assumed constant across clinics in Model I but may vary by clinic in Model II. Tables 2 and 3 compare results obtained using four procedures for fitting GLMMs, including the PQL2 procedure mentioned at the end of §2. Also shown for Model I are results for the "exact" conditional maximum likelihood (CML) analysis, based on convolutions of the non-central hypergeometric distributions that arise when one conditions on all four marginal totals in each table. [10, §2.5] The analog for Model II is the GLMM that adds a random effect to the log odds ratio parameter in each non-central hypergeometric distribution. This may be fitted by PQL using methods previously described.[5, §6.4] Some notable features of

TABLE 2. Estimates ± standard errors for Model I

Method		α_0	α_1	θ_0
NLMIXED	(ML)	-0.828±0.533	0.739±0.300	1.96±1.19
GLIMMIX	(PQL)	-0.784±0.537	0.724±0.296	2.03±1.26
MLwiN	(PQL)	-0.784±0.537	0.724±0.296	2.03±1.19
MLwiN	(PQL2)	-0.789±0.606	0.859±0.310	2.56±1.46
Hypergeometric	(CML)		0.756±0.303	

this comparison include: (*i*) the lack of any suggestion for a treatment by clinic interaction; (*ii*) the excellent agreement between the estimates and standard errors obtained by ML (adaptive quadrature) and PQL, especially for the variance component of the random intercept; and (*iii*) the fact that the PQL2 results are substantially different from the others. Note that the standard errors of the variance components estimated by the GLIMMIX and MLwiN implementations of PQL differ slightly. Otherwise the results were identical.

TABLE 3. Estimates ± standard errors for Model II

Method	α_0	α_1	θ_0	θ_1
NLMIXED (ML)	-0.830±0.535	0.746±0.323	1.97±1.20	0.02±0.32
GLIMMIX (PQL)	-0.791±0.538	0.749±0.333	2.04±1.27	0.12±0.41
MLwiN (PQL)	-0.791±0.538	0.749±0.333	2.04±1.15	0.12±0.37
MLwiN (PQL2)	-0.870±0.614	0.830±0.367	2.61±1.46	0.20±0.45
Hypergeometric	(PQL)	0.793±0.352		0.16±0.48

Table 4 reports results of a small simulation study designed to evaluate more systematically the performance of PQL in this setting.[4] For each of 10,000 simulations, 8 pairs of independent binomial observations $r_{ij} \sim$ binom(p_{ij}, n_{ij}), $i = 1, \ldots, 8$, $j = 1, 2$ were drawn with denominators n_{ij} chosen equal to those in the penultimate column of Table 1. The GLMM was specified by logit $p_{ij} = \alpha_0 + \alpha_1(2x_{ij} - 1) + b_i^0 + b_{ij}^1$ where $b_i^0 \sim \mathcal{N}(0, \theta_0)$ and $b_{ij}^1 \sim \mathcal{N}(0, \theta_1/2)$ were mutually independent sets of random effects. Thus the b_i^0 were random clinic effects, with roughly the same amount of clinic-to-clinic variation as for the data in Table 1, while the differences between b_{ij}^1 for $j = 1$ and $j = 2$ represented the variation in treatment effects (log odds ratios). Parameter settings were $\alpha_0 = 0$, $\theta_0 = 2$, $\alpha_1 = 0, 1,$ 2 and $\theta_1 = \text{Var}(b_{i1}^1 - b_{i2}^1) = 0, 0.5, 1, 2$. $\bar{\alpha}_1$ and $\bar{\theta}_1$ refer to the averages of the estimates of these two parameters over the 10,000 replications. The error rates refer to the proportion of replicates for which the 95% confidence interval for α_1 excluded the true value on the left or the right side.

The simulated data were analyzed using PQL as described above for the log odds ratio GLMM based on the non-central hypergeometric distribution. As with any mixed model, there was a tendency to over-estimate slightly the small (or null) values of the variance component since negative estimates were not allowed. The systematic underestimation of variance components often observed with clustered binary data (see §6 below) was not a problem here, probably because of the relatively large denominators and mid-range values for many of the binomial observations. PQL estimates of the regression coefficient α_1 and of the larger values of the variance component were remarkably unbiased. Error rates for interval estimation were quite satisfactory. Not shown here are corresponding results for the empirical transform (ET) method, which consisted of applying ordinary LMM methods to derived outcome variables. The derived variable was the logarithm of the observed odds ratio in each table, with 0.5 added to both cells whenever any marginal total of success or failure was zero, so as to avoid infinities. Conditional on the random effects, this outcome variable was treated as normally distributed with variance equal to the in-

TABLE 4. Results of the simulation study of PQL

True values		Estimates		Error rates	
θ_1	α_1	$\bar{\theta}_1$	$\bar{\alpha}_1 - \alpha_1$	Left	Right
	0	0.15	0.000	0.015	0.016
0.0	1	0.16	0.015	0.012	0.017
	2	0.18	0.030	0.013	0.018
	0	0.58	0.002	0.032	0.027
0.5	1	0.58	0.013	0.029	0.033
	2	0.60	0.023	0.018	0.034
	0	1.05	-0.003	0.030	0.032
1.0	1	0.96	-0.012	0.027	0.035
	2	1.04	0.002	0.024	0.038
	0	2.00	-0.016	0.026	0.031
2.0	1	1.98	0.000	0.030	0.032
	2	1.99	-0.000	0.025	0.029

Source: Breslow, Leroux and Platt [4]

verse of the sum of reciprocals of the cell frequencies. The ET estimates of both the variance component and the regression coefficient were seriously biased towards zero, so that the random effect predictors were similarly misbehaved.[4, pp. 57-58] A similar tendency of ET to underestimate the variance component was observed for simulated Poisson observations representing spatially correlated rates when the mean rates were very small.[4, pp. 58-59] Thus the recent recommendation that ET methods be used in preference to PQL in such situations appears to be unfounded.[30, p. 283]

5 Longitudinal Series of Counts

Our second example involves a series of counts of seizures recorded by 59 patients with epilepsy for each of four two-week periods that preceded clinic visits. Introduced by Thall and Vail [47], these data also have been used by numerous statisticians to illustrate methods for analysis of longitudinal data with discrete outcomes. Figure 2 plots the patient trajectories of the log counts, augmented by 0.5 to avoid infinities. Each trajectory starts with the log of the baseline count over the eight-week period before the study, which was divided by four for comparability. Other fixed covariates of interest included a binary treatment indicator, the logarithm of age in years, and either a binary indicator for the fourth visit or the visit number j after division by ten.

With y_{ij} now denoting the seizure count reported at the jth visit by the ith patient, assumed to have a Poisson distribution after condition-

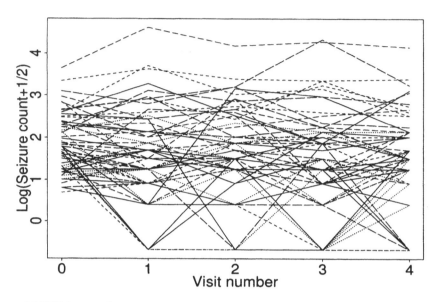

FIGURE 2. Epilepsy seizure counts at baseline and four follow-up periods.

TABLE 5. Estimates ± standard errors for Model III

Parameter	NLMIXED (ML)	GLIMMIX (PQL)	MLwiN (PQL)	MLwiN (PQL2)
	Regression coefficients			
Constant	-1.117±1.182	-1.256±1.220	-1.256±1.220	-1.335±1.239
Baseline*	0.884±0.131	0.872±0.136	0.872±0.136	0.881±0.138
Treatment	-0.933±0.401	-0.917±0.413	-0.917±0.413	-0.929±0.420
Bas*×Trt	0.338±0.203	0.331±0.210	0.331±0.210	0.336±0.213
Age*	0.484±0.347	0.472±0.358	0.472±0.359	0.481±0.364
Visit 4	-0.161±0.055	-0.161±0.055	-0.161±0.055	-0.161±0.055
	Variance component			
$\sqrt{\theta_0}$	0.503±0.059	0.524±0.062	0.524±0.059	0.529±0.060

* log transform

ing on the random effects, two models of interest were Model III: $\log \mathrm{E}(y_{ij}|b_i) = x_i^T \alpha + b_i^0$ and Model IV: $\log \mathrm{E}(y_{ij}|b_i) = x_i^T \alpha + b_i^0 + b_i^1 j/10$. Model IV was the more interesting in that it provided for a patient specific random slope and intercept, assumed to follow a bivariate normal distribution, to model the trends in the trajectories. Results of fitting these models using the NLMIXED and GLIMMIX procedures in SAS, and the PQL and PQL2 methods in MLwiN, are shown in Tables 5 and 6. There was remarkably good agreement in estimation of the regression coefficients and their standard errors. By contrast to the previous example, PQL2 produced regression coefficients slightly closer to those of ML than did PQL. The PQL2 estimates of the variance components, however, were slightly further from the ML estimates. The high (0.4 or so) within cluster (patient) correlation in the log epilepsy counts is reflected in the large, and highly statistically significant, estimates of variance components.

TABLE 6. Estimates ± standard errors for Model IV

Parameter	NLMIXED (ML)	GLIMMIX (PQL)	MLwiN (PQL)	MLwiN (PQL2)
		Regression coefficients		
Constant	-1.368±1.201	-1.267±1.215	-1.268±1.215	-1.361±1.241
Baseline*	0.885±0.131	0.870±0.135	0.870±0.135	0.882±0.138
Treatment	-0.929±0.402	-0.910±0.411	-0.910±0.411	-0.922±0.421
Bas*×Trt	0.338±0.204	0.330±0.209	0.330±0.209	0.335±0.214
Age*	0.477±0.354	0.463±0.357	0.463±0.357	0.472±0.364
Visit/10	-0.266±0.165	-0.264±0.157	-0.264±0.157	- 0.267±0.160
		Variance components		
$\sqrt{\theta_{00}}$	0.502±0.059	0.521±0.062	0.521±0.061	0.527±0.063
θ_{01}	0.003±0.089	0.002±0.090	0.002±0.088	0.005±0.091
$\sqrt{\theta_{11}}$	0.729±0.157	0.737±0.157	0.737±0.162	0.756±0.165

* log transform

6 Further Simulations with Binary Outcome Data

To further evaluate the bias of PQL estimates of variance components with binary outcome data, and assess the degree of correction afforded by CPQL, a new series of simulation experiments was run using a variant of a model originally proposed by Zeger and Karim [50] for clustered data. Each experiment involved K clusters of constant size n. Binary outcome variables y_{ij} for $i = 1, \ldots, K$ and $j = 1, \ldots, n$ were generated according to the hierarchical model

$$\text{logit}E(y_{ij}|b_i) = \alpha_0 + \alpha_1 t_{ij} + \alpha_2 x_i + \alpha_3 t_{ij} x_i + b_i,$$

where the t_{ij} were unit level covariates that were randomly generated from the uniform distribution on the interval $[-\frac{1}{2}, \frac{1}{2}]$, the x_i were subject level covariates of which the first half took the value 0 and the remainder the value 1, and the b_i were independent, normally distributed random effects with mean 0 and variance θ. The parameter values were $\alpha_0 = -0.5$, $\alpha_1 = 1$, $\alpha_2 = -1$, $\alpha_3 = 0.5$ and $\theta = 1$. The number K of clusters was 50 or 100 and the sample size n per cluster ranged between 2 and 40. Each experiment was replicated 200 times at each parameter setting.

The results in Figure 3 demonstrate the substantial bias in the PQL estimates. With matched pairs of binary outcome data, the true variance of the

FIGURE 3. Mean values of estimated variance component

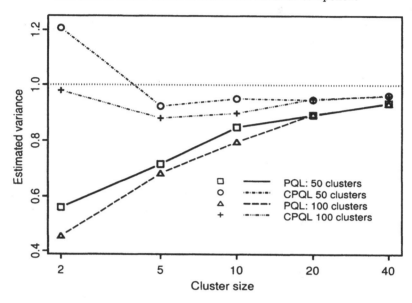

subject specific effects was underestimated by about a half.[6] Even with as many as 40 observations per cluster, the variance was still underestimated by 6%. The degree of bias was affected more by cluster size than by the number of clusters. Indeed, it was worse for $K = 100$ than for $K = 50$. When $\alpha_0 = -2.5$, the bias in $\hat{\theta}_p$ with $n = 40$ was closer to 10%.

CPQL substantially reduced the bias, overcorrecting with 50 clusters of size 2. However, the slow rates at which the averages of the PQL and CPQL estimates approached the true value 1 suggests that cluster sizes might need to be quite large to eliminate entirely the bias in the variance component. As noted previously [6, 24], the bias in the regression coefficients is unimportant once the variance components have been estimated correctly.

7 Higher Order Laplace Expansions

The integral in the expression (1) for the likelihood has dimensionality equal to the number of random effects and hence, for many problems of interest, increases with the sample size n. Shun and McCullagh [42] and Shun [41] noted that the standard Laplace approximation failed to have an asymptotic ($n \uparrow \infty$) justification in such circumstances, and derived a remainder term that improved its performance. Raudenbush, Yang and Yosef [39] developed a systematic approach to higher order Laplace expansions, and provided details for two-level models involving a series of clusters of independently distributed observations. Here we consider the simplest case, the GLMM with canonical link function where each cluster has a single random effect, in order to illustrate the potential of this approach.

Suppose then that the likelihood may be written

$$L(\alpha, \theta) = \prod_{i=1}^{K} L_i(\alpha, \theta) = \prod_{i=1}^{K} \frac{1}{\sqrt{2\pi}} \int \exp\left[\ell_i(\alpha, b_i) - \frac{1}{2\theta} b_i^2\right] db_i,$$

where K is the number of clusters, the b_i are K independently distributed random effects from a normal distribution with mean 0 and variance θ and the conditional log-likelihoods are

$$\ell_i(\alpha, b_i) = \frac{\phi}{a_i} \sum_{j=1}^{n_i} \{[y_{ij}\eta_{ij}^b - \delta(\eta_{ij}^b)] + \gamma(y_{ij}; \phi)\}$$

with $\eta_{ij}^b = x_{ij}^T \alpha + b_i$ denoting the linear predictor and n_i the number of observations in the ith cluster. Let $\bar{b}_i = \bar{b}_i(\alpha, \theta) = \arg\max[\ell_i(\alpha, b) - b^2/(2\theta)]$ denote the PQL estimate of the ith random effect and define

$$\bar{\ell}_i^{(k)} = \left(\frac{\partial}{\partial\beta}\right)^k \ell_i \Big|_{b=\bar{b}_i}$$

and

$$v_i = -\left[\bar{\ell}_i^{(2)} - \frac{1}{\theta}\right]^{-1} = \frac{\theta}{1 - \theta\bar{\ell}_i^{(2)}}.$$

Then, using a Taylor expansion,

$$L_i = \frac{e^{\bar{\ell}_i - \bar{b}_i^2/(2\theta)}}{\sqrt{2\pi\theta}} \int \exp\left[-\frac{1}{2v_i}(b - \bar{b}_i)^2 + R_i(b)\right] db,$$

where $R_i(b) = \sum_{k=3}^{\infty} T_{ki}(b)$ with $T_{ki}(b) = \bar{\ell}_i^{(k)}(b - \bar{b}_i)^k/k!$. It follows that

$$L_i = \sqrt{\frac{v_i}{\theta}} e^{\bar{\ell}_i - \bar{b}_i^2/(2\theta)} E_i\left[1 + R_i(b) + \frac{1}{2}R_i^2(b) + \frac{1}{3}R_i^3(b) + \cdots\right]$$

$$= \sqrt{\frac{v_i}{\theta}} e^{\bar{\ell}_i - \bar{b}_i^2/(2\theta)}\left[1 + E_i(T_{4i}) + E_i(T_{6i}) + \frac{1}{2}E_i(T_{3i}^2) + \cdots\right]$$

where $E_i = E_{\mathcal{N}(\bar{b}_i, v_i)}$ denotes expectation with respect to a normal distribution with mean $\bar{b}_i$ and variance v_i.

We evaluate the higher terms in this expansion, and note their asymptotic order in terms of $\theta \downarrow 0$ and the cluster-specific sample size $n \equiv n_i \uparrow \infty$:

$$E_i(T_{4i}) = \frac{\theta^2 \tilde{\ell}_i^{(4)}}{8[1 - \theta\tilde{\ell}_i^{(2)}]^2} = O(\theta^2) \times O\left(\frac{1}{n}\right)$$

$$E_i(T_{6i}) = \frac{\theta^3 \tilde{\ell}_i^{(6)}}{48[1 - \theta\tilde{\ell}_i^{(2)}]^3} = O(\theta^3) \times O\left(\frac{1}{n^2}\right)$$

$$\frac{1}{2}E_i(T_{3i}^2) = \frac{15\theta^3[\tilde{\ell}_i^{(3)}]^2}{72[1 - \theta\tilde{\ell}_i^{(2)}]^3} = O(\theta^3) \times O\left(\frac{1}{n}\right).$$

Quartic expansions, *i.e.*, those involving terms up to $E_i(T_{4i})$, were considered by several groups interested in approximations valid for small variance components. [43, 27, 6, 24] However, these are inadequate for larger values of θ no matter what the sample size in each cluster. Approximate inference based on terms up to sixth order, as shown, has been implemented for the logistic-normal model in version 5 of HLM.[38] Terms of all orders, for both univariate and multivariate normal random effects distributions, are available in principle.[39]

TABLE 7. Results of a simulation study of integral approximations

Para- meter	True value	PQL	GH-20	L-6
		Averages of estimates		
α_0	-1.200	-1.090	-1.205	-1.201
α_1	1.000	0.900	1.015	1.003
α_2	1.000	0.911	0.998	0.998
θ_{00}	1.625	1.275	1.655	1.635
θ_{01}	0.100	0.054	0.100	0.096
θ_{11}	0.250	0.161	0.256	0.267
		Mean squared errors		
α_0	-1.200	0.027	0.020	0.019
α_1	1.000	0.024	0.018	0.016
α_2	1.000	0.116	0.005	0.005
θ_{00}	1.625	0.152	0.063	0.056
θ_{01}	0.100	0.008	0.012	0.011
θ_{11}	0.250	0.113	0.007	0.008

Source: Raudenbush, Ying and Yosef [39]

Table 7 reports results of a simulation study of three estimators of paramaters in a logistic-normal random intercepts and slopes model with binary outcomes.[39] Here the $K=200$ clusters were intended to represent communities, in each of which $n = 20$ observations representing children were sampled. Both child and community level covariates were generated from normal distributions. The intercept (mean α_0) and slope (mean α_1) of the regression on the child level covariate were allowed to vary from community to community with variances θ_{00} and θ_{01}, respectively, and covariance θ_{01}. In addition to PQL, the estimation methods included 20 point Gauss-

Hermite quadrature using software developed by Hedeker and Gibbons [18] (GH-20) and the sixth order Laplace expansion as described above (L-6). Although the average estimation time for quadrature was substantially higher (720 seconds) than for the Laplace approximation (35 seconds), the latter method proved to be at least as accurate.

8 Conclusions

The implementation of the PQL algorithm in several commercial software packages has stimulated interest in the procedure and encouraged the use of GLMMs in a wide variety of scientific fields. This review was motivated by the desire to further evaluate the accuracy of the inferences that result from its use in settings that are typical of current practice.

PQL yields the standard REML estimates for normal theory, linear mixed models. In view of the correspondence between mixed models and smoothing splines, it therefore also provides correct inferences for normal theory, semiparametric linear mixed models where certain fixed covariate terms are replaced by nonparametric smooths.[25]

The illustrative analyses presented in §4 and §5, and simulations based on those analyses, suggest that PQL performs adequately for GLMMs with categorical outcomes provided that the nominally Poisson or binomial observations have distributions that are approximately Gaussian. Experience suggests that the algorithm provides reasonable approximations for Poisson outcomes provided that their means are generally greater than 5. An even lower cutoff may be adequate for many problems. With binomial outcomes, a rule of thumb might be that the expected numbers of "successes" and "failures" for each observation should also generally exceed 5. This means that the binomial denominators should be at least 10 for reponse probabilities in the midrange, with larger denominators needed if many of the probabilities were near 0 or 1. This is not all that different from standard guidelines for the practical adequacy of approximate inference procedures such as chi-squared tests for the analysis of contingency tables. However, one cannot hope to have a simple rule cover all contigencies.

For many of these situations where PQL performs well, application of the corresponding linear mixed model (LLM) to transformed outcome data likely will also be adequate. However, results [4] quoted at the end of §4 suggest that, for some sparse data situations, PQL will perform adequately whereas the empirical transform approach may not.

Where PQL has the greatest difficulty is for the analysis of binomial outcomes based on small denominators, especially binary outcomes. With clustered data, the critical feature is the number of conditionally independent binary observations per cluster. As the within cluster sample size increases, so does the information for prediction of the unobserved random effect. The within cluster sum of conditional deviances is then well approximated by a quadratic function of the random effect b, and the cluster's contribution to the likelihood (1) is well represented by its Laplace approximation. Lee and Nelder [22, 23] state asymptotic results that formalize this intuition.

As the simulations in §6 and similar evaluations by other authors demonstrate, however, the within cluster sample sizes may need to be quite large indeed before the asympotic results hold and the variance components are correctly estimated. Several groups have developed refinements or modifications to the PQL algorithm in an attempt to improve its performance in this setting. As shown in §6, multiplicative correction of the estimated variance components using CPQL can substantially improve performance in some situations. The PQL2 procedure available with MLwiN likewise improved performance in simulations conducted by its developers.[16, 37] An improved methodology for variance components has also been proposed for "h-likelihood" estimation, the generalization of PQL for HGLMs.[23]

One or more of these modifications should definitely be implemented when analyzing small clusters of binary outcome data using PQL. Since some uncertainty may remain as to whether or not significant bias persists, however, recourse should likely be made also to one of the presumptively more accurate methods developed during the past several years. The adaptive Gauss-Hermite quadrature procedure now available with SAS PROC NLMIXED should suffice for many multi-level, clustered data problems. It is still restricted, however, to situations where a very small number of correlated random effects is observed within each cluster. As illustrated in §7, the higher order Laplace methods developed by Raudenbush, Ying and Yosef [39] hold promise for the analysis of clustered data with higher dimensional random effects. Further commercial implementation of this approach would be desirable, as would implementation of the automated Monte Carlo EM algorithm [3] mentioned briefly in §2.

Finally, for time series, spatial statistics and crossed designs, where it is not possible to reduce the dimensionality of the integrations, approximation based on MCMC simulation is at present the only viable general approach. It is to be hoped that programs for maximum likelihood estimation using this approach will soon become available, as they have for Bayesian inference.

Acknowledgements:

This work was supported in part by USPHS grant 5-R01-CA40644. I am grateful to Kerrie Nelson for an extensive literature search that identified hundreds of papers on GLMM, PQL and their application.

9 REFERENCES

[1] A. Agresti and J. Hartzel. Strategies for comparing treatments on a binary response with multi-centre data. *Statistics in Medicine*, 19:1115–1139, 2000.

[2] P. J. Beitler and J. R. Landis. A mixed-effects model for categorical data. *Biometrics*, 41:991–1000, 1985.

[3] J. G. Booth and J. P. Hobert. Maximizing generalized linear mixed model likelihoods with an automated Monte Carlo EM algorithm. *Journal of the Royal Statistical Society, Series B*, 61:265–285, 1999.

[4] N. Breslow, B. Leroux, and R. Platt. Approximate hierarchical modelling of discrete data in epidemiology. *Statistical Methods in Medical Research*, 7:49–62, 1998.

[5] N. E. Breslow and D. G. Clayton. Approximate inference in generalized linear mixed models. *Journal of the American Statistical Association*, 88:9–25, 1993.

[6] N. E. Breslow and X. H. Lin. Bias correction in generalized linear mixed models with a single component of dispersion. *Biometrika*, 82:81–91, 1995.

[7] Z. Chen and L. Kuo. A note on the estimation of the multinomial logit model with random effects. *American Statistician*, 55:89–95, 2001.

[8] D. G. Clayton. Generalized linear mixed models. In W. R. Gilks, S. Richardson, and D. J. Spiegelhalter, editors, *Markov Chain Monte Carlo in Practice*, chapter 16, pages 275–301. Chapman and Hall, London, 1999.

[9] CYTEL Software Corporation. *EGRET for Windows*. CYTEL Software Corporation, Cambridge, MA, 1999.

[10] D. R. Cox and E. J. Snell. *Analysis of Binary Data, Second Edition*. Chapman and Hall, London, 1989.

[11] P. J. Davis and I. Polonsky. Numerical interpolation, differentiation and integration. In M. Abramowitz and I. A. Stegun, editors, *Handbook of Mathematical Functions*, chapter 25, pages 875–924. U.S. Government Printing Office, Washington, D.C., 1964.

[12] B. Engel and A. Keen. A simple approach for the analysis of generalized linear mixed models. *Statistica Neerlandica*, 48:1–22, 1994.

[13] C. J. Geyer. Practical Markov chain Monte Carlo. *Statistical Science*, 7:473–511, 1992.

[14] H. Goldstein. Nonlinear multilevel models, with an application to discrete response data. *Biometrika*, 78:45–51, 1991.

[15] H. Goldstein. *Multilevel Statistical Models*. Edward Arnold, London, 1995.

[16] H. Goldstein and J. Rasbash. Improved approximations for multilevel models with binary responses. *Journal of the Royal Statistical Society, Series A*, 159:505–513, 1996.

[17] S. Greenland. Hierarchical regression for epidemiologic analyses of multiple exposures. *Environmental Health Perspectives*, 102:33–39, 1994.

[18] D. Hedeker and R. D. Gibbons. MIXOR: A computer program for mixed-effects ordinal regression analysis. *Computer Methods and Programs in Biomedicine*, 49:157–176, 1996.

[19] C. R. Henderson. Best linear unbiased estimation and prediction under a selection model. *Biometrics*, 31:423–447, 1975.

[20] A. Y. C. Kuk and Y. W. Cheng. The Monte Carlo Newton-Raphson algorithm. *Journal of Statistical Computation and Simulation*, 59:233–250, 1997.

[21] A. Y. C. Kuk and Y. W. Cheng. Pointwise and functional approximations in Monte Carlo maximum likelihood estimation. *Statistics and Computing*, 9:91–99, 1999.

[22] Y. Lee and J. A. Nelder. Hierarchical generalized linear models (with discussion). *Journal of the Royal Statistical Society, Series B*, 58:619–678, 1996.

[23] Y. Lee and J. A. Nelder. Hierarchical generalised linear models: A synthesis of generalised linear models, random-effect models and structured dispersions. *Biometrika*, 88:987–1006, 2001.

[24] X. Lin and N. E. Breslow. Bias correction in generalized linear mixed models with multiple components of dispersion. *Journal of the American Statistical Association*, 91:1007–1016, 1996.

[25] X. Lin and D. Zhang. Inference in generalized additive mixed models by using smoothing splines. *Journal of the Royal Statistical Society, Series B*, 61:381–400, 1999.

[26] R. C. Littell, G. A. Milliken, W. W Stroup, and R. D. Wolfinger. *SAS System for Mixed Models*. SAS Institute Inc., Cary, N.C., 1996.

[27] Q. Liu and D. A. Pierce. A note on gauss-hermite quadrature. *Biometrika*, 81:624–629, 1994.

[28] P. McCullagh and J. A. Nelder. *Generalized Linear Models, Second Edition*. Chapman and Hall, London, 1989.

[29] C. E. McCulloch. Maximum likelihood algorithms for generalized linear mixed models. *Journal of the American Statistical Association*, 92:162–170, 1997.

[30] C. E. McCulloch and S. R. Searle. *Generalized, Linear, and Mixed Models*. Wiley, New York, 2001.

[31] C. A. McGilchrist. Estimation in generalized mixed models. *Journal of the Royal Statistical Society, Series B*, 56:61–69, 1994.

[32] K. J. McKonway, M. C. Jones, and P. C. Taylor. *Statistical Modelling using GENSTAT*. Arnold, London, 1999.

[33] R. B. Millar and T. J. Willis. Estimating the relative density of snapper in and around a marine reserve using a log-linear mixed-effects model. *Australian and New Zealand Journal of Statistics*, 41:383–394, 1999.

[34] J. Myles and D. Clayton. *GLMMGibbs: An R Package for Estimating Bayesian Generalised Linear Mixed Models by Gibbs Sampling*. Imperial Cancer Research Fund, London, 2001.

[35] J. A. Nelder and R. W. M. Wedderburn. Generalized linear models. *Journal of the Royal Statistical Society, Series A*, 135:370–384, 1972.

[36] J. Pinheiro and D. M. Bates. Approximations to the log-likelihood function in the nonlinear mixed-effects model. *Journal of Computational and Graphical Statistics*, 4:12–35, 1995.

[37] J. Rasbash, W. Browne, H. Goldstein, M. Yang, I. Plewis, M. Healy, G Woodhouse, D. Draper, I Langford, and T. Lewis. *A User's Guide to MLwiN*. Institute of Education, London, 2000.

[38] S. W. Raudenbush, A. S. Byrke, Y. F. Cheong, and R Congdon. *HLM 5: Hierarchical Linear and Nonlinear Modeling*. Scientific Software International, Lincolnwood, IL, 2000.

[39] S. W. Raudenbush, M. L. Yang, and M. Yosef. Maximum likelihood for generalized linear models with nested random effects via high-order, multivariate Laplace approximation. *Journal of Computational and Graphical Statistics*, 9:141–157, 2000.

[40] R. Schall. Estimation in generalized linear models with random effects. *Biometrika*, 78:719–727, 1991.

[41] Z. M. Shun. Another look at the salamander mating data: A modified Laplace approximation approach. *Journal of the American Statistical Association*, 92:341–349, 1997.

[42] Z. M. Shun and P. McCullagh. Laplace approximation of high-dimensional integrals. *Journal of the Royal Statistical Society, Series B*, 57:749–760, 1995.

[43] P. J. Solomon and D. R. Cox. Nonlinear component of variance models. *Biometrika*, 79:1–11, 1992.

[44] D. J. Spiegelhalter, A. Thomas, N. G. Best, and W. R. Gilks. *BUGS: Bayesian Inference using Gibbs Sampling, Version 0.30*. Medical Research Council Biostatistics Unit, Cambridge, 1994.

[45] SAS Institute Inc. Staff. The NLMIXED procedure. In *SAS/STAT User's Guide Version 8*, chapter 46, pages 2421–2504. SAS Publishing, Cary, NC, 2000.

[46] R. Stiratelli, N. Laird, and J. H. Ware. Random-effects models for serial observations with binary response. *Biometrics*, 40:961–971, 1984.

[47] P. F. Thall and S. C. Vail. Some covariance models for longitudinal count data with overdispersion. *Biometrics*, 46:657–671, 1990.

[48] R. Wolfinger. Laplace's approximation for nonlinear mixed models. *Biometrika*, 80:791–795, 1993.

[49] R. Wolfinger and M. O'Connell. Generalized linear mixed models: A pseudo-likelihood approach. *Journal of Statistical Computation and Simulation*, 48:233–243, 1993.

[50] S. L. Zeger and M. R. Karim. Generalized linear models with random effects; a Gibbs sampling approach. *Journal of the American Statistical Association*, 86:79–86, 1991.

Correlation and Marginal Longitudinal Kernel Nonparametric Regression

Oliver B. Linton, Enno Mammen, Xihong Lin and Raymond J. Carroll

London School of Economics and Heidelberg University and University of Michigan and Texas A&M University

ABSTRACT We consider nonparametric regression in a marginal longitudinal data framework. Previous work ([3]) has shown that the kernel nonparametric regression methods extant in the literature for such correlated data have the discouraging property that they generally do not improve upon methods that ignore the correlation structure entirely. The latter methods are called working independence methods. We construct a two-stage kernel-based estimator that asymptotically uniformly improves upon the working independence estimator. A small simulation study is given in support of the asymptotics.

1 Introduction

Nonparametric longitudinal regression in the marginal model using kernel methods has been investigated by a number of authors, see [2], [8], [9], [10] and [11], among others. Paper [8] estimates the covariance matrix of the correlated observations and use this in their kernel construction of the nonparametric regression estimate. The other papers effectively ignore the correlation structure entirely and "pretend" that the data are really independent, this being the so–called "working independence" method. Both [3] and [6] provided theoretical evidence in support of the working independence method. In fact, they showed that for many situations and different methods of kernel estimation, the working independence method is most efficient in terms of mean squared error. That is, for the kernel methods proposed in the literature, it is generally better to ignore the correlation structure entirely.

The purpose of this paper is to construct a kernel–type method that can take advantage of the correlations among the data. The method is a simple modification, and generalization to an arbitrary covariance matrix, of a method proposed by [6]. The resulting estimator is asymptotically more efficient than the working independence estimator.

The model for this paper is as follows. Suppose that there are $j = 1, ..., J$ time points, with responses Y_{ij} and covariates X_{ij}. Our basic assumption is that $E(Y_{ij}|X_{ij}) = E(Y_{ij}|X_{i1}, ..., X_{iJ})$, see [5]. Writing $\mathbf{Y}_i = (Y_{i1}, ..., Y_{iJ})^{\mathrm{T}}$ and similarly for $\mathbf{X}_i$ and $\mathbf{m}(\mathbf{X}_i) = m(X_{i1}), \cdots, m(X_{iJ})$, our model is that for an unknown function $m(\cdot)$,

$$\mathbf{Y}_i = \mathbf{m}(\mathbf{X}_i) + \mathbf{\Sigma}^{1/2}\boldsymbol{\epsilon}_i = \mathbf{m}(\mathbf{X}_i) + \mathbf{U}_i, \tag{1}$$

where $E(\mathbf{U}_i|\mathbf{X}_i) = 0$, $\mathrm{cov}(\mathbf{U}_i|\mathbf{X}_i) = \mathbf{\Sigma} = \{s_{jk}\}_{j,k}$, $\mathrm{cov}(\boldsymbol{\epsilon}_i|\mathbf{X}_i) = I_J$ and $\mathbf{\Sigma}^{1/2}$ is the symmetric square root of $\mathbf{\Sigma}$. Let $\mathbf{\Omega} = \mathbf{\Sigma}^{-1/2} = \{\omega_{jk}\}_{j,k}$ and let $\mathbf{\Lambda} = \mathrm{diag}(\mathbf{\Omega})$. Finally, let the marginal density of $(X_{ij})_i$ be $f_j(\cdot)$.

Because $\mathbf{\Sigma}$ can be estimated at parametric rates, which are faster than the rates available in nonparametric regression, for purposes of asymptotic theory we may assume without loss of generality that $\mathbf{\Sigma}$ is known. Since $\mathbf{\Sigma}$ is a $J \times J$ matrix, a root-n consistent estimate of it can be obtained by computing the sample covariance matrix of the residuals from a working independence smooth of the data.

The main idea of the two-stage estimator is to construct a linear transformation of $\mathbf{Y}$ and $\mathbf{m}(\mathbf{X})$ that has mean $\mathbf{m}(\mathbf{X})$ and diagonal covariance matrix, and to then apply working independence methods to this transformation. Specifically, for any function $g(\cdot)$, define

$$\mathbf{Z}_i(g) = \mathbf{Y}_i + \mathbf{\Lambda}^{-1}(\mathbf{\Omega} - \mathbf{\Lambda})\{\mathbf{Y}_i - \mathbf{g}(\mathbf{X}_i)\}. \tag{2}$$

Note that since $\mathbf{Z}_i(m) = \mathbf{m}(\mathbf{X}_i) + \mathbf{\Lambda}^{-1}\boldsymbol{\epsilon}_i$, (2) is one version of the required transformation.

The method we propose consists of two steps.

1. First assume working independence and fit the function $\widehat{m}_p(\cdot, h_p)$ using a kernel local polynomial method with bandwidth h_p and with the weights s_{jj}^{-1}. Without loss of generality the kernel function $K(\cdot)$ is a density function with variance one.

2. At the second step, run a local linear regression using working independence of $Z_{ij}\{\widehat{m}_p(\cdot, h_p)\}$ on X_{ij} with bandwidth h and with weights ζ_j, calling the result $\widehat{m}(\cdot, h, h_p)$. The weights ζ_j are arbitrary, but we show below that the optimal choice is $\zeta_j = \omega_{jj}^2$.

The method proposed here is essentially the same as that proposed by [6], with two exceptions: (a) our covariance structure is general, while theirs is restricted to the simple 1−way random effects model; and (b) more crucially, we allow the bandwidth at the first step to be different from the bandwidth at the second step. If one forces the two bandwidths to be identical, then as in [6], while the estimator often has a smaller variance than the working independence estimator, it has an extremely complex bias expression, and it need not have smaller mean squared error than the working independence estimator.

The paper is organized as follows. In Section 2, we state the main results. Section 3 gives the results of simulations that demonstrate that our method improves upon working independence in non–asymptotic situations. Section 4 gives concluding remarks. The proofs of the main results are sketched in a technical appendix.

2 Main Results

In this section, we state the main results. As a matter of notation, let $g^{(j)}(\cdot)$ be the jth derivative of a function $g(\cdot)$, and define $K_h(v) = h^{-1}K(v/h)$. All methods are based on working independence *local linear* kernel regression of some response R_{ij} on regressors X_{ij} with some weights W_{jj}. By this we mean that the function estimated at any value x is obtained by a weighted linear regression of the R_{ij} on the X_{ij} with weights $K_h(X_{ij} - x)W_{jj}$.

We state the results without conditions because they are standard, e.g., the regression function and density functions are thrice continuously differentiable, the density functions are positive on their support, etc. The essential condition is that (10) in the Appendix (Section 5.1) holds uniformly: conditions which would allow this are of the type used by [4].

By results in [3], to first order, the local linear regression weighted working independence estimator satisfies

$$\text{bias}\{\widehat{m}_p(\cdot, h_p)\} = (h_p^2/2)m^{(2)}(x); \tag{3}$$

$$\text{var}\{\widehat{m}_p(\cdot, h_p)\} = (nh_p)^{-1}\int K^2(x)dx \left\{\sum_{j=1}^{J} s_{jj}^{-1} f_j(x)\right\}^{-1}. \tag{4}$$

<u>Result 1</u> Assume that $h_p^3 = o(n^{-1/2})$ that $(nh_p)^{-1} = o(n^{-1/2})$, and that $h \propto n^{-1/5}$. Then to first order, the bias and variance of $\widehat{m}(\cdot, h, h_p)$ are given as follows:

$$\text{bias} = (h^2/2)m^{(2)}(x) \tag{5}$$

$$-(h_p^2/2)\left\{\sum_{j=1}^{J}\zeta_j f_j(x)\right\}^{-1}$$

$$\times \sum_{j=1}^{J}\sum_{k\neq j}^{J}\zeta_j(\omega_{jk}/\omega_{jj})f_j(x)E\left\{m^{(2)}(X_{ik})|X_{ij} = x\right\};$$

$$\text{var} = (nh)^{-1}\int K^2(x)dx \sum_{j=1}^{J}\zeta_j^2 f_j(x)/\omega_{jj}^2\left\{\sum_{j=1}^{J}\zeta_j f_j(x)\right\}^{-2}. \tag{6}$$

Let e_J be a vector of J–ones. Consider the variance components model $\Sigma = \sigma_1^2 e_J e_J^T + \sigma^2 I_J$ studied by [6]. They studied the case that $h_p = h$ and $\zeta_j = w_{jj}^2 \equiv w$, the last equivalence being a consequence of the form of Σ. They derived (5)–(6) in this special case. under some conditions, they showed that the variance (6) of their estimator was smaller than the variance of the working independence estimator (4). However, the complex nature of the bias expression (5) of their estimator as compared to that of the working independence estimator (3) meant that they could not show that the mean squared error of their estimator dominated that of the working independence estimator in any meaningful way.

Our next result shows that by undersmoothing the preliminary estimate, the two-stage estimator has the same simple, well–known bias expression as the working independence estimator, and for any Σ it has smaller variance, thus showing dominance in the mean squared error sense.

Result 2 Suppose that $h_p/h \to 0$ and that (6) is minimized by taking $\zeta_j = w_{jj}^2$. Then, to first order, the bias and variance of $\widehat{m}(x, h, h_p)$ are given as follows:

$$\text{bias} = (h^2/2)m^{(2)}(x); \tag{7}$$

$$\text{var} = (nh)^{-1} \int K^2(x)dx \left\{ \sum_{j=1}^{J} w_{jj}^2 f_j(x) \right\}^{-1}. \tag{8}$$

Since the bias expressions (3) and (7) are the same, comparing our method with the working independence estimator reduces to comparing the variance expressions (4) and (8). We show in the Appendix (Section 5.2) that for any arbitrary covariance structure Σ, our method always has smaller variance, i.e., $\text{var}\{\widehat{m}(x; h, h_p)\} \le \text{var}\{\widehat{m}_p(x; h)\}$, and hence smaller mean squared error. Our two-stage estimator hence is uniformly asymptotically dominant in terms of mean squared error compared to the regular kernel estimator.

If we compute the mean squared error at the optimal bandwidth for the working independence estimator using (3)–(4), and compare it to the mean squared error at the optimal bandwidth for the two–stage estimator using (7)–(8), we see that the asymptotic mean squared error efficiency of the working independence estimator relative to the two–stage estimator is

$$\left(\sum_{j=1}^{J} w_{jj}^2 / \sum_{j=1}^{J} s_{jj}^{-1} \right)^{4/5}. \tag{9}$$

3 Simulations

In this section, we present the results of simulations. The situation we consider is that the predictors X_{ij} for $i = 1, ..., n = 50, 100$ and $j = 1, ..., J = 3$

are independent uniform random variables on the interval $[-2, 2]$. Our theory predicts that our method will improve upon working independence. This will be seen to be the case numerically, as we now describe.

The common variance of the Y_{ij} was $\sigma_\epsilon^2 = 1$. We considered three correlation structures: exchangeable with common correlation $\rho = 0.6$, autoregressive with correlation $\rho = 0.6$, and unstructured where the correlation between measurements 1 and 2 and between measurements 2 and 3 is 0.80, and the correlation between units 1 and 3 is $\rho = 0.5$. The unstructured case was chosen because our theory predicts that it is for this case that the greatest gains in efficiency are possible when accounting for the covariance among observations. Specifically, using (9), the asymptotic mean squared error efficiency of the working independence estimator to the two-stage GLS estimator is 0.70, 0.67 and 0.38 in these three cases.

For simplicity, in the kernel calculations we assumed that it was known a priori that the variances of Y_{ij} were independent of j, so that no weighting was performed. The Epanechnikov kernel was used. At each stage of the calculations, we computed the bandwidth locally via EBBS ([7]). Undersmoothing in the two-stage estimator was achieved by multiplying the bandwidth by $(nJ)^{-2/15}$.

We estimated Σ by the following simple device: (a) form the residuals r_{ij} from a working independence fit; and (b) compute the covariance matrix of the residual vectors. We could have undersmoothed the working independence fit, but believe that the essential results would not have changes. If $\widehat{\Sigma}$ is the estimate so formed, the independence covariance matrix is simply $\widehat{\Sigma}_{indp} = \operatorname{diag}(\widehat{\Sigma})$.

Let $z = (x + 2)/4$. The functions chosen were Case 1 if $m(x) = \sin(2x)$; Case 2 if $m(x) = \sqrt{z(1-z)}\sin\{2\pi(1 + 2^{-3/5})/(z + 2^{-3/5})\}$; Case 3 if $m(x) = \sqrt{z(1-z)}\sin\{2\pi(1+2^{-7/5})/(z+2^{-7/5})\}$; Case 4 if $m(x) = \sin(8z - 4) + 2\exp\{-256(z - .5)^2\}$; Case 5 if $m(x) = H(100x) + H\{-100(x - .5)\}$, where $H(x) = 1/\{1 + \exp(-x)\}$. These cases are poorly fit by a quadratic polynomial.

The results are displayed in Tables 1–2, for $n = 50$ and $n = 100$, respectively. Here we compute the simulation mean squared errors of the estimators. The results for the two-stage GLS estimator with bandwidth estimated by EBBS at $n = 100$ are approximately what is predicted by theory for the exchangeable and autoregressive correlation structures, i.e., the MSE efficiency of working independence is approximately 70%. The same efficiencies occur for the unstructured case: generally around 60% efficiency when the theory predicts 38%. While this is somewhat disappointing, it still is clear evidence that the two-stage GLS method outperforms the working independence estimators.

	Autoregression				
	Case 1	Case 2	Case 3	Case 4	Case 5
KN(E), Work	8.81	8.94	9.78	10.34	10.69
KN(E), GLSU	6.90	6.96	7.82	7.97	8.45
	Exchangeable				
	Case 1	Case 2	Case 3	Case 4	Case 5
KN(E), Work	9.09	9.60	10.52	10.76	10.91
KN(E), GLSU	6.66	6.64	7.48	7.70	8.00
	Unstructured				
	Case 1	Case 2	Case 3	Case 4	Case 5
KN(E), Work	9.39	9.89	10.83	11.17	11.55
KN(E), GLSU	5.05	5.51	6.17	6.28	6.80

TABLE 1. For $n = 50$, $100\times$ MSE for simulations. KN = kernel, GLSU = our GLS method with an undersmoothed preliminary estimate. Work = Working independence. For kernels, the local bandwidth method EBBS was used to estimate the bandwidth. We considered three correlation structures: exchangeable with common correlation $\rho = 0.6$, autoregressive with correlation $\rho = 0.6$, and unstructured where the correlation between measurements 1 and 2 and between measurements 2 and 3 is 0.80, and the correlation between units 1 and 3 is $\rho = 0.5$.

4 Discussion

Our work was motivated by the fact ([3]) that currently existing methods for nonparametric kernel regression with correlated data do not account for the correlations in a sensible way. Indeed, these methods are often worse than simply ignoring the correlation structure entirely, i.e., than the working independence estimate.

Our main result is the construction of a two–stage kernel estimator that we have shown asymptotically uniformly improves upon the working independence estimator.

Interestingly, our proof shows that the *asymptotic* variance of the two-stage estimator can be calculated by applying standard methods to the derived variables $Z_{ij}\{\widehat{m}_p(\cdot, h_p)\}$ in the second stage of the regression. More precisely, having calculated the undersmoothed first–stage working independence estimator and having calculated the derived variables, both the estimator and its asymptotic variance can be computed as if the derived variables were actual independent observations.

We have described the methods for panel data, so that each individual unit has J observations. The methods have anticipated that the covariance matrix has no particular structure. In other longitudinal data problems, the number of observations per individual unit may depend on i, i.e., $J_i \leq J$ say. Our methods are easily extended to this case. What is required in this case is an estimate of the covariance matrix Σ_i of the J_i observations in the ith unit, and then (2) can be employed. Generally in such situations,

	Autoregression				
	Case 1	Case 2	Case 3	Case 4	Case 5
KN(E), Work	3.92	3.89	5.29	4.86	5.48
KN(E), GLSU	2.91	2.78	3.99	3.53	4.19
	Exchangeable				
	Case 1	Case 2	Case 3	Case 4	Case 5
KN(E), Work	3.91	4.29	5.07	5.11	5.67
KN(E), GLSU	2.73	3.20	3.80	3.81	4.48
	Unstructured				
	Case 1	Case 2	Case 3	Case 4	Case 5
KN(E), Work	3.93	4.04	4.89	5.11	5.49
KN(E), GLSU	2.10	2.17	2.62	2.79	3.26

TABLE 2. For $n = 100$, $100\times$ MSE for simulations. KN = kernel, GLSU = our GLS method with an undersmoothed preliminary estimate. Work = Working independence. For kernels, the local bandwidth method EBBS was used to estimate the bandwidth. We considered three correlation structures: exchangeable with common correlation $\rho = 0.6$, autoregressive with correlation $\rho = 0.6$, and unstructured where the correlation between measurements 1 and 2 and between measurements 2 and 3 is 0.80, and the correlation between units 1 and 3 is $\rho = 0.5$.

the covariance matrix is estimated in a structured way, as a function of a vector parameter γ, so that the covariance matrix $\Sigma_i(\gamma)$ is known up to the parameter γ, e.g., as exchangeable, autoregressive, etc. We believe but have not proved that the extension of our two–stage method to this case will still improve upon the working independence estimator.

Finally, we note an important technical point. In (2), the choice of Λ is crucial. While it is true that, for *any* diagonal matrix Λ, $Z_i(m) = \mathbf{m}(\mathbf{X}_i) + \Lambda^{-1}\epsilon_i$, our results are only true for our *particular* choice of Λ. The last step in the proof in Section 5.1 only holds for our choice.

5 Appendix

5.1 Sketch of Proof of Result 1

From [3], to terms of order $O_p\{h_p^3 + (nh_p)^{-1}\} = o_p(n^{-1/2})$, we have the asymptotic expansion

$$\widehat{m}_p(x, h_p) - m(x) = (h_p^2/2)m^{(2)}(x) + \left\{\sum_{j=1}^{J} s_{jj}^{-1} f_j(x)\right\}^{-1} \quad (10)$$

$$\times n^{-1} \sum_{i=1}^{n} \sum_{j=1}^{J} K_{h_p}(X_{ij} - x)U_{ij}s_{jj}^{-1}.$$

Now, $\widehat{m}(x, h, h_p)$ is the intercept when solving the local linear regression estimating equation

$$
0 = \sum_{i=1}^{n} \sum_{j=1}^{J} \left[\begin{array}{c} 1 \\ (X_{ij} - x)/h \end{array} \right] \zeta_j K_h(X_{ij} - x)
$$
$$
\times [Z_{ij} \{\widehat{m}_p(X_{ij}, h_p)\} - \alpha_0 - \alpha_1 (X_{ij} - x)/h].
$$

Define

$$
C_n = n^{-1} \sum_{i=1}^{n} \sum_{j=1}^{J} \zeta_j K_h(X_{ij} - x) \{1, (X_{ij} - x)/h\}^{\mathrm{T}} \{1, (X_{ij} - x)/h\}.
$$

Then by simple algebra, it can be shown that

$$
\widehat{m}(x, h, h_p) = (1,0) C_n^{-1} (B_{1n} + B_{2n});
$$
$$
B_{1n} = n^{-1} \sum_{i=1}^{n} \sum_{j=1}^{J} \zeta_j K_h(X_{ij} - x) \{1, (X_{ij} - x)/h\}^{\mathrm{T}} Z_{ij}(m);
$$
$$
B_{2n} = n^{-1} \sum_{i=1}^{n} \sum_{j=1}^{J} \left[\begin{array}{c} 1 \\ (X_{ij} - x)/h \end{array} \right] \zeta_j K_h(X_{ij} - x)
$$
$$
\times [Z_{ij} \{\widehat{m}_p(X_{ij}, h_p)\} - Z_{ij}(m)].
$$

Now, to terms of order $O_p(h^3)$,

$$
\begin{aligned}
Z_{ij}(m) &= m(X_{ij}) + \omega_{jj}^{-1} \epsilon_{ij} \\
&= m(x) + h m^{(1)}(x)\{(X_{ij} - x)/h\} \\
&\quad + (h^2/2) m^{(2)}(x)\{(X_{ij} - x)/h\}^2 + \omega_{jj}^{-1} \epsilon_{ij} \\
&= \{m(x), h m^{(1)}(x)\} \{1, (X_{ij} - x)/h\}^{\mathrm{T}} \\
&\quad + (h^2/2) m^{(2)}(x)\{(X_{ij} - x)/h\}^2 + \omega_{jj}^{-1} \epsilon_{ij}.
\end{aligned}
$$

By standard calculations, it is easily seen that

$$
(1,0) C_n^{-1} B_{1n} = m(x) + (h^2/2) m^{(2)}(x)
$$
$$
+ \left\{ \sum_{j=1}^{J} \zeta_j f_j(x) \right\}^{-1} n^{-1} \sum_{i=1}^{n} \sum_{j=1}^{J} (\zeta_j \epsilon_{ij}/\omega_{jj}) K_h(X_{ij} - x)
$$
$$
+ o_p\{h^2 + (nh)^{-1/2}\}.
$$

The mean of this expression is $m(x) + (h^2/2) m^{(2)}(x)$ and its variance is (6).

Note that

$$Z_{ij}\left\{\hat{m}_p(X_{ij}, h_p)\right\} - Z_{ij}(m) = \hat{m}_p(X_{ij}, h_p) - m(X_{ij})$$

$$-\omega_{jj}^{-1}\sum_{k=1}^{J}\omega_{jk}\left\{\hat{m}_p(X_{ik}, h_p) - m(X_{ik})\right\}.$$

Using (10), we can write $(1,0)C_n^{-1}B_{2n} = (1,0)C_n^{-1}(B_{2n1} - B_{2n2} + B_{2n3} - B_{2n4})$, where

$$(1,0)C_n^{-1}B_{2n1} = (h_p^2/2)\left\{\sum_{j=1}^{J}\zeta_j f_j(x)\right\}^{-1}$$

$$\times n^{-1}\sum_{i=1}^{n}\sum_{j=1}^{J}\zeta_j K_h(X_{ij} - x)m^{(2)}(X_{ij});$$

$$(1,0)C_n^{-1}B_{2n2} = (h_p^2/2)\left\{\sum_{j=1}^{J}\zeta_j f_j(x)\right\}^{-1}$$

$$\times n^{-1}\sum_{i=1}^{n}\sum_{j=1}^{J}\zeta_j K_h(X_{ij} - x)\sum_{k}\frac{\omega_{jk}}{\omega_{jj}}m^{(2)}(X_{ik});$$

$$(1,0)C_n^{-1}B_{2n3} = \left\{\sum_{j=1}^{J}\zeta_j f_j(x)\right\}^{-1} n^{-1}\sum_{i=1}^{n}\sum_{j=1}^{J}\zeta_j K_h(X_{ij} - x)$$

$$\times \left\{\sum_{j=1}^{J}s_{jj}^{-1}f_j(X_{ij})\right\}^{-1}$$

$$\times n^{-1}\sum_{\ell=1}^{n}\sum_{r=1}^{J}K_{h_p}(X_{\ell r} - X_{ij})U_{\ell r}s_{rr}^{-1};$$

$$(1,0)C_n^{-1}B_{2n4} = \left\{\sum_{j=1}^{J}\zeta_j f_j(x)\right\}^{-1} n^{-1}\sum_{i=1}^{n}\sum_{j=1}^{J}\zeta_j K_h(X_{ij} - x)$$

$$\times \omega_{jj}^{-1}\sum_{k=1}^{J}\omega_{jk}\left\{\sum_{j=1}^{J}s_{jj}^{-1}f_j(X_{ik})\right\}^{-1}$$

$$\times n^{-1}\sum_{\ell=1}^{n}\sum_{r=1}^{J}K_{h_p}(X_{\ell r} - X_{ik})U_{\ell r}s_{rr}^{-1}.$$

It is easily seen that to order $o_p\{h^2 + (nh)^{-1/2}\}$

$$(1,0)C_n^{-1}(B_{2n1} - B_{2n2}) = -(h_p^2/2)\left\{\sum_{j=1}^{J}\zeta_j f_j(x)\right\}^{-1}$$

$$\times \sum_{j=1}^{M} \sum_{k \neq j}^{M} (\zeta_j \omega_{jk}/\omega_{jj}) E\left\{ m^{(2)}(X_{ik})|X_{ij} = x \right\}.$$

It is tedious but straightforward to show that

$$(1,0)C_n^{-1}(B_{2n3} - B_{2n4}) = o_p\{h^2 + (nh)^{-1/2}\},$$

completing the proof.

5.2 Proof of $\mathrm{var}\{\widehat{m}(x; h, h_p)\} \leq \mathrm{var}\{\widehat{m}_p(x; h)\}$

Denote by $\mathbf{A}$ any $J \times J$ positive definite symmetric matrix. Let $\mathbf{A} = \{a_{ij}\}$, $\mathbf{B} = \mathbf{A}^{1/2} = \{b_{ij}\}$ and $\mathbf{C} = \mathbf{A}^{-1/2} = \{c_{ij}\}$. We first show that $\sum_{i=1}^{J} c_{ii}^2 \geq \sum_{i=1}^{J}(1/a_{ii})$.

Since for any $1 \leq i \leq J$, $a_{ii} = \sum_{j=1}^{J} b_{ij}^2$, we have $b_{ii}^2 \leq a_{ii}$. Since $\mathbf{B}$ is a positive definite matrix, the standard matrix theory gives $c_{ii}b_{ii} \geq 1$ ([1], page 403). It follows that $c_{ii} \geq 1/b_{ii} \geq 1/\sqrt{a_{ii}}$, i.e., $c_{ii} \geq 1/\sqrt{a_{ii}}$. Hence $\sum_{i=1}^{J} c_{ii}^2 \geq \sum_{i=1}^{J}(1/a_{ii})$.

Define $\mathbf{A} = \boldsymbol{f}^{-1/2}\boldsymbol{\Sigma}\boldsymbol{f}^{-1/2}$, where $\boldsymbol{f} = \mathrm{diag}\{f_1(x), \cdots, f_J(x)\}$. Then the diagonal elements of $\mathbf{A}$ are $a_{ii} = s_{ii}/f_j(x)$. Now $\mathbf{C} = \mathbf{A}^{-1/2} = \boldsymbol{f}^{1/4}\boldsymbol{\Sigma}^{-1/2}\boldsymbol{f}^{1/4}$. The diagonal elements of $\mathbf{C}$ are $c_{ii} = w_{ii}f_i(x)^{1/2}$. Using the above results, we have $\sum_{i=1}^{J} w_{ii}^2 f_i(x) \geq \sum_{i=1}^{J} s_{ii}^{-1} f_i(x)$. It follows immediately from equations (4) and (8) that $\mathrm{var}\{\widehat{m}(x; h, h_p)\} \leq \mathrm{var}\{\widehat{m}_p(x; h)\}$. This completes the proof.

Acknowledgments: This research was supported by grants from the National Science Foundation (SBR-9730282), the Deutsche Forschungsgemeinschaft (Project MA-1026/6-2) National Cancer Institute (CA-57030 and CA-76404) and the National Institute of Environmental Health Sciences (P30-ES09106).

6 REFERENCES

[1] F. A. Graybill. *Matrices with Applications in Statistic.* Wadsworth & Brooks/Cole, 1983.

[2] D. R. Hoover, J. A. Rice, C. O. Wu, and Y. Yang. Nonparametric smoothing estimates of time–varying coefficient models with longitudinal data. *Biometrika*, 85:809–822, 1998.

[3] X. Lin and R. J. Carroll. Nonparametric function estimation for clustered data when the predictor is measured without/with error. *Journal of the American Statistical Association*, 95:520–534, 2000.

[4] J. S. Marron and W. Härdle. Random approximations to some measures of accuracy in nonparametric curve estimatio. *Journal of Multivariate Analysis*, 20:91–113, 1986.

[5] M. S. Pepe and D. Couper. Modeling partly conditional means with longitudinal data. *Journal of the American Statistical Association*, 92:991–998, 1997.

[6] A. Ruckstuhl, A. H. Welsh, and R. J. Carroll. Nonparametric function estimation of the relationship between two repeatedly measured variables. *Statistica Sinica*, 10:51–71, 2000.

[7] D. Ruppert. Empirical-bias bandwidths for local polynomial nonparametric regression and density estimatio. *Journal of the American Statistical Association*, 92:1049–1062, 1997.

[8] T. A. Severini and J. G. Staniswalis. Quasilikelihood estimation in semiparametric models. *Journal of the American Statistical Association*, 89:501–511, 1994.

[9] C. J. Wild and T. W. Yee. Additive extensions to generalized estimating equation methods. *J. Royal Statist. Soc. B*, 58:711–725, 1996.

[10] C. O. Wu, C. T. Chiang, and D. R. Hoover. Asymptotic confidence regions for kernel smoothing of a varying coefficient model with longitudinal data. *Journal of the American Statistical Association*, 93:1388–1402, 1998.

[11] S. L. Zeger and P. J. Diggle. Semi-parametric models for longitudinal data with application to cd4 cell numbers in hiv seroconverters. *Biometrics*, 50:689–699, 1994.

Analysis of Multivariate Monotone Missing Data by A Pseudolikelihood Method

Gong Tang, Roderick J. A. Little and Trivelore E. Raghunathan

ABSTRACT We consider analysis of multivariate data with a monotone pattern of missing values, where the missingness depends on the underlying value of the missing variable. Maximum likelihood and estimating-equation-based methods, based on selection models, require specifying the functional form of the missing-data mechanism. Pattern-mixture models are useful for multivariate monotone missing data with two patterns but difficult to generalize to data with more than two patterns. Pseudolikelihood selection models can obtain consistent estimates of complete-data model parameters without specifying the missing-data mechanism. We extend this method to a class of more general missing-data mechanisms and illustrate its utility using data from a schizophrenia trial.

1 Introduction

In recent years there has been enormous development in methods for statistical inference from longitudinal studies with missing data caused by design or attrition over time. Statistical methods have been developed for a wide variety of study designs, types of measurements (quantitative or qualitative), study objectives and missing-data mechanisms. In general, the literature can be classified into likelihood-based and non-likelihood-based approaches. In the likelihood framework, the joint distribution of outcomes and missing-data mechanisms are specified, and inference is based on the likelihood function. The likelihood can be based on selection models or pattern-mixture-models, depending on how the joint distribution is factored. Little (1995) provides a general review of much of this literature, including the work of Diggle and Kenward (1994), Little (1993, 1994), Mori, Woolson and Woodsworth (1994), Schluchter (1992), Wu and Bailey (1989), and Wu and Carroll (1988).

In the non-likelihood-based approaches of Robins, Rotnitzky and Zhao (1994, 1995), Rotnitzky, Robins and Scharfstein (1998), and Scharfstein, Rotnitzky, and Robins (1999), the joint distribution of the outcomes is assumed to follow a non-parametric or semi-parametric model, and a parametric or semi-parametric model is assumed for the missing-data mechanism. Estimating equations are then constructed based on these model assumptions.

Consider multivariate missing data where the variables $Y_1, ..., Y_K$ can be arranged so that if Y_j is missing for an observation, then Y_k is also missing for that observation, for $k = j+1, ..., K$. Such a missing-data pattern is called monotone (Little and Rubin, 2002). Suppose the missingness of one outcome only depends on its underlying value, so the missing data are not missing at random. Maximum likelihood based on selection models and non-likelihood-based methods (Robins et al., 1994, 1995) for such missing data require models that specify the functional form of the missing-data mechanism. However, the underlying true functional form is often not well understood in practice, and misspecification of the missingness mechanism often leads to biased estimates. For monotone missing data with two patterns, pattern-mixture models yield valid inference without specifying the mechanism if the model parameters are identifiable (Little & Wang, 1996). However, extension of this approach to general multivariate monotone missing data with such non-MAR mechanisms is difficult, and currently there is no well-established pattern-mixture model for this problem.

Tang, Little and Raghunathan (2003) proposed pseudolikelihood selection models for multivariate missing data to make inference on the complete-data model without specifying the functional form of response-dependent mechanisms. Here we present simulation results from this method and extend it to a general class of mechanisms. In the next section, we describe the assumed data structure and approaches to statistical inference. Data from a schizophrenia trial are used to illustrate the pseudolikelihood method.

2 Multivariate monotone missing data

We consider analysis of multivariate monotone missing data $\{x_i, y_i\}$, $i = 1, ..., n$, where $X = (X_1, ..., X_q)^T$ are fully-observed covariates and $Y = (Y_1, ..., Y_K)^T$ are outcomes. We assume that Y are observed in a monotone pattern, that is, Y_{k+1} is missing if Y_k is missing, $k = 1, ..., K - 1$. Let R_i denote the missing-data indicator, its value indicating the number of observed response variables for subject i, $i = 1, ..., n$. For example, if $R_i = k$, then $\{y_{i1}, ..., y_{ik}\}$ are observed but $\{y_{i,k+1}, ..., y_{iK}\}$ are missing, $k = 1, ..., K - 1$. For complete cases, $R = K$. The primary interest is the conditional distribution of Y given X or the marginal distribution of Y. With the conditional distribution of Y given X estimated and the empirical distribution of X obtained from the observed data, the marginal distribution of Y can then be estimated. Even if the marginal distribution of Y is the primary interest, we may wish to model the conditional distribution of Y given X in order to incorporate auxillary information from X when Y has missing values. Throughout this paper, we use $[\cdot]$ to denote a generic distribution, $pr[\cdot]$ the probability of an event, and $p(\cdot)$ a density function.

Multivariate monotone missing data are prevalent in longitudinal studies with dropouts. As an example, we consider data from a phase III trial comparing different drug regimes in the treatment of chronic schizophrenia (Diggle, 1998). In this multi-center, double-blinded trial, 523 patients were randomized to six treatments: placebo, haloperidol 20 mg and risperidone at four different dose levels. Haloperidol is a standard therapy and risperidone is a novel chemical compound with useful pharmacological characteristics. The primary outcome was the total score obtained on the positive and negative symptom rating scale (PANSS), measuring psychotic disorder. The score was recorded at weeks -1, 0, 1, 2, 4, 6, and 8, where -1 refers to selection into the trial and 0 to baseline. A reduction of 20% in the mean score was regarded as demonstrating a clinical improvement. The primary interest was to compare three treatment groups, placebo, haloperidol and risperidone, with respect to the average reduction in PANSS scores at week 8, had the outcome been observed for all the patients in the study.

Only 269 of the 523 patients had outcomes observed at all the seven time points. Three patients had no observation at baseline and are excluded from the analysis. For simplicity we also discard 3 out of 251 incomplete cases with intermittent missing values, yielding a monotone pattern of missing data. Twenty-nine of 88 cases (33%) in the placebo group, 41 of 87 (47%) in the haloperidol group and 199 of 345 (58%) in the risperidone groups were complete. Exploratory data analysis (Diggle, 1998) suggests that patients with higher PANSS scores tend to have higher probability of dropout at each time point.

Let (x_i, y_i, R_i) denote the values of X, Y and R for observation i, and assume independence across observations. Two generic likelihood-based approaches for missing data are selection models and pattern-mixture models (Little and Rubin 2002; Glynn, Laird, and Rubin, 1986). They differ in the way they factor joint distribution of the complete data (X, Y) and the missing-data mechanism R. Selection models factor the joint distribution as product of a distribution for the hypothetical complete data and a distribution for the mechanism given the hypothetical complete data:

$$p(x_i, y_i, R_i; \theta, \psi) = p(x_i, y_i; \theta)p(R_i|x_i, y_i, \psi), \qquad (1)$$

where θ and ψ are model parameters.Pattern-mixture models stratify data by missing-data patterns and model the distribution of the complete data within each pattern:

$$p(x_i, y_i, R_i; \delta, \gamma) = p(x_i, y_i|R_i, \delta)p(R_i; \gamma), \qquad (2)$$

where δ and γ are model parameters.

The selection modeling approach is more common in literature, and more natural when interest concerns parameters of the entire population. Data are missing at random (MAR) (Little and Rubin, 2002; Rubin, 1976) if:

$$pr[R_i = k | x_i, y_i, R_i \geq k] = w_k(x_i, y_{i1}, ..., y_{ik}), \qquad (3)$$
$$k = 1, ..., K - 1; \ i = 1, ..., n,$$

where $\{x_i, y_{i1}, ..., y_{ik}\}$ are observed data for subject i; $w_k(\cdot)'s$ are functions with range $[0, 1]$. When the data are MAR and θ is distinct from ψ, the mechanism is ignorable for maximum likelihood inference based on selection models of the form (1) (Rubin 1976). If the missing-data mechanism not only depends on observed data but also on missing data, it is called not missing at random (NMAR) (Rubin, 1976). When the mechanism is not MAR, maximum likelihood for selection models (Diggle and Kenward, 1994) requires specifying the functional form of the mechanism, and inferences are vulnerable to misspecification of this mechanism.

3 Pattern-mixture models for multivariate missing data

Pattern-mixture models are more natural when interest concerns the population strata defined by missing-data pattern. Some parameters for incomplete patterns need to be identified by prior information or parametric restrictions, which result from assumptions about the missing-data mechanism. For some non-MAR mechanisms, pattern-mixture models are simpler to fit and do not require specifying the form of the missing-data mechanism (Little 1993, 1994; Little and Wang 1996).

Superficially, it appears that the pattern-mixture method of Little and Wang (1996) can be extended to monotone data with more than two patterns, as is the case in the MAR analysis of monotone missing data in Anderson (1957). However, this extension is problematic because some model parameters are identified by equating distributions across patterns and this procedure often leads to inconsistent model structures. A simple example is a trivariate monotone missing data set of (Y_1, Y_2, Y_3) with missing-data mechanism:

$$pr[R = 1 | Y_1, Y_2, Y_3] = w_1(Y_2) \qquad (4)$$
$$pr[R = 2 | Y_1, Y_2, Y_3, R \geq 2] = w_2(Y_3) \qquad (5)$$

where $w_1(\cdot)$ and $w_2(\cdot)$ are arbitrary functions. A typical pattern-mixture model assumes that given $R = r$, $[Y_1, Y_2, Y_3]$ is trivariate normal, $r = 1, 2, 3$. However, (4) implies that:

$$[Y_1, Y_3 | Y_2, R = 1] = [Y_1, Y_3 | Y_2, R > 1] \qquad (6)$$

The left hand of (6) is a normal distribution and the right hand of (6) is a mixture of two normal distributions. Equating these distributions requires stronger assumptions than we are willing to make. This example shows that pattern-mixture models have limited flexibility for general multivariate monotone missing data.

A simple modification of the pattern-mixture method is to create moment restrictions, instead of parameter restrictions on some parametric models, from missing-data mechanism (4) and (5). For instance, in the above example, let $\phi^{(r)}$ be the first and second moments of the complete data within pattern $R = r$, $r = 1, 2, 3$. Since the complete data are observed for $R = 3$, $\phi^{(3)}$ is estimated by sample moments in that pattern. Missing-data assumption (5) implies that:

$$[Y_1, Y_2 | Y_3, R = 3] = [Y_1, Y_2 | Y_3, R = 2] \tag{7}$$

If we assume that the left hand and the right hand of (7) are approximately normal, then (7) can be regarded as restrictions on moments, that is, $\phi_{12.3}^{(2)} = \phi_{12.3}^{(3)}$, where $\phi_{12.3}^{(r)}$ includes regression coefficients and residual variance calculated based on $\phi^{(r)}$. Then the pattern-mixture method of Little and Wang (1996) can be used to estimate $\phi^{(2)}$ based on the subset $[R > 1]$. Similarly, if we assume that the left hand and the right hand of (6) are approximately normal, we have $\phi_{13.2}^{(1)} = \phi_{13.2}^{(23)}$, where $\phi_{13.2}^{(23)}$ represents the set of the regression coefficients and residual variance of $[Y_1, Y_3 | Y_2, R > 1]$. From the first step, $\phi_{13.2}^{(23)}$ is estimated based on estimates of $\phi^{(3)}$ and $\phi^{(2)}$, and the sample proportions of $R = 2$ and $R = 3$. Since Y_1 is observed for pattern $R = 1$, $\phi^{(1)}$ is then estimated by the marginal moments of Y_1 and estimate of $\phi_{13.2}^{(1)}$, obtained in the second step.

This approach method looks promising but has some pitfalls. In order to validate those moment restrictions, some conditional regressions are required to be approximately normal, which is inconsistent with the pattern-mixture model. The following example based on a simulated data shows that this method fails to supply consistent estimates of sample moments.

A random sample of $N(\mu_1, \sigma_{11})$ of size n was simulated for Y_1. Then Y_2 and Y_3 were simulated as:

$$\begin{pmatrix} y_2 \\ y_3 \end{pmatrix} = \begin{pmatrix} \beta_{20.1} & \beta_{21.1} & 0 \\ \beta_{30.12} & \beta_{31.12} & \beta_{32.12} \end{pmatrix} \begin{pmatrix} 1 \\ y_1 \\ y_2 \end{pmatrix} + \begin{pmatrix} \epsilon_1 \\ \epsilon_2 \end{pmatrix}$$

where $\epsilon_1 \sim N(0, \sigma_{22.1})$ and $\epsilon_2 \sim N(0, \sigma_{33.12})$.

The dropout mechanism was:

$$pr[R = 1 | Y_1, Y_2, Y_3] = \Phi(\psi_0 + \psi_1 Y_2)$$
$$pr[R = 2 | Y_1, Y_2, Y_3] = \Phi(\psi_0 + \psi_1 Y_3)$$

where, $\Phi(\cdot)$ is the cumulative distribution function of the standard normal distribution, (ψ_0, ψ_1) are constants.

For the simulated data, $n = 300$, $(\mu_1, \sigma_{11}) = (3, 1)$, $(\beta_{20.1}, \beta_{21.1}, \sigma_{22.1}) = (0.1, 1.1, 1)$, $(\beta_{30.12}, \beta_{31.12}, \beta_{32.12}, \sigma_{22.1}) = (0.1, 0.1, 1.1, 1)$, and $(\psi_0, \psi_1) = (-4.2, 1)$. Two methods were used to estimate the first and second moments of data: analysis based on date before deletion (BD) and the method based on moment restrictions (MMR). The following table displays the estimates of the first and second moments of some variables in incomplete patterns:

Table 1: moment estimates of some variables in
incomplete patterns: MMR versus BD

Parameters	MMR	BD
$\mu_3^{(2)}$	5.62	5.20
$\sigma_{33}^{(2)}$	1.10	0.66
$\mu_2^{(1)}$	5.16	5.22
$\sigma_{22}^{(1)}$	1.09	1.29
$\mu_3^{(1)}$	6.16	6.12
$\sigma_{33}^{(1)}$	2.16	2.35

where $\mu_i^{(r)}$ and $\sigma_{ii}^{(r)}$ are the mean and variance of Y_i within pattern $R = r$, $i, r = 1, 2, 3$; respectively.

Although moment estimates of parameters other than $\sigma_{33}^{(2)}$ from MMR are quite close to the sample moments from BD, the MMR estimate of $\sigma_{33}^{(2)}$ seems severely biased. This is supported by further simulation studies. According to assumptions (4) and (5), even if the complete data are normal, $[Y_1, Y_2, Y_3 | R > 1]$ is no longer normal though $[Y_1, Y_3 | Y_2, R > 1]$ is still a normal regression according to (6). The resulting sample of $[Y_1, Y_2 | Y_3, R > 1]$ is not normal and the natural extension of the pattern-mixture method of Little and Wang (1996) to more than two patterns yields a biased estimate of $\phi^{(2)}$. This problem motivates the search for a robust procedure for multivariate monotone missing data with missingness depending only on the missing variables, that avoids a parametric specification of the missing data mechanism, and yields consistent estimates of parameters of interest. The pseudo-likelihood method of Tang, Little and Raghunathan (2003), which we now describe, meets this objective.

4 A pseudolikelihood method

Consider first multivariate monotone missing data with two patterns: $\{x_i, y_i\}$, $i = 1, ..., n$, where both x_i and y_i are vectors of variables, y_i's are observed for $i = 1, ..., m$, and missing for $i = m + 1, ..., n$. Models for the complete data and the missing-data mechanism are as follows:

$$p(x, y; \theta, \alpha) = f(x; \alpha)g(y|x; \theta) \tag{8}$$

$$pr[M = 1|x, y] = w(x, y; \psi) = w(y; \psi), \tag{9}$$

where $f(\cdot)$ and $g(\cdot)$ are density functions of the marginal distribution of X and the conditional distribution of Y given X, respectively; M the missing-data indicator: $M_i = 1$ if y_i is missing and 0 otherwise; $w(\cdot)$ an arbitrary function with range $[0, 1]$; α is the set of parameters for the marginal distribution of X, θ the set of regression parameters of interest, ψ the set of parameters for the missing-data mechanism, and these parameters are distinct from each other. Under the following pseudolikelihood method, the distribution of $f(\cdot)$ can be parametric or non-parametric, as discussed later in this section. The conditional density $g(y|x; \theta)$ is from a parametric family. If a normal density is assumed, then θ includes the regression coefficients and the residual variance. Initially we assume that the missing-data mechanism only depends on Y, as in (9). Extensions to more general mechanisms involving the covariate will be discussed in section 6.

Under the missing-data mechanism (9), the complete cases are a random sample from the conditional distribution of X given Y. To avoid modeling the missing-data mechanism, the pseudolikelihood method (Tang et al., 2003) makes inferences based on the corresponding conditional likelihood. Three cases can be distinguished:

(a) If the parametric form of $f(\cdot)$ and $\alpha = \alpha_0$ are known, the estimate $\hat{\theta}$ is the value of θ that maximizes

$$L_2(\theta; \alpha_0) = \prod_{i=1}^{m} \frac{g(y_i|x_i; \theta)}{p(y_i; \theta, \alpha_0)} \propto \prod_{i=1}^{m} p(x_i|y_i; \theta, \alpha_0), \tag{10}$$

with $p(y; \theta, \alpha)$ being the marginal density function of y:

$$p(y; \theta, \alpha) = \int g(y|x, \theta) \, dF(x; \alpha),$$

where $F(x; \alpha)$ is the cumulative distribution function of X.

(b) If the parametric form of $f(\cdot)$ is known but α_0 is unknown, then a consistent estimator of α, say $\hat{\alpha}$, is estimated by maximizing

$$L_1(\alpha) = \prod_{i=1}^{n} f(x_i; \alpha),$$

then the estimate $\hat{\theta}$ of θ is the value that maximizes $L_2(\theta; \hat{\alpha})$.

(c) If $f(\cdot)$ is treated as non-parametric, the estimate $\hat{\theta}$ is the value of θ that maximizes $L_2(\theta; F_n(x))$, where

$$L_2(\theta; F_n(x)) = \prod_{i=1}^{m} \frac{g(y_i|x_i, \theta)}{\int g(y_i|x, \theta) \, dF_n(x)}$$

and $F_n(x) = \frac{1}{n}\sum_{i=1}^{n} I(x \le x_i)$ is the empirical distribution of X, where x and $x_i's$ are vectors.

Model parameters are identifiable and the pseudolikelihood estimate is consistent under some regularity conditions. When $g(y|x,\theta)$ is a normal regression, θ is identifiable when the number of continuous variables that X contains is no less than the dimension of Y. Intuitively, under such a condition, parameters of $[Y|X]$ are uniquely determined by the format of $[X|Y]$, which can be *empirically* estimated from the complete cases since complete cases are a random sample from $[X|Y]$ under assumption (9).

Let PL0, PL1 and PL2 denote maximum pseudolikelihood estimates under scenarios (a), (b) and (c), respectively. Also, let

$$l(\theta,\alpha) = I\{M = 0\}\{\log g(y|x,\theta) - \log \int g(y|x,\theta)f(x;\alpha)\,dx\},$$

$$S(\alpha) = \log f(x;\alpha).$$

Under some regularity conditions, all these estimates are consistent. The PL0 and PL1 estimates of θ are asymptotically normal with variances Σ_0 and Σ_1, respectively (Tang et al., 2003), where:

$$\Sigma_0 = \frac{1}{n}E(-l_{\theta\theta})^{-1}E(l_\theta l_\theta^T)E(-l_{\theta\theta})^{-1} \tag{11}$$

$$\Sigma_1 = \frac{1}{n}E(-l_{\theta\theta})^{-1}\{E(l_\theta l_\theta^T) - E(l_{\theta\alpha})E(-S_{\alpha\alpha})^{-1}E(l_{\alpha\theta})\}E(-l_{\theta\theta})^{-1}. \tag{12}$$

The asymptotic properties of the PL2 estimate are still under investigation. We suspect that the PL2 estimate is also asymptotically normal with a formula conjectured in Tang et al. (2003). As implied by (11) and (12), the PL1 estimate is more efficient than the PL0 estimate. Simulation studies (Tang et al., 2003) suggest that the PL2 estimate, which makes the weakest distribution assumptions for the covariate X, is even more efficient than the PL1 estimate. In the following, we refer to the PL2 estimate as the PL estimate without causing any confusion.

Sometimes, when more information is available about the mechanism, the method can be extended to the cases where the dimension of X is less than the dimension of Y. For example, suppose the mechanism just depends on a sub-vector of Y, say Y_1:

$$pr[R = 1|x, y_1, y_2] = w(y_1, y_2; \psi) = w(y_1; \psi),$$

and the number of continuous variables which X contains is no less than the dimension of Y_1. This may happen in drop-out data, for example when Y_2 is missing if and only if Y_1 is missing. Then a modified pseudolikelihood method can be used for inference about θ without specifying $w(\cdot)$. Let:

$$\tilde{L}_1(\alpha) = \prod_{i=1}^{n} f(x_i; \alpha)$$

$$\tilde{L}_2(\alpha, \theta) = \prod_{i=1}^{m} \frac{g(y_{i1}, y_{i2}|x_i, \theta)}{p(y_{i1}; \theta, \alpha)},$$

where $p(y_1; \theta, \alpha)$ is the marginal density function of y_1:

$$p(y_1; \theta, \alpha) = \int \int g(y_1, y_2|x, \theta) f(x; \alpha) \, dy_2 \, dx$$

$$= \int \int g(y_1, y_2|x, \theta) \, dy_2 \, dF(x; \alpha)$$

If the functional form $f(\cdot)$ is known, the pseudolikelihood estimate of θ is:

$$\hat{\theta} = \arg\max_\theta \tilde{L}_2(\theta, \hat{\alpha}), \quad \text{where } \hat{\alpha} = \arg\max_\alpha \tilde{L}_1(\alpha).$$

When $f(\cdot)$ is unknown, then the estimate is:

$$\hat{\theta} = \arg\max_\theta \tilde{L}_2(F_n(x), \theta)$$

$$= \arg\max_\theta \prod_{i=1}^{m} \frac{\phi(y_{i1}, y_{i2}|x_i, \theta)}{\int \int p(y_{i1}, y_2|x, \theta, \alpha) \, dy_2 \, dF_n(x)},$$

where $F_n(x)$ is the empirical distribution of X. Under some regularity conditions, this pseudolikelihood estimate is consistent.

Since this pseudolikelihood method does not require assumptions on the distribution of the covariates, it can be extended to multivariate monotone missing data with more than two patterns (Tang et al., 2003). Consider multivariate monotone missing data $\{X, Y_1, ..., Y_K\}$, where the missingness of response variables depends only on their underlying values:

$$pr[R = k - 1|X, Y_1, ..., Y_K, R \geq k - 1] = w_k(Y_k), \quad k = 2, ..., K, \quad (13)$$

where $w_k(\cdot)$'s are arbitrary functions. We assume that interest concerns the conditional distribution of the responses Y given the covariates X. This conditional distribution can be factored as:

$$[Y|X, \theta] = [Y_1, ..., Y_K|X, \theta]$$

$$= [Y_1|X, \theta_1] \prod_{k=2}^{K} [Y_k|X, Y_1, ..., Y_{k-1}, \theta_k], \quad k = 1, ..., K \quad (14)$$

Corresponding to this factorization, parameters are grouped into K distinct subsets: $\{\theta_1, \theta_2, ..., \theta_K\}$. Suppose that the conditional distributions in (14) have the following density functions:

$$[Y_1|X, \theta_1] \sim g_1(y_1|x, \theta_1)$$
$$[Y_k|X, Y_1, ..., Y_{k-1}, \theta_k] \sim g_k(y_k|x, y_1, ..., y_{k-1}, \theta_k), \quad k = 2, ..., K \quad (15)$$

where $g_k(\cdot)$'s are known parametric density functions and $\theta = \{\theta_1, ..., \theta_K\}$ are parameters of interest.

Based on assumption (13), we have the following property (Tang et al., 2003):

$$[Y_k|X, Y_1, ..., Y_{k-1}, R \geq k-1] = [Y_k|X, Y_1, ..., Y_{k-1}], \quad k = 3, ..., K. \quad (16)$$

Let $F_{k-1}(x, y_1, ..., y_{k-1})$ denote the empirical distribution of $[X, Y_1, ..., Y_{k-1}|R \geq k-1]$, and:

$$L_1(\theta_1) = \prod_{i=1}^{n} g_1(y_{i1}|x_i, \theta_1)$$

and

$$L_k(\theta_k) = \prod_{R_i \geq k-1} \frac{g_k(y_{ik}|x, ..., y_{i,k-1}, \theta_k)}{\int g_k(y_{ik}|x, y_1, ..., y_{k-1}, \theta_k)\, dF_{k-1}(x, y_1, ..., y_{k-1})} \quad (17)$$

with $k = 2, ..., K$. In fact, the integration in the denominator of (17) is just the average value of $g_k(y_{ik}|x, y_1, ..., y_{k-1}, \theta_k)$, as a function of $(x, y_1, ..., y_{k-1})$, over the subset $[R \geq k-1]$.

Theorem (Tang et al., 2003): Under some regularity conditions, the pseudo-likelihood estimates $\hat{\theta} = \{\hat{\theta}_1, ..., \hat{\theta}_K\}$ given by:

$$\hat{\theta}_k = \arg \max_{\theta_k} L_k(\theta_k), \quad k = 1, ..., K$$

are consistent estimates of $\theta = \{\theta_1, ..., \theta_K\}$.

The required regularity conditions include dimension requirements and some uniform convergence properties. These estimates are suspected to be asymptotically normal though analytical results are not available at this time.

5 Simulation results

In Tang et al. (2003), simulation results are presented for the pseudolikelihood method applied to bivariate monotone data. We conducted two simulation studies ton trivariate monotone missing data to compare the performance of the pseudolikelihood method with other methods. For simplicity, suppose that there is no covariate and complete data $Y = \{Y_1, Y_2, Y_3\}$ were generated from a trivariate normal distribution:

$$[Y_1] \sim N(\mu_1, \sigma_{11})$$
$$[Y_2|Y_1] \sim N(\beta_{20.1} + \beta_{21.1}Y_1, \sigma_{22.1})$$
$$[Y_3|Y_1, Y_2] \sim N(\beta_{30.12} + \beta_{31.12}Y_1 + \beta_{32.12}Y_2, \sigma_{33.12})$$

with $(\mu_1, \sigma_{11}) = (0, 1)$, $\phi_{2.1} = (\beta_{20.1}, \beta_{21.1}, \sigma_{22.1}) = (-1, 1, 1)$, and $\phi_{3.12} = (\beta_{30.12}, \beta_{31.12}, \beta_{32.12}, \sigma_{33.12}) = (1, 1, 1, 1)$.

In the first simulation study, missing values of Y_2 and Y_3 were generated using the probit model

$$pr[R = k - 1 | X, Y, R \geq k - 1] = \Phi(\psi_0 + \psi_1 Y_k), \quad k = 2, 3, \qquad (18)$$

where $\psi = (\psi_0, \psi_1) = (-0.5, 1)$, $\Phi(\cdot)$ is the cumulative distribution function of the standard normal distribution.

Since Y_1 is fully observed, efficient estimates of (μ_1, σ_{11}) are given by maximizing the likelihood function based on the marginal distribution of Y_1. Hence we focus on estimation of $\phi_{2.1}$ and $\phi_{3.12}$. Under mechanism (18), 1000 data sets with sample size 300 were simulated. In average, the number of complete cases is 136 and there are about 191 cases with both Y_1 and Y_2 observed. These data sets were analyzed by the following methods: Complete-data analysis on the data before deletion of the missing values (BD), ignorable maximum likelihood (IML), full maximum likelihood (ML) which assumes the mechanism (18) with ψ unknown, and pseudolikelihood (PL). The computations for the PL method were based on a hybrid of Newton-Raphson and Quasi-Newton algorithms (Press et al., 1992) with the complete-case estimate as the initial value. When the sample size and number of complete cases were fairly large, this hybrid algorithm converged within around 30 iterations. If the sample size and number of complete cases are small, like the PANSS data set analyzed later in section 6, initial values need to be chosen carefully in order to achieve convergence. The empirical bias and standard deviation (S.D.) of each method over the 1000 data sets are displayed in Table 2. Note that (a) the IML method is seriously biased for this nonignorable mechanism; (b) the ML and PL methods have negligible bias; and (c) the PL method is less precise than ML, as one would expect given that it does not assume knowledge of the functional form of the mechanism (13).

Table 2. Simulation results from four methods on 1000 replicates
with selection following (18)
(a) Empirical bias (empirical S.D.)($\times 10^3$) of estimates for $\phi_{2.1}$

Method	$\beta_{20.1}$	$\beta_{21.1}$	$\sigma_{22.1}$
BD	2 (59)	-2 (60)	-8 (83)
IML	-262 (61)	-173 (66)	-182 (81)
ML	2 (74)	1 (70)	-8 (115)
PL	3 (83)	3 (83)	-1 (134)

(b) Empirical bias (empirical S.D.)($\times 10^3$) of estimates for $\phi_{3.12}$

Method	$\beta_{30.12}$	$\beta_{31.12}$	$\beta_{32.12}$	$\sigma_{33.12}$
BD	2 (80)	-2 (80)	4 (56)	-11 (82)
IML	-593 (152)	-150 (113)	-134 (85)	-160 (102)
ML	5 (160)	-4 (116)	5 (84)	-11 (131)
PL	3 (177)	-3 (122)	4 (91)	-11 (141)

In the second simulation study, the missing data were created using the following model:

$$pr[R = k - 1|X, Y, R \geq k - 1] = \Phi(\xi_0 + \xi_1 Y_k + \xi_2 Y_k^2), \quad k = 2, 3 \quad (19)$$

with $\xi = (\xi_1, \xi_2, \xi_3) = (-4, -1, 1)$. Again, 1000 data sets were simulated. The number of complete cases averaged 121 and the number of cases with Y_1 and Y_2 observed averaged 177. These data sets were also analyzed by BD, IML, ML and PL, with ML based on the misspecified model (18). The empirical bias and standard deviation (S.D.) of each method over the 1000 data sets are displayed in Table 3.

Table 3. Simulation results from four methods on 1000 replicates
with selection following (19)
(a) Empirical bias (empirical S.D.)($\times 10^3$) of estimates for $\phi_{2.1}$

Method	$\beta_{20.1}$	$\beta_{21.1}$	$\sigma_{22.1}$
BD	1 (57)	1 (58)	-9 (83)
IML	538 (56)	-405 (66)	-411 (58)
ML	443 (130)	-324 (101)	-385 (97)
PL	-7 (113)	10 (105)	13 (201)

(b) Empirical bias (empirical S.D.)($\times 10^3$) of estimates for $\phi_{3.12}$

Method	$\beta_{30.12}$	$\beta_{31.12}$	$\beta_{32.12}$	$\sigma_{33.12}$
BD	1 (84)	-3 (83)	1 (61)	-13 (79)
IML	-182 (89)	-346 (105)	-352 (100)	-357 (74)
ML	-306 (267)	-418 (175)	-473 (262)	-237 (483)
PL	3 (0.113)	5 (154)	9 (138)	-4 (190)

The simulation results Table 3 show that the pseudolikelihood estimates still have negligible bias. The ML method is now seriously biased, reflecting misspecification of the missing-data mechanism (19).

6 Extension and a sensitivity analysis

In this section we consider an extension of the pseudolikelihood method to multivariate monotone missing data $\{X, Y_1, ..., Y_K\}$ with the more general class of mechanisms:

$$pr[R = k - 1|x, y, R \geq k - 1] = w_k(y_k + g_k(x, y_1, ..., y_{k-1})), \quad k = 2, ...K \quad (20)$$

where $g_k(\cdot)'s$ are known functions and $w_k(\cdot)'s$ are arbitrary. Useful mechanisms include cases with $g_k(x, y_1, ..., y_{k-1}) = \lambda y_{k-1}$, where λ reflects the relative weight of the last observed response to the current response in the missing-data mechanism. The estimation procedure is applied to transformed data, $\{X, Y_1 + \lambda X\}$ for example, and the results are transformed back to the original variables. In practice, observed data do not supply information about the functional forms of $g_k(\cdot)'s$ or the value of λ. Hence we recommend a sensitivity analysis to assess the impact of a variety of choices of $g_k(\cdot)'s$ or λ on inferences for the parameters of interest.

We revisit the schizophrenia trial referred in section 2 and illustrate our method on a subset of the data. The primary interest of this trial is the effect of placebo, haloperidol and risperidone on reducing PANSS score at week 8 from the baseline level. Exploratory analysis (Diggle, 1998) showed that the observed mean response decreases over time within each treatment group. The overall reduction in mean response within each active treatment group (haloperidol or risperidone) ranges from about 70 to 90, which suggests that these active treatments have resulted in a clinical improvement. However, these observed means were calculated based on subjects who had not dropped out at each time point. Exploratory analysis (Diggle, 1998) suggests that patients with higher PANSS scores are less reluctant to stay in the trial, so the above results based on observed values are likely to overstate the effect of the treatments.

To illustrate the pseudolikelihood method, we apply it to the data at baseline (Y_1), week 4 (Y_2) and week 8 (Y_3). We assume the following model for the missing-data mechanism:

$$pr[R = k - 1 | X, Y_1, ..., Y_K, R \geq k - 1] = w_k(Y_k + \lambda Y_{k-1}) \qquad (21)$$

with $\lambda = 0$, 0.5, 1, 2, and 9. The conditional distribution of (Y_2, Y_3) given Y_1 follows a normal regression for each treatment arm. Two methods: IML and PL with various values of λ that are mentioned above, are compared. From each method and each treatment arm, the regression parameters of $[Y_2|Y_1]$ and $[Y_3|Y_1, Y_2]$ are estimated and the mean of PANSS score at week 8 is estimated by estimated regression coefficients and the sample mean of Y_1. Although the primary interest is the mean of Y_3, we feel that it is appropriate to model the conditional distribution $[Y_2, Y_3|Y_1]$ when the data have missing values and the missing-data mechanism is suspected not to be MCAR. Table 4 displays the estimated means of week 8 PANSS score for each treatment arm from IML and PL, for a range of assumed values of λ. Standard errors (S.E.'s) are calculated based on 100 bootstrap samples, and are displayed in the parentheses. Since the number of complete cases in the placebo arm is small (29), the program did not converge for about 5 out of 100 of the bootstrap samples. It is suspected that such divergence was caused by bad choices of initial values, resulting in overflow during computation. For simplicity, these samples were replaced by newly generated bootstrap samples.

Table 4: means of PANSS and their S.E.s at Week 8
under MAR or alternative assumptions (21)

$\frac{1}{\lambda}$	Placebo	Haloperidol	Risperidone
∞	95.0 (7.2)	95.3 (6.8)	76.7 (1.7)
2	91.8 (6.5)	90.3 (5.9)	76.0 (1.6)
1	91.0 (5.6)	88.3 (5.2)	75.7 (1.5)
1/2	89.9 (4.8)	86.6 (4.6)	75.4 (1.4)
1/9	88.5 (4.1)	83.8 (4.7)	75.0 (1.4)
IML	86.5 (3.6)	83.6 (3.5)	74.8 (1.4)

The sensitivity analyses suggest that, as the mechanism depends more on the last observed response than the current response, i.e., $\frac{1}{\lambda}$ goes to 0, estimates of improvement in PANSS scores tend to be larger for the placebo and haloperidol groups; estimate of improvement for the risperidone group maintains the same magnitude. Risperidone performs consistently better than the other two treatments, and is close to clinical improvement with about 17% deduction on the PANSS score. As we expected, when the mechanism primarily depends on the last observed data, e.g., $1/\lambda = 1/9$, the pseudolikelihood estimate is close to the IML estimate.

In order to draw conclusions about this study, we need to explore various possible mean structures. For example, Diggle (1998) models the trajectory of mean PANSS scores as quadratic curves over time. Other tools, like random-effects models (Laird and Ware, 1982), can be applied to exploit the repeated-measures nature of this data set.

7 Discussion

Selection modeling is a standard approach to the analysis of multivariate data with a monotone missing-data pattern. Unless the data are MAR, selection models have the drawback that they require specification of the functional form of the missing-data. Usually this functional form is not well understood in practice, even if we have some idea about the set of variables on which the mechanism depends. Misspecification of the mechanism can lead to biased estimates, as shown in the simulations in Table 3.

Pattern-mixture models are useful for multivariate monotone missing data with two patterns (Little and Wang, 1996), but as we have shown, extension to monotone missing data with more than two patterns is problematic because the implied identities for distributions across sets of patterns often lead to intractable model structures.

Like pattern-mixture models, pseudolikelihood selection models can provide robustness within a class of non-MAR mechanisms by not requiring specification of the functional form of the mechanism, and these methods are more readily extended to more than two patterns. In particular, in this paper we extend this method to a multivariate missing data with a monotone missing-data pattern. The PL method is useful when investigators have good reasons to believe that the missingness is determined by either the missing data or a known linear combination of the missing data and the observed data, but they do not wish to specify the form of the *link* functions between the missing-data mechanism and the hypothetical complete data.

Although the PL method is inferior to maximum likelihood with a correctly specified mechanism, it is robust and valid for a general class of mechanisms, and can be close to fully efficient when the correlation between the observed variables and missing variables is strong.

In the estimation procedure, model parameters θ are grouped into K sets of parameters: $\theta_1, ..., \theta_K$. The form of the asymptotic correlations between these parameters is not transparent and is still under investigation.

Acknowledgements

This research is supported by the National Science Foundation under Grant No. DMS-9803720.

References

Anderson, T.W. (1957). Maximum likelihood estimation for the multivariate normal distribution when some observations are missing. *Journal of the American Statistical Association*, 52, 200-203.

Diggle, P.J. (1998). Dealing with missing values in longitudinal studies. *Statistical Analysis of Medical Data: New Developments*, Editors: Everitt, B.S. and Dunn, G. New York: Oxford University Press.

Diggle, P.J. and Kenward, M.G. (1994). Informative Dropout in Longitudinal Data Analysis. *Applied Statistics*, 43, 49-94.

Glynn, R., Laird, N.M., and Rubin, D.B. (1986). Selection modeling versus mixture modeling with nonignorable nonresponse, in *Drawing Inferences from Self-Selected Samples*, H. Wainer, ed. Springer-Verlag, New York, 119-146.

Laird, N.M. and Ware, J.H. (1982). Random-effects models for longitudinal data. *Biometrics*, 37, 383-390.

Little, R.J.A.(1993). Pattern-Mixture Models for Multivariate Incomplete Data. *Journal of the American Statistical Association*, 88, 125-134.

Little, R.J.A. (1994). A Class of Pattern-Mixture Models for Normal Missing Data. *Biometrika*, 81, 471-483.

Little, R.J.A. (1995). Modeling the Dropout Mechanism in Repeated-Measures Studies. *Journal of the American Statistical Association*, 90, 1112-1121.

Little, R.J.A. and Wang, Y-X (1996). Pattern-Mixture Models for Multivariate Incomplete Data with Covariates. *Biometrics*, 52, 98-111.

Little, R.J.A and Rubin, D.B. (2002). *Statistical Analysis with Missing Data*, 2nd. Edition. New York: John Wiley.

Mori, M., Woodworth, G.G., and Woolson, R.F. (1992). Application of Empirical Bayes Inference to Estimation of Rate of Change in the Presence of Informative Right Censoring. *Statistics in Medicine*, 11, 621-631.

Robins, J.M., Rotnitzky, A., and Zhao, L.P. (1994). Estimation of Regression Coefficients When Some Regressors are not Always Observed. *Journal of the American Statistical Association*, 89, 846-866.

Robins, J.M., Rotnitzky, A., and Zhao, L.P. (1995). Analysis of Semiparametric Regression Models for Repeated Outcomes in the Presence of Missing Data. *Journal of the American Statistical Association*, 90, 106-121.

Rotnitzky, A., Robins, J.M., and Scharfstein, D.O. (1998). Semiparametric Regression for Repeated Outcomes with Non-Ignorable Non-Response. *Journal of the American Statistical Association*, 93, 1321-1339.

Rubin, D.B. (1976). Inference and missing data. *Biometrika*, 63, 581-592.

Scharfstein, D.O., Rotnitzky, A., and Robins, J.M. (1999). Adjusting for Nonignorable Drop-Out Using Semiparametric Nonresponse Models. *Journal of the American Statistical Association*, 94, 1096-1120.

Schluchter, M.D. (1992). Methods for the Analysis of Informatively Censored Longitudinal Data. *Statistics in Medicine*, 11, 1861-1870.

Tang, G., Little, R.J.A., and Raghunathan, T.E. (2003). Analysis of Multivariate Missing Data with Nonignorable Nonresponse. *Biometrika*, 90, 747-764.

Quantile Regression for Correlated Observations

Li Chen[1], Lee-Jen Wei[2], and Michael I. Parzen[3]

[1] Division of Biostatistics, University of Minnesota, Minneapolis, MN 55414
[2] Department of Biostatistics, Harvard University, Boston, MA 02115
[3] Graduate School of Business, University of Chicago, Chicago, IL 60637

ABSTRACT We consider the problem of regression analysis for data which consist of a large number of independent small groups or clusters of correlated observations. Instead of using the standard mean regression, we regress various percentiles of each marginal response variable over its covariates to obtain a more accurate assessment of the covariate effect. Our inference procedures are derived using the generalized estimating equations approach. The new proposal is robust and can be easily implemented. Graphical and numerical methods for checking the adequacy of the fitted quantile regression model are also proposed. The new methods are illustrated with an animal study in toxicology.

1 Introduction

Although quite a few useful parametric and semi-parametric regression methods are available for analyzing correlated observations, they can only be used to evaluate the covariate effect on the *mean* of the response variable (Laird and Ware, 1982; Liang and Zeger, 1986). To obtain a global picture about the covariate effect on the distribution of the response variable, one may use the quantile regression model. Specifically, let τ be a constant between 0 and 1, Y be the response variable and x be the corresponding $(p+1) \times 1$ covariate vector. Given x, let the 100τth percentile of Y be $\beta_\tau' x$, where β_τ is an unknown $(p+1) \times 1$ parameter vector and may depend on τ. Inference procedures for β_τ with a set of properly chosen τ's would provide much more information about the effect of x on Y than their counterparts based on the usual mean regression model (Mosteller and Tukey, 1977). For independent observations, inference procedures for β_τ have been proposed, for example, by Bassett and Koenker (1978, 1982), Koenker and Bassett (1978, 1982) and Parzen et al. (1994). When $\tau = 1/2$, which corresponds to the median regression model, the celebrated L_1 estimator which minimizes the sum of the absolute residuals is consistent for $\beta_{0.5}$ (Bloomfield and Steiger, 1983).

Recently, Jung (1996) proposed an interesting quasi-likelihood equation approach for median regression models with dependent observations. However, his method assumes a known relationship between the median and the density function of the response variable. The variance estimate of his estimator for the regression parameter appears to be rather sensitive to this assumption. Moreover, Jung's optimal estimating equations may have multiple roots and, therefore, the estimator for β_τ may not be well-defined.

In this paper, we present a simple and robust procedure to make inferences about β_τ without imposing any parametric assumption on the density function of the response variable or on the dependent structure among those correlated observations. Furthermore, our estimating functions are monotonic component-wise and the resulting estimator for the regression parameter can be easily obtained through well-established linear programming techniques. The new proposal is illustrated with an animal study in toxicology.

2 Inferences for Regression Parameters

In this section, we derive regression methods for analyzing data that consist of a large number of independent small groups or clusters of correlated observations. Let Y_{ij} be the continuous response variable for the jth measurement in the ith cluster, where $i = 1, ..., n; j = 1, .., K_i$, where K_i is relatively small with respect to n. Let x_{ij} be the corresponding covariate vector. Furthermore, assume that the 100τth percentile of Y_{ij} is $\beta_\tau' x_{ij}$. The observations within each cluster may be dependent, but (Y_{ij}, x_{ij}) and $(Y_{i'j'}, x_{i'j'})$ are independent when $i \neq i'$. Note that the distribution function $F_{\tau ij}(\cdot)$ of the error term $(Y_{ij} - \beta_\tau' x_{ij})$ is completely unspecified and may involve x_{ij}.

Suppose that we are interested in β_τ for a particular τ. If all the observations $\{(Y_{ij}, x_{ij})\}$ are mutually independent, the following estimating functions are often used to make inferences about β_τ:

$$W_\tau(\beta) = n^{-1/2} \sum_{i=1}^{n} \sum_{j=1}^{K_i} x_{ij}\{I(Y_{ij} - \beta' x_{ij} \leq 0) - \tau\}, \qquad (1)$$

where $I(\cdot)$ is the indicator function. For the aforementioned correlated observations, (1) are estimating functions based on the "independence working model" (Liang and Zeger, 1986) and the expected value of $W_\tau(\beta_\tau)$ is 0. Therefore, a solution $\hat{\beta}_\tau$ to the equations $W_\tau(\beta) = 0$, would be a reasonable estimate for β_τ. The consistency of $\hat{\beta}_\tau$ can be easily established using similar arguments for the case of independent observations. In practice, $\hat{\beta}_\tau$ can be obtained by minimizing

$$\sum_{i=1}^{n} \sum_{j=1}^{K_i} \rho_\tau(Y_{ij} - \beta' x_{ij}), \qquad (2)$$

where $\rho_\tau(v)$ is τv if $v > 0$, and $(\tau - 1)v$, if $v \leq 0$ (Koenker and Bassett, 1978). This optimization problem can be handled by linear programming techniques

(Barrodale and Roberts, 1973). An efficient algorithm developed by Koenker and D'Orey (1987) is available in Splus to obtain a minimizer $\hat{\beta}_\tau$ for (2). Using a similar argument given in Chamberlain (1994) for the case of independent observations, one can show that for the present case, the distribution of $n^{1/2}(\hat{\beta}_\tau - \beta_\tau)$ goes to a normal distribution as $n \to \infty$. The corresponding covariance matrix is $A_\tau^{-1}(\beta_\tau) \mathrm{var}\{W_\tau(\beta_\tau)\}\{A_\tau^T(\beta_\tau)\}^{-1}$, where $A_\tau(\beta)$ is the expected value of the derivative of $W_\tau(\beta)$ with respect to β. For the heteroskedastic quantile regression model considered here, it is difficult to estimate the covariance matrix because $A_\tau(\beta)$ may involve the unknown underlying density functions. Complicated and subjective nonparametric functional estimates are needed to estimate the variance directly.

Recently, Parzen et al. (1994) developed a general resampling method which can be used to approximate the distribution of $(\hat{\beta}_\tau - \beta_\tau)$ without involving any complicated and subjective nonparametric functional estimation. To apply this resampling method to the case with correlated observations, let

$$U_\tau = n^{-1/2} \sum_{i=1}^{n} \left[\sum_{j=1}^{K_i} x_{ij}\{I(y_{ij} - \tilde{\beta}_\tau' x_{ij} \leq 0) - \tau\} \right] Z_i,$$

where $\{Z_i, i = 1, ...n\}$ is a random sample from the standard normal population, y and $\tilde{\beta}_\tau$ are the observed values of Y and $\hat{\beta}_\tau$, respectively. Note the only component that is random in U_τ is Z_i. It is straightforward to show that the unconditional distribution of $W_\tau(\beta_\tau)$ and the conditional distribution of U_τ converge to the same limiting distribution. Let $w_\tau(\beta)$ be the observed $W_\tau(\beta)$. Define a random vector β_τ^* such that $w_\tau(\beta_\tau^*) = -U_\tau$. Then, the unconditional distribution of $(\hat{\beta}_\tau - \beta_\tau)$ can be approximated by the conditional distribution of $(\beta_\tau^* - \tilde{\beta}_\tau)$. The adequacy of using the distribution of $(\beta_\tau^* - \tilde{\beta}_\tau)$ to approximate the unconditional distribution of $(\hat{\beta}_\tau - \beta_\tau)$ has been addressed by Parzen et al. (1994) through extensive simulation studies. Furthermore, the distribution of β_τ^* can be estimated using a large random sample $\{u_{\tau m}, m = 1, ..., M\}$ generated from U_τ. For each realized $u_{\tau m}$, we obtain a solution of $\beta_{\tau m}^*$, by solving the equation $w(\beta_{\tau m}^*) = -u_{\tau m}$, $m = 1, .., M$. The covariance matrix of $\hat{\beta}_\tau$ can then be estimated by the empirical distribution function based on $\{\beta_{\tau m}^*, m = 1, ..., M\}$, for example, by $\sum_{m=1}^{M}(\beta_{\tau m}^* - \tilde{\beta}_\tau)(\beta_{\tau m}^* - \tilde{\beta}_\tau)^T/M$. The standard bootstrap method can also be used for estimating the variance of the regression parameters. For independently identically distributed correlated observations, the validity of the bootstrap approach has been demonstrated by van der Vaart and Wellner (1996). However, few data exist on how well the method works for the general quantile regression model.

In order to use existing statistical software (for example, Koenker and D'Orey, 1987) to solve the equation $w_\tau(\beta) = -u$, one may artificially create an extra data point (y^*, x^*), where x^* is $n^{1/2}u/\tau$ and y^* is an extremely large number such that $I(y^* - \beta'x^* \leq 0)$ is always 0. Let $w_\tau^*(\beta) = w_\tau(\beta) + n^{-1/2}x^*\{I(y^* - \beta'x^* \leq 0) - \tau\}$. Then, solving the equation $w_\tau(\beta) = u$ is equivalent to solving the equation $w_\tau^*(\beta) = 0$.

To illustrate the above method, we use an animal study in developmental toxicity evaluation of Dietary Di(2-ethylhexyl)phthalate (DEHP), a widely used plasticizing agent, in timed-pregnant mice (Tyl et al; 1988). DEHP was administered in the diet on days 6 through 15 of gestation with dose levels of 0, 44, 91, 191 and 292 (mg/kg/day). On the 17th gestational day, the maternal animals were sacrificed and all the fetuses were examined. One of the major outcomes for the study is the fetal body weight. The investigators would like to know whether DEHP has a negative effect on the fetal body weight. Since the sex of the fetus is expected to be correlated with the weight, an adjustment from this covariate in the analysis is needed. Here, the litter is the cluster and each live fetus is a member of the cluster. Furthermore, Y_{ij} is the weight and x_{ij} is a 3×1 vector, where the first component is one, the second one is the dose level, and the third one is the sex indicator for the fetus. For the animal study data, there are total of 108 clusters and the cluster sizes range from 2 to 16. With the aforementioned quantile regression, estimates for β_τ and the corresponding estimated standard errors obtained based on the estimating functions (1) are reported in the third and fourth columns in Table 1. The estimated standard error is obtained using the new method with 500 resampling samples.

Table 1. Estimates for quantile regression for the DEHP study

Quantile	Coefficient		Standard Error		
			New Method	Paired-BS	Heqf-BS
0.05	Intercept	0.80	0.049	0.047	0.049
	Dose*	-0.048	0.015	0.014	0.013
	Sex	-0.019	0.028	0.027	0.027
0.25	Intercept	0.97	0.023	0.021	0.017
	Dose*	-0.048	0.013	0.012	0.007
	Sex	-0.038	0.010	0.010	0.011
0.50	Intercept	1.03	0.021	0.022	0.015
	Dose*	-0.039	0.012	0.012	0.005
	Sex	-0.036	0.094	0.091	0.082
0.75	Intercept	1.10	0.026	0.026	0.015
	Dose*	-0.028	0.014	0.013	0.007
	Sex	-0.045	0.011	0.010	0.008
0.95	Intercept	1.20	0.027	0.023	0.018
	Dose*	-0.030	0.013	0.012	0.006
	Sex	-0.047	0.012	0.009	0.010

* Estimates for dose effect are for per 100 unit increase.

For comparison, Table 1 also gives the estimated standard errors with two heteroskedastic bootstrap procedures. The first procedure is the paired bootstrap (denoted as paired-BS) method (Efron, 1982, p.36), where the (x_{ij}, y_{ij}) pair is resampled. Specifically, we resampled the clusters to accommodate the dependency and heteroskedasticity. The second procedure is the empirical quantile function bootstrap (denoted as Heqf-BS) method proposed by Koenker (1994), where the full quantile regression process β_τ is resampled. Specifically, for each bootstrap realization of n observations, n vectors of p-dimensions from the estimated regression quantile process $\hat{\beta}_\tau$ are drawn. The bootstrapped observation y_{ij} is then the inner product of the design row x_{ij} and the corresponding ith draw from the regression quantile process. This procedure again accommodate certain forms of dependency and heteroskedasticity. The standard error estimated by bootstrap methods are based on 500 bootstrap samples. The results from the paired-BS is similar to those obtained from our resampling procedure. The results from the Heqf-BS are smaller than those obtained from our resampling procedure.

For any given set of percentiles, say, $\{\tau_k, k = 1, .., K\}$, one may obtain a simultaneous confidence interval for a particular component η_{τ_k} of $\beta_{\tau_k}, k = 1, ..., K$. More specifically, consider a class of estimating functions $\{W_{\tau_k}(\beta_{\tau_k}), k = 1, ..., K\}$ and the corresponding $\{U_{\tau_k}, k = 1, .., K\}$, where the random sample $\{Z_i, i = 1, ..., n\}$ is now shared by all the U_{τ_k}'s. Let $\{\beta^*_{\tau_k}, k = 1, ..., K\}$, be the solutions to the simultaneous equations $\{w_{\tau_k}(\beta^*_{\tau_k}) = -U_{\tau_k}, k = 1, .., K\}$. Then, the joint distribution of $\{(\hat{\beta}_{\tau_k} - \beta_{\tau_k}), k = 1, ..., K\}$ can be approximated by that of $\{(\beta^*_{\tau_k} - \tilde{\beta}_{\tau_k}), k = 1, .., K\}$. To obtain a $(1 - \alpha)$ confidence band for η_{τ_k}, we first find a critical value c_α such that

$$\Pr(\sup_k \{\hat{\sigma}_{\tau_k}^{-1} | \eta^*_{\tau_k} - \tilde{\eta}_{\tau_k}|\} \leq c_\alpha) = 1 - \alpha,$$

where $\eta^*_{\tau_k}$ and $\tilde{\eta}_{\tau_k}$ are the corresponding components of $\beta^*_{\tau_k}$ and $\tilde{\beta}_{\tau_k}$, respectively; $\hat{\sigma}^2_{\tau_k}$ is the variance estimate of $\hat{\eta}_{\tau_k}$, obtained through the above resampling method. A confidence band of $\{\eta_{\tau_k}, k = 1, ..., K\}$ is then

$$\hat{\eta}_{\tau_k} \pm c_\alpha \hat{\sigma}_{\tau_k}, k = 1, ..., K.$$

For the animal study example, if we let $K = 5$ with $\tau_1 = 0.05, \tau_2 = 0.25, \tau_3 = 0.5, \tau_4 = 0.75$, and $\tau_5 = 0.95$, then a 95% confidence band, displayed in the dashed lines, for the dose effect is given in Figure 1. The corresponding critical value is 2.38 based on 1000 simulations. For comparison, we also provide corresponding pointwise confidence intervals, displayed in the solid lines. The simultaneous confidence intervals in the figure are not too different from their pointwise counterparts. Naturally, the confidence band would become wider if K gets larger.

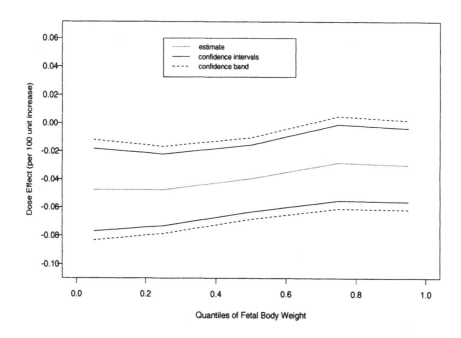

Fig. 1. Confidence intervals and band for dose effect

A very useful application of the above flexible modeling is to make prediction of the τth quantiles of the distribution of the fetal body weight. Figure 2(a) shows the point estimates of fetal body weight for males with various dosing levels, and Figure 2(b) gives the corresponding predicted weights for females. These plots are quite informative, for example, one may readily conclude that with a 20% chance the weight of a male whose mother was treated with the highest dose is less than 0.77 grams. On the other hand, if the mother were not exposed to DEHP, the corresponding weight would be 0.91 grams.

If the effect of a particular covariate, say ξ_k of β_{τ_k}, is about the same across the set of quantiles $\tau_k, k = 1, ..., K$, one may want to combine $\hat{\xi}_k$'s, obtained from $\hat{\beta}_{\tau_k}$'s, to make inferences about the common parameter ξ. To this end, consider an "optimal" linear combination $\hat{\xi} = \sum_{i=1}^{K} a_k \hat{\xi}_k$, where $a = (a_1, ..., a_K)' = \Gamma^{-1}e/\{e'\Gamma^{-1}e\}$, $e = (1, ..., 1)'$ is a K-dimensional vector and Γ is a $K \times K$ covariance matrix of $\hat{\xi}_k$'s. Note that asymptotically, $\hat{\xi}$ has the smallest variance among all the linear combinations of $\hat{\xi}_k$'s (Wei and Johnson, 1985). Note that even if the covariate effects of ξ_k are unequal across different quantiles, in practice one may still combine the $\hat{\xi}_k$'s to draw a conclusion about the "average effect" of the covariate provided that there are no qualitative differences among the $\hat{\xi}_k$'s. For the DEHP study example, if the dose effects are about the same for τ_1 through τ_5, then the common dose effect (per 100 unit increase) is $\hat{\xi} = -0.041$ with an estimated standard error of 0.01.

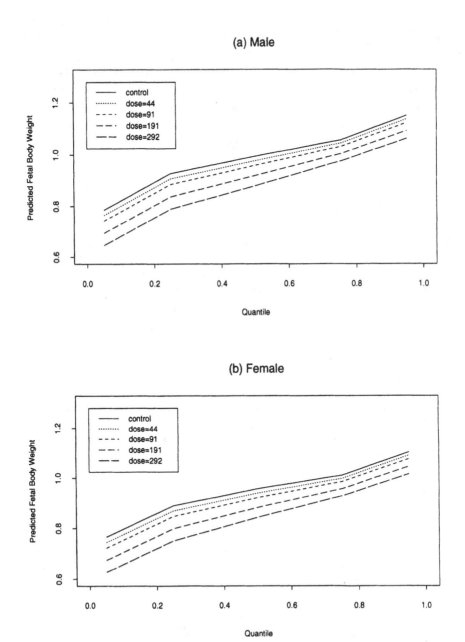

Fig. 2. Predicting fetal body weight for the DEHP study with various dosing levels

3 Simulation Studies

To examine the performance of the proposed resampling method, we conducted simulation studies for median regression. In the simulation studies, we generated 500 samples $\{(Y_{ij}, x_{ij}), i = 1, ..., 50; j = 1, 2\}$ from the following linear model: $Y_{ij} = \beta_{0.5} x_{ij} + e_i + \varepsilon_{ij}$, where $\beta_{0.5} = 1$, $\{x_{ij}\}$ is a realization of a random sample from the uniform variable on $(0, 1)$, e_i is the standard normal variable. Two models for ε_{ij} are considered: (a) ε_{ij} is a normal variable with mean 0 and variance 0.5; (b) ε_{ij} is a normal variable with mean 0 and variance proportional to x_{ij}. For each simulated sample, the distribution of $(\beta_{0.5}^* - \tilde{\beta}_{0.5})$ was estimated based on 500 samples from $U_{0.5}$. The standard and percentile methods (Efron and Tibshirani, 1986, pp. 67-70) were then used to construct confidence intervals of the regression coefficient corresponding to x_{ij}. The empirical coverage probabilities and estimated average lengths for these intervals are summarized in Table 2 for the model with constant variance and in Table 3 for the model with heteroskedastic variance. For comparison we also report the results based on the paired bootstrap method and the empirical quantile function bootstrap method in the tables. In general, the resampling procedure performs well. The paired bootstrap method also performs well, but the empirical quantile function bootstrap method has lower coverage probabilities. These findings are consistent with those in the paper by Koenker (1994).

We also performed simulation studies on the performance of the new method with variable cluster size. We generated 500 samples $\{(Y_{ij}, x_{ij}), i = 1, ..., 50; j = 1, K_i\}$ from the above linear model. The cluster size K_i was randomly chosen from any numbers between 2 and 10. Again, for each of the 500 simulations, 500 resampling samples were used. Table 4 displays the empirical coverage probability and the estimated mean length for median regression with Gaussian error of mean 0 and either constant or heteroskedastic variance. As demonstrated in the table, the new method performs well in the case of variable cluster sizes. The computing time for each of these simulation studies was approximately 12 minutes on a Sun Solaris II machine.

Table 2. Empirical coverage probabilities (ECP) and estimated mean lengths (EML) for Gaussian error with mean 0 and variance 0.5 for median regression

Confidence level	New Method		Paired-BS		Heqf-BS	
	ECP	EML	ECP	EML	ECP	EML
0.95	S 0.95	1.28	0.93	1.25	0.88	1.06
	P 0.95	1.23	0.94	1.19	0.91	1.03
0.90	S 0.91	1.06	0.89	1.04	0.84	0.85
	P 0.90	1.01	0.89	0.99	0.85	0.82

S: standard method; P: percentile method

Table 3. Empirical coverage probabilities (ECP) and estimated mean lengths (EML) for Gaussian error with mean 0 and heteroskedastic variance for median regression

Confidence level		New Method ECP EML		Paired-BS ECP EML		Heqf-BS ECP EML	
0.95	S	0.93	1.22	0.92	1.19	0.90	1.08
	P	0.93	1.17	0.92	1.13	0.91	1.04
0.90	S	0.89	1.02	0.89	1.00	0.81	0.81
	P	0.89	0.98	0.90	0.96	0.82	0.78

S: standard method; P: percentile method

Table 4. Empirical coverage probabilities (ECP) and estimated mean lengths (EML) for Gaussian error with mean 0 and either constant or heteroskedastic variance for median regression for variable cluster size

Confidence level		Constant variance ECP EML		Heteroskedastic variance ECP EML	
0.95	S	0.94	1.16	0.95	1.19
	P	0.95	1.13	0.95	1.18
0.90	S	0.92	0.99	0.91	0.99
	P	0.90	0.97	0.91	0.98

S: standard method; P: percentile method

The set of estimating functions $W_\tau(\beta)$ in (1) is a special case of the functions $\tilde{W}_\tau$ considered by Jung for estimating β_τ, where

$$\tilde{W}_\tau(\beta) = n^{-1/2} \sum_{i=1}^{n} R_i \begin{pmatrix} I(Y_{i1} - \beta' x_{i1} \leq 0) - \tau \\ \vdots \\ I(Y_{iK_i} - \beta' x_{iK_i} \leq 0) - \tau \end{pmatrix}$$

and R_i is a $K_i \times K_i$ matrix which may involve $x_{ij}, j = 1, ..., K_i$ and β. Under some regularity conditions on R_i, a root to the equation $\tilde{W}_\tau(\beta) = 0$, is consistent (Jung, 1996). In theory, the inclusion of R_i, which accounts for the dependence among the correlated measurements, may achieve greater efficiency than the procedures based on (1). However, if R_i depends on β, the equation $\tilde{W}_\tau(\beta) = 0$ may have multiple roots. Furthermore, empirically we have found that such efficiency improvement is quite small if there is any. For example, in the simulation study using models (a) and (b) mentioned above, the mean squared errors (MSE) are estimated. Jung's optimal estimating function given in his Section 6 was used for comparison. Jung's variance estimate for β_τ is derived by assuming a specific relationship between the median and the dispersion of the response variable. If this assumption is violated, his inference procedure may not be valid.

The MSE for our estimator and Jung's are displayed in Table 5 for $\beta_{0.5}$. Also displayed in Table 5 are the simulated MSEs when the covariate x_{ij} is discrete. Specifically, $\{x_{ij}\}$ is a realization of a random sample from the Bernoulli (0.5) distribution. As seen in Table 5, if the variance of ε_{ij} in the above linear model is proportional to x_{ij}, but we assume that the variance of ε_{ij} is constant for Jung's method, the loss of efficiency of Jung's method compare to the independent working model of the new method ranges from 30% to 54%. We were not able to make comparisons for quantiles other than the median because Jung's method was developed for median regression.

Table 5. Mean MSEs for the new method and Jung's method

Sample	Distribution			MSE		MSE ratio
size	x_{ij}	e_i	ε_{ij}	Jung	New	(Jung/New)
50	Ber(0.5)	N(0,1)	N(0,.5)	0.050	0.049	1.01
			N(0,.5)x_{ij}	0.065	0.050	1.30
	Uni(0,1)	N(0,1)	N(0,.5)	0.060	0.058	1.02
			N(0,.5)x_{ij}	0.066	0.048	1.34
100	Ber(0.5)	N(0,1)	N(0,.5)	0.033	0.032	1.04
			N(0,.5)x_{ij}	0.040	0.030	1.32
	Uni(0,1)	N(0,1)	N(0,.5)	0.043	0.042	1.03
			N(0,.5)x_{ij}	0.042	0.028	1.54

4 Model Checking

If the deterministic portion of the fitted quantile regression model is correctly specified, the inference procedures discussed in Section 2 are valid even when the error term $(Y - \beta'_\tau x)$ in the model depends on the covariates. For the aforementioned animal study example, the crucial modeling assumption is that the 100τth percentile of the response variable is linearly related to the covariates. The plot, given in Figure 3, of the ordinary residuals against the dose level for median regression offers little information on the adequacy of the fitted quantile regression model. The difficulty with using such plots for model checking is that we simply have no knowledge about the behavior of those individual correlated residuals even under the simple additive quantile regression model.

Consider the random components $\{e_{\tau ij}(\beta), j = 1, ..., K_i; i = 1, ..., n\}$ in the estimating function (1), where $e_{\tau ij}(\beta) = I(Y_{ij} - \beta'x_{ij} \leq 0) - \tau$. The quantities $\{e_{\tau ij}(\hat{\beta}_\tau)\}$ resemble ordinary residuals in linear models. For example, $\sum_{i=1}^{n}\sum_{j=1}^{K_i} e_{\tau ij}(\hat{\beta}_\tau) = 0$, and under the fitted model, for large n, $E\{e_{\tau ij}(\hat{\beta}_\tau)\} = 0$. Note that $e_{\tau ij}(\hat{\beta}_\tau)$ is either $1 - \tau$ or $-\tau$. Therefore, it is difficult to use such individual "quantile residuals" graphically to examine the adequacy of the assumed quantile regression model. Here, we show how to use cumulative sums of quantile residuals to examine the model assumption graphically and numerically (see Lin, Wei and Ying, 2002, for a general review on this approach of model checking). First, consider the following process:

$$V_{\tau l}(\beta; t) = n^{-1/2} \sum_{i=1}^{n} \sum_{j=1}^{K_i} e_{\tau ij}(\beta) I(x_{lij} \leq t),$$

where $t \in R$, $l = 1, ..., p$, and $x_{ij} = (1, x_{1ij}, ..., x_{pij})'$. If the 100τth percentile of Y_{ij}, given x_{ij}, is $\beta_\tau' x_{ij}$, we expect $V_{\tau l}(\hat{\beta}_\tau; t)$ to behave approximately like a Gaussian process. One may plot the observed $v_{\tau l}(\tilde{\beta}_\tau; t)$ of $V_{\tau l}(\hat{\beta}_\tau; t)$ to see if it is an unusual realization of a zero-mean normal process. For the animal study, the above process $v_{\tau l}(\cdot)$ is plotted against the dose level $\{x_{1ij}\}$ and is displayed in the solid curves in Figure 4.

Next, the solid curves in Figure 4 are compared with the null distribution of $V_{\tau l}(\hat{\beta}_\tau; t)$. In the Appendix, we show that this null distribution can be approximated by the conditional distribution of $V_{\tau l}^*(t)$:

$$n^{-1/2} \sum_{i=1}^{n} \left[\sum_{j=1}^{K_i} \{I(y_{ij} - \tilde{\beta}_\tau' x_{ij} \leq 0) - \tau\} I(x_{lij} \leq t) \right] Z_i + v_{\tau l}(\beta_\tau^*; t) - v_{\tau l}(\tilde{\beta}_\tau; t),$$

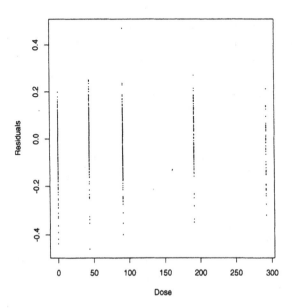

Fig. 3. Ordinary residuals against dose level for median regression

where $\{Z_i, i = 1, \ldots, n\}$ is the random sample which generates U_τ in Section 2. Note that the process $\{V_{\tau l}^*(t)\}$ can be easily simulated. First, we generate a random sample $\{Z_i\}$. For this particular sample, we obtain u_τ, β_τ^* and then a realization $\{v_{\tau l}^*(t)\}$. For the animal data, 30 such realizations, displayed by the dotted curves, against the dose level are presented in Figure 4. The solid curves do not seem to be unusual with respect to their dotted counterparts.

One can also plot the cumulative sums of $\{e_{\tau ij}(\hat{\beta}_\tau)\}$ against the predicted values $\{\hat{\beta}_\tau' x_{ij}\}$ based on the process:

$$S_\tau(\hat{\beta}_\tau; t) = n^{-1/2} \sum_{i=1}^{n} \sum_{j=1}^{K_i} e_{\tau ij}(\hat{\beta}_\tau) I(\hat{\beta}_\tau' x_{ij} \le t).$$

In the Appendix, we show that the null distribution of the process can be approximated by the conditional distribution of $S_\tau^*(t)$:

$$n^{-1/2} \sum_{i=1}^{n} \left[\sum_{j=1}^{K_i} \{I(y_{ij} - \tilde{\beta}_\tau' x_{ij} \le 0) - \tau\} I(\tilde{\beta}_\tau' x_{ij} \le t) \right] Z_i + s_\tau(\beta_\tau^*; t) - s_\tau(\tilde{\beta}_\tau; t),$$

where s_τ is the observed S_τ. Thirty realizations displayed by dotted curves generated from $S_\tau^*(t)$ are given in Figure 5. Again, comparing with those dotted curves the solid curves of the observed $s_\tau(\tilde{\beta}_\tau; t)$ do not seem atypical.

If we fit the above animal study data with log(dose) instead of using the original dose level for the median regression model (1), the curves based on $\{v_{0.5,1}(\tilde{\beta}_{0.5}; t)\}$ and $\{v_{0.5,1}^*(t)\}$ against dose level are given in Figure 6. This model does not seem to fit the data well.

Figures 4 and 5 provide much more information regarding the adequacy of the fitted additive quantile regression model than the usual residual plot in Figure 3. One may make the above graphical procedures even more objective by supplementing it with some numerical values that measure how extreme the observed $\{v_{\tau l}(t)\}$ and $\{s_\tau(t)\}$ are under the fitted model. For example, let $G_{\tau l} = \sup_t |V_{\tau l}(\hat{\beta}_\tau; t)|$ and $g_{\tau l}$ be its observed value. Then the probabilities $p_{\tau l} = Pr(G_{\tau l} \ge g_{\tau l})$ would be reasonable candidates for such numerical measures. These probabilities can be estimated by simulating $\{V_{\tau l}^*(t)\}$. For the solid curves in Figure 4, estimates of such p-values based on 500 realizations of $\sup_t\{V_{\tau l}^*(t)\}$ are 0.694, 0.346 and 0.906 for τ being 0.25, 0.50 and 0.75, respectively. For Figure 5, the corresponding p-values are 0.998, 0.676 and 0.994, respectively. For Figure 6, the p-value is 0.056.

One can also plot the partial sums of $\{e_{\tau ij}(\hat{\beta}_\tau)\}$ against a covariate variable which is not included in the fitted model to assess if it is an important predictor. Although the diagnostic plots against individual explanatory variables in Figures 4, 5 and 6 are useful for checking the adequacy of the assumed model, they may not be able to detect, for example, the existence of high-order interaction terms in the model. To tackle this problem, one may consider a high dimensional residual plot based on the following multi-parameter process:

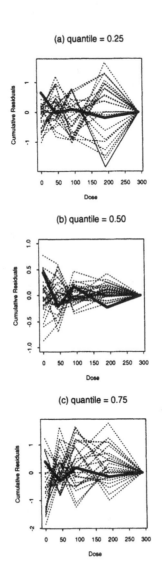

Fig. 4. Cumulative sums of residuals against dose level

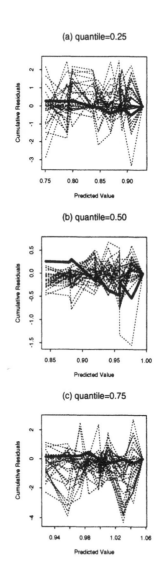

Fig. 5. Cumulative sums of residuals against predicted value

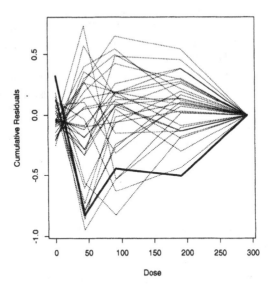

Fig. 6. Cumulative sums of residuals against dose level by fitting a median regression model with logarithm of dose level

$$\mathbf{V}_\tau(\hat{\beta}_\tau;\mathbf{t}) = n^{-1/2}\sum_{i=1}^{n}\sum_{j=1}^{K_i}\{I(Y_{ij}-\hat{\beta}_\tau' x_{ij}\leq 0)-\tau\}\begin{pmatrix} I(x_{1ij}\leq t_1)\\ \vdots\\ I(x_{pij}\leq t_p)\end{pmatrix}$$

where $\mathbf{t}=(t_1,...,t_p)'$. If the 100τth percentile of Y, given x, is $\beta_\tau'x$, we would expect that the partial-sum process $\{\mathbf{V}_\tau(\hat{\beta}_\tau;\mathbf{t})\}$ to fluctuate about 0. Let $\mathbf{v}_\tau(\hat{\beta}_\tau;\mathbf{t})$ be the observed $\mathbf{V}_\tau(\hat{\beta}_\tau;\mathbf{t})$. Using similar arguments in the Appendix, one can show that the null distribution of $\mathbf{V}_\tau(\hat{\beta}_\tau,\mathbf{t})$ may be approximated by that of $\mathbf{V}_\tau^*(\mathbf{t})$, where

$$\mathbf{V}_\tau^*(\mathbf{t}) = n^{-1/2}\sum_{i=1}^{n}[\sum_{j=1}^{K_i}\{I(y_{ij}-\tilde{\beta}_\tau' x_{ij}\leq 0)-\tau\}\begin{pmatrix} I(x_{1ij}\leq t_1)\\ \vdots\\ I(x_{pij}\leq t_p)\end{pmatrix}]Z_i$$

$$+\mathbf{v}_\tau(\beta_\tau^*;\mathbf{t})-\mathbf{v}_\tau(\tilde{\beta}_\tau;\mathbf{t}).$$

Again, the distribution of $\mathbf{V}_\tau^*$ can be easily obtained through simulation. Presumably one may compare the observed $\mathbf{v}_\tau(\tilde{\beta}_\tau;\mathbf{t})$ with a number of realizations generated from $\mathbf{V}_\tau^*(\mathbf{t})$ in a high-dimensional plot to see if there is a lack-of-fit of the assumed model. Unfortunately, this may not be feasible if $p > 2$. On the other hand, numerical lack of fit tests can be easily constructed based on the process $\mathbf{V}_\tau(\hat{\beta}_\tau; \mathbf{t})$. For example, a large value of $\sup_{\mathbf{t}} \|\mathbf{V}_\tau(\hat{\beta}_\tau; \mathbf{t})\|$ suggests that the fitted model may be misspecified. Using the above simple additive quantile regression model to fit the animal study data with three covariates, the p-values of this sup-type test based on 500 realizations from $\mathbf{V}_\tau^*(\mathbf{t})$ are 0.71, 0.34 and 0.93 for τ being $0.25, 0.5$ and 0.75 respectively. It can be shown that this sup-type statistic gives an omnibus test. That is, the test is consistent against a general alternative. An omnibus test, however, may not be very powerful against some particular alternatives. In practice, we recommend that both numerical and graphical methods proposed here should be used for model checking.

5 Remarks

The new procedure can be used to analyze data comprised of a group of repeated measurements over time. This type of correlated data is often encountered in medical studies. It is important to note that for such repeated measurements, our method is valid when the missing observations are missing completely at random. For the usual mean regression problem, several methods have been proposed to analyze the longitudinal data which are subject to informative censoring (Wu and Carroll, 1988; Baker, Wax and Patterson, 1993; Rotnitzky and Robins, 1995). Recently, Lipsitz, Fitzmaurice, Molenberghs and Zhao (1997) proposed a set of weighted estimating equations for quantile regression to handle the data whose missing observations are missing at random. Their novel proposal, however, does not have theoretical justification. It would be interesting to investigate if the resampling method discussed in the present paper is applicable to those weighted estimating functions.

We proposed a graphical method for checking the adequacy of the assumed quantile regression model. More work is clearly needed in this area. Recently, a goodness of fit process for quantile regression analogous to the conventional R^2 statistic of least squares regression has been introduced for independent observations (Koenker and Machado, 1999). Their related tests are based on some sup-type statistics. They mentioned it is possible to expand the test to Cramer-von-Mises forms, where the test would be based on an integral of the square of the regression quantile process over τ. It would be useful to study if the methods can be extended to handle the quantile regression with correlated observations.

Acknowledgments: The authors are grateful to Dr. Robert Gray for his helpful comments on this paper and to Dr. Paul Catalano for providing the dataset.

Appendix

We will give a heuristic justification of using the distribution of $\{V_{\tau l}^*(t)\}$ to approximate that of $\{V_{\tau l}(\hat{\beta}_\tau; t)\}$. With a minor modification of Theorem 1 in Lai and Ying (1988), one can show that there exists a deterministic row vector $A(t)$ such that

$$V_{\tau l}(\hat{\beta}_\tau; t) = V_{\tau l}(\beta_\tau; t) + A(t)n^{1/2}(\hat{\beta}_\tau - \beta_\tau) + o(1), \quad \text{a.s.}$$

Also,

$$v_{\tau l}(\beta_\tau^*; t) = v_{\tau l}(\tilde{\beta}_\tau; t) + A(t)n^{1/2}(\beta_\tau^* - \tilde{\beta}_\tau) + o(1). \tag{A.1}$$

Recall that $\hat{\beta}_\tau$ is a solution to the estimating equations: $W_\tau(\beta) = 0$. It follows from the argument in Appendix 2 of Parzen et al. (1994) that $n^{1/2}(\hat{\beta}_\tau - \beta_\tau) \approx C_\tau W_\tau(\beta_\tau)$, where C_τ is a deterministic matrix. Hence the limiting distribution of $\{V_{\tau l}(\hat{\beta}_\tau; t)\}$ is the same as that of

$$n^{-1/2} \sum_{i=1}^{n} \left[\sum_{j=1}^{K_i} \{I(y_{ij} - \tilde{\beta}_\tau' x_{ij} \leq 0) - \tau\} I(x_{lij} \leq t) \right] Z_i + A(t)C_\tau U_\tau. \tag{A.2}$$

On the other hand, the random vector β_τ^* is a solution to $w_\tau(\beta_\tau^*) = -U_\tau$. Again, from the argument in Appendix 2 of Parzen et al. (1994), $n^{1/2}(\beta_\tau^* - \tilde{\beta}_\tau) = C_\tau U_\tau + o(1)$. This, coupled with (A.1), gives

$$v_{\tau l}(\beta_\tau^*; t) - v_{\tau l}(\tilde{\beta}_\tau; t) = A(t)C_\tau U_\tau + o(1). \tag{A.3}$$

From (A.2) and (A.3), we obtain the desired asymptotic equivalence.

Next, we show that $S_\tau(\hat{\beta}_\tau; t)$ and $S_\tau^*(t)$ have the same limiting distribution. Taking linear expansion of $S_\tau(\hat{\beta}_\tau; t)$ at β_τ we can approximate $S_\tau(\hat{\beta}_\tau; t)$ by $S_\tau(\beta_\tau; t) + D(t)n^{1/2}(\hat{\beta}_\tau - \beta_\tau)$ with a deterministic row vector $D(t)$. Likewise, we can approximate $s_\tau(\beta_\tau^*; t) - s_\tau(\tilde{\beta}_\tau; t)$ by $D(t)n^{1/2}(\beta_\tau^* - \tilde{\beta}_\tau)$, where the slope remains the same because β_τ^* and $\tilde{\beta}_\tau$ are close to β_τ. Thus

$$S_\tau(\hat{\beta}_\tau; t) = n^{-1/2} \sum_{i=1}^{n} \sum_{j=1}^{K_i} e_{\tau ij}(\beta_\tau) I(\beta_\tau' x_{ij} \leq t) + D(t)C_\tau n^{-1/2} \sum_{i=1}^{n} \sum_{j=1}^{K_i} e_{\tau ij}(\beta_\tau) x_{ij}$$

$$+ o(1),$$

and

$$S_\tau^*(t) = n^{-1/2} \sum_{i=1}^{n} \left[\sum_{j=1}^{K_i} e_{\tau ij}(\tilde{\beta}_\tau) I(\tilde{\beta}_\tau' x_{ij} \leq t) \right] Z_i$$

$$+ D(t)C_\tau n^{-1/2} \sum_{i=1}^{n} \left[\sum_{j=1}^{K_i} e_{\tau ij}(\tilde{\beta}_\tau) x_{ij} \right] Z_i + o(1).$$

By comparing the preceding two approximations, it is clear that $S_\tau(\hat{\beta}_\tau; t)$ and $S_\tau^*(t)$ converge to the same limiting distribution.

References

Baker, S. G., Wax, Y. and Patterson, B. (1993). Regression analysis of grouped survival data: Informative censoring and double sampling. *Biometrics* **49**, 379–390.

Barrodale, I. and Roberts, F. (1973). An improved algorithm for discrete L_1 linear approximations. *SIAM, Journal of Numerical Analysis* **10**, 839–848.

Bassett, G. Jr. & Koenker, R. (1978). Asymptotic theory of least absolute error regression, *J. Am. Statist. Assoc.* **73**, 618–622.

Bassett, G. Jr. and Koenker, R. (1982). An empirical quantile function for linear models with iid errors, *J. Am. Statist. Assoc.* **77**, 407–415.

Bloomfield, P. & Steiger, W. L. (1983). Least Absolute Deviations: Theory, Applications, and Algorithms. Birkhauser, Boston, Mass.

Chamberlain, G. (1994). Quantile regression, censoring and the structure of wages. In *Proceedings of the Sixth World Congress of the Econometrics Society* (eds. C. Sims and J.J. Laffont). New York: Cambridge University Press.

Efron B. & Tibshirani, R. (1986). Bootstrap methods for standard errors, confidence intervals, and other measures of statistical accuracy. *Statist. Sci.* **1**, 54–75.

Jung, S. (1996). Quasi-likelihood for median regression models. *J. Am. Statist. Assoc.* **91**, 251–257.

Koenker, R. (1994). Confidence intervals for regression quantiles. *Proc. of the 5th Prague Symp. on Asymptotic Stat.*, 349–359, Springer-Verlag.

Koenker, R. and Bassett, G. Jr. (1978). Regression quantiles. *Econometrica* **84**, 33–50.

Koenker, R. and Bassett, G. Jr. (1982). Tests of linear hypotheses and L_1 estimation. *Econometrica* **50**, 1577–1584.

Koenker, R. and D'Orey, V. (1987). Computing regression quantiles. *Applied Statistics* **36**, 383–393.

Koenker, R. and Machado, J. A. F. (1999). Goodness of fit and related inference processes for quantile regression. *J. Am. Statist. Assoc.* **94**, 1296–1310.

Lai, T. L. and Ying, Z. (1988). Stochastic integrals of empirical-type processes with applications to censored regression. *Journal of Multivariate Analysis* **27**, 334–358.

Laird, N. M. and Ware, J. H. (1982). Random-effects models for longitudinal data. *Biometrics* **38**, 963–974.

Liang, K. Y. and Zeger, S. L. (1986). Longitudinal data analysis using generalized linear models. *Biometrika* **73**, 13–22.

Lin, D. Y., Wei, L. J. and Ying, Z. (2002). Model-checking techniques based on cumulative residuals. *Biometrics* **58**, 1–12.

Lipsitz, S. R., Fitzmaurice, G. M., Molenberghs, G. and Zhao, L. P. (1997). Quantile regression models for longitudinal data with drop-out: Application to CD4 cell counts of patients infected with the human immunodeficiency virus. *Applied Statistics* **46**, 463–476.

Mosteller, F. and Tukey, J. W. (1977). *Data Analysis and Regression: A Secondary Course in Statistics.* Addison-Wesley.

Parzen, M. I., Wei, L. J. and Ying, Z. (1994). A resampling method based on pivotal estimating functions. *Biometrika* **81**, 341–350.

Portnoy, S. (1992). A regression quantile based statistic for testing non-stationary errors. In *Nonparametric Statistics and Related Topics*, ed. by A.Saleh, 191–203.

Rotnitzky, A. and Robins, J. M. (1995). Semi-parametric regression estimation in the presence of dependent censoring. *Biometrika* **82**, 805–820.

Tyl, R.W., Price, M. C., Marr, M. C. and Kimmel, C. A. (1988). Developmental toxicity evaluation of dietary di(2-ethylhexyl)phthalate in Fisher 344 rats and CD-1 mice. *Fundamental and Applied Toxicology* **10**, 395–412.

van der Vaart, A. and Wellner, J. A. (1996). Weak Convergence and Empirical Processes, Springer.

Wei, L. J. and Johnson, W. E. (1985). Combining dependent tests with incomplete repeated measurements, *Biometrika* **72**, 359–364.

Wu, M. C. and Carroll, R. J. (1988). Estimation and comparison of changes in the presence of informative right censoring by modeling the censoring process. *Biometrics* **44**, 175–188.

Small Sample Inference for Clustered Data

Ziding Feng, Thomas Braun and Charles McCulloch

Cancer Prevention Research Program, Fred Hutchinson Cancer Research Center, 1100 Fairview Ave.N. MP-702, Seattle, WA 98109-1024; Department of Biostatistics, University of Michigan, Ann Arbor, MI 48108; and Department of Epidemiology and Biostatistics, 500 Parnassus, 420 MU-W, San Francisco, CA 94143-0560

ABSTRACT   When the number of independent units is not adequate to invoke large sample approximations in clustered data analysis, a situation that often arises in group randomized trials (GRTs), valid and efficient small sample inference becomes important. We review the current methods for analyzing data from small numbers of clusters, namely methods based on full distribution assumptions (mixed effect models), semi-parametric methods based on Generalized Estimating Equations (GEE), and non-parametric methods based on permutation tests.

KEY WORDS: Correlated data; group randomized trials; linear mixed models; Generalized Estimating Equations (GEE); permutation tests; small sample inference.

1 Introduction

Clustered data from studies where a small number of independent clusters are involved are common. A most important example appears in group randomized trials (GRTs), a family of clinical trials in which treatment is randomly allocated to groups of individuals and, as a consequence, all individuals in the same group receive the same treatment. Motivation for a public health strategy delivered to groups may be due to feasibility constraints or to reduce expenses, as with media campaigns, or to increase the likelihood of subjects adopting the strategy by encouraging them to seek the support of others in their group. Examples of such studies include the Community Intervention Trial for Smoking Cessation (COMMIT) (Gail et al., 1992), which examined the benefit of community smoking cessation strategies, and the Working Well Trial (WWT) (Sorensen et al., 1996), which studied the effects of worksite interventions regarding smoking cessation and diet on employee health. Because adding more communities into the study is far more expensive than surveying more individuals within the community, the most cost efficient design is to have a relatively large number of individuals per community and a relatively small number of communities. However, we now have a small sample problem with regard to inference. For example, COMMIT randomized 22 communities into two treatment conditions, though smoking outcomes were collected from a cohort of 500 baseline smokers per community.

Clustered data from a small number of clusters also arises in longitudinal studies when a small number of individuals (e.g., a couple of dozen) are included in the study, even though the number of repeated measures collected per individual, and therefore the total number of observations, could be relatively large.

Clustered data analysis using linear mixed models has a long history (Harville, 1977; Laird and Ware, 1982; Jennrich and Schluchter, 1986; and others) and has been further popularized by the recent extension to generalized linear mixed models (GLMM) (Breslow and Clayton, 1993; Schall, 1991; McGilchrist, 1994; McCulloch, 1994, 1997; McCulloch and Searle, 2001; and others). Since its introduction by Liang and Zeger (1986), GEE has been widely used for clustered data as an alternative to mixed effect models because GEE only needs to specify the mean structure of the data and the marginal interpretation of the parameters is appealing in some situations. The inference for ML and REML estimates under linear mixed models and GLMMs, as well as estimates under GEE are all based on asymptotic normality of the estimates.

The inadequacy of a large sample approximation for inference for small sample clustered data has long been recognized for ML and REML estimates under linear mixed models (Kackar and Harville, 1984) and for estimates in GEE (Emrich and Piedmonte, 1992; Sharples and Breslow, 1992; Park, 1996; and others). Feng et al. (1996) and Evans et al. (2001) compared REML and GEE estimates and their standard errors for fixed effects and variance parameters, respectively, under a GRT setting. Except for rather simple settings such as one- and two-way random effects models (Kackar and Harville, 1984), small sample inference for clustered data has, until recently, been understudied. In this paper we will summarize what has been done and what remains to be done in small sample inference for clustered data, although we do not intend to give an exhaustive survey. Section 2 summarizes recent advances in small sample inference for likelihood based inference for linear mixed models, section 3 surveys GEE small sample corrections, section 4 presents recent work on permutation based inference, which is followed by discussion and summary in section 5.

2 Small Sample Inference for Linear Mixed Model

Consider the linear mixed model in its marginal form for a vector of observations $Y \sim N(X\beta; \Sigma)$, where β is the $p \times 1$ regression parameter vector and X is the $N \times p$ design matrix. The structure of the covariance matrix Σ as a function of an r-dimensional variance parameter σ depends on the experimental settings and is usually of block-diagonal form, with block corresponding to independent units such as communities in GRTs or subjects in longitudinal studies.

2.1 Correction Based on Wald Statistic (Kenward and Rodger)

Kenward and Roger address the small sample testing situation by starting with the Wald statistic and deriving improved estimates of the variance of the plug-in estimator and the degrees of freedom to use when comparing the Wald statistic to an F-distribution. Kenward and Rodger's correction is based on two concepts. First, let $\hat{\beta} = \Phi(\hat{\sigma})X'\Sigma(\hat{\sigma})^{-1}Y$ where $\Phi(\sigma) = (X'\Sigma(\sigma)^{-1}X)^{-1}$. $\Phi(\sigma)$ is the covariance matrix not of $\hat{\beta}$ but of $\Phi(\sigma)X'\Sigma(\sigma)^{-1}Y$. Therefore, $\text{var}(\hat{\beta}) = \Phi + \Lambda$ where Λ is the extra variation due to plugging in $\hat{\sigma}$ for σ. Note that $\Lambda > 0$ even if $\hat{\Phi}$ is unbiased for Φ. Second, $\hat{\Phi}$ is usually a biased estimator of $\Phi(\sigma)$.

To adjust for the added variance component Λ, Kackar and Harville (1984) showed that

$$\Lambda \approx \Phi \left\{ \sum_{i=1}^{r} \sum_{j=1}^{r} W_{ij}(Q_{ij} - P_i \Phi P_j) \right\} \Phi, \tag{1}$$

where $P_i = X'\frac{\partial \Sigma^{-1}}{\partial \sigma_i}X$, $Q_{ij} = X'\frac{\partial \Sigma^{-1}}{\partial \sigma_i}\Sigma\frac{\partial \Sigma^{-1}}{\partial \sigma_j}X$, and W_{ij} is the (i,j)-th element of $W = \text{Cov}(\hat{\sigma})$.

To adjust for the bias of $\hat{\Phi}$, Kenward and Rodger showed that

$$E(\hat{\Phi}) \approx \Phi + 0.5 \sum_{i=1}^{r} \sum_{j=1}^{r} W_{ij} \frac{\partial^2 \Phi}{\partial \sigma_i \partial \sigma_j}. \tag{2}$$

Combining (1) and (2), we have a small sample approximation to $\text{var}(\hat{\beta})$

$$\hat{\Phi}_A = \hat{\Phi} + 2\hat{\Phi} \left\{ \sum_{i=1}^{r} \sum_{j=1}^{r} W_{ij}(Q_{ij} - P_i \hat{\Phi} P_j - .25 R_{ij}) \right\} \hat{\Phi},$$

where $R_{ij} = X'\Sigma^{-1}\frac{\partial^2 \Sigma}{\partial \sigma_i \partial \sigma_j}\Sigma^{-1}X$, and $\Sigma(\hat{\sigma})$ is substitued for Σ in the equation.

Using our improved estimate for $\text{var}(\hat{\beta})$, we can approximate the distribution of the Wald statistic $\hat{F} = \frac{1}{l}(\hat{\beta} - \beta)'L(L'\hat{\Phi}_A L)^{-1}L'(\hat{\beta} - \beta)$ for testing $H_0 : L\beta = 0$ as follows (L is an $l \times p$ fixed matrix). If we assume that $\hat{F}$ has an approximate F-distribution, an approach similar to Satterthwaite (1941) is to equate the first two moments of $\lambda \hat{F}$ and $F(l, m)$, where l is the known numerator degrees of freedom and m is the unknown denominator degrees of freedom. Setting $E(\lambda \hat{F}) = m/(m-2)$ and $\text{var}(\lambda \hat{F}) = 2(\frac{m}{m-2})^2 \frac{l+m-2}{l(m-4)}$ and solving for λ and m, we get

$$m = 4 + (l+2)/(l\rho - 1),$$

where $\rho = \frac{var(\hat{F})}{2(E(\hat{F}))^2}$, and

$$\lambda = \frac{m}{E(\hat{F})(m-2)}.$$

Kenward and Rodger have also provided approximation formulas for $E(\hat{F})$ and $\text{var}(\hat{F})$. Kenward and Rodger's procedure has been implemented in SAS PROC MIXED and we forsee it will be widely used in the future.

2.2 Correction Based on Likelihood Ratio (Zucker et al.)

Though likelihood ratio (LR) statistics and Wald statistics are asymptotically equivalent, it is generally agreed that LR is preferable. Moreover, higher order asymptotic theory exists for the LR (Bartlett, 1937), which is the motivation behind Zucker et al. (2000).

A Bartlett correction is easier to implement when the parameters of interest are orthogonal to the nuisance parameters. Without loss of generality, let β_1 be the parameter of interest and $\gamma = (\beta_2, ..., \beta_{p-1})'$. Zucker et al. first transforms $(\beta_1, \gamma, \sigma)$ to $\theta = (\beta_1, \xi, \sigma)$, where

$$\xi = \gamma + \beta_1 (\tilde{X}' \Sigma^{-1}(\sigma) \tilde{X})^{-1} \tilde{X}' \Sigma^{-1}(\sigma) x_1,$$

x_1 is the first column of X, and $\tilde{X}$ is the remaining columns of X. In a linear mixed model, σ is usually assumed to be orthogonal to the mean and therefore no transformation is needed. We denote $\psi = \beta_1$ and $\phi = (\xi, \sigma)$.

We denote the log-profile-likelihood $L(\psi, \phi^*(\psi))$ as $M(\psi)$, where $\phi^*(\psi)$ is the maximum likelihood estimate of ϕ for a fixed ψ. Let $W(\psi_0) = 2(M(\hat{\psi}) - M(\psi_0))$ be the usual LR statistic for testing $\psi = \psi_0$. Bartlett's correction procedure first expands $E(W(\psi)) = (d - d_0)[1 + A(\theta) + O(n^{-3/2})]$, where d and d_0 are the dimensions of the parameter space under the full model and the reduced model, respectively. The Bartlett-corrected statistic is

$$\tilde{W}(\psi_0) = [1 + A(\psi_0, \phi^*(\psi_0))]^{-1} W(\psi_0).$$

With a Bartlett correction, not only does $\tilde{W}(\psi_0)$ have expectation $d - d_0$ (in our example, β_1 is a scalar so $d - d_0 = 1$), the expectation of a Chi-squared distribution with $d - d_0$ degrees of freedom, with error rate $O(n^{-3/2})$, but all higher order cumulants match that of a Chi-squared distribution as well. As a result, a correction on the first moment improves the whole distribution, due to the special property of the LR. To contrast the correction by Kenward and Rodger on the Wald statistic is only for the first two moments.

Unfortunately, $A(\theta)$ is quite tedious to calculate, involving the fourth-order derivatives of the log-likelihood with respect to the parameters. Letting F denote the set of indices in θ corresponding to ξ and letting G denote the set of indices corresponding to elements of σ, Zucker et al. (2000) provided an expression for $A(\theta)$:

$$
A(\theta) = -.5\lambda_{11}^{-1} \sum_{r,s\in G} \lambda^{rs}\lambda_{11rs} + .25\lambda_{11}^{-2} \sum_{r,s\in G} \lambda^{rs}\lambda_{11r}\lambda_{11s}
$$
$$
-.5\lambda_{11}^{-1} \sum_{r,s\in G}\sum_{t,u\in F} \lambda^{rs}\lambda^{tu}\lambda_{11r}\lambda_{stu},
$$

where λ_{rs} is the (r,s)-th element of the expected second-derivative matrix, λ^{rs} are corresponding elements of the inverse matrix, and λ_{stu} and λ_{11rs} are third and fourth-order derivatives defined by Zucker et al.

Zucker et al. provided Fortran code for the model fitting and computation of $A(\theta)$ for linear mixed models with fairly general structure for Σ. That code is available at

http://www.blackwellpublishers.co.uk/rss/

An alternative likelihood based small sample improvement technique is due to Lyons and Peters (2000). They applied Skovgaard's modified directed likelihood statistic to mixed linear models. A comparison of these three competing procedures would be useful.

2.3 GLMM

A Generalized Linear Mixed Model (GLMM) has the form $g(\mu_i) = X\beta + Zb_i$, where g is a link function (e.g., logit), μ_i is the mean vector of the i-th independent unit, and b_i is the random effect for i-th unit. Therefore, a linear mixed model is a special case of GLMM when g is the identity link function. McCulloch and Searle (2001) gives an extensive survey of this subject.

It is obvious now that the small sample correction, even for linear mixed models, involves very tedious calculations. The parallel correction for GLMM is currently not available. Therefore, for non-normal data, there is an urgent need for small-sample corrections before the popular GLMM procedures can be used in small sample settings with some confidence.

Furthermore, Bartlett correction, even if worked out for discrete data, may not necessarily lead to improvement in small sample inference. Frydenberg and Jensen (1989) showed by numerical analysis that the error rate of the corrected LR statistic has about the same order as the uncorrected LR statistic. The similar error rates occur because the central regularity assumption for Bartlett's correction is that the LR statistic can be written as a function of a random variable having a valid continuous Edgeworth expansion to a certain order. This assumption holds in general with most continuous data (Chandra and Ghosh, 1979), but not for discrete data.

Therefore, to improve likelihood ratio based inference for small samples, we may need to take other routes. In their paper, Zucker et al. also explored a Cox-Reid adjusted LR statistic (Cox and Reid, 1987). The performance was similar to the conventional LR in a random slope example but showed significant improvement in a crossover example. Whether the Cox-Reid method suffers the same drawback in discrete data as Bartlett's correction needs further investigation.

3 Small Sample Inference for GEE

GEE is a marginal regression procedure widely used for clustered data (Liang and Zeger, 1986). The expectation, μ_{ij}, of the observed response, y_{ij}, for the j-th observation in the i-th cluster, is related to covariate X_{ij} through $g(\mu_{ij}) = X'_{ij}\beta$. The variance and working covariance matrix for correlated responses within the i-th cluster are $\phi v(\mu_{ij})$ and $V_i = \phi A_i^{1/2} R_i(\alpha) A_i^{1/2}$ respectively, where $A_i = \text{diag}(v(\mu_{i1}), ..., v(\mu_{in_i}))$. GEE estimates, $\hat{\beta}$, are given by the solution to the estimating equations:

$$\sum_{i=1}^{K} D'_i V_i^{-1} S_i = 0,$$

where $D_i = \partial\mu_i/\partial\beta$, $S_i = Y_i - \mu_i$, and Y_i and μ_i are vector of y_{ij} and μ_{ij} for i-th cluster. Liang and Zeger (1986) proposed a sandwich estimator to estimate the covariance matrix of $\hat{\beta}$

$$V_S = \left(\sum_{i=1}^{K} D'_i V_i^{-1} D_i\right)^{-1} \left(\sum_{i=1}^{K} D'_i V_i^{-1} S_i S'_i V_i^{-1} D_i\right) \left(\sum_{i=1}^{K} D'_i V_i^{-1} D_i\right)^{-1},$$

where β and α are replaced by their estimates $\hat{\beta}$ and $\hat{\alpha}$. $V_M = \left(\sum_{i=1}^{K} D'_i V_i^{-1} D_i\right)^{-1}$ is a model based covariance estimator of $\text{var}(\hat{\beta})$ if the variance and covariance of Y are correctly specified.

A number of studies indicate that in small samples, GEE tends to have type I error larger than the target for inference on cluster level fixed effects (Emrich and Piedmonte, 1992; Sharples and Breslow, 1992; Park, 1993; Feng et al., 1996; and others). In a variety of GRT settings, Evans et al. (2001) compared the REML and GEE estimates of fixed effects and variance parameters and found GEE under-estimates the variance parameters and their standard errors in small samples. In general, GEE is not recommended for analyses of GRTs (Feng et al., 2001) due to its poor small sample properties.

3.1 Correction on Bias in Variance Estimates (Mancl and DeRouen)

The motivation of Mancl and DeRouen (2001) is that $\hat{S}_i\hat{S}'_i$ under-estimates $\text{Cov}(Y_i)$. They showed that $E(\hat{S}_i\hat{S}'_i) \approx (I_i - H_{ii})\text{Cov}(Y_i)(I_i - H'_{ii})$ where I_i is $n_i \times n_i$ identity matrix with n_i the number of observations for i-th cluster, and $H_{ij} = D_i \left(\sum_{l=1}^{K} D'_l V_l^{-1} D_l\right)^{-1} D'_j V_j^{-1}$ so a bias-corrected covariance estimator is

$$\text{var}_{BC}(\hat{\beta}) = \left(\sum_{i=1}^{K} D'_i V_i^{-1} D_i\right)^{-1}$$

$$\times \left(\sum_{i=1}^{K} D'_i V_i^{-1}(I_i - H_{ii})^{-1}\hat{S}_i\hat{S}'_i(I_i - H'_{ii})^{-1}V_i^{-1}D_i\right)\left(\sum_{i=1}^{K} D'_i V_i^{-1} D_i\right)^{-1} \quad (3)$$

Mancl and DeRouen found through simulations that this bias correction is not enough to bring the test size to nominal level. As a solution, they use an ad-hoc F-test for the Wald statistic with degrees of freedom $K - p$, where p is the number of regression parameters.

3.2 Correction on Variability in Variance Estimates (Pan and Wall)

Pan and Wall (2001) adjust the degree of freedom of the Wald statistic in a more formal way, similar in the spirit of Kenward and Rodger. The first idea is to simplify the problem by treating the model-based estimator V_M as constant and estimate the mean and variance of the middle piece of the sandwich estimator V_S using unbiased sample moment estimators. Let $P_i = \text{vec}\left(D'_i V_i^{-1} S_i S'_i V_i^{-1} D_i\right)$, where $\text{vec}(U)$ is a vector formed by stacking the columns of U below one another. The mean, Q, and covariance matrix, T, of $\sum_{i=1}^{K} P_i/K = \bar{P}$, can be consistently estimated by $\hat{Q} = \bar{P}$ (i.e., $\bar{P}$ itself) and $\hat{T} = \sum_{i=1}^{K}(P_i - \bar{P})(P_i - \bar{P})'/K(K-1)$. Now the covariance matrix of $\text{vec}(V_S)$ is estimated by

$$\widehat{\text{Cov}}(\text{vec}(V_s)) = K^2(V_M \otimes V_M)\hat{T}(V_M \otimes V_M),$$

where $\otimes$ is the Kronecker product operation.

In order to create an approximation to a scaled t or F statistic, let us consider a simple test of only one parameter with $H_0 : \beta_k = 0$. We can equate the consistent estimate of the mean and variance of the corresponding element V_{Sk} in V_s, namely the elements in the estimates of the mean of $\text{vec}(V_S)$, $K(V_M \otimes V_M)\bar{P}$, and the element in $\widehat{\text{Cov}}(\text{vec}(V_s))$ respectively, corresponding to β_k, denoted as σ_k and τ_k respectively, with the mean and variance of the scaled chi-squared distribution $c\chi_d^2$. In other words, set $cd = \sigma_k$ and

$2c^2d = \tau_k$, and solve for c and d. Solving these equations leads to $c = \tau_k/2\sigma_k$ and $d = 2\sigma_k^2/\tau_k$. Then the scaled t is:

$$t = \frac{\hat{\beta}_k/\sqrt{\sigma_k}}{\sqrt{V_{Sk}/cd}} = \frac{\hat{\beta}_k}{\sqrt{V_{Sk}}},$$

which is the same test statistic as that for the usual z-test using V_{Sk} except using t_d as the reference distribution.

Similarly we can use a scaled F for the Wald statistic $W = \hat{\beta}' V_S^{-1} \hat{\beta}$, where β is a p-dimensional vector, using

$$\frac{\nu - p + 1}{\nu p} W \approx F(p, \nu - p + 1),$$

instead of using χ_p^2. This correction comes from approximating W by Hotelling's T^2 with numerator degrees of freedom p and an unknown denominator degrees of freedom $\nu - p + 1$. The scaling factor ν is determined by minimizing the sum of squared errors between all elements of the empirical covariance matrix of νV_S and its asymptotic covariance matrix, that of a Wishart distribution with degrees of freedom ν. Pan and Wall provide details. Note that unlike the one-dimensional case, this scaled statistic is not the same as the original W.

By comparing their approach to that of Mancl and DeRouen, Pan and Wall found additional bias correction on the sandwich estimate is not necessary after their correction. This is intuitive because the scaling process automatically takes the bias of the sandwich estimate into account.

3.3 Other Related Work

Fay and Graubard (2001) used another bias correction for the middle part of V_S, $\hat{U}_i \hat{U}_i'$, where $\hat{U}_i = D_i' V_i^{-1} S_i$. By assuming the working covariance matrix V_i is proportionally equal to the true covariance matrix, they showed that $E(\hat{U}_i \hat{U}_i') \approx (I_p - V_m \hat{\Omega}_i)$, where $\hat{\Omega}_i = -\partial \hat{U}_i/\partial \beta = D_i' V_i^{-1} D_i$. Therefore the adjusted sandwich estimator is

$$V_a = V_M \left(\sum_{i=1}^{K} H_i \hat{U}_i \hat{U}_i' H_i \right) V_M, \tag{4}$$

where $H_i = (I_p - V_m \hat{\Omega}_i)^{-1/2}$. By comparing (4) to (3), we can see (4) made the correction on $\hat{U}_i \hat{U}_i'$ while (3) made the correction on $\hat{S}_i \hat{S}_i'$. Fay and Graubard also proposed a F-test for testing $H_0 : C'\beta = C'\beta_0$ where the denominator degrees of freedom of this F distribution is estimated.

The early work on the small sample correction for the sandwich estimate was in econometric literature by MacKinnon and White (1985), who proposed jackknife sandwich estimates. The early work on the small sample correction for GEE appears to be an unpublished Fred Hutchinson Cancer Center Technical Report by Thornquist and Anderson (1992). For Gaussian data they showed that one needs to use both an unbiased estimate for $\text{Cov}(\hat{\beta})$ and a corrected degrees of freedom to bring the type I error to the nominal level. The bias-corrected covariance estimators turn out to be MIVQUE (Rao, 1971). Kauermann and Carroll (2001) derived small-sample properties of the efficiency of the sandwich estimate and proposed an adjustment that depends on normal distribution quantiles and the variance of the sandwich variance estimate.

4 Small Sample Inference Using Permutation Test

Another way to deal with small sample clustered data is to use a permutation test on the cluster means which, under certain assumptions discussed below, will maintain a nominal level. Maritz and Jarrett (1983) and Gail et al. (1992) used this permutation-based approach for clustered data. In particular, Gail and his co-workers popularized the use of permutation methods in GRTs in a series papers. The suggestion of applying the permutations to the covariate adjusted cluster residual means makes the procedure quite flexible and potentially as efficient as mixed models and GEE while retaining certain degree of robustness.

The simplest permutation-based inference for clustered data is, by permuting the unadjusted cluster means, to form the null permutation distribution for hypothesis testing or a permutation test-based confidence interval (Edgington, 1987; Good, 1994). If a matched pair design is used for GRTs, the permutations are performed within each pair of clusters.

The validity of the permutation test, i.e. type I error rate is at the target nominal level, requires an assumption of exchangeability (also known as "symmetry"). This assumption means that under the null hypothesis, the distribution of the statistics to be permuted remains the same for all permutations. This is true under the "strong" null hypothesis, i.e., no treatment effect on any cluster response, but is not true in general under the "weak" null hypothesis, i.e., no treatment effect on average. This concept was originally proposed by Neyman et al. (1935). Testing an intervention effect under the "weak" null hypothesis is important since a rejection of the "strong" null hypothesis may simply mean intervention produces a positive effect in some clusters (communities) but negative effect in other clusters, with no improvement on average.

Gail et al. (1996) studied the properties of permutation tests for GRTs and found permutation tests are very robust even under the weak null hypothesis. The permutation test usually has a near-nominal level unless the number of clusters is quite unbalanced between two treatment arms *and* the cluster means have unequal variances. A design which balances cluster sizes across treatment arms will eliminate serious imbalance although unequal variances could be the result of the intervention. In particular, a pair-matched design, especially if the cluster size is used as one of the matching criteria, will effectively be balanced and therefore be more robust than an unbalanced, unpaired design under the weak null hypothesis.

4.1 Covariate Adjustment (Gail et al.)

Gail et al. (1988, 1996) made an important extension to permutation-based inference on treatment effects by allowing for adjustment of individual and cluster level covariates. This extension makes permutation-based inference potentially as flexible and efficient as GEE or GLMM while retaining a nominal type I error rate.

Let $h(\mu_{jk}) = h(\beta_0 + Z_j\beta_1 + X_{jk}\beta_2)$ be the regression model for the k-th individual in the j-th cluster with individual-level covariates X_{jk} and cluster-level covariates Z_j, containing no treatment indicator. This model contains no random effects and can be fit by traditional maximum likelihood estimation to obtain the predicted response $\hat{y}_{jk}$.

Under the strong null hypothesis, the residual $r_{jk} = y_{jk} - \hat{y}_{jk}$ is independent of treatment because $\hat{y}_{jk}$ is a function only of covariates, which are independent of treatment by randomization, and of y_{jk}, which is independent of treatment by hypothesis. Therefore, we can permute the cluster mean residuals r_j instead of the unadjusted cluster means y_j to form the permutation distribution. The test and test-based confidence intervals are based on this permutation distribution.

Extensive simulation studies by Gail et al. (1996) showed that sizes are very near nominal levels even if we misspecify the regression function $h(.)$ or the number of individuals per clusters varies, as long as the number of clusters is balanced between treatment arms. The gain in statistical power by individual-level covariate adjustment is usually modest unless the covariate effect is big, the distribution of the covariate is unbalanced, and between-cluster variance not explained by individual-level covariates is small compared to within-cluster variance.

The adjustment by cluster-level covariates is more challenging because such an adjustment consumes the cluster level degrees of freedom. Because we have a small number of clusters, the validity of the permutation test based on cluster means or adjusted cluster mean residuals could be seriously impacted. Suppose, for example, the number of cluster level covariates is equal or larger than the number of clusters, the residual cluster means will have no variation and permutation test is not meaningful. Therefore, we recommend not adjusting on cluster-level covariates, but instead using important cluster-level covariates as matching variables. Note that in a matched pair design, the number of permutations is much smaller than that for an unpaired design, reflecting the restriction imposed by using matching variables.

4.2 Weighted Permutation (Braun and Feng)

Although maximum likelihood estimation and GEE both have some optimality properties, less is known about permutation tests. For example, are permutation tests on cluster means or adjusted residuals as proposed by Gail et al. (1996) most powerful? Intuitively, we can see here is room for improvement, for no matter how cluster sizes vary, the same weight is used for each cluster. One would think weighted permutation tests compared to unweighted permutation tests would parallel weighted least squares to unweighed least squares, or weighted t-tests to unweighted t-tests. One may think a natural weight is the cluster size. However, the observations within cluster are correlated and do not represent independent pieces of information. Therefore, when the between cluster variance is large, or equivalently the intracluster correlation is large, weighting by cluster size will lose power. Therefore, there should be an optimality criterion for selecting weights. This is the rationale of Braun and Feng (2001).

Lehmann and Stein (1949) proved that for N independent observations from an exponential family, n_1 observations in treatment group 1 and n_2 in group 2, the statistic leading to the most powerful permutation test is

$$h(Y) = \exp\{[\sum_{i=1}^{n_1}(Y_i\theta_1 - b(\theta_1)) + \sum_{j=1}^{n_2}(Y_{n_1+j}\theta_2 - b(\theta_2))]/a(\phi) + \sum_{i=1}^{N}c(Y_i;\phi)\},$$

which is the joint density of all N observations under the alternative, evaluated at the observed values Y. Dropping terms which are invariant under permutations, one can simplify $h(Y)$ to $\bar{y}_1$.

Define a linear mixed model $Y_{ik} = \beta_0 + X_{ik}\beta + T_i\delta + u_i + e_{ij}$, where β_0 is intercept parameter, X_{ik} is a covariate vector for the k-th subject, β is the vector of covariate effect parameters, T_i represents the treatment assignment for the ith cluster, δ is the intervention effect parameter, u_i is a realized value of the random cluster effect, and e_{ij} is the within cluster error. We assume u_i and e_{ij} are normally distributed with mean zero and variances τ^2 and σ^2, respectively. Braun and Feng (2001) showed that the statistic leading to the most powerful permutation test is

$$\sum_i T_i W_i \sum_k \epsilon_{ik},$$

with $\epsilon_{ik} = Y_{ik} - (\lambda + X_{ik}\beta)$ and $W_i = (\sigma^2 + n_i\tau^2)^{-1}$, if the nuisance parameters (all parameters except δ) are known. This statistic is easily interpreted as a weighted sum of cluster errors, with weights equal to the inverse of the total variance for each cluster. Braun and Feng suggest replacing the nuisance parameters by their consistent estimates. Compared to the test proposed by Gail et al. (1996), we now permute weighted cluster mean residuals.

This concept of weighting can be extended to GEE, in which we permute the quasi-score statistic

$$\sum_i \{T_i D_i V_i^{-1}[Y_i - \mu_i]\} \,|_{\delta=0}, \tag{5}$$

where T_i is a scalar 1 or -1 representing the intervention assignment of the ith cluster, and Y_i and μ_i are the corresponding $(n_i \times 1)$ vectors of outcomes and their expected values, respectively. D_i is the corresponding $(1 \times n_i)$ vector whose k^{th} element is $(\partial \eta_{ik}/\partial \mu_{ik})^{-1}$, and V_i is an $(n_i \times n_i)$ covariance matrix of the ith cluster, with non-zero elements off its diagonal. To perform a permutation test of $\delta = 0$, we would compare the observed value of (5) to its distribution of values under every permutation of the intervention assignments, with a large value of (5) corresponding to a large intervention effect.

Braun and Feng (2001) showed by simulations that the weighted permutation tests do increase the power compared to unweighted permutation tests. The gain in power is largest when the between cluster variance is near zero, a situation often seen in GRTs.

4.3 More on Validity

It should be emphasized that the common perception that a permutation test is always exact is incorrect. It is only true under the strong null hypothesis. Note that the permutation process scrambles all clusters together and reassigns the treatment labels. Doing so it assumes equal variances of the original observations under the null hypothesis, an assumption true only under the strong null hypothesis. As a result one way to assess how much a permutation test could deviate from an exact type I error rate is to compare the variance of the statistic under the permutation distribution to the variance under a specific model, such as a mixed effect model. If the two variances are similar, the permutation test is likely to have a near-nominal level; otherwise, it will not. This approach has been used by Gail et al. (1996) and Romano (1990). The permutation test is more likely to be at a nominal level when the number of clusters is balanced across treatment arms. This result is similar to a two sample t-test that assumes equal variances, but the true variances are unequal between the two groups. Validity of the t-test is maintained because the denominator of the t-statistic will converge to the correct variance under a balanced design and is therefore properly standardized. Whether the weighted permutation test will be more robust or less robust than the unweighted permutation test needs further investigation.

5 Summary and Discussion

The first recommendation for investigators when planning a study with clustered data is to include an adequate number of clusters. Usually when the number of clusters is larger than 20, asymptotic approximations are reliable. In GRTs, investigators are often fooled by the large number of individuals and small observed between cluster variance, often not statistically different from zero. Surprisingly, we have observed large number of such cases, both in literature and at NIH Study Section grant review. Simpson et al. (1995) reviewed primary prevention trials involving the allocation of identifiable groups that were published between 1990 and 1993 in the *American Journal of Public Health* and in *Preventive Medicine*. They found that fewer than 20% dealt with these issues adequately in their sample-size calculations and that less than 57% dealt with them adequately in their analysis. Therefore, statisticians should guard against the temptation to analyze such data as independent non-clustered data.

In analysis, if an assumption of normality is tenable, both procedures of Kenward and Rodger and Zucker et al. have quite firm theoretical justifications. A comparison between the two will be very useful. For discrete data, currently the small sample adjustment procedures in GEE are a bit more ad-hoc compared to that of likelihood-based methods in a linear mixed model. It seems that Pan and Wall's method requires less assumptions, but using the fourth moments could make the procedure sensitive to outliers. Both Pan and Wall and Fay and Graubard adjusted the impact of variability in estimating covariance, which seems more important than the bias correction for covariance, in order to bring the size of the corresponding hypothesis test to a nominal level.

Permutation based tests for clustered data also need further investigation. First, how can we make the permutation test more robust under the weak null hypotheses? Second, what is the best way to adjust for nuisance parameters? Gail et al. (1996) estimated nuisance parameters under the null hypothesis, making the residuals independent of the treatment. On the other hand, covariate parameter estimators are consistent when estimated under the alternative but not consistent in general under the null hypothesis. Braun and Feng (2001) used the MLEs under the alternative, which are consistent estimators for nuisance parameters. However, under the weak null hypothesis, using MLE under the alternative hypothesis may be more subject to incorrect type I error rates than using estimates under the null hypothesis. One referee made a good point that in the score statistic, the nuisance parameters are always estimated under the null. Therefore, if permuting the score statistic is employed, the nuisance parameters should be estimated under the null.

Finally, comparisons between small sample inference procedures for mixed models, for GEE, and for permutation tests will tell us whether utilizing the distribution information will benefit small sample inference, and if it does, how much. We should also compare the performance of these three classes of procedures when the distribution assumptions are incorrect or when the strong null hypothesis does not hold. To date, no such comparisons have been made. All procedures discussed in this review were published after 1996 and most are within the last two years or in press. It is evident that small sample methods for clustered data is an important and active area of research.

REFERENCES

Barlett MS (1937) Properties of sufficiency and statistical tests. *Proceedings of the Royal Society, A,* 160:268-282.

Braun T and Feng Z (2001) Optimal permutation tests for the analysis of group randomized trials. *Journal of the American Statistical Association,* 96:1424-1432.

Breslow NE, Clayton DG (1993) Approximate Inference in Generalized Linear Mixed Models. *Journal of the American Statistical Association,* 88:9-25.

Chandra T and Ghosh J (1979) Valid asymptotic expansions for the likelihood ratio statistic and other perturbed chi-square variables. *Sankhya A,* 41:22-47.

Cox DR and Reid N (1987) Parameter orthogonality and approximate conditional inference 9with discussion) *Journal of the Royal Statistical Society Series B,* 49:1-39.

Donner A, Eliasziw M, Klar N (1994) A comparison of methods for testing homogeneity of proportions for teratologic studies. *Statistics in Medicine,* 13:479-93.

Donner A, Klar N (2000) *Design and Analysis of Cluster Randomization Trials In Health Research.* New York, Oxford University Press.

Edgington ES (1987) *Randomization Tests* Marcel Decker, New York.

Emrich L, Piedmonte M (1992) On some small sample properties of generalized estimating equation estimates for multivariate dichotomous outcomes. *Journal of Statistical Computation and Simulationa,* 41:19-29.

Evans B, Feng Z, Peterson AV (2001) A comparison of generalized linear mixed model procedures with estimating equations for variance and covariance parameter estimation in longitudinal studies and group randomized trials. *Statistics in Medicine,* 20:3353-3373.

Fay M, Graubard B (2001) Small-sample adjustment for Wald-type tests using sandwich estimators. *Biometrics,* 57:1198-1206.

Feng Z, McLerran D, Grizzle J (1996) A comparison of statistical methods for clustered data analysis with Gaussian error. *Statistics in Medicine,*

15:1793-806.

Feng Z, Diehr P, Peterson A, McLerran D (2001) Selected statistical issues in group randomized trials. *Annual Review of Public Health*, 22:167-87.

Frydenberg M and Jensen J (1989) Is the 'improved likelihood ratio statistic' really improved in the discrete case? *Biometrika*, 76:655-662.

Gail MH, Tan WY, and Piantadosi S (1988) Tests for no treatment effect in randomized clinical trials, *Biometrika*, 75:57-64.

Gail MH, Byar DP, Pechacek TF, Corle DK (1992) Aspects of statistical design for the Community Intervention Trial for Smoking Cessation (COMMIT). *Controlled Clinical Trials*, 123:6-21.

Gail MH, Mark SD, Carroll R, Greeen S, Pee D (1996) On design considerations and randomization-based inference for community intervention trials. *Statistics in Medicine*, 15:1069-92.

Good P *Permutation Tests* (1994) Springer-Verlag, New York.

Harville D (1977). Maximum likelihood approaches to variance component estimation and to related problems. *Journal of the American Statistical Association*, 72:320-340.

Jennrich R and Schluchter M (1986). Unbalanced repeated-measures models with structured covariance matrices. *Biometrics*, 42:805-820.

Kackar A and Harville D (1984) Approximations for standard errors of estimators of fixed and random effects in mixed linear models. *Journal of the American Statistical Association*, 79:853-862.

Kauermann G, Carroll R (2001) A note on the efficiency of sandwich covariance matrix estimation. *Journal of the American Statistical Association*, 96:1387-1396.

Kenward M and Roger J (1997) Small sample inference for fixed effects from restricted maximum likelihood. *Biometrics*, 53:983-997.

Laird N and Ware J (1982). Random-effects models for longitudinal data. *Biometrics*, 38:963-974.

Lehmann EL and Stein C (1949) On the theory of some non-parametric hypotheses. *The Annals of Mathematical Statistics*, 20:28-45.

Liang KY, Zeger SL (1986) Longitudinal Data Analysis Using Generalized Linear Models. *Biometrika*, 73:13-22.

Lyons B, Peters D (2000) Applying Skovgaard's modified directed likelihood statistic to mixed linear models. *Journal of Statistical Computation and Simulations*, 65:225-242.

MacKinnon JG, White H (1985) Some heteroscedasticity-consistent covariance matrix estimators with improved finite sample properties. *Journal of Econometrics*, 29:305-325.

Mancl L and DeRouren T (2001) A covariance estimator for GEE with improved small-sample properties. *Biometrics*, 57:126-134.

Maritz J, Jarrett R (1983) The use of statistics to examine the association between fluoride in drinking water and cancer death rates. *Applied Statistics*, 32:97-101.

McCulloch CE (1994) Maximum likelihood variance components estimation for binary data. *Journal of the American Statistical Association*, 89:330-35.

McCulloch CE (1997) Maximum likelihood algorithms for generalized linear mixed models. *Journal of the American Statistical Association*, 92:162-70.

McCulloch CE and Searle SR (2001) *Generalized, Linear, and Mixed Models*. New York, Wiley.

McGilchrist CA. (1994) Estimation in Generalized Mixed Models. *Journal of the Royal Statistical Society Series B*, 56:61-69

Murray DM (1998) *Design and Analysis of Group-Randomized Trials*. New York, Oxford University Press.

Neyman J, Iwaskiewicz K, and Kolodziejczyk T (1935) Statistical problems in agricultural experimentation. *Journal of the Royal Statistical Society*, 2:107-180.

Pan W and Wall M (2002) Small-sample adjustments in using the sandwich variance estimator in generalized estimating equations. *Statistics in*

Medicine, 21:1429-1441.

Park T (1993) A Comparison of the Generalized Estimating Equation Approach with the Maximum Likelihood Approach for Repeated measurements. *Statistics in Medicine,* 12:1723-1732.

Rao CR (1971) Minimum variance quadratic unbiased estimation of variance components. *Journal of Multivariate Analysis,* 1:445-56.

Romano J (1990) On the behavior of randomization tests without a group invariance assumption, *Journal of the American Statistical Association,* 85:686-692.

Satterthwaite F (1941) Synthesis of variance. *Psychometrika,* 6:309-316.

Schall R (1991) Estimation in Generalized Linear Models with Random Effects. *Biometrika,* 40:917-927.

Sharples K, Breslow N (1992) Regression analysis of correlated binary data: some small sample results for the estimating equation approach. *Journal of Statistical Computation and Simulations,* 42:1-20.

Sorensen G, Thompson B, Glanz K, Feng Z, Kinne S, DiClemente C, Emmons K, Heimendinger J, Probart C, Lichtenstein E, for Working Well Trial (1996) Work site-based cancer prevention: primary results form the Working Well Trial. *American Journal of Public Health,* 86:939-947.

Thornquist M, Anderson G (1992) Small sample properties of generalized estimating equations in group-randomized designs with gaussian response. Technical Report, Fred Hutchinson Cancer Research Center.

Zucker D, Lieberman O, and Manor O (2000) Improved small sample inference in the mixed linear model: Bartlett correction and adjusted likelihood. *Journal of the Royal Statistical Society Series B,* 62:827-838.

Some Applications of Indirect Inference to Longitudinal and Repeated Events Data

Wenxin Jiang and Bruce W. Turnbull

Department of Statistics, Northwestern University, Evanston, IL 60208, USA and School of Operations Research and Department of Statistical Science, 227 Rhodes Hall, Cornell University, Ithaca, NY 14853, USA

Key words and phrases: Asymptotic normality; bias correction; consistency; efficiency; estimating equations; generalized method of moments; indirect inference, indirect likelihood; measurement error; naive estimators; overdispersion; quasi-likelihood; random effects; robustness.

ABSTRACT

In this paper we illustrate the so-called "indirect" method of inference, originally developed from the econometric literature, with analyses of three biological data sets involving longitudinal or repeated events data. This method is often more convenient computationally than maximum likelihood estimation when handling such model complexities as random effects and measurement error, for example; and it can also serve as a basis for robust inference with less stringent assumptions on the data generating mechanism.

The first data set involves times of recurrences of skin tumors in individual patients in a clinical trial. The methodology is applied in a regression analysis to accommodate random effects and covariate measurement error. The second data set concerns prevention of mammary tumors in rats and is analyzed using a Poisson regression model with overdispersion. The third application is to longitudinal data on epileptic seizures and analyzed using indirect inference based on low order moments.

Address for correspondence: Bruce Turnbull, School of Operations Research and Industrial Engineering, 227 Rhodes Hall, Cornell University, Ithaca, NY 14853-3801, USA.

E-mail: turnbull@orie.cornell.edu

1 INTRODUCTION

Methods of "indirect inference" have been developed and used in the field of econometrics where they have proved valuable for parameter estimation in highly complex models. This article recasts the basic technique in a likelihood-flavored approach and illustrates some applications in biostatistics, in particular for longitudinal and repeated events data.

This general technique, termed *indirect inference* (Gourieroux, Monfort and Renault, 1993), was motivated by complex dynamic financial models where the technique of indirect inference provides a computationally tractable alternative to the method of maximum likelihood (ML). In the biostatistical applications that we will consider, on the other hand, we place more focus on obtaining estimates that are robust to misspecification of the underlying model, in addition to ease of computation.

We begin by illustrating the steps involved in the indirect method by a simple pedagogic example.

2   EXAMPLE: MULTINOMIAL GENETIC DATA

Dempster, Laird and Rubin (1977, Sec.1) fit some phenotype data of Rao (1973, p.369) to a genetic linkage model of Fisher (1946, p.303). The sample consists of $n = 197$ progeny which are distributed multinomially into four phenotypic categories according to probabilities from an intercross model M of the genotypes AB/ab $\times$ AB/ab: $(\frac{1}{2} + \frac{1}{4}\theta, \frac{1}{4}(1 - \theta), \frac{1}{4}(1 - \theta), \frac{1}{4}\theta)$ for some $\theta \in [0, 1]$. The corresponding observed counts are

$$\mathbf{y} = (y_1, y_2, y_3, y_4) = (125, 18, 20, 34).$$

For the first step, we define an intermediate statistic as a naive estimate of θ from a "convenient" but misspecified model M' in which it is wrongly assumed that $\mathbf{y}$ is drawn from a four-category multinomial distribution with probabilities $(\frac{1}{2}s, \frac{1}{2}(1 - s), \frac{1}{2}(1 - s), \frac{1}{2}s)$. This corresponds to a backcross of the genotypes AB/ab $\times$ ab/ab. This naive or 'auxiliary' model M' is convenient because the naive maximum likelihood estimate is simply calculated as $\hat{s} = (y_1 + y_4)/n = (125 + 34)/197 = 0.8071$. In the second step we derive a 'bridge relation' which relates the "naive parameter" s (the large sample limit of $\hat{s}$) to the true parameter θ. Here the bridge relation is $s = (1 + \theta)/2$ since, under the true model, this is the almost sure limit of $\hat{s}$ as $n \to \infty$. The third step is to invert the bridge relation to obtain the adjusted estimate $\hat{\theta} = 2\hat{s} - 1 = (y_1 + y_4 - y_2 - y_3)/n = 0.6142$. Of course, in this case, the maximum likelihood estimate (MLE) based on the true model, $\hat{\theta}_{ML}$ say, can be computed explicitly as

$$\hat{\theta}_{ML} = (y_1 - 2y_2 - 2y_3 - y_4 + \sqrt{(y_1 - 2y_2 - 2y_3 - y_4)^2 + 8ny_4})/(2n) = 0.6268,$$

which can be obtained directly from solving the score equation. Alternatively, the EM algorithm can be used as in Dempster et al. (1977, Sec.1). The MLE $\hat{\theta}_{ML}$ is biased, unlike the adjusted estimator $\hat{\theta}$, but has smaller variance than $\hat{\theta}$. We have Var $\hat{\theta} = 4$ Var $\hat{s} = 4s(1 - s)/n$, which can be estimated as $4\hat{s}(1-\hat{s})/n = 0.0032$. This compares with the estimate of the asymptotic estimate (avar) of $\hat{\theta}_{ML}$ of 0.0026, obtained from the sample Fisher information. The asymptotic efficiency of $\hat{\theta}$ relative to $\hat{\theta}_{ML}$, is therefore estimated to be $0.0026/0.0032 = 0.81$. The loss of efficiency is due to model misspecification; $\hat{s}$ is not sufficient under model M.

When $\hat{\theta}$ is not efficient, a general method for obtaining an asymptotically fully efficient estimator $\tilde{\theta}$ is via a one-step Newton-Raphson correction or "efficientization" e.g. see Le Cam (1956), White (1994, page 137) or Lehmann and Casella (1998, p.454). Specifically, since $\hat{\theta}$ is consistent and asymptotically normal, the estimator

$$\tilde{\theta} = \hat{\theta} - \{\partial_{\hat{\theta}} S(\hat{\theta})\}^{-1} S(\hat{\theta}), \tag{1}$$

where $S(\cdot)$ is the true score function, is asymptotically the same as the ML estimate, and hence achieves full efficiency. For complicated likelihoods, the one-step efficientization method, which requires the evaluation of $S(\hat{\theta})$ and $\partial_{\hat{\theta}} S(\hat{\theta})$ only once, can greatly reduce the computational effort compared to that for $\hat{\theta}_{ML}$. In our genetic linkage example the true log-likelihood function is

$$L = Y_1 \log(\frac{1}{2} + \frac{\theta}{4}) + (Y_2 + Y_3) \log(\frac{1}{4} - \frac{\theta}{4}) + Y_4 \log(\frac{\theta}{4}).$$

First and second order derivatives of L can easily be evaluated, leading to the following one-step correction estimator:

$$\tilde{\theta} = \hat{\theta} + \frac{Y_1(2+\hat{\theta})^{-1} - (Y_2+Y_3)(1-\hat{\theta})^{-1} + Y_4\hat{\theta}^{-1}}{Y_1(2+\hat{\theta})^{-2} + (Y_2+Y_3)(1-\hat{\theta})^{-2} + Y_4\hat{\theta}^{-2}} = 0.6271.$$

This estimate is closer to the MLE $\hat{\theta}_{ML} = 0.6268$ and has the same asymptotic variance of 0.0026, Thus we have obtained a consistent and asymptotically efficient estimate.

Another way to increase efficiency is to incorporate more information into the intermediate statistic. For example, all information in the data is incorporated if we instead define intermediate statistic $\hat{s} = (y_1/n, y_2/n, y_3/n)^T$ [the last cell frequency is determined by $(1 - \hat{s}_1 - \hat{s}_2 - \hat{s}_3)$]. Here $q = \dim(\hat{s}) = 3 > 1 = p = \dim(\theta)$. The new bridge relation is

$$s = s(\theta) = \left(\frac{1}{2} + \frac{1}{4}\theta, \frac{1}{4}(1-\theta), \frac{1}{4}(1-\theta)\right).$$

If we use the generalized method of moments (see e.g. Hansen 1982, Matyas, 1999) and choose v to be an estimate of the asymptotic variance $\widehat{var}(\hat{s})$ of $\hat{s}$ with the jkth element being $(\hat{s}_j\delta_{jk} - \hat{s}_j\hat{s}_k)/n$ (δ_{jk} is the Kronecker delta), then the adjusted estimate or the minimum chi-square estimate (Ferguson 1958) is $\hat{\theta} = \arg\min_\theta H(\theta)$ where $H(\theta) = \{\hat{s} - s(\theta)\}^T v^{-1}\{\hat{s} - s(\theta)\}$. This leads to the adjusted estimate

$$\hat{\theta} = \left(Y_1^{-1} + Y_2^{-1} + Y_3^{-1} + Y_4^{-1}\right)^{-1}\left(-2Y_1^{-1} + Y_2^{-1} + Y_3^{-1}\right) = 0.6264,$$

which is closer to the ML estimator. The asymptotic variance (avar) of $\hat{\theta}$ can be estimated by $\widehat{var}(\hat{\theta}) = 2(\nabla_\theta^2 H)^{-1}|_{\theta=\hat{\theta}}$, where $\nabla_\theta^2 H$ is the Hessian of the objective function $H(\theta)$ (see Jiang and Turnbull 2003, Proposition 1). In this example, upon evaluation, we obtain:

$$\widehat{var}(\hat{\theta}) = \frac{16}{n^2}\left(Y_1^{-1} + Y_2^{-1} + Y_3^{-1} + Y_4^{-1}\right)^{-1} = 0.0029.$$

The avar estimate now is very close to that of the ML estimator. In fact, here $\hat{\theta}$ is fully efficient because now it is based on an intermediate statistic $\hat{s}$ that is sufficient under model M. The discrepancy between the avar estimates arises because of the finite sample size.

3 INDIRECT INFERENCE

3.1 The Basic Approach

Suppose we have a data set consisting of n independent units. The essential ingredients of the indirect approach, when reformulated in a likelihood-flavored treatment, are as follows.

- There is a hypothesized true model M for data generation, with distribution $P^{(\theta)}$ which depends on an unknown parameter θ of interest which is of dimension p.
- One first computes an *intermediate* or *auxiliary* statistic $\hat{s}$ of dimension $q \geq p$, which is asymptotically normal with mean $s(\theta)$, say, under model M.
- An *indirect likelihood* $L(\theta|\hat{s})$ is then constructed based on the normal approximation, so that, apart from an additive constant,

$$-2\log L(\theta|\hat{s}) = \{\hat{s} - s(\theta)\}^T v^{-1}\{\hat{s} - s(\theta)\} = H(\theta), \text{ say}, \qquad (2)$$

where v is a consistent estimate of the asymptotic variance $\widehat{var}(\hat{s})$. A typical choice might be the 'robust' or 'sandwich formula', when $\hat{s}$ solves an estimating equation (see e.g. Carroll, Ruppert and Stefanski 1995, Section A.3).
- This indirect likelihood is then maximized to generate an indirect maximum likelihood estimate (*indirect MLE*) or *adjusted* estimate $\hat{\theta}(\hat{s})$ for θ. In the case when the dimension (q) of the intermediate statistic equals that (p) of the parameter θ and $s(\theta)$ is invertible, it can be seen from (2) that maximization of the indirect likelihood is equivalent to solving the "bridge" or "binding" equation $s(\theta) = \hat{s}$ for θ, because then (2) can be made zero.

In the "indirect" analysis of the example of Section 2, the true model M is the multinomial one with cell probabilities: $(\frac{1}{2} + \frac{1}{4}\theta, \frac{1}{4}(1 - \theta), \frac{1}{4}(1 - \theta), \frac{1}{4}\theta)$. In the initial approach, the intermediate statistic is $\hat{s} = (y_1 + y_4)/n$ and the indirect likelihood $L(\theta|\hat{s})$ is given by

$$-2\log L(\theta|\hat{s}) = \frac{n}{\hat{s}(1 - \hat{s})}\left(\hat{s} - \frac{1 + \theta}{2}\right)^2.$$

Finally the adjusted estimate is $\hat{\theta} = 2\hat{s} - 1$.

In this approach, the data are first summarized by the intermediate statistic. Its asymptotic mean is referred to as the *auxiliary parameter*. The auxiliary parameter is related to the original parameter by a relation $s = s(\theta)$, termed the *bridge relation* or *binding function*.

The starting point is the choice of an intermediate statistic $\hat{s}$. This can be chosen as some set of sample moments, or the solution of some estimating equations, or the ML estimator (MLE) based on some convenient model M′, say, termed the *auxiliary* (or *naive*) model. If the last, then the model M′ is a simpler but misspecified or partially misspecified model. The choice of an intermediate statistic $\hat{s}$ is not necessarily unique; however in any given situation there is often a natural one to use.

In general, the indirect MLE has a set of properties similar to those of the usual MLE:

- It is a consistent and asymptotically normal estimate for θ. Its asymptotic variance is estimable by the inverse of the Hessian matrix of $-\log(\text{indirect likelihood})$, i.e. $\widehat{var}(\hat{\theta}) = 2(\nabla_\theta^2 H)^{-1}|_{\theta=\hat{\theta}}$ with H given by (2).
- Hence $(-2)\log(\text{indirect likelihood ratio})$ can be used in the same way as the usual chi-squared test to assess goodness of fit when comparing nested models.
- The indirect MLE is asymptotically efficient relative to estimators constructed by smooth mappings of the same intermediate statistic.

These are summarized in Jiang and Turnbull (2003, Proposition 1), see also the references in Section 3.3.

When different intermediate statistics are used, the asymptotic efficiency can be different. The indirect MLE in general is not as efficient as the MLE based on the true model M, although there are situations that can be identified where the efficiency will be high, as in the example of Section 4.2. Jiang and Turnbull (2003) provide further discussions on efficiency and on determination of the auxiliary parameter; they also justify the asymptotic properties of the indirect MLE stated above.

3.2 Why Consider the Indirect Method?

This indirect approach offers the following advantages:

1. *Ease of computation.* The indirect method is typically computationally simpler and more convenient. For example, when $\hat{s}$ is based on some simplified model M', it can often can be computed with available standard computer software,

2. *Informativeness on the effect of model misspecification.* When $\hat{s}$ is a 'naive estimate' obtained from a naive model M' neglecting certain model complexities, the approach is very informative on the effect of model misspecification — the bridge relation $s = s(\theta)$ provides a dynamic correspondence between M' and M. For example, in errors-in-variable regression, such a relation is sometimes termed an 'attenuation relation' (see e.g., Carroll, Ruppert and Stefanski 1995, Chapter 2), and tells how regression coefficients can be underestimated when neglecting the measurement error in a predictor.

3. *Robustness.* The validity of the inference based on an intermediate statistic essentially relies on the correct specification of its asymptotic mean. This is typically a less demanding assumption than the correct specification of a full probability model, which would be generally needed for a direct likelihood inference to be valid. Therefore inferences based on the adjusted estimate $\hat{\theta}$ can remain valid despite some departure of the data generation mechanism from the hypothesized true model M.

3.3 Bibliography and Notes

The above very brief exposition of the indirect method of inference represents a summary of results that have appeared in the econometric and statistical literature in varying forms and generality and tailored for various applications. Examples include: the generalized method of moments (GMM: Hansen 1982); the method of linear forms and minimum χ^2 (Ferguson 1958); the regular best asymptotic normal estimates that are functions of sample averages (Chiang 1956, Theorem 3); simulated method of moments and indirect inference [McFadden (1989), Pakes and Pollard (1989), Gourieroux *et al.* (1993), Gallant and Tauchen (1996, 1999) Gallant and Long (1997)]. Applications of GMM in the settings of generalized estimating equations from biostatistics are discussed in Qu, Lindsay and Li (2000).

The theory of properties of estimators obtained from misspecified likelihoods goes back at least as far as Cox (1962), Berk (1966) and Huber (1967) and is summarized in the comprehensive monograph by White (1994). The use of $\hat{s}$ (based on an auxiliary model M') in indirect inference about θ (under model M) appears recently in the field of econometrics to treat complex time series and dynamic models, see, e.g., Gourieroux et al. (1993) and Gallant and Tauchen (1996, 1999); as well as in the field of biostatistics to treat regression models with random effects and measurement error, see e.g., Kuk (1995),

Turnbull, Jiang and Clark (1997), and Jiang *et al.* (1999). This bibliography is far from exhaustive. A thorough review and a synthesis of the methods of indirect inference are given in Jiang and Turnbull (2003). In a recent paper, Genton and Ronchetti (2003) discuss robust indirect inference with bounded influence.

4 THREE DATA SETS

Below we illustrate the application of indirect inference with three analyses: a recap of some analyses on repeated events data from the NPC trial (Clark *et al.* 1996; Turnbull *et al.* 1997; Jiang *et al.* 1999) where random effect and covariate measurement error are present; analysis of a carcinogenicity data set utilizing a Poisson regression model with random effects (over-dispersion); an analysis on epileptic seizure data illustrating indirect inference based on first order moments. The first and second use estimates from a naive model M′ as intermediate statistics. The third uses sample moments and leads to a goodness-of-fit test.

4.1 Intensity Regression Model for Repeated Events Data with Frailties and Covariate Measurement Error: Skin Cancer Data

Clark et al. (1996) have described the results of the "Nutritional Prevention of Cancer" (NPC) trial. This trial, begun in 1983, studied the long-term safety and efficacy of a daily 200μg nutritional supplement of selenium (Se) for the prevention of cancer. It was a double-blind, placebo-controlled randomized clinical trial with $n = 1312$ patients accrued and followed for up to about ten years. Here we shall consider a particular primary endpoint — namely squamous cell carcinoma (SCC) of the skin. The results for this endpoint are of particular interest because Clark et al. (1996) found a negative (but not statistically significant, P = 0.15) effect of selenium (Se) supplementation. This was opposite to previous expectations, and contrasted sharply with findings of highly significant positive benefits of the selenium supplementation in preventing a number of other types of cancers. However in their analysis, Clark et al. used only data on the time to *first* occurrence of SCC in each subject and employed a Cox model that ignored patient heterogeneity (i.e. that assumed a common baseline hazard) and ignored that some explanatory covariates were measured with error.

Here we will consider the recurrences of SCC over time, measured from date of randomization, for patients $i = 1, ..., n$ as n i.i.d. discrete point processes $\{Y_i(t)\}$. Here $Y_i(t)$ is the observed number of recurrences for patient i on day t (usually zero or one). Time t is measured in days on a discrete time scale $t = 1, \ldots, K$, where $K = 4618$ days, the longest followup time. The indicator variable $H_i(t)$ is one if patient i is still on study ("at risk") on day t and zero otherwise. For illustration purposes, we will consider only two explanatory variables, namely treatment assignment indicator a and baseline Se level x. The latter is an important predictor, measured prior to randomization in each patient, but is contaminated with measurement error so that the observed value is recorded as z not x. For our base model M, we postulate only a multiplicative model for the observed mean response:

$$E[Y_i(t)] = H_i(t)\psi_i\lambda(t)\exp(a_i\gamma + x_i\beta), \text{ for all } i = 1, 2, \ldots, n, \ t = 1, \ldots, K.$$
(3)

Here the $\{\psi_i\}$ represent subject-specific random effects which modulate the nonparametric baseline mean rate $\lambda(t)$. Without loss of generality we may take $E[\psi_i] = 1$. This random effect or "frailty" factor is introduced to model the effect of 'unexplained heterogeneity' of patients perhaps induced by omitting covariates, unused, unmeasured or undreamed of. Here the true parameter of interest is $\theta = (\gamma, \beta, \lambda(\cdot))$, where $\lambda(\cdot) = (\lambda(1), \ldots, \lambda(K))$.

This is clearly a complex model, particularly because the frailties $\{\psi_i\}$ are unobserved, and only the surrogate z_i is observed in place of x_i. Jiang et al. (1999) proposed an indirect inference approach based on the auxiliary model M' given by nonhomogeneous Poisson process model with multiplicative intensity $m(t)\exp(a_ig + z_ib)$. Note M' is simpler; it ignores the presence of frailties and measurement error. This leads to consideration of the intermediate statistic $\hat{s} = (\hat{g}, \hat{b}, \hat{m}(\cdot))$. Here $(\hat{g}, \hat{b})^T$ is the Cox (1972) partial likelihood estimate and $\hat{m}(t)$ is a discrete intensity estimate for $\lambda(t)$ that corresponds to the Nelson Aalen estimate of the cumulative intensity (see Andersen et al. 1993, Sec.VII.2.1). Standard computer software can be employed to compute these estimates — e.g. in Splus Release 6 (Insightful Corp. 2001). The auxiliary or 'naive' estimator $\hat{s}$ is computed ignoring both the random effect (by taking ψ_i to be its mean 1) and the measurement error (by taking x_i to be z_i). The dimensionality of $\hat{s}$ and θ are equal and so the $\hat{\theta}$ can be obtained from the bridge relation $s = s(\theta)$. Jiang et al. (1999) used a Gaussian additive noise model for the measurement error effect. This implies the pairs (z_i, x_i) are i.i.d. bivariate normal with $var(z_i) = \sigma_z^2$ and $var(x_i) = cov(x_i, z_i) = \sigma_x^2$. An external validation data set was used to justify this model and also to obtain estimates of the parameters σ_z^2 and σ_x^2. They go on to find the auxiliary or 'naive' parameter $s = (g, b, m(\cdot))$, the asymptotic mean of $\hat{s}$, leading to the bridge relations:

$$g = \gamma, \quad b = (\sigma_x^2/\sigma_z^2)\beta, \quad m(t) = \lambda(t)\exp\{0.5\beta^2\sigma_z^{-2}\sigma_x^2(\sigma_z^2 - \sigma_x^2)\}.$$

This bridge relation is then inverted to obtain a consistent adjusted estimator $\hat{\theta}$ for the true parameter $\theta = (\gamma, \beta, \lambda(\cdot))$. Robust sandwich variance estimates were used to obtain standard errors. Details of the calculations are given by Jiang et al. (1999). The results are summarized in lines 1a and 1b of Table 1.

Note that there is a qualitative difference between the estimates of treatment effect: in the general model M, the treatment is no longer statistically

Table 1. Statistical analyses for several models of NPC trial SCC data

Model	Treatment estimate (s.e.)	Baseline Se estimate (s.e.)
1) Semi-parametric		
a) Naive (Model M′)	$\hat{g}=0.117$ (0.059)	$\hat{b}_1=-0.690$ (0.146)
b) Adjusted (Model M)	$\hat{\gamma}=0.117$ (0.125)	$\hat{\beta}_1=-2.076$ (0.963)
2) Constant Intensity		
a) Naive (Model M′)	$\hat{g}=0.122$ (0.059)	$\hat{b}_1=-0.725$ (0.145)
b) Adjusted (Model M)	$\hat{\gamma}=0.122$ (0.125)	$\hat{\beta}_1=-2.181$ (0.963)

significant. The results based on model M (line 1b) are robust against mis-specifications of models on the response $\{Y_i(t)\}$– only a very general model for the mean need be postulated (cf. Lawless and Nadeau 1995). Assumptions on higher moments, such as those that might be imposed by the Poisson distribution, are not needed for valid inference.

In an earlier paper, for data based on interim data for the same study, Turnbull et al. (1997) used an indirect approach for model M, but where the intensity $\lambda(t)$ was constant over time. The corresponding auxiliary model M′ then reduces to a negative binomial regression, for which again standard software is available, e.g. procedure 'nbreg' in STATA 5.0 (StataCorp 1997). For our data set, the results are displayed in Lines 2a and 2b of Table 1. The results are similar to those in Lines 1a and 1b, as would be expected if the much simpler constant intensity function is adequate; the semiparametric model is not needed. However, the indirect method is still needed to accommodate the random effects and measurement error features. Turnbull et al. (1997) also consider estimation of variance of the random effects. Jiang et al. (1999) also discuss a situation with frailty but no covariate measurement error.

4.2 Poisson Regression with Overdispersion: Animal Carcinogenicity Data

We use carcinogenicity data presented by Gail, Santner and Brown (1980) from an experiment conducted by Thompson et al. (1978) to illustrate our method for treating a Poisson regression model with random effects (overdispersion). Forty-eight female rats who remained tumor-free after sixty days of pre-treatment of a prevention drug (retinyl acetate) were randomized with equal probability into two groups. In Group 1 they continued to receive treatment ($Z = 1$), in Group 2 they received placebo ($Z = 0$). All rats were followed for an additional 122 days and palpated for mammary tumors twice a week. The objective of the study was to estimate the effect of the preventive treatment (Z) on number of tumors (Y) diagnosed.

In the model M, given Z and ϵ, Y is assumed to be Poisson with mean $e^{\alpha+Z\beta+\epsilon}$. Here Z is observed but ϵ represents an unobserved random effect assumed normal with zero mean and constant variance σ^2, independent of Z. This unobserved random effect or "unexplained heterogeneity" could be caused by omitted covariates. We observe n i.i.d. pairs $W_i = (Y_i, Z_i)$, $i = 1, \ldots, n$. The likelihood for the observed data involves integration over ϵ and is difficult to compute. (However it is possible – see below.) Instead we start by taking the indirect approach with an auxiliary statistic $\hat{s} = (\hat{a}, \hat{b}, \hat{t}^2)^T$, where $(\hat{a}, \hat{b})$ are the regression coefficient estimates maximizing a naive log-likelihood $R = \sum_1^n \{Y_i(a+Z_ib) - e^{a+Z_ib}\}$, and $\hat{t}^2 = n^{-1}\sum_{i=1}^n Y_i^2$ is the second sample moment. Here the auxiliary parameter is $s = (a, b, t^2)^T$, whereas the true parameter to be estimated is $\theta = (\alpha, \beta, \sigma^2)^T$. The use of the naive log-likelihood R corresponds to a simplified model M′ in which the presence of the random effect ϵ is neglected. The second sample moment is included in the intermediate statistic to provide information for estimation of the variance parameter. Therefore $\hat{s}$ is solved from the estimating equation $G(\mathbf{W}, s) = 0$, where (formally) $G = (n^{-1}\partial_a R, n^{-1}\partial_b R, \hat{t}^2 - t^2)^T$ or

$$G = n^{-1}\sum_{i=1}^n g_i \equiv n^{-1}\sum_{i=1}^n (Y_i - e^{a+Z_ib}, \ Z_i(Y_i - e^{a+Z_ib}), \ Y_i^2 - t^2)^T.$$

The solution $\hat{s} = (\hat{a}, \hat{b}, \hat{t}^2)^T$ can be computed easily. For the rat carcinogenicity data we obtain the auxiliary estimates $\hat{a} = 1.7984$; $\hat{b} = -0.8230$; $\hat{t}^2 = 31.875$. The asymptotic variance $var(\hat{s})$ can be estimated by the sandwich formula (see e.g. Carroll, Ruppert and Stefanski 1995, Section A.3)

$$v = (\nabla_s G)^{-1}\widehat{var}(G)(\nabla_s G)^{-T}|_{s=\hat{s}}$$

where $\widehat{var}(G) = n^{-2}\sum_{i=1}^n g_i g_i^T|_{s=\hat{s}}$, $\nabla_s G$ is a 3×3 matrix with elements $(\nabla_s G)_{jk} = \partial_{s_k} G_j, j, k = 1, 2, 3$, and $A^{-T} = (A^{-1})^T$ for a generic matrix A.

The indirect likelihood $L(\theta|\hat{s})$, up to an additive constant, satisfies

$$-2\log L(\theta|\hat{s}) = \{\hat{s} - s(\theta)\}^T v^{-1}\{\hat{s} - s(\theta)\},$$

where $s(\theta)$ is the asymptotic mean or large sample almost sure limit of $\hat{s}$. Since $\hat{s}$ solves the estimating equation $G = 0$, its limit is the solution of the limiting estimating equation $F(\theta, s) = E_{\mathbf{W}|\theta}G(\mathbf{W}, s) = 0$, which can be explicitly solved to obtain $s = s(\theta)$. This yields the bridge equation:

$$s = (a, b, t^2)^T$$
$$= s(\theta) = \left(\alpha + \sigma^2/2, \ \beta, \ \frac{1}{2}(1 + e^\beta)e^{\alpha+\frac{1}{2}\sigma^2} + \frac{1}{2}(1 + e^{2\beta})e^{2(\alpha+\sigma^2)}\right)^T.$$

Because $\dim(s) = \dim(\theta) = 3$ and $s(\theta)$ is a smooth invertible mapping, the indirect MLE $\hat{\theta} = \arg\max_\theta L(\theta|\hat{s})$ can be obtained by solving $\hat{s} = s(\theta)$, which gives the adjusted estimates $\hat{\theta} = (\hat{\alpha}, \hat{\beta}, \hat{\sigma}^2) = s^{-1}(\hat{s})$. Thus $\hat{\beta} = \hat{b}$, and $\hat{\alpha} = \hat{a} - \hat{\sigma}^2/2$ where $\hat{\sigma}^2 = \log\left\{\frac{2\hat{t}^2 - e^{\hat{a}}(1+e^{\hat{b}})}{e^{2\hat{a}}(1+e^{2\hat{b}})}\right\}$. For the rat data, this leads to adjusted estimates $\hat{\alpha} = 1.6808(0.1589)$; $\hat{\beta} = -0.8230(0.1968)$; $\hat{\sigma} = 0.4850(0.1274)$.

The estimated standard errors shown in parentheses are obtained using the delta method formula: $\widehat{var}(\hat{\theta}) = (\nabla_\theta s)^{-1} v (\nabla_\theta s)^{-T}|_{\theta=\hat{\theta}}$, and then taking the square roots of the 3 diagonal elements of this matrix. It is noted that this delta method expression is equivalent to deriving the variance by

$$\{-\nabla_\theta^2 \log L(\theta|\hat{s})\}^{-1}|_{\theta=\hat{\theta}}$$

based on the 'indirect likelihood Fisher information', where ∇_θ^2 represents the Hessian. This is because that the jkth element of the Hessian is, for $j, k = 1, 2, 3$,

$$\{-\nabla_\theta^2 \log L(\theta|\hat{s})\}_{jk}|_{\theta=\hat{\theta}} = -\partial_{\theta_j}\partial_{\theta_k}\log L(\theta|\hat{s})|_{\theta=\hat{\theta}}$$
$$= (\partial_{\theta_j} s^T) v^{-1}(\partial_{\theta_k} s)|_{\theta=\hat{\theta}} - (\partial_{\theta_j}\partial_{\theta_k} s^T) v^{-1}(\hat{s} - s)|_{\theta=\hat{\theta}}$$
$$= (\partial_{\theta_j} s^T) v^{-1}(\partial_{\theta_k} s)|_{\theta=\hat{\theta}} + 0$$
$$= \{\widehat{var}(\hat{\theta})^{-1}\}_{jk}.$$

If we wish to obtain the MLE of $\theta = (\alpha, \beta, \sigma^2)$ based on model M, then it can be found by a somewhat tedious iterative numerical maximization of the true likelihood which involves numerical integration over the distribution of ϵ. These estimates are: $\hat{\alpha}_{ML} = 1.6717$ (0.1560); $\hat{\beta}_{ML} = -0.8125$ (0.2078); $\hat{\sigma}_{ML} = 0.5034$ (0.0859). For the MLEs, the estimated standard errors are based on the inverse of the Fisher information matrix, evaluated at the corresponding estimate values.

The estimated standard errors suggest that the efficiency of indirect estimation of the treatment effect parameter β is high here in this example. Related results (Cox, 1983; Jiang et al, 1999) show that such high efficiency is achievable if the follow-up times are about the same across different subjects (which is true here), or if the overdispersion is small. Also it should be noted that the adjusted estimator $\hat{\beta}$ is robust, in the sense that it remains consistent, essentially as long as the mean function $E(Y|Z, \epsilon)$ is correctly specified and ϵ and Z are independent. (Its standard error estimate from the sandwich formula is also model-independent and robust.) In particular, the consistency property does not depend on the specification of a complete probability model, namely that Y is Poisson and ϵ is normal. Thus the indirect estimator enjoys a robustness advantage over the MLE.

The indirect approach, although formulated from the different perspective of using naive model plus method of moments, is intimately related to the work of Breslow (1990) based on quasi-likelihood and method of moments. Breslow used a different linear combination of Y_i's based on quasi-likelihood (Wedderburn, 1974; McCullagh and Nelder, 1989), which enjoy general efficiency properties among linear estimating equations. However, (i) our approach can be interpreted as basing inference on the simple moments $n^{-1}\sum Y_i$, $n^{-1}\sum Z_i Y_i$ and $n^{-1}\sum Y_i^2$ (which can be easily seen from the estimating equation $G = 0$), and (ii) our approach shows clearly, by the use of bridge relations, the sensitivity and robustness of parameter estimates to the omission of over-dispersion in modeling. Also note that here we used a log-normal distribution to model the random effects and the variance parameter also enters the mean model (unconditional on ϵ), whereas Breslow (1990) focused on the examples such as ones with gamma multiplicative random effects in which the mean model does not change. For the only comparable parameter β (the treatment effect), the Breslow method (from his equations (1), (2) and (7)) gives exactly the same answer as our adjusted analysis: $\hat{\beta}_{\text{Breslow}} = -0.8230(0.1968)$. This is because, for this special two-group design, both methods essentially use the log(frequency ratio) to estimate the treatment effect.

4.3 Loglinear Regression Model for Longitudinal Count Data: Epileptic Seizures Data

We consider seizures data from a clinical trial of 59 epileptics carried out by Leppik et al. (1985) and presented in Table 2 of Thall and Vail (1990). The data set is also reproduced in Diggle, Liang and Zeger (1994, Table 1.5). For each patient, the number of epileptic seizures was recorded during a baseline period of eight weeks. Patients were then randomized to treatment with the anti-epileptic drug progabide, or to placebo. The number of seizures was then recorded in four consecutive two-week intervals. As in Thall and Vail (1990, p.666) and Diggle et al. (1994, p.166), we will also remove the outlier record of patient #207 in the following analysis. (Analysis can be carried out in entirely similar way if we include this observation.) We will use this data set to illustrate estimation and goodness-of-fit tests in the context of indirect inference.

Let Y_{ij} be the number of epileptic seizures the i-th patient has in the j-th period [$j=0$ (baseline), 1, 2, 3, 4]. Define $z_i=1$ if the i-th patient is in the treatment group, 0 if placebo; and τ_j to be the length of the jth period. Hence $\tau_0 = 8, \tau_1 = \ldots = \tau_4 = 2$. A saturated log-linear structure for the mean response has the form:

$$\log \mathrm{E}(Y_{ij}) = \log(\tau_j) + \mu_j + \gamma_j z_i, \text{ for } i = 1, 2, \ldots, n; \ j = 0, \ldots, 4. \quad (4)$$

This log-linear specification really does not make any assumption to the means because it allows different and arbitrary trends for the rates of seizures in the two groups of patients — there are 10 cell means and 10 parameters. We make no further distributional assumptions e.g. concerning variances; indeed we may expect there to be extra-Poisson variation.

For our model M we will take the reduced model of a constant mean rate of seizures after randomization dependent on treatment, as proposed by Diggle et al. (1994, p.167), i.e.:

Model M: $\mu_1 = \mu_2 = \mu_3 = \mu_4 = \mu_0 + \beta_0; \quad \gamma_1 = \gamma_2 = \gamma_3 = \gamma_4 = \gamma_0 + \alpha_0.$

The parameter vector is $\theta = (\mu_0, \gamma_0, \beta_0, \alpha_0)$. Here μ_0 represents an intercept term, β_0 represents the effect of time (pre- versus post-randomization), γ_0 the effect of treatment, and α_0 the time-treatment interaction.

We will consider indirect inference based on the intermediate statistic $\hat{s} = (\bar{y}_{0,0}, ..., \bar{y}_{0,4}; \bar{y}_{1,0}..., \bar{y}_{1,4})^T$, where $\bar{y}_{z,j}$ is the average of number of seizures in treatment group z in time period j ($z = 0, 1; j = 0, ..., 4$). Here these ten cell means are:

$$\hat{s} = (30.79, 9.36, 8.29, 8.79, 7.96; \ 27.63, 5.47, 6.53, \dot{6}.00, 4.83)^T.$$

The auxiliary parameter s is the asymptotic mean of $\hat{s}$; in fact

$$s = E(\hat{s}|\theta)$$
$$= (8e^{\mu_0}, 2e^{\mu_0+\beta_0}, 2e^{\mu_0+\beta_0}, 2e^{\mu_0+\beta_0}, 2e^{\mu_0+\beta_0};$$
$$8e^{\mu_0+\gamma_0}, 2e^{\mu_0+\beta_0+\gamma_0+\alpha_0}, 2e^{\mu_0+\beta_0+\gamma_0+\alpha_0}, 2e^{\mu_0+\beta_0+\gamma_0+\alpha_0}, 2e^{\mu_0+\beta_0+\gamma_0+\alpha_0})^T.$$

In the model M, the parameter vector $\theta = (\mu_0, \gamma_0, \beta_0, \alpha_0)$ to be estimated has dimension $p = 4$ while the dimension of the auxiliary statistic $\hat{s}$ is $q = 10$. Following the development in Section 3.1, we obtain the indirect MLE $\hat{\theta}$ and its standard error (s.e.) by minimization and second order derivatives of the objective function

$$-2\log L(\theta|\hat{s}) = \{\hat{s} - E(\hat{s}|\theta)\}^T v^{-1}\{\hat{s} - E(\hat{s}|\theta)\}. \tag{5}$$

Here v, the robust variance matrix estimate, is a 10×10 matrix of the block diagonal form:

$$\begin{pmatrix} v_0 & 0 \\ 0 & v_1 \end{pmatrix}.$$

The elements of the 5×5 submatrix v_0 are given by

$$(v_0)_{jj'} = \frac{1}{n_0(n_0 - 1)} \sum_{i:z_i=0} (Y_{ij} - \bar{y}_{0,j})(Y_{ij'} - \bar{y}_{0,j'}), \quad j, j' = 0, 1, 2, 3, 4.$$

Similarly the elements of v_1 are

$$(v_1)_{jj'} = \frac{1}{n_1(n_1 - 1)} \sum_{i:z_i=1} (Y_{ij} - \bar{y}_{1,j})(Y_{ij'} - \bar{y}_{1,j'}), \quad j, j' = 0, 1, 2, 3, 4.$$

Here $n_0 = 28$ the number of patients on placebo and $n_1 = 30$ the number of patients on progabide (excluding patient # 207). Carrying out the computation we get

$$v_0 = \begin{pmatrix} 24.33 & 7.03 & 6.33 & 6.75 & 5.82 \\ 7.03 & 3.67 & 2.31 & 2.69 & 1.86 \\ 6.33 & 2.31 & 2.38 & 2.83 & 1.74 \\ 6.75 & 2.69 & 2.83 & 7.69 & 2.70 \\ 5.82 & 1.86 & 1.74 & 2.70 & 2.08 \end{pmatrix}$$

and

$$v_1 = \begin{pmatrix} 10.07 & 1.79 & 1.66 & 2.14 & 1.53 \\ 1.79 & 1.11 & 0.49 & 0.89 & 0.64 \\ 1.66 & 0.49 & 1.05 & 0.96 & 0.58 \\ 2.14 & 0.89 & 0.96 & 1.81 & 0.87 \\ 1.53 & 0.64 & 0.58 & 0.87 & 0.61 \end{pmatrix}.$$

The minimization of (5) can be done directly using computer software, e.g. MATLAB (MathWorks, 2000) or subroutine E04JAF in NAG (Numerical Algorithms Group, 2001). Alternatively, by pooling post-randomization responses for each treatment and a reparametrization, the problem can be transformed to one of minimizing a generalized *linear* least squares criterion, for which an explicit solution can written down. The results are summarized in column (a) of Table 2.

Table 2. Log-linear regression coefficients and robust standard errors (in parentheses) for epileptic seizure data using (a) indirect MLE method and (b) GEE with exchangeable correlation. The GEE estimates are from Diggle et al. (1994, Table 8.10).

Variable	(a) Indirect estimate	(b) GEE estimate
Intercept (μ_0)	1.32 (0.23)	1.35 (0.16)
Time (β_0)	0.06 (0.11)	0.11 (0.12)
Treatment (γ_0)	−0.14 (0.28)	−0.11 (0.19)
Time×treatment (α_0)	−0.39 (0.21)	−0.30 (0.17)

For comparison, Table 2 column (b) also displays the results of Diggle et al. (1994, Table 8.10) who used GEE estimates based an exchangeable correlation. Qualitatively, the results are very similar, namely a nonsignificant treatment effect and a modestly significant interaction between treatment and time. Both GEE and indirect estimation are robust – they depend only on the mean model (M) and not on distributional assumptions concerning the $\{Y_{ij}\}$. Note that, theoretically, the indirect method estimator is guaranteed to be fully efficient among estimators that are smooth functions of $\hat{s}$. The GEE estimator can be less efficient asymptotically depending on the choice of working covariance matrix.

In addition, the indirect likelihood approach leads naturally to a test for goodness-of-fit of the model M which postulated a constant seizure rate by treatment post-randomization. This is not directly available in the GEE approach. When evaluated at the indirect MLE $\hat{\theta}$, the indirect likelihood leads to a test statistic value $- \sup_\theta 2 \log L(\theta|\hat{s}) = 10.1008$. This is to be compared with the percentiles of the χ_6^2 distribution because the dimension of the parameter space is reduced from 10 in the unconstrained saturated model to 4 in the constant rate model M. The P-value is 0.1205 and there is no significant evidence against the constant rate model M.

ACKNOWLEDGMENTS

The authors were partially supported by a grant from the U.S. National Institutes of Health and a grant from the National Science Foundation.

REFERENCES

Andersen, P. K., Borgan, O., Gill, R. D. and Keiding, N. (1993). *Statistical Models Based on Counting Processes.* New York: Springer-Verlag,

Berk, R.H. (1966). Limiting behavior of posterior distributions when the model is incorrect. *Ann. Math. Statist.*, **37**, 51-58.

Breslow, N. (1990). Tests of hypotheses in overdispersed Poisson regression and other quasi-likelihood models. *J. Am. Statist. Assoc.* **85**, 565-571.

Carroll, R. J., Ruppert, D. and Stefanski, L. A. (1995). *Measurement Error in Nonlinear Models.* London: Chapman and Hall.

Chiang, C. L. (1956). On regular best asymptotically normal estimates. *Ann. Math. Statist.*, **27**, 336-351.

Clark, L.C., Combs, G. F., Turnbull, B.W., Slate, E.H., Chalker, D.K., Chow, J., Davis, L.S., Glover, R.A., Graham, G.F., Gross, E.G., Krongrad, A., Lesher, J.L., Park, H.K., Sanders, B.B., Smith, C.L., Taylor, J.R. and the Nutritional Prevention of Cancer Study Group. (1996) Effects of Selenium Supplementation for Cancer Prevention in Patients with Carcinoma of the Skin: A Randomized Clinical Trial. *J. Am. Med. Ass.*, 276 (24), 1957-1963. (Editorial: p1984-5.)

Cox, D.R. (1962). Further results on tests of separate families of hypotheses. *J. R. Statist. Soc.* B, **24**, 406-424.

Cox, D.R. (1972). Regression models and life-tables (with discussion). *J. R. Statist. Soc.* B, **34**, 187-207.

Cox D. R. (1983). Some remarks on overdispersion. *Biometrika*, 70, 269-274.

Dempster, A. P., Laird, N. M. and Rubin, D. B. (1977). Maximum Likelihood from Incomplete Data via the EM Algorithm (with discussion). *J. R. Statist. Soc. B*, **39**, 1-38 .

Diggle, P. J., Liang, K. -Y. and Zeger, S. L. (1994). *Analysis of Longitudinal Data*, Clarendon Press, Oxford.

Ferguson, T. S. (1958). A method of generating best asymptotic normal estimates with application to the estimation of bacterial densities. *Ann. Math. Statist.*, **29**, 1046-1062.

Fisher, R.A. (1946). *Statistical Methods for Research Workers, 10th edn.* Edinburgh: Oliver and Boyd.

Gail, M. H., Santner, T.J. and Brown, C.C. (1980). An analysis of comparative carcinogenesis experiments based on multiple times to tumor. *Biometrics*, **36**, 255-266.

Gallant, A. R. and Long, J. R. (1997). Estimating stochastic differential equations efficiently by minimum chi-squared. *Biometrika*, **84**, 125-141.

Gallant, A. R. and Tauchen, G. (1996). Which moments to match? *Econometric Theory*, **12**, 657-681.

Gallant, A. R. and Tauchen, G. (1999). The relative efficiency of method of moments estimators. *J. of Econometrics*, **92**, 149-172.

Genton, M. G. and Ronchetti E. (2003). Robust indirect inference. *J. Am. Statist. Assoc.* **98**, 67-76.

Gourieroux, C., Monfort, A. and Renault, E. (1993). Indirect inference. *J. of Appl. Econometrics* **8S**, 85-118.

Hansen, L. P. (1982). Large sample properties of generalised method of moments estimators. *Econometrica*, **50**, 1029-1054.

Huber, P.J. (1967). The behavior of maximum likelihood estimates under nonstandard conditions. In *Procceedings of the Fifth Berkeley Symposium on Probability and Statistics I*, pp.221-233. Berkeley: Univ. of California Press.

Insightful Corporation (2001), *S-PLUS 6* Seattle, Washington.

Jiang, W. and Turnbull, B. W. (2003). The indirect method — robust inference based on intermediate statistics. *Technical Report No. 1377, School of Operations Research, Cornell University*, Ithaca NY.

  Available at http://www.orie.cornell.edu/trlist/trlist.html

Jiang, W., Turnbull, B. W. and Clark, L. C. (1999). Semiparametric Regression Models for Repeated Events with Random Effects and Measurement Error. *J. Am. Statist. Ass.*, **94** 111-124.

Kuk, A. Y. C. (1995). Asymptotically unbiased estimation in generalised linear models with random effects. *J. R. Statist. Soc. B*, **57**, 395-407.

Lawless J.F. and Nadeau, C. (1995) Some simple robust methods for the analysis of recurrent events. *Technometrics*, **37**, 158-168.

Le Cam, L. (1956). On the Asymptotic Theory of Estimation and Testing Hypotheses. *Proceedings of the Third Berkeley Symposium on Mathematical Statistics and Probability* **1**, pp. 129-156. Berkeley: Univ. of California Press.

Lehmann, E.L. and Casella, G. (1998). *Theory of Point Estimation*, 2nd edn. New York: Springer.

Leppik, I.E. et al. (1985). A double-blind crossover evaluation of progabide in partial seizures. *Neurology*, **35**, 285.

MathWorks, Inc. (2000). MATLAB Version 6. The MathWorks Inc., Natick, Massachussets.

Matyas, L., Ed. (1999). *Generalized Method of Moments Estimation*. Cambridge: Cambridge University Press.

McCullagh, P. and Nelder, J. A. (1989). *Generalized Linear Models*. New York: Chapman and Hall.

McFadden, D. (1989). A method of simulated moments for estimation of discrete response models without numerical integration. *Econometrica*, **57**, 995-1026.

Numerical Algorithms Group (2001). NAG Fortran Algorithms, Mark 20. Numerical Algorithms Group, Oxford, UK.

Pakes, A. and Pollard, D. (1989). Simulation and the asymptotics of optimization estimators. *Econometrica*, **57**, 1027-57.

Qu, A., Lindsay, B. G. and Li, B. (2000). Improving generalised estimating equations using quadratic inference functions. *Biometrika*, **87**, 823-836.

Rao C. R. (1973). *Linear Statistical Inference and its Applications*, 2nd edn. New York: Wiley.

StataCorp (1997). *Stata Statistical Software, Release 5.0* Stata Corporation, College Station, Texas.

Thall, P.F. and Vail, S.C. (1990). Some covariance models for longitudinal count data with overdispersion. *Biometrics*, **46**, 657-71.

Thompson, H. F., Grubbs, C. J., Moon, R. C. and Sporn, M. B. (1978). Continual requirement of retinoid for maintenance of mammary cancer inhibition. *Proceedings of the Annual Meeting of the American Association for Cancer Research*, **19**, 74.

Turnbull, B.W., Jiang, W. and Clark, L.C. (1997). Regression models for recurrent event data: parametric random effects models with measurement error. *Statist. in Med.*, **16**, 853-64.

Wedderburn, R. W. M. (1974). Quasi-likelihood, generalized linear models and the Gauss-Newton method. *Biometrika*, **61**, 439-447.

White, H. (1994). *Estimation, Inference and Specification Analysis*. Cambridge: Cambridge University Press.

On Characterizing Joint Survivor Functions by Minima

David Oakes

Department of Biostatistics and Computational Biology, University of Rochester Medical Center, 601 Elmwood Avenue Box 630, Rochester NY 14642, U.S.A., email: oakes@bst.rochester.edu

ABSTRACT   We consider some consequences of the fact that the joint survivor function of a bivariate random variable (T_1, T_2) is characterized by the collection of univariate survivor functions of the random variables $\min(\lambda_1 T_1, \lambda_2 T_2)$ for positive λ_1 and λ_2. Specifically, we consider the use of data on minima or combinations of minima to estimate the dependence parameter in Hougaard's positive stable frailty model with known marginals.

1 Introduction

It is well known that the joint distribution of the random variable (T_1, T_2) is characterized by the set of univariate distributions of all linear combinations $\lambda_1 T_1 + \lambda_2 T_2$, for real λ_1 and λ_2 The proof is an immediate consequence of the uniqueness theorem for characteristic functions. Less well known, though even easier to prove, is the following analogous result regarding minima:

"Theorem 1". The joint survivor function $S(t_1, t_2) = \mathrm{pr}(T_1 > t_1, T_2 > t_2)$ of a bivariate non-negative random variable (T_1, T_2) is characterized by the collection of univariate survivor functions $S_{\lambda_1, \lambda_2}(t) = \mathrm{pr}(T_{\lambda_1, \lambda_2} > t)$, for $\lambda_1 > 0, \lambda_2 > 0$, where $T_{\lambda_1, \lambda_2} = \min(\lambda_1 T_1, \lambda_2 T_2)$.

Proof. For $t_1 t_2 > 0$ we have, simply,

$$S(t_1, t_2) = \mathrm{pr}(t_2 T_1 > t_1 t_2, t_1 T_2 > t_1 t_2) = \mathrm{pr}(T_{t_2, t_1} > t_1 t_2),$$

and the result for $t_1 = 0$ or $t_2 = 0$ follows by continuity.

Suppose now that we have data from Hougaard's (1986) positive stable bivariate frailty model with unit exponential marginals. The joint survivor function is

$$S(t_1, t_2) = \exp\{-(t_1^\phi + t_2^\phi)^\alpha\}, \tag{1}$$

where $0 < \alpha < 1$ and $\phi = 1/\alpha$. In this model Kendall's coefficient of concordance is $\tau = 1 - \alpha$, with $\alpha = 1$ corresponding to independence between T_1

and T_2 and $\alpha = 0$ to complete dependence, $T_1 = T_2$. See e.g. Oakes (1989). Note that (1) is less restrictive than it appears: by making the transformation $T_1' = -\log S_1(T_1)$ and $T_2' = -\log S_2(T_2)$ we can transform data from a bivariate distribution of the form

$$S(t_1, t_2) = \exp(-[\{-\log S_1(t_1)\}^\phi + \{-\log S_2(t_2)\}^\phi]^\alpha), \qquad (2)$$

which has arbitrary marginals $S_1(t_1) = \mathrm{pr}(T_1 > t_1)$ and $S_2(t_2) = \mathrm{pr}(T_2 > t_2)$, to data from (1).

Given data from (1), the parameter α can be estimated by maximum likelihood in the usual way. Oakes and Manatunga (1992) calculated the Fisher information matrix for the five-parameter model obtained by parameterizing the marginal survivor functions $S_1(t_1)$ and $S_2(t_2)$ in (2) as Weibull distributions. For the single parameter model (1), the unit Fisher information $I(\alpha)$ for α is

$$\phi^2 \left(-\frac{2}{3} + \frac{\pi^2}{9} \right) - \phi + 2\frac{K_0}{\phi} + \left\{ \phi^3 + \phi^2 + (K_0 - 1)\phi - 2K_0 + \frac{K_0}{\phi} \right\} E_1(\phi - 1)e^{\phi - 1}, \quad (3)$$

where $K_0 = (15 - \pi^2)/18$ and $E_1(\phi)$ is the exponential integral. A simpler estimate of α in (1) may be found by maximizing the likelihood from the $T_{1,1} = \min(T_1, T_2)$, which are exponential with parameter 2^α. The asymptotic variance of this estimator is just $(-\log 2)^2 = 2.0\tilde{8}1$ which is, of course, very much greater than the reciprocal of (3). In the present note we investigate how much closer we may get to this lower bound by appropriately combining the information from $T_{1,1}$ with that from $T_{1,\lambda}$ and $T_{\lambda,1}$.

2 Calculations

The distribution of $T_{\lambda,1}$ is exponential with parameter $\rho_\lambda = (1 + \lambda^\phi)^\alpha$. The maximum likelihood estimator $\hat{\alpha}_{\lambda,1}$ of α from the data on $T_{\lambda,1}$ is obtained by solving the equation $\rho_\lambda = n / \sum T_{\lambda,1}$. The asymptotic variance of $\hat{\alpha}_{\lambda,1}$ is

$$\lim_{n \to \infty} n\mathrm{var}(\hat{\alpha}_{\lambda,1}) = \left(\frac{\partial}{\partial \alpha} \log \rho_\lambda \right)^{-2}. \qquad (4)$$

We also have

$$\frac{\partial}{\partial \alpha} \log \rho_\lambda = \log(1 + \theta) - \frac{\theta}{\theta + 1} \log \theta = f(\theta),$$

say, where $\theta = \lambda^{-\phi}$. It is easily seen that $f(\theta) = f(1/\theta)$ and that $f(\theta)$ has a unique maximum at $\theta = 1$. It follows that the natural choice $\lambda = 1$ is optimal if only a single estimator $\hat{\alpha}_{\lambda,1}$ is to be used.

We now consider the possibility of combining the estimator $\hat{\alpha}_{1,1}$ with estimators $\hat{\alpha}_{\lambda,1}$ and $\hat{\alpha}_{1,\lambda}$. To calculate the covariances among $\hat{\alpha}_{1,1}$, $\hat{\alpha}_{1,\lambda}$ and $\hat{\alpha}_{\lambda,1}$ we may use the representation

$$T_1 = U^\alpha Z, \quad T_2 = (1 - U)^\alpha Z$$

of (T_1, T_2) in terms of independent random variables U, with a uniform distribution over $(0,1)$, and Z, with the mixed gamma density $f(z) = (1 - \alpha + \alpha z) \exp(-z)$. See for example, Lee (1979) and Oakes and Manatunga (1992). We have

$$T_{\lambda,1} = [\min\{\lambda U^\alpha, (1 - U)^\alpha\}]Z.$$

So

$$E(T_{\lambda,1} T_{1,1}) = E\{E(T_{\lambda,1} T_{1,1} | Z)\} =$$

$$E[\min\{\lambda U^\alpha, (1 - U)^\alpha\} \min\{U^\alpha, (1 - U)^\alpha\}]E(Z^2).$$

However $E(Z^2) = 2 + 4\alpha$ and the first integral can be expressed as a sum of incomplete beta integrals and calculated by univariate numerical integration. A similar expression holds for $E(T_{1,\lambda} T_{\lambda,1})$.

Writing

$$n\rho_{\lambda,1}^{-1} = \sum T_{\lambda,1},$$

it is clear that the asymptotic covariances between $\hat{\rho}_{\lambda,1}, \hat{\rho}_{1,\lambda}$ and $\hat{\rho}_{1,1}$ can be easily calculated. This yields the asymptotic covariances γ_1 between $\hat{\alpha}_{1,1}$ and $\hat{\alpha}_{1,\lambda}$ or $\hat{\alpha}_{\lambda,1}$, and γ_λ between $\hat{\alpha}_{\lambda,1}$ and $\hat{\alpha}_{1,\lambda}$. Finally, writing ν_1 and ν_λ for the asymptotic variances of $\hat{\alpha}_{1,1}$ and $\hat{\alpha}_{\lambda,1}$ respectively, the variance of the linear combination

$$(1 - c)\hat{\alpha}_{1,1} + \frac{c}{2}(\hat{\alpha}_{\lambda,1} + \hat{\alpha}_{1,\lambda}) \tag{5}$$

of the three estimators is

$$(1 - c)^2 \nu_1 + \frac{c^2}{2}\nu_\lambda + 2c(1 - c)\gamma_1 + \frac{c^2}{2}\gamma_\lambda.$$

The optimal choice of c (for a given λ) is

$$c = \frac{\nu_1 - \gamma_1}{\nu_1 + \frac{1}{2}\nu_\lambda - 2\gamma_1 + \frac{1}{2}\gamma_\lambda}.$$

3 Results

The table below compares the asymptotic variances of the maximum likelihood estimator, calculated from $I(\alpha)$, the simple estimator $\hat{\alpha}_{1,1}$ and of the optimal combination (5) of the three estimators, for varying choices of λ. Not shown is the asymptotic variance of the combination $(\alpha_{1,\lambda} + \alpha_{\lambda,1})/2$, which was found to exceed that of $\alpha_{1,1}$ for $\lambda \neq 1$.

α	$1/I(\alpha)$	ν_1	$\lambda = 2$	$\lambda = 5$	$\lambda = 10$	$\lambda = 100$
0.2	0.0278	2.081	0.065	0.054	0.054	0.054
0.3	0.062	2.081	0.199	0.124	0.119	0.118
0.4	0.109	2.081	0.476	0.239	0.212	0.204
0.5	0.165	2.081	0.907	0.422	0.345	0.310
0.6	0.228	2.081	1.385	0.694	0.530	0.435
0.7	0.291	2.081	1.758	1.050	0.782	0.581
0.8	0.341	2.081	1.973	1.438	1.095	0.753
0.9	0.354	2.081	2.063	1.771	1.438	0.951

The following conclusions may be drawn from this table. First, it appears that there is no finite optimum value of λ for any value of α. Across each row of the table, the variances appear to decrease to a non-zero limiting asymptote as $\lambda \to \infty$. Secondly, very substantial recovery of information is possible by combining the three estimators of α. This is most evident in the first row of the table, where the variance of the best combined estimator is only one fortieth that of the simple estimator, and is within a factor of two of the variance of the maximum likelihood estimator. Thirdly, the larger the value of α the larger the value of λ needed to provide useful efficiency gain by using the combined estimator over the simpler estimator.

4 Discussion

For bivariate data (T_1, T_2) subject to censoring by a bivariate censoring variable (C_1, C_2), the cumulative hazard functions for T_1 and T_2 can be estimated by the usual Nelson-Aalen procedure. The cumulative hazard function for the minimum $T_{1,1}$ can be estimated consistently from the data $X_{1,1} = \min(T_{1,1}, C_{1,1})$ and $\Delta_{1,1} = 1(T_{1,1} < C_{1,1})$, where $C_{1,1} = \min(C_1, C_2)$. Note that this may necessitate the discarding of some information if $C_1 \neq C_2$ a.s.

When $S_1(t) = S_2(t)$ in Hougaard's model (2), the ratio of the integrated hazard functions for $T_{1,1}$ and T_1 (or T_2) is just 2^α. In the context of developing a method for combining stratified and unstratified log-rank tests for bivariate censored data, Feng and Oakes (2002) used the corresponding sample ratios (evaluated at a series of specified values of t) as simple non-iterative estimators of α. Simulation studies suggested that these estimators worked well even with substantial censoring. The work reported here was motivated by an effort to improve this estimator. Note that the entire procedure may be applied to data from (2), even with $S_1(t) \neq S_2(t)$, after preliminary integrated hazard transformations aplied to the data on T_1 and, separately, to the data on T_2. The properties of this approach in this semiparametric context require further investigation. A referee has pointed out that with censored data we will in practice be restricted to the use of values of λ that are not too far from unity.

The approach to parameter estimation does depend heavily on the assumption of the positive stable frailty model (2). For other bivariate distributions the relationship between the integrated hazard functions for the marginal distributions and for the minimum will differ. Of course, Theorem 1 still applies.

Theorem 1 also shows how an estimator of a bivariate survivor function may be constructed from data subject to censoring in both components. To estimate $S(t_1, t_2)$ we may simply evaluate the univariate Kaplan -Meier estimator from the data on $T_{t_2, t_1} = \min(t_2 T_1, t_1 T_2)$ at $t = t_1 t_2$. This proposal may be new, although the estimator will be closely related to path-dependent estimators proposed by Campbell and Folges (1982) and others. It has the virtues of consistency and of possessing a simple variance estimate, but is unlikely to be as efficient as those for example of Dabrowska (1989) and Prentice and Cai (1992).

Finally, Theorem 1 sheds some light on the success of accelerated life formulations of covariate effects to resolve the identifiability problem in competing risks data, see Lin, Robins and Wei (1996).

Acknowledgements

I thank Changyong Feng for useful discussions. This work was supported in part of grant CA-52572 from the National Cancer Institute.

References

Campell, G. & Foldes, A. (1982). Large sample properties of nonparametric bivariate estimators with censored data. In *Nonparametric Statistical Inference*, Colloq. Math. Soc. Janos Bolyai 32, Ed. B.V. Gnedenko, M.L. Puri, and I. Vincze, pp 103-21. Amsterdam: North Holland.

Dabrowska, D, (1988). Kaplan-Meier estimate on the plane. *Ann. Statist.* **16**, 1475-89.

Feng, C. & Oakes, D. (2002). Combining Stratified and Unstratified Log-Rank Tests in Matched Pair Data. *Unpublished Manuscript.* (Student Travel Awardee, Biometric Society ENAR Meeting, Crystal City, March 2002).

Hougaard, P. (1986). A class of multivariate failure time distributions. *Biometrika* **73**, 671-8.

Lee, L. (1979). Multivariate distributions having Weibull properties. *J. Mult. Anal.* **9**, 267-77.

Lin, D. Y., Robins, J. M. & Wei, L. J. (1996). Comparing two failure time distributions in the presence of dependent censoring. *Biometrika* **83**, 381-93.

Oakes, D. (1989). Bivariate survival models induced by frailties. *J. Am. Statist. Assoc.* **93**, 487-93.

Oakes, D. & Manatunga, A. K. (1992). Fisher information for a bivariate extreme value distribution. *Biometrika* **79**, 827-32.

Prentice, R. L. & Cai, J. (1992). Covariance and survivor function estimation using censored multivariate failure time data. *Biometrika* **79**, 495-512. Correction (1993), **80**, 711-2.

Nonparametric Estimation of the Bivariate Survivor Function

Ross L. Prentice, Zoe Moodie and Jianrong Wu

Division of Public Health Sciences, Fred Hutchinson Cancer Research Center, Seattle, WA 98109-1024, USA and Department of Biostatistics, St. Jude Children's Research Hospital, Memphis, TN 38105 E-mail: rprentic@fhcrc.org, zmoodie@scharp.org, jianrong.wu@stjude.org

ABSTRACT   Nonparametric estimators of the bivariate survivor function have the potential to provide a basic tool for the display and comparison of survival curves, analogous to the Kaplan-Meier estimator for univariate failure time data. Available nonparametric estimators include estimators that plug empirical estimators of single and double failure hazard rates into survivor function representations, and versions of nonparametric maximum likelihood estimators (NPMLE) that address uniqueness problems. In this paper we consider candidate bivariate survivor function estimators that arise either from representations of the survivor function in terms of the marginal survivor functions and double failure hazard, or in terms of the double failure hazard only for a suitably truncated version of the data. The former class of estimators includes the Dabrowska (1988) and Prentice-Cai (1992) estimators, for which a marginal hazard-double failure hazard representation leads to suggestions for several new estimators. The estimators in this class tend to incorporate substantial negative mass, but corresponding proper estimators can be obtained by defining a restricted estimator that is either equal to the unrestricted estimator, or is as close as possible to the unrestricted estimator without violating non-negativity constraints. The second class of estimators includes an estimator arising from the simple empirical double failure hazard, as well more efficient estimators that redistribute singly censored observations within the strips of a partition of the risk region, following Van der Laan's (1996) repaired NPMLE, as well as related adaptive estimators. These and selected other estimators are compared in simulation studies, leading to a synthesis of available estimation techniques, and to suggestions for future research.

KEY WORDS: Bivariate hazard function; Bivariate survivor function; Nonparametric; Maximum likelihood; Peano series.

1 Introduction

The Kaplan-Meier (1958) survivor function estimator, and closely related Nelson-Aalen estimator of the cumulative hazard function, provide basic tools for the display and analysis of univariate censored failure time data. Their uses include a role in censored data rank tests to compare survival distributions, and in Cox (1972) regression and other regression generalizations. However, the identification of an estimator that can fulfill a corresponding role for paired failure times, or multivariate failure times more generally, has been a long standing, vexing statistical problem.

Convenient, efficient estimators of a bivariate survivor function would be of value in diverse application areas. These include, for example, the analysis of disease occurrence data among twins; the analysis of time to event data involving paired organs; study of the relationship of a treatment or intervention to two (or more) health outcomes jointly in a clinical trial; study of the strength of dependence between disease risk among pairs of family members in genetic epidemiology; and the analysis of group randomized clinical trials, or even multicenter clinical trials with individual randomization. In some of these settings the principal interest resides in the assessment of treatment or intervention effects in relation to failure time outcomes with dependencies between the failure times in a pair or cluster serving as nuisance parameters, the existence of which may affect the efficiency of treatment contrasts. In other settings, such as twin studies or genetic epidemiology studies, characterization of the nature of dependence between failure times in a pair may be a principal study goal.

There are other reasons for attempting to understand this estimation problem. One of these is the so-called auxiliary data problem. Specifically if interest resides in a particular failure time variate which may be heavily censored while there are available one or more correlated failure time variates with lesser censorship, one can ask whether it is possible to materially strengthen the analysis of data on the principal outcome by making use of the correlated outcome data. In a clinical trial, for example a primary prevention trial or a screening trial, there may be a designated primary failure time outcome which the intervention is hypothesized to affect favorably, but such outcome may occur only in a small fraction of the study cohort during trial follow-up. However, there may be more proximate and frequent outcomes that are correlated with the true outcome, and in some cases can even be thought of as precursors to the true outcome event. The biomedical research community places great hope in the utility of such biomarker precursors, but practical nonparametric methods for their use in 'true endpoint' analyses remain to be developed. Such methods will depend directly on nonparametric survivor function estimators and their implied marginal survivor function estimators.

It is not difficult to obtain strongly consistent nonparametric estimators of the bivariate survivor function. The earliest such estimators, due to Campbell and Földes (1982), used the factorization

$$p(T_1 > t_1, T_2 > t_2) = p(T_1 > t_1)p(T_2 > t_2 \mid T_1 > t_1), \qquad (1)$$

or the corresponding factorization reversing the roles of the failure time variates $T_1 > 0$ and $T_2 > 0$, and inserted Kaplan-Meier estimators for each factor. While easy to compute, these estimators do not have good efficiency properties. There are many other 'path-dependent' estimators that can be defined by writing the survival probability at (t_1, t_2) as a connected sequence of horizontal or vertical lines from $(0,0)$ to (t_1, t_2) and inserting empirical estimators for the conditional probabilities for each such line segment. But these estimators will have differing, and typically poor, efficiency properties. Such estimators will also tend to assign negative mass in the presence of censoring, a feature of many available bivariate survivor function estimators. Bickel et al (1993, pp. 289-292) provide a technical view of this estimation problem by noting that there are many nonparametric estimators that are asymptotically linear but not asymptotically equivalent, and hence that may have differing asymptotic efficiency properties.

A number of approaches have been considered in the search for bivariate survivor function estimators having desirable efficiency and other properties. These include an approach that plugs empirical estimators of the single and double failure hazard functions into survivor function representations; nonparametric maximum likelihood and related self-consistency approaches; inverse censoring probability weighted approaches; and, recently, a double failure hazard plug-in approach. Subsequent sections will review the status of estimators arising from these various approaches, and numerical comparisons among a number of them will be presented. We begin with a discussion of survivor function representations.

2 Survivor Function Representation

2.1 Univariate Survivor Function Representation and Estimation

The distribution of a univariate (continuous, discrete, or mixed) failure time $T > 0$ can be characterized by its survivor function $F(t) = p(T > t)$, or by its (cumulative) hazard function $\Lambda(t) = \int_0^t \Lambda(du)$ where, here and subsequently, Stieltjes integrals are used, and where $\Lambda(du) = -F(du)/F(u^-)$ is the hazard at time $T = u$. Writing $F(du) = -F(u^-)\Lambda(du)$ and integrating both sides of the equation from zero to t gives the Volterra integral equation

$$F(t) = 1 - \int_0^t F(u^-)\Lambda(du) \qquad (2)$$

linking the survivor and hazard functions. This Volterra equation has a unique solution that can be written in equivalent product integral or Peano series forms (Gill and Johansen, 1990) as

$$F(t) = \prod_{u \le t} \{1 - \Lambda(du)\} \tag{3}$$

$$= 1 + \sum_{n=1}^{\infty} \int_{0 < u_1 < u_2 < \cdots < u_n \le t} \prod_{\ell=1}^{n} \{-\Lambda(du_\ell)\} \tag{4}$$

Now consider survivor function estimation. An independent censoring assumption allows the survivor function to be identifiable within the support of the observed time $X = T \wedge C$ where C is a potential censoring time. Also let $\delta = [T = X]$ be the censoring indicator that takes value one if the observation is uncensored and value zero if censored, and let $G(t) = p(C > t)$. The reason for expressing F in terms of Λ is because Λ can be readily estimated in the presence of independent right censoring. Specifically the Nelson-Aalen estimator is given by

$$\hat{\Lambda}(t) = \int_0^t \hat{\Lambda}(du)$$

where the empirical estimator $\hat{\Lambda}(du)$ is ratio of the number of failures to the size of the risk set at time $T = u$. Inserting this estimator into the product integral representation (3) gives

$$\hat{F}(t) = \prod_{t_i \le t} \left(1 - \frac{d_i}{r_i}\right), \tag{5}$$

the familiar Kaplan-Meier estimator, where the ordered uncensored failure times have been denoted $t_1 < t_2 < \cdots < t_I$ where d_i is the number of failures at $T = t_i$ and where r_i is the number of study subjects at risk for failure just prior to time t_i; that is, at t_i^-. Note that the corresponding Peano series estimator formed by plugging $\hat{\Lambda}$ into (4) is obtained by expanding the product in (5). The Kaplan-Meier estimator is strongly consistent, it converges weakly to a Gaussian process with $n^{\frac{1}{2}}$ rate of convergence, and it is nonparametric efficient provided only that the estimation is restricted to a time period $[0, \tau]$ such that $F(\tau)G(\tau) > 0$ or equivalently to a time period such that $p(X > \tau) > 0$, and that F and G are continuous from the right with left hand limits (eg. Andersen et al, 1993). Specifically, the strong consistency and weak convergence properties of $\hat{\Lambda}$ can be derived using empirical process theory, and the corresponding properties for (5) follow from the continuous compact differentiability of the product integral transformation (3) or the Peano series transformation (4) using a functional delta argument.

The estimator (5) was originally developed using a nonparametric maximum likelihood NPML argument (Kaplan and Meier, 1958). The likelihood contribution from a pair (X, δ) is $F(X)$ if X is censored and $-F(dX) = F(X^-) - F(X)$ if X is uncensored. The likelihood is the product of these contributions over the n observations. It can be maximized by placing mass at the uncensored failures, as well as beyond the largest observed X value, if such value is censored. The partially maximized likelihood can hence be written

$$L = \prod_{i=0}^{I} \{F(t_i^-) - F(t_i)\}^{n_i^1} \; F(t_i)^{n_i^0}$$

where $n_i^1 = d_i$ is the number of uncensored failures at $T = t_i$, and n_i^0 is the number of censored times in $[t_i, t_{i+1}), i = 1, \cdots, I$ where $t_0 = 0$ and $t_{I+1} = \infty$. Maximizing L by rewriting it in terms of discrete hazards at each failure time, or by requiring the mass assignments $p_i = F(t_i^-) - F(t_i), i = 1, \ldots I$ and $p_{I+1} = F(t_I)$ to sum to unity, give the Kaplan-Meier estimator (5). Note that any mass $\hat{F}(t_I) > 0$ is to be placed beyond the largest censored observation, but its distribution is otherwise not defined by the NPML procedure.

A less familiar development of (5) builds on the fact that $H(t) = F(t)G(t)$ is the 'survivor' function for the observed $X = T \wedge C$ variate, so that H is readily nonparametrically estimated by the empirical estimator that assigns mass $1/n$ to each observation on X. Under the usual convention that failures precede censoring if the two are tied, this empirical estimator $\hat{H}$ gives expressions

$$\hat{F}(t) = 1 - \sum_{x_i \leq t} \frac{\hat{p}(C \geq x_i, T = x_i)}{\hat{p}(C \geq x_i)} = 1 - \frac{1}{n} \sum_{x_i \leq t} m_i^1 / \hat{G}(x_i^-)$$

$$\text{and } \hat{G}(t) = 1 - \sum_{x_i \leq t} \frac{\hat{p}(C = x_i, T > x_i)}{\hat{p}(T > x_i)} = 1 - \frac{1}{n} \sum_{x_i \leq t} m_i^0 / \hat{F}(x_i)$$

where $x_1 < x_2 < \cdots$ are the ordered observed X values. A simple inductive argument, starting with $G(x_1^-) = 1$ then yields

$$\hat{F}(t) = \prod_{x_i \leq t} \left(\frac{s_i - m_i^1}{s_i}\right) \text{ and } \hat{G}(t) = \prod_{x_i \leq t} \left(\frac{s_{i+1}}{s_i - m_i^1}\right)$$

where m_i^1 and m_i^0 are the numbers of uncensored and censored values equal to x_i and $s_i = n - \sum_{j<i}(m_j^1 + m_j^0)$ is the size of the risk set at x_i. Note that this estimator of F is identical to (5).

2.2 Bivariate Survivor Function Representation

The distribution of a pair of (continuous, discrete, or mixed) failure times $T_1 > 0, T_2 > 0$ can also be characterized by the survivor function $F(t_1, t_2) = p(T_1 > t_1, T_2 > t_2)$. Note that failure time variates that place mass along lines (e.g., along $T_1 = T_2$) that are not parallel to the coordinate axes are excluded from consideration. The natural hazard function corresponding to F, sometimes referred to as the double failure hazard function, can be written

$$\Lambda(t_1, t_2) = \int_0^{t_1} \int_0^{t_2} \Lambda(du_1, du_2)$$

where the hazard rate at (u_1, u_2) is given by $\Lambda(du_1, du_2) = F(du_1, du_2)/F(u_1^-, u_2^-)$. Integrating

$$\int_0^{t_1} \int_0^{t_2} F(du_1, du_2) = \int_0^{t_1} \int_0^{t_2} F(u_1^-, u_2^-) \Lambda(du_1, du_2)$$

gives the inhomogeneous Volterra integral equation

$$F(t_1, t_2) = F_1(t_1) + F_2(t_2) - 1 + \int_0^{t_1} \int_0^{t_2} F(u_1^-, u_2^-) \Lambda(du_1, du_2) \qquad (6)$$

which has been attributed to Peter Bickel (eg. Dabrowska, 1988), where $F_1(t_1) = F(t_1, 0)$ and $F_2(t_2) = F(0, t_2)$ are the marginal survivor functions. This expression shows that a survivor function F is determined by its marginal survivor (or hazard) functions, and its double failure hazard function. In fact, (6) has a unique Peano series solution (Gill and Johansen, 1990; Gill, Van der Laan and Wellner, 1995) that can be written

$$F(t_1, t_2) = \psi(t_1, t_2) + \int_0^{t_1} \int_0^{t_2} \psi(s_1^-, s_2^-) P\{(s, t]; \Lambda\} \Lambda(ds_1, ds_2) \qquad (7)$$

where the Peano series factor is given by

$$P\{(s, t]; \Lambda\} = 1 + \sum_{n=1}^{\infty} \int_{s < u_1 < \cdots < u_n \le t} \prod_{i=1}^{n} \Lambda(du_{1i}, du_{2i}),$$

where $s = (s_1, s_2) < u_i = (u_{1i}, u_{2i})$ implies $s_1 < u_{1i}$ and $s_2 < u_{2i}$, and $\psi(t_1, t_2) = F_1(t_1) + F_2(t_2) - 1$. It follows, for example, that if one begins with Kaplan-Meier estimators $\hat{F}_1$ and $\hat{F}_2$ of the marginal survivor functions that the problem of estimating F nonparametrically can be reduced to that of estimating Λ nonparametrically. Note, however, that a positive answer to the auxiliary data problem described above would require marginal survivor function estimators that differ from Kaplan-Meier estimators.

3 Plug-In Estimators of the Bivariate Survivor Function and Simulation Comparison

3.1 Existing Estimators as Peano Series Estimators

Because of independent censoring one observes $X_1 = T_1 \wedge C_1, X_2 = T_2 \wedge C_2$, $\delta_1 = [T_1 = X_1]$, and $\delta_2 = [T_2 = X_2]$ where C_1 and C_2, assumed to be independent of (T_1, T_2), are potential censoring times for T_1 and T_2 respectively. Let $G(t_1, t_2) = p(C_1 > t_1, C_2 > t_2)$ denote the censoring 'survivor' function. We assume that F and G are right continuous functions with left hand limits and wish to estimate F over a region $[0_1, \tau_1] \times [0_1, \tau_2]$ where $F(\tau_1, \tau_2)G(\tau_1, \tau_2) > 0$.

Denote by $t_{11}, t_{12}, \cdots, t_{1I}$ the ordered uncensored T_1 failures, and by $t_{21}, t_{22}, \cdots, t_{2J}$ the ordered uncensored T_2 failures from a sample of size n. At a point (t_{1i}, t_{2j}) in the grid formed by these uncensored values let r_{ij}, d_{ij}, d_{1ij} and d_{2ij} denote the size of the risk set, the number of double (T_1 and T_2) failures, the number of T_1 failures, and the number of T_2 failures, respectively. That is,

$$r_{ij} = \#\{X_{1\ell} \geq t_{1i}, X_{2\ell} \geq t_{2j}\}, \quad d_{ij} = \#\{X_{1\ell} = t_{1i}, X_{2\ell} = t_{2j}, \delta_{1\ell} = \delta_{2\ell} = 1\},$$
$$d_{1ij} = \#\{X_{1\ell} = t_{1i}, X_{2\ell} \geq t_{2j}, \delta_{1\ell} = 1\}, \text{ and}$$
$$d_{2ij} = \#\{X_{1\ell} \geq t_{1i}, X_{2\ell} = t_{2j}, \delta_{2\ell} = 1\}$$

as ℓ ranges from 1 to n over the n data points. Bickel's Volterra estimator of F arises by inserting Kaplan-Meier estimators $\hat{F}_1$ and $\hat{F}_2$ into (7), along with the empirical hazard estimator

$$\hat{\Lambda}_{11}(t_1, t_2) = \int_0^{t_1} \int_0^{t_2} \hat{\Lambda}_{11}(du_1, du_2)$$

where $\hat{\Lambda}_{11}(du_1, du_2)$ is zero except at failure time grid points (t_{1i}, t_{2j}) where $d_{ij} > 0$, when it takes value $\hat{\Lambda}_{11}(dt_{1i}, dt_{2j}) = d_{ij}/r_{ij}$. The resulting estimator of $\hat{F}$ is a step function defined at all points in the risk region. For any step function estimator of this type the mass assigned at a grid point (t_{1i}, t_{2j}) in the risk region can be written, using (6), as

$$\hat{F}(\Delta t_{1i}, \Delta t_{2j}) = \hat{F}(t_{1i}^-, t_{2j}^-) - \hat{F}(t_{1i}^-, t_{2j}) - \hat{F}(t_{1i}, t_{2j}^-) + \hat{F}(t_{1i}, t_{2j})$$
$$= \hat{F}(t_{1i}^-, t_{2j}^-)\hat{\Lambda}(\Delta t_{1i}, \Delta t_{2j})$$

giving the simple recursive calculation

$$\hat{F}(t_{1i}, t_{2j}) = \hat{F}(t_{1i}^-, t_{2j}) + \hat{F}(t_{1i}, t_{2j}^-) - \hat{F}(t_{1i}^-, t_{2j}^-)\{1 - \hat{\Lambda}(\Delta t_{1i}, \Delta t_{2j})\}.$$

The Volterra estimator defined by $\{\hat{F}_1, \hat{F}_2, \hat{\Lambda}_{11}\}$ has been shown (Gill et al, 1995) to be strongly consistent, weakly convergent to a Gaussian process, and to support bootstrap procedures. However, unlike certain other plug-in estimators (Dabrowska, 1988; Prentice and Cai, 1992) this estimator is not nonparametric efficient under the complete independence of T_1, T_2, C_1 and C_2. In fact, Gill et al (1995) summarize its asymptotic efficiency properties by stating that the Volterra estimator is 'much inferior' to these other estimators.

The plug-in estimators of Dabrowska and Prentice-Cai rely on representations other than (7) for F, and also bring in empirical estimates of the single failure hazard functions Λ_1 and Λ_2 defined by

$$\Lambda_1(t_1, t_2) = \int_0^{t_1} \Lambda_1(du_1, t_2) \text{ and } \Lambda_2(t_1, t_2) = \int_0^{t_2} \Lambda_2(t_1, du_2)$$

where

$$\Lambda_1(du_1, u_2^-) = -F(du_1, u_2^-)/F(u_1^-, u_2^-)$$

and

$$\Lambda_2(u_1^-, du_2) = -F(u_1^-, du_2)/F(u_1^-, u_2^-).$$

These empirical estimators $\hat{\Lambda}_1$ and $\hat{\Lambda}_2$ are step functions determined by values

$$\hat{\Lambda}_1(\Delta t_{1i}, t_{2j}^-) = d_{1ij}/r_{ij} \text{ and } \hat{\Lambda}_2(t_{1i}^-, \Delta t_{2j}) = d_{2ij}/r_{ij}$$

at failure time grid points in the risk region. The Dabrowska (1988) estimator arises from Kaplan-Meier margins and plugging the empirical estimators $\{\hat{\Lambda}_{11}, \hat{\Lambda}_1, \hat{\Lambda}_2\}$ into a product integral representation for the ratio $F(t_1, t_2)/\{F_1(t_1)F_2(t_2)\}$. It is a step function that takes value

$$\hat{F}(t_{1i}, t_{2j}) = \hat{F}_1(t_{1i})\hat{F}_2(t_{2j})$$
$$\times \prod_{\substack{t_{1\ell} \le t_{1i} \\ t_{2m} \le t_{2j}}} \left[1 + \frac{\hat{\Lambda}_{11}(\Delta t_{1\ell}, \Delta t_{2m}) - \hat{\Lambda}_1(\Delta t_{1\ell}, t_{2m}^-)\hat{\Lambda}_2(t_{1\ell}^-, \Delta t_{2m})}{\{1 - \hat{\Lambda}_1(\Delta t_{1\ell}, t_{2m}^-)\}\{1 - \hat{\Lambda}_2(t_{1\ell}^-, \Delta t_{2m})\}}\right] \quad (8)$$

at each failure time grid point (t_{1i}, t_{2j}) in the risk region.

The Prentice-Cai (1992) estimator involves plugging these same empirical hazards into a Peano series representation of the ratio of F to the product of its margins. It can be written

$$\hat{F}(t_{1i}, t_{2j}) = \hat{F}_1(t_{1i})\hat{F}_2(t_{2j})$$
$$\times \left[1 + \sum_{n=1}^{i \wedge j} \sum_{t_{1\ell_1} < \cdots < t_{1\ell_n} \le t_{1i}} \sum_{t_{2m_1} < \cdots < t_{2m_n} \le t_{2j}} \prod_{s=1}^{n} \hat{B}(\Delta t_{1\ell_s}, \Delta t_{2m_s})\right], \quad (9)$$

where

$$\hat{B}(\Delta t_{1\ell}, \Delta t_{2m})$$
$$= \{\{1 - \hat{\Lambda}_1(\Delta t_{1\ell}, t_{2m}^-)\}\{1 - \hat{\Lambda}_2(t_{1\ell}^-, \Delta t_{2m})\}\}^{-1} \{\hat{\Lambda}_{11}(\Delta t_{1\ell}, \Delta t_{2m})$$
$$- \hat{\Lambda}_1(\Delta t_{1\ell}, t_{2m}^-)\hat{\Lambda}_2(0, \Delta t_{2m}) - \hat{\Lambda}_1(\Delta t_{1\ell}, 0)\hat{\Lambda}_2(t_{1\ell}^-, \Delta t_{2m})$$
$$+ \hat{\Lambda}_1(\Delta t_{1\ell}, 0)\hat{\Lambda}_2(0, \Delta t_{2m})\}$$

It is interesting to consider the relationship between (8), (9) and the Volterra estimator that arises by inserting $\{\hat{F}_1, \hat{F}_2, \hat{\Lambda}_{11}\}$ into (7). All three are based on representations that hold universally, so that each estimator could be recast in the form of the other estimators. Specifically, since each uses Kaplan-Meier margins it is possible to rewrite (8) and (9) as a plug-in estimator of the form (7) with a suitable choice of estimator of the hazard function Λ. In order to do so define

$$\hat{L}_1(t_1, t_2) = \int_0^{t_1} \hat{L}_1(\Delta u_1, t_2) \text{ and } \hat{L}_2(t_1, t_2) = \int_0^{t_2} \hat{L}_2(t_1, \Delta t_2)$$

where $\hat{L}_1(\Delta t_{1i}, t_{2j}^-) = -\hat{F}(\Delta t_{1i}, t_{2j}^-)/\hat{F}(t_{1i}^-, t_{2j}^-)$
and $\hat{L}_2(t_{1i}^-, \Delta t_{2j}) = -\hat{F}(t_{1i}^-, \Delta t_{2j})/\hat{F}(t_{1i}^-, t_{2j}^-)$
at grid points in the risk region, and zero otherwise. Beginning with the Kaplan-Meier marginal mass assignments note that $\hat{L}_1(\Delta t_{1i}, t_{2j}^-)$ is the mass that remains to be assigned along $T_1 = t_{1i}$ at or beyond (t_{1i}, t_{2j}) expressed as a fraction of the total mass $\hat{F}(t_{1i}^-, t_{2j}^-)$ that remains to be assigned at (t_{1i}, t_{2j}), while $\hat{L}_2(t_{1i}^-, \Delta t_{2j})$ has a similar interpretation along $T_2 = t_{2j}$. In comparison the corresponding empirical hazard rates $\hat{\Lambda}_1(\Delta t_{1i}, t_{2j}^-)$ and $\hat{\Lambda}_2(t_{1i}^-, \Delta t_{2j})$ do not acknowledge the Kaplan-Meier marginal mass assignments, nor the mass assignments at earlier times along $T_1 = t_{1i}$ or $T_2 = t_{2j}$.

Following a little algebra, the Dabrowska estimator (8) mass assignments can be written

$$\hat{F}(\Delta t_{1i}, \Delta t_{2j}) = \hat{F}(t_{1i}^-, t_{2j}^-)\left[\hat{L}_1(\Delta t_{1i}, t_{2j}^-)\hat{L}_2(t_{1i}^-, \Delta t_{2j})\right.$$

$$+ \frac{\{1 - \hat{L}_1(\Delta t_{1i}, t_{2j}^-)\}\{1 - \hat{L}_2(t_{1i}^-, \Delta t_{2j})\}}{\{1 - \hat{\Lambda}_1(\Delta t_{1i}, t_{2j}^-)\}\{1 - \hat{\Lambda}_2(t_{1i}^-, \Delta t_{2j})\}}$$

$$\left. \times \{\hat{\Lambda}_{11}(\Delta t_{1i}, \Delta t_{2j}) - \hat{\Lambda}_1(\Delta t_{1i}, t_{2j}^-)\hat{\Lambda}_2(t_{1i}^-, \Delta t_{2j})\}\right]. \quad (10)$$

Hence if this estimator were viewed as a plug-in estimator from (7) the implied hazard rate estimator $\hat{\Lambda}(\Delta t_{1i}, \Delta t_{2j})$ would equal the term in square brackets; that is, $\hat{F}(\Delta t_{1i}, \Delta t_{2j})/\hat{F}(t_{1i}^-, t_{2j}^-)$, from (10). This hazard rate estimator can be viewed as starting with a local independence specification to which an adjustment is made if there is evidence, based on the value of $\hat{\Lambda}_{11}(\Delta t_{1i}, \Delta t_{2j}) - \hat{\Lambda}_1(\Delta t_{1i}, t_{2j}^-)\hat{\Lambda}_2(t_{1i}^-, \Delta t_{2j})$, of departure from local independence.

Similarly from (9), noting that $\hat{L}_1(\Delta t_{1i}, 0) = \hat{\Lambda}_1(\Delta t_{1i}, 0)$ and $\hat{L}_2(0, \Delta t_{2j}) = \hat{\Lambda}_2(0, \Delta t_{2j})$, one can write

$$\hat{F}(\Delta t_{1i}, \Delta t_{2j}) = \hat{F}(t_{1i}^-, t_{2j}^-)$$

$$\times \left[\hat{\Lambda}_{11}(\Delta t_{1i}, \Delta t_{2j}) + \hat{L}_1(\Delta t_{1i}, 0)\{\hat{L}_2(t_{1i}^-, \Delta t_{2j}) - \hat{\Lambda}_2(t_{1i}^-, \Delta t_{2j})\}\right.$$

$$\left. + \hat{L}_2(0, \Delta t_{2j})\{\hat{L}_1(\Delta t_{1i}, t_{2j}^-) - \hat{\Lambda}_1(\Delta t_{1i}, t_{2j}^-)\}\right] \qquad (11)$$

so that the Prentice-Cai estimator (9) can be viewed as a Peano series estimator for F in which $\hat{F}_1$ and $\hat{F}_2$ are inserted along with an estimator of Λ that adjusts the empirical estimator $\hat{\Lambda}_{11}$ according to whether the remaining mass to be assigned along $T_1 = t_{1i}$ differs from its corresponding empirical quantity and according to whether the remaining mass along $T_2 = t_{2j}$ differs from its empirical quantity.

It is interesting to note that if $\hat{\Lambda}_1(\Delta t_{1i}, t_{2j}^-)$ and $\hat{\Lambda}_2(t_{1i}^-, \Delta t_{2j})$ were replaced by the single failure hazards that acknowledge the preceding mass assignments, then both (10) and (11) would reduce to

$$\hat{F}(\Delta t_{1i}, \Delta t_{2j})/\hat{F}(t_{1i}^-, t_{2j}^-) = \hat{\Lambda}_{11}(\Delta t_{1i}, \Delta t_{2j}),$$

and the corresponding survivor function estimators would reduce to the Volterra estimator with its comparably poor efficiency properties. In fact, if $\hat{L}_1$, and $\hat{L}_2$ are used to define single failure hazard rates the three estimators will always be identical if a common estimator of the double failure hazard is used. The better efficiency properties of (8) and (9) versus Bickel's Volterra estimator point to the value of using a hazard estimator $\hat{\Lambda}$ that releases mass at a grid point (t_{1i}, t_{2j}) not only based on the empirical hazard d_{ij}/r_{ij}, but also on the basis of an excess of residual mass along $T_1 = t_{1i}$ or $T_2 = t_{2j}$ or both, at or beyond (t_{1i}, t_{2j}). The empirical estimator $\hat{\Lambda}_{11}$ is a rather poor choice of hazard rate estimators in that it pays no attention to the marginal or earlier mass assignments. As a result, for example, if there are no failures along a given row or column in the failure time grid the entire Kaplan-Meier marginal mass must be pushed out beyond the risk region. To compensate relatively large amounts of mass must be assigned (by $\hat{\Lambda}_{11}$) at the (double) failures within the risk region, typically requiring substantial negative mass beyond the risk region along the rows or columns through the uncensored failures. This poor correspondence between $\hat{\Lambda}_{11}$ as an estimator of Λ and the Kaplan-Meier estimators $\hat{F}_1$ and $\hat{F}_2$ provides an explanation for the relatively poor efficiency properties of the Bickel Volterra estimator. In comparison, the Dabrowska and Prentice-Cai estimators acknowledge $\hat{F}_1$ and $\hat{F}_2$ by estimating Λ via (10) and (11) in a manner that achieves nonparametric efficiency under complete independence. These estimators are also strongly consistent, converge weakly to Gaussian processes, and support bootstrap procedures (Dabrowska, 1988, 1989; Prentice and Cai, 1992; Gill et al, 1995). However, these estimators also incorporate negative mass and are not fully efficient away from complete independence. Hence there is reason to seek estimators that are better in these respects. Before suggesting some potential new plug-in estimators we will give some simulation results to illustrate the difference between the estimators thus far mentioned in respect to negative mass assignment and moderate sample size estimation efficiency.

Failure times (T_1, T_2) were generated under both an independence model $F(t_1, t_2) = F_1(t_1) F_2(t_2)$, and Clayton's (1978) model

$$F(t_1, t_2) = \{F_1(t_1)^{-\theta} + F_2(t_2)^{-\theta} - 1\}^{-\theta^{-1}},$$

with $\theta = 4$ implying a fairly strong positive dependence between T_1 and T_2. In either case the marginal distributions were unit exponential and the censoring variables C_1 and C_2 were independent and exponentially distributed with expectation 0.5, so that there is a two-thirds probability of censoring for each of T_1 and T_2. Sample sizes $n = 30, 60$ and 120 were considered with 500 simulation runs at each configuration.

Table 1 shows sample means and sample standard deviations for the Campbell-Földes estimator $\hat{F}_{CF}$ based on (1), the Bickel estimator $\hat{F}_B$ based on inserting $\hat{F}_1, \hat{F}_2$ and $\hat{\Lambda}_{11}$ into (7), the Dabrowska estimator $\hat{F}_D$ given by (8) and the Prentice-Cai estimator $\hat{F}_{PC}$ given by (9). Since Kaplan-Meier marginal survivor functions are used by all estimators summary statistics are given at values (70,70), (70,55) and (55,55) for (percent T_1 survival, percent T_2 survival) that are away from the margins but not so far into the tails to yield an unacceptable number of empty risk sets. Table 1 also shows the average amount of negative mass assigned by each estimator, both within the failure time risk region (m_I) and along half lines beyond the risk region (m_0).

An impressive feature from Table 1 is the apparent near unbiasedness of all four estimators, even at sample size $n = 30$, where there are but 10 expected failures for each of T_1 and T_2. Also from the sample standard deviations one can see that the relative efficiency of the four estimators is similar under the independence and Clayton models, with the Prentice-Cai estimator having the smallest sample standard deviation and the Campbell-Földes estimator the largest sample standard deviation in each configuration. For example compared to the Prentice-Cai estimator the Campbell-Földes estimator has estimated efficiency of about 40% at $n = 30$ and about 55% at $n = 120$, at percentiles (55,55) for (T_1, T_2). The Bickel and Dabrowska estimators have intermediate sample standard deviations, with those for the Bickel estimator being slightly the smaller at $n = 30$, and those for the Dabrowska estimator being smaller and very similar to the Prentice-Cai sample standard deviations at $n = 120$. Compared to the Prentice-Cai estimator the Bickel estimator has an estimated efficiency of about 65-70% under both sample configurations and each sample size at (T_1, T_2) percentiles of (55,55). As noted previously the Dabrowska and Prentice-Cai estimators are known to be nonparametric efficient under the independence configuration of Table 1. Indeed their performances are nearly identical by $n = 120$. The somewhat larger sample standard deviations for the Dabrowska as compared to the Prentice-Cai estimator at small sample sizes (eg. $n = 30$) may reflect some small sample noise in the Dabrowska mass assignment procedure (10).

Note also from Table 1 that all four estimators assign substantial negative mass, and that the average total negative mass assigned evidently does not decrease as sample size increases, as was previously noted by Pruitt (1991) for the Dabrowska estimator. The sample standard deviations in Table 1 at each sample size tend to vary inversely with the amount of negative mass $(m_I + m_0)$ assigned by the estimator. Hence a modification that eliminates negative mass may be helpful in the identification of a survivor function estimator having good efficiency.

3.2 Some Candidate Plug-In Bivariate Survivor Function Estimators

The perspective that differences between $\hat{L}_1$ and $\hat{\Lambda}_1$, and between $\hat{L}_2$ and $\hat{\Lambda}_2$, should be acknowledged in specifying a hazard function estimator, and the strongly consistent specifications (10) and (11) as examples, provide a context for defining new candidate hazard function estimators $\hat{\Lambda}$. Such estimators, in conjunction with Kaplan-Meier margins, then give new Peano-series survivor function estimators $\hat{F}$ using (7). Note, however, that consistency or other asymptotic properties have not been established for the candidate survivor function estimators introduced in this section.

One may hypothesize that the ratio in the Dabrowska mass assignments (10) is a noise factor that contributes to the excess variance at small sample sizes noted in Table 1. If this ratio is replaced by unity one obtains a Dabrowska-like estimator $\hat{F}_{D1}$ that arises from a hazard rate estimator

$$\hat{\Lambda}_{D1}(\Delta t_{1i}, \Delta t_{2j}) = \hat{\Lambda}_{11}(\Delta t_{1i}, \Delta t_{2j}) + \hat{L}_1(\Delta t_{1i}, t_{2j}^-)\hat{L}_2(t_{1i}^-, \Delta t_{2j})$$
$$- \hat{\Lambda}_1(\Delta t_{1i}, t_{2j}^-)\hat{\Lambda}_2(t_{1i}^-, \Delta t_{2j}). \tag{12}$$

A modification of (12) would use a hazard rate at grid point (t_{1i}, t_{2j}) that augments the empirical hazard $\hat{\Lambda}_{11}(\Delta t_{1i}, \Delta t_{2j}) = d_{ij}/r_{ij}$ according to (12) but with $\hat{L}_1(\Delta t_{1i}, t_{2j}^-)$ replaced by $\hat{L}_1(\Delta t_{1i}, t_{2j}^-) - \hat{\Lambda}_{11}(\Delta t_{1i}, \Delta t_{2j})$ the residual T_1 hazard along $T_1 = t_{1i}$ beyond t_{2j}, and similarly with each of $\hat{L}_2(t_{1i}^-, \Delta t_{2j}), \hat{\Lambda}_1(\Delta t_{1i}, t_{2j}^-)$ and $\hat{\Lambda}_2(t_{1i}^-, \Delta t_{2j})$ shifted by $\hat{\Lambda}_{11}(\Delta t_{1i}, \Delta t_{2j})$ to acknowledge the empirical (double) hazard at (t_{1i}, t_{2j}). This modification would give a Dabrowska-like survivor function estimator $\hat{F}_{D2}$ that arises using (7) and a hazard rate estimator

$$\hat{\Lambda}_{D2}(\Delta t_{1i}, \Delta t_{2j}) = \hat{\Lambda}_{11}(\Delta t_{1i}, \Delta t_{2j})\{1 - \hat{L}_1(\Delta t_{1i}, t_{2j}^-) - \hat{L}_2(t_{1i}^-, \Delta t_{2j})$$
$$+ \hat{\Lambda}_1(\Delta t_{1i}, t_{2j}^-) + \hat{\Lambda}_2(t_{1i}^-, \Delta t_{2j})\} + \hat{L}_1(\Delta t_{1i}, t_{2j}^-)\hat{L}_2(t_{1i}^-, \Delta t_{2j})$$
$$- \hat{\Lambda}_1(\Delta t_{1i}, t_{2j}^-)\hat{\Lambda}_2(t_{1i}^-, \Delta t_{2j}). \tag{13}$$

The term in curly brackets in (13) can be viewed as a first order approximation to the ratio in (10). As such one may expect $\hat{F}_{D2}$ to have properties closer to those of the Dabrowska estimator $\hat{F}_D$, than does $\hat{F}_{D1}$.

The Prentice-Cai mass assignment procedure (11) can also be used to suggest some new candidate hazard estimators and Peano series survivor function estimators. For example, it seems natural to consider weighting the differences between residual and empirical single failure hazards at (t_{1i}, t_{2j}) not by the respective Kaplan-Meier hazards $\hat{L}_1(\Delta t_{1i}, 0)$ and $\hat{L}_2(0, \Delta t_{2j})$, but rather by the 'current' hazards $\hat{L}_1(\Delta t_{1i}, t_{2j}^-)$ and $\hat{L}_2(t_{1i}^-, \Delta t_{2j})$, giving a Prentice-Cai like estimator $\hat{F}_{PC1}$ using (7) and hazard rate estimator

$$\hat{\Lambda}_{PC1}(\Delta t_{1i}, \Delta t_{2j}) = \hat{\Lambda}_{11}(\Delta t_{1i}, \Delta t_{2j})$$
$$+ \hat{L}_2(t_{1i}^-, \Delta t_{2j})\{\hat{L}_1(\Delta t_{1i}, t_{2j}^-) - \hat{\Lambda}_1(\Delta t_{1i}, t_{2j}^-)\}$$
$$+ \hat{L}_1(\Delta t_{1i}, t_{2j}^-)\{\hat{L}_2(t_{1i}^-, \Delta t_{2j}) - \hat{\Lambda}_2(t_{1i}^-, \Delta t_{2j})\} \quad (14)$$

Alternatively, along the lines of (13), one could use as weights the residual single failure hazard rate estimators beyond (t_{1i}, t_{2j}) giving $\hat{F}_{PC2}$ based on (7) and the hazard rate estimator

$$\hat{\Lambda}_{PC2}(\Delta t_{1i}, \Delta t_{2j}) = \hat{\Lambda}_{11}(\Delta t_{1i}, \Delta t_{2j})\{1 - \hat{L}_1(\Delta t_{1i}, t_{2j}^-) - \hat{L}_2(t_{1i}^-, \Delta t_{2j})$$
$$+ \hat{\Lambda}_1(\Delta t_{1i}, t_{2j}^-) + \hat{\Lambda}_2(t_{1i}^-, \Delta t_{2j})\}$$
$$+ \hat{L}_2(t_{1i}^-, \Delta t_{2j})\{\hat{L}_1(\Delta t_{1i}, t_{2j}^-) - \hat{\Lambda}_1(\Delta t_{1i}, t_{2j}^-)\}$$
$$+ \hat{L}_1(\Delta t_{1i}, t_{2j}^-)\{\hat{L}_2(t_{1i}^-, \Delta t_{2j}) - \hat{\Lambda}_2(t_{1i}^-, \Delta t_{2j})\} \quad (15)$$

Table 2 presents simulation summary statistics for these four new estimators, using the same samples that were used to produce Table 1. Summary statistics for the Dabrowska and Prentice-Cai estimators, $\hat{F}_D$ and $\hat{F}_{PC}$, are repeated from Table 1 to facilitate comparisons. One can see that the Dabrowska-like estimators $\hat{F}_{D1}$ and $\hat{F}_{D2}$ have apparently reduced the small sample variance compared to the Dabrowska estimator and have sample standard deviations very similar to those for the Prentice-Cai estimator. Also, both estimators $\hat{F}_{D1}$ and $\hat{F}_{PC1}$ tend to be biased upward, indicating excessive mass assignments within the risk region, under both the independence and Clayton model configurations, at small sample sizes. This upward bias appears to be essentially absent for the $\hat{F}_{D2}$ and $\hat{F}_{PC2}$ estimators supporting the value of the adjustment factor (in curly brackets) in (13) and (15). These simulations point to $\hat{F}_{PC}, \hat{F}_{D2}$ and $\hat{F}_{PC2}$ as candidate survivor function estimators of good small sample behavior. In fact there is little to distinguish these estimators based on Table 2.

4 Nonparametric Maximum Likelihood and Related Estimators

4.1 Previous and Ongoing Developments

There is a considerable literature on the generalization of nonparametric maximum likelihood and related self-consistency (Efron, 1967) approaches from univariate to bivariate survivor function estimation. The contribution to the likelihood for F corresponding to an observation $(X_1, \delta_1), (X_2, \delta_2)$ can be written

$$F(dX_1, dX_2)^{\delta_1\delta_2}\{-F(dX_1, X_2)\}^{\delta_1(1-\delta_2)}\{-F(X_1, dX_2)\}^{(1-\delta_1)\delta_2}$$
$$\times F(X_1, X_2)^{(1-\delta_1)(1-\delta_2)}$$

and the overall likelihood is the product of such terms over n pairs of failure time data. This likelihood can be maximized by placing all mass at (uncensored data) grid points in the failure time risk region or along grid half lines beyond the risk region with the possibility of some additional mass within the intersection of the quadrant formed by the doubly censored observations. The resulting partially maximized likelihood function can be written

$$L = \prod_{i=0}^{I}\prod_{j=0}^{J}\left\{ p_{ij}^{n_{ij}^{11}}\,(p_{i\cdot} - \sum_{m=0}^{j}p_{im})^{n_{ij}^{10}}(p_{\cdot j} - \sum_{\ell=0}^{i}p_{\ell j})^{n_{ij}^{01}}(1 - \sum_{\ell=0}^{i}p_{\ell\cdot} - \sum_{m=0}^{j}p_{\cdot m}\right.$$
$$\left. + \sum_{\ell=0}^{i}\sum_{m=0}^{j}p_{\ell m})^{n_{ij}^{00}}\right\}, \tag{16}$$

where $n_{ij}^{v_1 v_2} = \#\{X_1 = t_{1i}, X_2 = t_{2j}, \delta_1 = v_1, \delta_2 = v_2\}$ for $v_1\varepsilon\{0,1\}$ and $v_2\varepsilon\{0,1\}$ following a left or downward shifting of the censored X-values to their nearest uncensored X-value, and where $t_{10} = t_{20} = 0$. Also $p_{ij} = F(\Delta t_{1i}, \Delta t_{2j})$ is the mass assignment at (t_{1i}, t_{2j}) in the risk region, and $p_{i\cdot} = -F(\Delta t_{1i}, 0)$ and $p_{\cdot j} = -F(0, \Delta t_{2j})$ are the marginal mass assignments along $T_1 = t_{1i}$ and $T_2 = t_{2j}$ respectively. Campbell (1981) showed that L is convex in its parameters, but that there may be likelihood flat spots, in which case a unique NPMLE will not be available. This uniqueness problem is most easily illustrated in the special case in which T_1, but not T_2, is subject to censoring, so that $n_{ij}^{10} \equiv n_{ij}^{00} \equiv 0$, and in which failure times are absolutely continuous. In this special case maximization of the (multinomial) likelihood (16) gives a mass assignment of $1/n$ to each uncensored observation ($n_{ij}^{11} = 1$) and to the half line formed by each singly censored observation ($n_{ij}^{01} = 1$) but does not otherwise determine an estimator of F. Note that this lack of uniqueness of the NPMLE typically extends well inside the failure time risk region and, hence, is qualitatively more problematic than that attending the univariate NPMLE. The bivariate nonparametric likelihood L suffers from involving more parameters than the data can distinguish using standard likelihood methods (Robins and Ritov, 1997). Bivariate censoring tends to ease the uniqueness problems as there is then a preference for placing mass not only at the uncensored failures, but also at the points of intersection of singly censored rays in opposing directions, or on the intersections of singly censored rays with quadrants formed by doubly censored observations. However, multiple thorny uniqueness problems persist even if there is substantial censoring on both T_1 and T_2, and (16) can be very difficult to maximize numerically. For example the mass assignments at the intersection points of the singly censored rays may be mutually very highly dependent and the identification of the subset of those points to receive zero mass may be a very delicate matter (eg. Prentice, 1999). Gentleman and Vandal (2001) have done some nice work using graph theoretic representation of the data to identify the sets for which an NPML procedure determines a unique estimator, and to calculate the corresponding mass assignments.

There are at least two reasons to try to repair the NPML estimators. First, it may be possible to identify estimators that improve on the efficiency and negative mass aspects of the above plug-in estimators. Secondly, these estimators, all use Kaplan-Meier margins, and hence do not allow one to address the auxiliary data problem. Toward a viable NPMLE-like development one can reduce the number of parameters by imposing smoothing conditions, or by reducing the data somewhat through imposing additional censorship. For example, Tsai, Leurgans and Crowley (1986) add survivor function smoothness assumptions leading to a survivor function estimator that involves a kernel density estimator. R.C. Pruitt in an unpublished 1991 Dept. of Statistics, University of Minnesota Technical Report (#543) proposed an estimator, also involving kernel estimation, which solves an approximation to self-consistency equations. These estimators require bandwidth specification in addition to smoothness assumptions, and their moderate sample size performance is evidently not particularly good. For example, M.J. Van der Laan, in a 1996, CWI, Amsterdam Technical Report proves strong consistency and $n^{1/2}$ convergence to a Gaussian distribution for Pruitt's estimator, but he notes that this estimator is not asymptotically efficient and that its moderate sample performance is often not as good as that of the Dabrowska or Prentice-Cai estimators.

Van der Laan (1996), in an important paper, considered a modified NPML procedure in which one imposes additional censorship and interval censors each of T_1 and T_2 according to fixed partitions of $[0, \tau_1]$ and $[0, \tau_2]$, with (τ_1, τ_2) in the support of the distribution of (X_1, X_2). The resulting modified NPML estimator was shown to be asymptotically unique, consistent and convergent at a $n^{1/2}$ rate to a Gaussian process. Moreover, if the partition bandwidth was allowed to go to zero slowly enough the estimator was also shown to be nonparametric efficient. In particular, Van der Laan's work also shows the potential to improve upon Kaplan-Meier marginal survivor functions. For example, if T_1 and T_2 are very strongly dependent, and T_1 but not

T_2 is subject to censoring, then the nonparametric efficient lower bound for estimating F, and hence for the marginal survivor function F_1, is essentially that for the underlying uncensored data. Note, however, that Van der Laan's method involves some data reduction, the specification of partitions, and an iterative calculation via the E-M algorithm. In simulation studies (Van der Laan, 1997) the repaired NPMLE showed moderate sample size performance that tended to be better than the Dabrowska and Prentice-Cai estimators near the margins, but not in the tail of the distribution, and then only away from the complete independence special case where these other estimators are also nonparametric efficient.

4.2 Some Additional Approaches to NPML Estimation

Certain alternative modifications of a NPML procedure were entertained with a view toward simple computations and desirable moderate sample size properties. These involve the maximization of a sequence of likelihoods over the uncensored data grid points in the failure time region with additional common censoring imposed at each grid point in turn. This sequential imposition of additional censoring allows the mass assignments to be considered individually giving a straightforward, though iterative, approach to calculation. These approaches additionally involve the specification of Kaplan-Meier margins. These efforts have not lead to 'estimators' with better small sample performance than the best of the plug-in estimators of earlier sections, and hence their presentation will be brief. Note also that asymptotic properties have not been developed for these NPML candidates.

First suppose that a survivor function estimator is developed by scanning over the grid points in the risk region such that a point (t_{1i}, t_{2j}) is considered only after the preceding points $(t_{1,i-1}, t_{2j})$ and $(t_{1i}, t_{2,j-1})$ have been considered. For example one could scan across rows from the bottom (or columns from the left) in the risk region. The calculations at (t_{1i}, t_{2j}) involves maximizing a likelihood of the form (16) with common additional censoring at (t_{1i}, t_{2j}) with all mass assignments $p_{\ell m}$, for $\ell \leq i$ and $m \leq j$, $(\ell, m) \neq (i, j)$ fixed by the earlier maximizations. Beginning with Kaplan-Meier margins this sequential NPML procedure involves maximizing the likelihood for a 2×2 table at each grid point (t_{1i}, t_{2j}). The 2×2 table is determined by the numbers of pairs where T_1 equals or exceeds t_{1i}, and T_2 equals or exceeds t_{2j}, from among the r_{ij} pairs at risk. The marginal cell probabilities for this table are determined by the Kaplan-Meier marginal mass assignments, and by the mass assignments at earlier grid points, as for $\hat{L}_1(\Delta t_{1i}, t_{2j}^-)$ and $\hat{L}_2(t_{1i}^-, \Delta t_{2j})$ in the preceeding sections. Given that the cell probabilities add to one, this likelihood involves the single parameter p_{ij}, constrained so that all cell probabilities in the table are non-negative. The resulting NPML-like estimator is readily calculated. However, simulation studies of the type leading to Table 1 reveal a strong upward bias in the survivor function estimators under the independence of T_1 and T_2. For example at (T_1, T_2) percentiles of (55,55) the survivor function estimate averaged about 0.4, compared to the target value of 0.303 at each of $n = 30, 60$ and 120. This bias evidently derives from inappropriate mass assignment when one or both of d_{1ij} or d_{2ij} are zero. For example if $d_{1ij} = d_{2ij} = 0$ the likelihood maximization assigns the maximal mass to (t_{1i}, t_{2j}) that is consistent with the table marginal probabilities. In view of the fixed marginal probabilities such excessive mass assignment lead to an overestimation of the corresponding survivor function.

A grouped data version of this sequential NPML idea was considered toward avoiding the bias just noted. The grouping used was adaptive in that a likelihood function with additional censorship at a grid point (t_{1i}, t_{2j}) was maximized only if $d_{1ij} > 0$ and $d_{2ij} > 0$ and the resulting mass assignment was spread among points $(t_{1\ell}, t_{2m})$ with $\ell \leq i$ and $m \leq j$ to which mass had not been previously assigned. Once again the process was initiated by specifying Kaplan-Meier margins, and the risk region was scanned in a manner that (t_{1i}, t_{2j}) was considered for an NPML assignment only after all points to the left and downward had likewise been considered.

To be specific, suppose that one proceeds along rows (or columns) in the risk region to identify 'informative' points having $d_{1ij} > 0$ and $d_{2ij} > 0$. At any such point there will be a maximum index $u = u(i, j) \leq i$ such that p_{uj} has yet to be specified, and a maximum index $v = v(i, j)$ such that p_{iv} has yet to be specified. Denote by $\hat{P}_{1ij}$ the total mass that remains to be assigned along columns $T_1 = t_{1u}$ up through $T_1 = t_{1i}$ and by $\hat{P}_{2ij}$ the corresponding remaining mass along rows $T_2 = t_{2v}$ up to $T_2 = t_{2j}$. Also denote by

$$\hat{Q}_{ij} = 1 - \sum_{\ell=1}^{u-1} \hat{p}_{\ell \cdot} - \sum_{m=1}^{v-1} \hat{p}_{\cdot m} + \sum_{\ell=1}^{u-1}\sum_{m=1}^{v-1} \hat{p}_{\ell m} - \sum_{\ell=u}^{i}\sum_{m=v}^{j} \hat{p}_{\ell m} \gamma_{\ell m}$$

the mass that remains to be assigned at or beyond (t_{1u}, t_{2v}), where $\hat{p}_{\ell \cdot}$ and $\hat{p}_{\cdot m}$ are the column and row Kaplan-Meier mass assignments and $\gamma_{ij} = 1$ if mass has already been assigned at $(t_{1\ell}, t_{2m})$ and $\gamma_{\ell m} = 0$ otherwise. The grouped data likelihood to be maximized at (t_{1i}, t_{2j}) can now be written

$$L_{ij} = P_{ij}^{d_{ij}} (\hat{P}_{1ij} - P_{ij})^{d_{1ij} - d_{ij}} (\hat{P}_{2ij} - P_{ij})^{d_{2ij} - d_{ij}}$$
$$\times (\hat{Q}_{ij} - \hat{P}_{1ij} - \hat{P}_{2ij} + P_{ij})^{r_{ij} - d_{1ij} - d_{2ij} + d_{ij}}$$

where P_{ij} is the new mass to be assigned at or before (t_{1i}, t_{2j}) as a result of this maximization. L_{ij} is readily maximized subject to the constraints

$$0 \vee (\hat{P}_{1ij} + \hat{P}_{2ij} - \hat{Q}_{ij}) \leq P_{ij} \leq \hat{P}_{1ij} \wedge \hat{P}_{2ij}$$

using a modified Newton-Raphson procedure. The manner of distributing the resulting mass $\hat{P}_{ij}$ among the grid points in the grouping region needs to acknowledge the remaining mass along the affected rows and columns, but is otherwise undetermined. The maximum mass that can be assigned in this region is $\hat{P}_{1ij} \wedge \hat{P}_{2ij}$ as occurs by proceeding along rows (or columns) in the grouping region and assigning maximum allowable mass at each point. The grouped data estimator was implemented by assigning a fraction $\hat{P}_{ij}/\hat{P}_{1ij} \wedge \hat{P}_{2ij}$ of this maximal mass at each point in the grouping region.

Table 3 shows simulation summary statistics for this grouped data NPML estimator $(\tilde{F}_{GD})$ in the same format as previous tables. The Prentice-Cai estimator is also included for comparison. Evidently the grouping has been responsive to the bias problem noted for the previous NPML-type estimator. In fact, the summary statistics for the two proper survivor function estimators $\tilde{F}_{GD}$ and $\hat{F}_{PC}$ are quite similar. There is a suggestion, however, of a tiny bias with $\tilde{F}_{GD}$ that persists as the sample size becomes larger, possibly due to the manner of spreading the grouped data mass $\hat{P}_{ij}$ among points in the grouping region. Whether or not such bias is real or can be remedied, Table 3 provides no evidence that an NPML approach that uses Kaplan-Meier margins, and that bases survivor function estimates on data available when all pairs have been followed through (t_1, t_2) or to earlier failure or censoring, can improve materially on the Prentice-Cai estimator. A larger number of simulations (1000) is used in Table 3 compared to previous tables in order to illustrate the apparent slight bias of $\tilde{F}_{GD}$.

5 Inverse Censoring Probability Weighted Estimators

From Section 2 another expression for the nonparametric efficient Kaplan-Meier estimator is given by

$$\hat{F}(t) = 1 - \frac{1}{n} \sum_{t_i < t} \frac{d_i}{\hat{G}(t_i^-)}$$

where $t_1 < t_2 < \ldots$ are the ordered uncensored failure times, d_i is the number of failures at t_i and $\hat{G}(t)$ is a complementary Kaplan-Meier estimator of the censoring probability at time t.

Estimators of this type have also been considered in the bivariate situation. Once can rewrite (6) as

$$F(t_1, t_2) = F_1(t_1) + F_2(t_2) - 1$$
$$+ \int_0^{t_1} \int_0^{t_2} \frac{p\{X_1\varepsilon(u_1, u_1 + du_1), X_2\varepsilon(u_2, u_2 + du_2), \delta_1 = 1, \delta_2 = 1)}{G(u_1^-, u_2^-)}$$

suggesting the survivor function estimator

$$\hat{F}(t_1, t_2) = \hat{F}_1(t_1) + \hat{F}_2(t_2) - 1 + \sum_{t_{1i} \le t_1} \sum_{t_{2j} \le t_2} \frac{(d_{ij}/n)}{\hat{G}(t_{1i}^-, t_{2j}^-)} \qquad (17)$$

where $\hat{F}_1$ and $\hat{F}_2$ are Kaplan-Meier estimators and $\hat{G}$ is a strongly consistent estimator of the censoring distribution function G. Burke (1988) considered the right hand summation in (17) as an estimator of the distribution function, and he showed the strong consistency of that estimator provided a strongly consistent estimator of G is inserted. Note, however, that if one inserts the empirical estimator $\hat{F}(t_{1i}^-, t_{2j}^-)\hat{G}(t_{1i}^-, t_{2j}^-) = r_{ij}/n$ into (17) one obtains

$$\hat{F}(t_1, t_2) = \hat{F}_1(t_1) + \hat{F}_2(t_2) - 1 + \int_0^{t_1}\int_0^{t_2} \hat{F}(u_1^-, u_2^-)\hat{\Lambda}_{11}(du_1, du_2)$$

which determines the Bickel Volterra estimator. Hence survivor function estimators of the form (17) cannot be expected to have very good efficiency properties due to the poor correspondence between the implied (double failure) hazard estimator and the estimators of the marginal survivor functions. The efficiency properties of the corresponding distribution function will also be comparably poor for the same reason. In fact, simulation summary statistics for distribution function estimators were examined for all the estimators considered in Tables 1-2. For example, the sample standard deviations for the Bickel distribution function estimator were considerably larger than for the Prentice-Cai estimator under both the independence and Clayton models.

Robins, Rotnitski and Van der Laan (2000) also consider estimation procedures of the inverse censoring probability form. Because the censoring survivor function G can be estimated uniformly at a $n^{1/2}$ rate, even if inefficiently, by estimators of the type considered in Section 3 (e.g., Dabrowska, Prentice-Cai or Bickel estimators) it follows from their theory of locally efficient estimating equations that efficient estimators can be given under semiparametric specifications of F (e.g., Clayton model). Moreover, this type of locally efficient estimator is also available for higher dimensional survivor function estimation problems. See Ritov and Robins (1997) for a related estimation procedure in a broad class of semiparametric models. Their arguments indicate that nonparametric estimators of F that achieve the nonparametric variance bound uniformly may not exist in the absence of further assumptions (e.g., smoothness assumptions), and even if such assumptions hold that convergence to asymptotic distributions may be painfully slow.

6 Hazard-Based Nonparametric Survivor Function Estimators

The plug-in estimators studied in Section 3 arose from the fact that F is determined by its marginal survivor functions and (double failure) hazard function. The negative mass assigned by these estimators arose from a lack of compatability between estimators of $\{F_1, F_2\}$ and that for Λ. The type of truncation used by Van der Laan in developing his repaired NPMLE replaces mass along half lines beyond the truncation region $[0, \tau_1] \times [0, \tau_2]$ by mass on the boundary $T_1 = \tau_1$ or $T_2 = \tau_2$, where (τ_1, τ_2) is such that $F(\tau_1, \tau_2)G(\tau_1^-, \tau_2^-) > 0$. The truncation procedure leads to unit mass being assigned to $[0, \tau_1] \times [0, \tau_2]$ without altering $F(t_1, t_2)$ for any $(t_1, t_2)\varepsilon[0, \tau_1) \times [0, \tau_2)$.

As shown in Prentice, Moodie and Wu (2003), the distribution for the truncated failure time variables has a representation in terms of the (double failure) hazard only, so that the search for good survivor function estimators reduces to a search for good hazard function estimators alone. This formulation obviates the need to specify marginal survivor functions, and provides an approach to survivor function estimation that avoids negative mass, and that may yield plug-in estimators having good efficiency properties.

Specifically, one can write, for the truncated variates,

$$F(t_1^-, t_2^-) = \{1 - \Lambda(\Delta t)\}^{-1} P\{(t, \tau); \alpha\} / P\{(0, \tau); \alpha\}$$

where the Peano series P is defined as in (7) except that $t < u_i$ implies $t_1 \le u_{1i}, t_2 \le u_{2i}$ and $(t_1, t_2) \ne (u_{1i}, u_{2i})$, and $\alpha(dt_1, dt_2) = \Lambda(dt_1, dt_2)/\{1 - \Lambda(\Delta t_1, \Delta t_2)\}$. The compact differentiability of the Peano series transformation implies that such properties of strong consistency, weak convergence to a Gaussian process, and applicability of bootstrap procedures for estimators of F, follow from the corresponding property for estimators of Λ.

The authors also consider some choices for Λ estimator. The simple empirical estimator $\hat{\Lambda}_E$ for the truncated data is an obvious candidate, but the corresponding estimator $\hat{F}_E$ is inefficient due to an underutilization of the singly censored data. Van der Laan's approach of partitioning each of $[0, \tau_1]$ and $[0, \tau_2]$ and assigning singly censored observations nonparametrically within strips in either direction yields a class of redistributed empirical hazard estimators $\hat{\Lambda}_{RE}$ and survivor function estimators $\hat{F}_{RE}$ that can address this efficiency issue. One can also define adaptive versions, $\hat{\Lambda}_{AE}$ and $\hat{F}_{AE}$ of these redistributed empirical estimators by allowing the partitions of $[0, \tau_1]$ and $[0, \tau_2]$ to be defined, for example, by sample percentiles of the distribution of uncensored observations, though asymptotic properties for such adaptive estimators have yet to be developed.

The calculation of a (truncated) survivor function estimator $\hat{F}$ from the corresponding hazard function estimator $\hat{\Lambda}$ is straightforward. Following truncation of the data with (τ_1, τ_2) in the risk region $\hat{\Lambda}$ will specify positive hazards λ_ℓ at selected points $(t_{1\ell}, t_{2\ell}), \ell = 1, \dots, s$ within the grid formed by uncensored T_1 and T_2 observations. For example these points can be ordered by scanning across rows, starting from the bottom of the failure time grid in which case $(t_{1s}, t_{2s}) = (\tau_1, \tau_2)$ and $\hat{\lambda}_s = 1$. The corresponding mass assignments $\hat{p}_\ell, \ell = 1, \dots, s$ can be obtained as solution $\hat{\underline{p}} = \hat{A}^{-1}\underline{1}$ to a set of s linear equations where the $s = s$ matrix $\hat{A} = A(\hat{\Lambda})$ has ones below the main diagonal, reciprocal hazards $\lambda_\ell^{-1}, \ell = 1, \dots, s$ on the main diagonal, and zeros or ones above the main diagonal. The fact that $\hat{p}_\ell > 0, \ell = 1, \dots, s$ shows that the noniterative survivor function estimator

$$\hat{F}(t_1, t_2) = \sum_{\{\ell \mid t_{1\ell} > t_1 \text{ and } t_{2\ell} > t_2\}} \hat{p}_\ell$$

avoids negative mass, provided only that $\hat{\lambda}_\ell > 0, \ell = 1, \dots, s$ with $\hat{\lambda}_s = 1$.

Table 4 shows simulation results for $\hat{F}_E$ and for specific choices of partitions for $\hat{F}_{RE}$ and $\hat{F}_{AE}$, in the same format as Tables 1 and 2. The Prentice-Cai estimator $\hat{F}_{PC}$ is also included for comparison. The same simulation configurations are used as for the previous tables except that, for simplicity, T_2 is not subject to censoring. The estimator $\hat{F}_{RE}$ is, in fact, just Van der Laan's repaired NPMLE, and the Peano series formulation provides a non-iterative approach to its calculation under these censoring conditions. Note also that both $\hat{F}_{RE}$ and $\hat{F}_{AE}$ involve a data reduction wherein additional censorship is imposed by reducing each potential censoring time to its nearest smaller partition point. Lack of censorship on T_2 implies that no data reduction is needed, and hence represents a best case scenario in this respect, for these redistributed estimators. The truncation points in these simulations was defined so that $F_1(\tau_1) = F_2(\tau_2) = 0.55$. Samples having empty risk sets at (τ_1, τ_2) were omitted from summary statistics. This meant dropping 34 of the 500 runs at $n = 30$ under the independence model, and two of the 500 runs at $n = 30$ under the Clayton model.

In these simulations the elements of the fixed partition of $[0, \tau_2]$ for $\hat{F}_{RE}$ were $\{0, -\log(.6), -\log(.55)\}$ at $n = 30$; $\{0, -\log(.78), -\log(.56), -\log(.55)\}$ at $n = 60$; and $\{0, -\log(.85), -\log(.70), -\log(.55), -\log(.55)\}$ at $n = 120$. In each case other choices of partition elements were considered, with quite similar simulation results provided the corresponding strips did not become too narrow, in which case sample standard deviations tended to increase.

For the adaptive empirical estimator $\hat{F}_{AE}$ various choices of number of double failures per strip were considered. The summary statistics in Table 4 are based on 10 such failures at $n = 30$, 7 at $n = 60$ and 5 at $n = 120$. An approach that uses a fixed number (e.g., 5) of double failures per strip, or a slowly increasing number as sample size increases seems sensible in defining this adaptive estimator.

None of the estimators shown in Table 4 show evidence of bias at the selected (t_1, t_2) values. The empirical-hazard based estimator, $\hat{F}_E$, has unacceptable efficiency relative to $\hat{F}_{PC}$. The fixed-strip redistributed empirical estimator, $\hat{F}_{RE}$, also shows some additional sampling variation relative to $\hat{F}_{PC}$ at small sample sizes, but this difference evidently disappears by $n = 120$. Similarly the adaptive redistributed estimator is somewhat noisy at $n = 30$, but has summary statistics very similar to $\hat{F}_{PC}$ and $\hat{F}_{RE}$ at $n = 120$.

Though not shown in Table 4 similar comparisons prevail along the margins for T_1 and T_2. The simple empirical estimator $\hat{F}_E$ has comparable sample standard deviations to the other estimators for estimating the marginal survivor function for T_1, but poor efficiency under these simulation conditions for estimating the T_2 marginal survivor function. Especially at the larger sample sizes $\hat{F}_{RE}$ and $\hat{F}_{AE}$ had similar sample standard deviations to those for $\hat{F}_{PC}$ along both margins, but neither provided any substantial improvement, compared to $\hat{F}_{PC}$, for estimating the T_1 marginal survivor function.

7 Plug-In Estimators Restricted to Avoid Negative Mass

Van der Laan's repaired NPMLE and the closely related hazard-based estimators just described place all mass on the double failure for the truncated failure time variates. In fact, Van der Laan's work shows that efficient nonparametric survivor function estimation is possible while placing all mass on the uncensored failures. This realization stimulates consideration of plug-in estimators of the type illustrated in Section 3, that are restricted to avoid negative mass. Specifically, an 'estimator' $\tilde{F}$ corresponding to an unrestricted estimator $\hat{F}$ can be defined recursively by

$$
\tilde{F}(t_1,t_2) = \begin{cases}
0 \vee \{\tilde{F}(t_1^-,t_2) + \tilde{F}(t_1,t_2^-) - \tilde{F}(t_1^-,t_2^-)\} \\
\qquad \text{if } \hat{F}(t_1,t_2) < 0 \vee \{\tilde{F}(t_1^-,t_2) + \tilde{F}(t_1,t_2^-) - \tilde{F}(t_1^-,t_2^-)\} \\
\tilde{F}(t_1^-,t_2) \wedge \tilde{F}(t_1,t_2^-) \\
\qquad \text{if } \hat{F}(t_1,t_2) > \tilde{F}(t_1^-,t_2) \wedge \tilde{F}(t_1,t_2^-) \\
\hat{F}(t_1,t_2) \\
\qquad \text{otherwise.}
\end{cases}
$$

Table 5 shows simulation summary statistics for restricted estimators $\tilde{F}_D$, $\tilde{F}_{D2}$, $\tilde{F}_{PC}$ and $\tilde{F}_{PC2}$ that correspond to the estimators behaving best in Table 3, under the simulation configuration of Table 4 (censoring on T_1 only). Summary statistics for $\hat{F}_{PC}$ are also given for comparison.

The striking feature of Table 5 is the nearly identical performance of each of the four estimators that have been restricted to avoid negative mass, and the unrestricted estimator $\hat{F}_{PC}$. In effect, these restricted estimators place the mass that would be assigned by the corresponding unrestricted estimator at a failure time grid point as close as possible to the uncensored observation in the grid formed by the uncensored T_1 and T_2 failures, while acknowledging the Kaplan-Meier margins, and while avoiding negative mass. These simulations suggest that plug-in estimators, based on $\{\hat{F}_1, \hat{F}_2, \hat{\Lambda}\}$ may be able to be corrected to avoid negative mass without adversely affecting moderate or large sample performance. Simulation results (not shown) were similar with censoring on both T_1 and T_2, with the restrictions evidently providing some improvement in efficiency in small samples.

It would be interesting to determine whether choices of marginal survivor function estimators other than Kaplan-Meier could be constructed, perhaps through likelihood maximization, that would yield further improvement in the efficiency of these restricted plug-in estimators.

8 Summary

Various approaches to nonparametric estimation of the bivariate survivor function have been reviewed, and some proposals for new estimators have been given. The estimators due to Dabrowska (1988) and Prentice-Cai (1992) are easily calculated and have very good small sample performance. A distracting feature of these estimators is their propensity to assign negative mass, even for large sample sizes. From our numerical work it appears that a simple restriction can avoid negative mass without adversely affecting other properties, though asymptotic properties for these restricted estimators has yet to be developed.

The plug-in estimators just mentioned are not fully efficient away from the independence of T_1 and T_2, in part because the Kaplan-Meier marginals that these estimators used are not generally nonparametric efficient if the two failure times are dependent. To date, estimation procedures that have potential to improve efficiency, and to address the auxiliary data problem, are more complicated numerically and appear, at best, to yield modest efficiency gains unless the dependency between T_1 and T_2 is very strong and sample sizes are very large. Within this class Van der Laan's (1996) repaired NPMLE has the ability to achieve full asymptotic efficiency. Van der Laan's estimators can also be derived using a hazard-based approach, avoiding an iterative calculation in important special cases. If one is willing to impose semiparametric constraints on the joint survivor function then nonparametric estimators that are efficient under the assumed semiparametric model and consistent elsewhere can be defined and are expected to have good moderate sample performance (Robins et al, 2000).

Some additional estimators of F are available under specialized censoring schemes. For example Lin and Ying (1993) and Tsai and Crowley (1998) discuss inverse censoring probability weighted estimators of the bivariate survivor function under univariate censoring ($C_1 = C_2 = C$). Such restriction on the censoring scheme evidently does not materially simplify the challenge of identifying efficient estimators of F having good moderate sample performance.

The problem of nonparametric bivariate survivor function estimation is of practical importance and, as well, provides a stimulating context for the development and comparison of statistical estimation and inference strategies.

Acknowledgment

The author would like to thank Mark Mason for computational support. This work was supported by grant CA53996 from the National Institutes of Health and by an NSERC fellowship.

References

Andersen, P.K., Borgan, O., Gill, R.D., and Keiding, N. (1992). *Statistical Models Based on Counting Processes*, Springer-Verlag, New York.

Bickel, P.J., Klaasen, A.J., Ritov, Y., and Wellner, J.A. (1993). *Efficient and Adaptive Estimation for Semi-Parametric Models.* Johns Hopkins University Press.

Burke, M.D. (1988). Estimation of a bivariate distribution function under random censorship. *Biometrika* **75**, 379-382.

Campbell, G. (1981). Nonparametric bivariate estimation with randomly censored data. *Biometrika* **68**, 417-422.

Campbell, G., and Földes, A. (1982). Large-sample properties of nonparametric bivariate estimators with censored data. In *Nonparametric Statistical Inference*, B.V. Gredenko, M.L. Puri, and I. Vineze, eds., pp.103-122, North-Holland, Amsterdam.

Clayton, D.G. (1978). A model for association in bivariate life tables and its application in epidemiological studies of familial tendency in chronic disease incidence. *Biometrika* **65**, 141-151.

Cox, D.R. (1972). Regression models and life tables (with discussion). *Journal of the Royal Statistical Society* B **34**, 187-220.

Dabrowska, D.M. (1988). Kaplan-Meier estimate on the plane. *Annals of Statistics* **16**, 1475-1489.

Dabrowska, D.M. (1989). Kaplan-Meier estimate on the plane: weak convergence, LIL, and the bootstrap. *J. Multivariate Anal.* **29**, 308-325.

Efron, B. (1967). The two sample problem with censored data. Proc. Fifth Berkeley Symposium in Mathematical Statistics IV, pp.831-853, Prentice-Hall, New York.

Gentleman, R. and Vandal, A.C. (2001). Computational Algorithms for Censored Data Problems Using Intersection Graphs. *Journal of Computational and Graphical Statistics* **10**, 403-421.

Gill, R.D. and Johansen, S. (1990). A survey of product integration with a view towards application in survival analysis. *Annals of Statistics* **18**, 1501-1555.

Gill, R.D., Van der Laan, M.J., and Wellner, J.A. (1995). Inefficient estimators of the bivariate survival function for three models. *Ann. Inst. H. Poincaré Prob. Statist.* **31**, 547-597.

Kaplan, E.L. and Meier, P. (1958). Nonparametric estimation from incomplete observations. *Journal of the American Statistical Association* **53**, 457-481.

Lin, D.Y. and Ying, Z. (1993). A sample nonparametric estimator of the bivariate survival function under univariate censoring. *Biometrika* **80**, 573-581.

Prentice, R.L. and Cai, J. (1992). Covariance and survivor function estimation using censored multivariate failure time data. *Biometrika* **79**, 495-512.

Prentice, R.L., Moodie, Z. and Wu, J.(2003). Hazard-based nonparametric estimation of the bivariate survivor function. In press, *J.Roy.Statist.Soc.B.*

Prentice, R.L. (1999). Nonparametric maximum likelihood estimation of the bivariate survivor function. *Statistics in Medicine* **18**, 2517-2527.

Pruitt, R.C. (1991). On negative mass assigned by the bivariate Kaplan-Meier estimator. *Annals of Statistics* **19**, 443-453.

Robins, J.M. and Ritov, Y. (1997). Toward a curse of dimensionality appropriate (CODA) asymptotic theory for semi-parametric models. *Statistics in Medicine* **16**, 285-319.

Robins, J.M., Rotnitski, A. and Van der Laan, M. (2000). Commentary on 'on profile likelihood' by S.A. Murphy and A.W. Van der Vaart. *Journal of American Statistical Association* **95**, 477-482.

Tsai, W.Y., Leurgans, S. and Crowley, J. (1986). Nonparametric estimator of a bivariate survival function in the presence of censoring. *Annals of Statistics* **14**, 1351-1365.

Tsai, W.Y. and Crowley, J. (1998). A note on nonparametric estimators of the bivariate survival function under univariate censoring. *Biometrika* **85**, 573-580.

Van der Laan, M.J. (1996). Efficient estimation in the bivariate censoring model and repairing NPMLE. *Annals of Statistics* **24**, 596-627.

Van der Laan, M.J. (1997). Nonparametric estimators of the bivariate survival function under random censoring. *Statistica Neerlandica* **51**, 178-200.

Table 1

Simulation summary statistics for certain nonparametric estimators of the bivariate survivor function, based on 500 simulations at each sample size and sampling configuration

Sample Size	Estimator*	Independence Model					Clayton Model				
		T_1 and T_2 Percent Survival			Negative Mass[o]		T_1 and T_2 Percent Survival			Negative Mass[o]	
		(70,70)	(70,55)	(55,55)	m_I	m_0	(70,70)	(70,55)	(55,55)	m_I	m_0
	True $F(t_1,t_2)$	.490	.385	.303			.608	.516	.468		
30	$\hat{F}_{CF}$	.495 (.140)+	.394 (.178)	.301 (.209)	0.85	0.25	.603 (.131)	.516 (.172)	.448 (.206)	0.63	0.28
	$\hat{F}_B$	.498 (.120)	.389 (.136)	.306 (.161)	0	0.34	.611 (.113)	.518 (.133)	.467 (.164)	0	0.44
	$\hat{F}_D$	.498 (.122)	.388 (.141)	.303 (.167)	0.42	0.10	.611 (.114)	.520 (.138)	.469 (.179)	0.38	0.17
	$\hat{F}_{PC}$	.499 (.116)	.393 (.126)	.323 (.133)	0.21	0.11	.607 (.110)	.512 (.123)	.462 (.134)	0.20	0.15
60	$\hat{F}_{CF}$	.491 (.097)	.390 (.123)	.310 (.141)	1.11	0.30	.606 (.094)	.519 (.119)	.468 (.131)	0.85	0.31
	$\hat{F}_B$	.490 (.080)	.389 (.094)	.308 (.114)	0	0.44	.608 (.081)	.519 (.096)	.468 (.118)	0	0.54
	$\hat{F}_D$	.490 (.080)	.390 (.092)	.307 (.115)	0.58	0.12	.609 (.078)	.521 (.090)	.474 (.111)	0.54	0.20
	$\hat{F}_{PC}$	.490 (.079)	.389 (.089)	.312 (.095)	0.32	0.15	.607 (.077)	.517 (.088)	.466 (.093)	0.29	0.18
120	$\hat{F}_{CF}$	.492 (.066)	.392 (.081)	.314 (.088)	1.37	0.35	.607 (.062)	.521 (.076)	.468 (.086)	1.08	0.35
	$\hat{F}_B$	.490 (.056)	.389 (.067)	.304 (.077)	0	0.54	.606 (.053)	.516 (.063)	.462 (.079)	0	0.62
	$\hat{F}_D$	.491 (.055)	.390 (.064)	.308 (.070)	0.74	0.15	.607 (.052)	.518 (.059)	.468 (.068)	0.66	0.22
	$\hat{F}_{PC}$	.491 (.055)	.389 (.064)	.307 (.065)	0.43	0.18	.606 (.051)	.516 (.058)	.463 (.065)	0.38	0.21

* At $n = 30$ $\hat{F}$ values are based on 497, 480 and 425 runs with non-empty risk sets under the independence model, and 499, 488 and 455 runs having non-empty risk sets under the Clayton model at the (70,70), (70,55) and (55,55) percentiles respectively. Corresponding counts at $n = 60$ were 500, 497 and 468 under independence, and 500, 499 and 490 under the Clayton model. At $n = 120$ the counts were 500, 500 and 494 under independence, and 500, 500 and 498 under the Clayton model.

+ Entries are the sample means of $\hat{F}$ values, along with sample standard deviations in parentheses.

o The entries under m_I and m_0 are the average across simulations of the total amount of negative mass assigned by the estimator inside the risk region, and along half lines outside the risk region, respectively.

Table 2
Simulation summary statistics for some potential new plug-in estimators of the bivariate survivor function, based on 500 simulations at each sample size and sample configuration

Sample Size	Estimator*	Independence Model					Clayton Model				
		T_1 and T_2 Percent Survival			Negative Mass°		T_1 and T_2 Percent Survival			Negative Mass°	
		(70,70)	(70,55)	(55,55)	m_1	m_0	(70,70)	(70,55)	(55,55)	m_1	m_0
	True $F(t_1,t_2)$	.490	.385	.303			.608	.516	.468		
30	$\hat{F}_D$	.498 (.122)+	.388 (.141)	.303 (.167)	0.42	0.10	.611 (.114)	.520 (.138)	.469 (.179)	0.38	0.17
	$\hat{F}_{D1}$	.505 (.115)	.405 (.124)	.343 (.131)	0.23	0.35	.620 (.109)	.531 (.127)	.493 (.159)	0.21	0.36
	$\hat{F}_{D2}$	.497 (.116)	.388 (.125)	.318 (.125)	0.16	0.06	.600 (.110)	.501 (.124)	.444 (.134)	0.12	0.11
	$\hat{F}_{PC}$	.499 (.116)	.393 (.126)	.323 (.133)	0.21	0.11	.607 (.110)	.512 (.123)	.462 (.134)	0.20	0.15
	$\hat{F}_{PC1}$	.507 (.115)	.408 (.128)	.346 (.141)	0.27	0.49	.626 (.110)	.540 (.128)	.506 (.152)	0.29	0.50
	$\hat{F}_{PC2}$	.499 (.116)	.391 (.126)	.321 (.131)	0.19	0.09	.606 (.110)	.510 (.123)	.456 (.134)	0.16	0.14
60	$\hat{F}_D$	.490 (.080)	.390 (.092)	.307 (.115)	0.58	0.12	.609 (.078)	.521 (.090)	.474 (.111)	0.54	0.20
	$\hat{F}_{D1}$	.494 (.087)	.397 (.088)	.327 (.093)	0.34	0.35	.613 (.077)	.526 (.089)	.483 (.099)	0.28	0.38
	$\hat{F}_{D2}$	.489 (.079)	.388 (.088)	.311 (.090)	0.26	0.10	.602 (.078)	.511 (.089)	.457 (.093)	0.20	0.17
	$\hat{F}_{PC}$	.490 (.079)	.389 (.089)	.312 (.095)	0.32	0.15	.607 (.077)	.517 (.088)	.466 (.093)	0.29	0.18
	$\hat{F}_{PC1}$	.495 (.079)	.398 (.088)	.326 (.097)	0.40	0.47	.617 (.077)	.530 (.089)	.490 (.136)	0.38	0.49
	$\hat{F}_{PC2}$	.490 (.079)	.391 (.088)	.311 (.092)	0.29	0.11	.606 (.077)	.515 (.089)	.463 (.105)	0.26	0.19
120	$\hat{F}_D$	.491 (.055)	.390 (.064)	.308 (.070)	0.74	0.15	.607 (.052)	.516 (.059)	.468 (.068)	0.66	0.22
	$\hat{F}_{D1}$	.493 (.054)	.393 (.063)	.315 (.064)	0.45	0.37	.609 (.052)	.520 (.059)	.471 (.067)	0.36	0.37
	$\hat{F}_{D2}$	.490 (.054)	.389 (.063)	.307 (.063)	0.38	0.13	.604 (.052)	.513 (.059)	.458 (.065)	0.29	0.21
	$\hat{F}_{PC}$	.491 (.055)	.389 (.064)	.307 (.065)	0.43	0.18	.606 (.051)	.516 (.058)	.463 (.065)	0.38	0.21
	$\hat{F}_{PC1}$	.493 (.054)	.394 (.063)	.315 (.065)	0.53	0.47	.611 (.051)	.522 (.059)	.474 (.069)	0.44	0.44
	$\hat{F}_{PC2}$	.491 (.054)	.389 (.063)	.307 (.064)	0.41	0.14	.605 (.052)	.515 (.059)	.461 (.074)	0.37	0.22

* See footnote * of Table 1.

° The entries under m_1 and m_0 are the average across simulations of the total amount of negative mass assigned by the estimator inside the risk region, and along half lines outside the risk region, respectively.

+ Entries are the sample means of $\hat{F}$ values, along with sample standard deviations in parentheses.

Table 3

Simulation summary statistics for a grouped data NPML estimator ($\tilde{F}_{GD}$) of the bivariate survivor function based on 1000 simulations at each sample size and sample configuration

Sample Size	Estimator*	Independence Model T_1 and T_2 Percent Survival			Clayton Model T_1 and T_2 Percent Survival		
		(70,70)	(70,55)	(55,55)	(70,70)	(70,55)	(55,55)
	$F(t_1, t_2)$	.490	.385	.303	.608	.516	.468
30	$\tilde{F}_{GD}$ (grouped data)	.505 (.111)+	.404 (.123)	.334 (.124)	.602 (.109)	.501 (.125)	.434 (.129)
	$\hat{F}_{PC}$ (Prentice-Cai)	.499 (.113)	.395 (.126)	.322 (.133)	.610 (.109)	.516 (.125)	.466 (.134)
60	$\tilde{F}_{GD}$	.494 (.077)	.396 (.087)	.323 (.088)	.595 (.076)	.503 (.089)	.440 (.094)
	$\hat{F}_{PC}$	.491 (.077)	.390 (.090)	.311 (.094)	.605 (.073)	.515 (.086)	.462 (.093)
120	$\tilde{F}_{GD}$	.496 (.056)	.397 (.062)	.319 (.066)	.596 (.056)	.509 (.063)	.452 (.068)
	$\hat{F}_{PC}$	.492 (.056)	.390 (.063)	.308 (.066)	.607 (.055)	.518 (.060)	.468 (.064)

* At $n = 30$ $\hat{F}$ values are based on 997, 969 and 866 runs having non-empty risk sets at (T_1, T_2) percentiles of (70,70), (70,55) and (55,55) under the independence model, and 998, 985 and 920 under Clayton model. Corresponding numbers are (1000, 993, 940) and (1000, 999, 972) at $n = 60$; and (1000, 1000, 990) and (1000, 1000, 997) at $n = 120$.

+ Entries are the sample mean and sample standard deviation in parentheses of $\hat{F}$ values.

Table 4

Simulation summary statistics for certain nonparametric estimators of the bivariate survivor function, based on 500 simulations at each configuration, with censoring on T_1 only

Sample Size	Estimator	Independence Model T_1 and T_2 Percent Survival			Clayton Model T_1 and T_2 Percent Survival		
		(70,70)	(70,55)	(55,55)	(70,70)	(70,55)	(55,55)
	True $F(t_1,t_2)$	.490	.385	.303	.608	.516	.468
30	$\hat{F}_{PC}$	.487 (.107)*	.384 (.100)	.301 (.109)	.601 (.099)	.513 (.098)	.461 (.114)
	$\hat{F}_E$	.495 (.143)	.397 (.136)	.313 (.127)	.602 (.125)	.514 (.136)	.467 (.139)
	$\hat{F}_{RE}$	.493 (.127)	.394 (.104)	.313 (.109)	.601 (.110)	.516 (.098)	.470 (.111)
	$\hat{F}_{AE}$	.496 (.138)	.391 (.096)	.311 (.103)	.601 (.113)	.517 (.097)	.471 (.111)
60	$\hat{F}_{PC}$	.487 (.074)	.384 (.072)	.306 (.080)	.605 (.068)	.513 (.067)	.468 (.076)
	$\hat{F}_E$	.484 (.099)	.377 (.098)	.301 (.095)	.605 (.084)	.507 (.100)	.466 (.103)
	$\hat{F}_{RE}$	.487 (.084)	.384 (.073)	.306 (.081)	.605 (.075)	.514 (.071)	.472 (.078)
	$\hat{F}_{AE}$	.496 (.093)	.384 (.072)	.306 (.081)	.606 (.076)	.514 (.067)	.472 (.074)
120	$\hat{F}_{PC}$	.492 (.054)	.384 (.051)	.301 (.057)	.610 (.050)	.518 (.050)	.468 (.056)
	$\hat{F}_E$	.494 (.067)	.381 (.069)	.298 (.067)	.610 (.062)	.516 (.070)	.468 (.070)
	$\hat{F}_{RE}$	.492 (.055)	.384 (.052)	.300 (.058)	.610 (.050)	.519 (.051)	.470 (.055)
	$\hat{F}_{AE}$	.497 (.059)	.384 (.051)	.301 (.057)	.611 (.053)	.519 (.050)	.470 (.055)

* Entries are sample means of $\hat{F}$, along with sample standard deviations in parentheses.

Table 5

Simulation summary statistics for restricted versions of selected plug-in estimators considered in Table 2, based on 1000 simulations at each sample size and sample configuration

Sample Size	Estimator	Independence Model T_1 and T_2 Percent Survival			Clayton Model T_1 and T_2 Percent Survival		
		(70,70)	(70,55)	(55,55)	(70,70)	(70,55)	(55,55)
	True $F(t_1, t_2)$	.490	.385	.303	.608	.516	.468
30	$\hat{F}_{PC}$	.494 (.098)*	.392 (.094)	.315 (.107)	.608 (.096)	.519 (.093)	.466 (.107)
	$\tilde{F}_D$	.498 (.096)	.395 (.092)	.318 (.104)	.602 (.096)	.517 (.092)	.454 (.106)
	$\tilde{F}_{D2}$	.495 (.096)	.391 (.092)	.310 (.104)	.595 (.098)	.506 (.094)	.441 (.108)
	$\tilde{F}_{PC}$	.497 (.096)	.394 (.093)	.315 (.106)	.602 (.096)	.516 (.093)	.455 (.107)
	$\tilde{F}_{PC2}$	.497 (.096)	.395 (.092)	.317 (.103)	.600 (.096)	.514 (.093)	.450 (.107)
60	$\hat{F}_{PC}$	.491 (.069)	.388 (.067)	.305 (.078)	.606 (.068)	.517 (.066)	.465 (.076)
	$\tilde{F}_D$	.494 (.068)	.390 (.067)	.308 (.076)	.604 (.068)	.516 (.066)	.457 (.076)
	$\tilde{F}_{D2}$	.492 (.068)	.387 (.067)	.304 (.075)	.600 (.068)	.510 (.066)	.449 (.076)
	$\tilde{F}_{PC}$	.493 (.068)	.389 (.067)	.306 (.077)	.605 (.068)	.516 (.066)	.459 (.076)
	$\tilde{F}_{PC2}$	.494 (.068)	.390 (.067)	.308 (.075)	.603 (.068)	.515 (.066)	.454 (.076)
120	$\hat{F}_{PC}$	.493 (.050)	.389 (.049)	.306 (.054)	.609 (.049)	.519 (.047)	.469 (.053)
	$\tilde{F}_D$	.495 (.050)	.391 (.048)	.309 (.053)	.608 (.050)	.519 (.047)	.466 (.053)
	$\tilde{F}_{D2}$	.494 (.050)	.390 (.048)	.307 (.053)	.606 (.050)	.516 (.047)	.461 (.053)
	$\tilde{F}_{PC}$	.494 (.050)	.389 (.049)	.306 (.054)	.609 (.049)	.519 (.047)	.468 (.053)
	$\tilde{F}_{PC2}$	.495 (.050)	.391 (.048)	.307 (.053)	.608 (.050)	.518 (.047)	.464 (.053)

* Entries are sample means, with sample standard deviations in parentheses.

A Semiparametric Regression Model for Panel Count Data: When Do Pseudo-likelihood Estimators Become Badly Inefficient?

Jon A. Wellner[1], Ying Zhang[2], and Hao Liu[3]

[1] Statistics, University of Washington   `jaw@stat.washington.edu`
[2] Statistics, University of Central Florida   `zhang@pegasus.cc.ucf.edu`
[3] Biostatistics, University of Washington   `hliu@u.washington.edu`

Summary. We consider estimation in a particular semiparametric regression model for the mean of a counting process under the assumption of "panel count" data. The basic model assumption is that the conditional mean function of the counting process is of the form $E\{\mathbb{N}(t)|Z\} = \exp(\theta' Z)\Lambda(t)$ where Z is a vector of covariates and Λ is the baseline mean function. The "panel count" observation scheme involves observation of the counting process $\mathbb{N}$ for an individual at a random number K of random time points; both the number and the locations of these time points may differ across individuals.

We study maximum pseudo-likelihood and maximum likelihood estimators $\widehat{\theta}_n^{ps}$ and $\widehat{\theta}_n$ of the regression parameter θ. The pseudo-likelihood estimators are fairly easy to compute, while the full maximum likelihood estimators pose more challenges from the computational perspective. We derive expressions for the asymptotic variances of both estimators under the proportional mean model. Our primary aim is to understand when the pseudo-likelihood estimators have very low efficiency relative to the full maximum likelihood estimators. The upshot is that the pseudo-likelihood estimators can have arbitrarily small efficiency relative to the full maximum likelihood estimators when the distribution of K, the number of observation time points per individual, is very heavy-tailed.

Outline

1 Introduction

Our goal in this paper is to study efficiency aspects of two types of estimators for a particular semiparametric model for *panel count data*. Panel count data arise in many fields including demographic studies, industrial reliability, and clinical trials; see for example KALBFLEISCH AND LAWLESS (1985), GAVER AND O'MUIRCHEARTAIGH (1987), THALL AND LACHIN (1988), THALL (1988), SUN AND KALBFLEISCH (1995), and WELLNER AND ZHANG (2000) where the estimation of either the intensity of event recurrence or the mean function of a counting process with panel count data was studied. Many applications involve covariates whose effects on the underlying counting process are of interest. While there is considerable work on regression modeling for recurrent events based on continuous observations (see, for example LAWLESS AND NADEAU (1995), COOK, LAWLESS, AND NADEAU (1996), and LIN, WEI, YANG, AND YING (2000)), regression analysis with panel count data for counting processes has just started recently. SUN AND WEI (2000) proposed estimating equation methods, while ZHANG (1998) and ZHANG (2002) proposed a pseudo-likelihood method for studying the multiplicative mean model (1) with panel count data.

Here is a description of the model and the observation scheme. Suppose that $\mathbb{N} = \{\mathbb{N}(t) : t \geq 0\}$ is a univariate counting process. In many applications, it is important to estimate the expected number of events $E\{\mathbb{N}(t)|Z\}$ which will occur by the time t, conditionally on a covariate vector Z.

In this paper we consider the proportional mean regression model given by

$$\Lambda(t|Z) \equiv E\{\mathbb{N}(t)|Z\} = e^{\theta' Z} \Lambda(t) , \tag{1}$$

where the monotone increasing function Λ is the *baseline mean function*. The parameters of primary interest are θ and Λ.

The observation scheme we want to study is as follows: suppose that we observe the counting process $\mathbb{N}$ at a random number K of random times

$$0 \equiv T_{K,0} < T_{K,1} < \cdots < T_{K,K}.$$

We write $\underline{T}_K \equiv (T_{K,1}, \ldots, T_{K,K})$, and we assume that $(K, \underline{T}_K | Z) \sim G(\cdot | Z)$ is conditionally independent of the counting process $\mathbb{N}$ given the covariate vector Z. We further assume that $Z \sim H$ on R^d, but we will make no further assumptions about G or H (modulo mild integrability and boundedness requirements).

The data for each individual will consist of

$$X = (Z, K, \underline{T}_K, \mathbb{N}(T_{K,1}), \ldots, \mathbb{N}(T_{K,K})) \equiv (Z, K, \underline{T}_K, \underline{\mathbb{N}}_K). \qquad (2)$$

We will assume that the data consist of $X_1, \ldots, X_n$ i.i.d. as X.

To derive useful estimators for this model we will often assume, in addition to (1), that the counting process $\mathbb{N}$, conditionally on Z, is a non-homogeneous Poisson process. But our general perspective will be to study the estimators and other procedures when the Poisson assumption *fails to hold* and we assume *only* that the proportional mean assumption (1) holds.

Such a program was carried out for estimation of Λ without any covariates for this panel count observation model by WELLNER AND ZHANG (2000). Briefly, WELLNER AND ZHANG (2000) studied both the maximum likelihood estimator $\widehat{\Lambda}_n$ and the pseudo-maximum likelihood estimator $\widehat{\Lambda}_n^{ps}$ of Λ. They showed that both estimators are consistent in $L_2(\mu)$ where μ is the measure defined (in terms of the observation process) by

$$\mu(B) = \sum_{k=1}^{\infty} P(K = k) \sum_{j=1}^{k} P(T_{k,j} \in B | K = k).$$

WELLNER AND ZHANG (2000) also succeeded in showing (under additional smoothness and boundedness assumptions) that

$$n^{1/3}(\widehat{\Lambda}_n^{ps}(t_0) - \Lambda_0(t_0)) \to_d \left\{ \frac{\sigma^2(t_0)\Lambda_0'(t_0)}{2G'(t_0)} \right\}^{1/3} 2\mathbb{Z}$$

where $\sigma^2(t) = Var[\mathbb{N}(t)]$, $G'(t) = \sum_{k=1}^{\infty} P(K = k) \sum_{j=1}^{k} G'_{k,j}(t)$, and $\mathbb{Z} = \operatorname{argmax}\{W(t) - t^2\}$ for a two-sided Brownian motion process W starting at 0. They also proved a corresponding result for a "toy estimator" version of the maximum likelihood estimator $\widehat{\Lambda}_n$ under the Poisson process assumption, and made efficiency comparisons between the two estimators based on Monte-Carlo studies.

The outline of the rest of the present paper is as follows: In section 2, we describe two methods of estimation, namely *maximum pseudo-likelihood estimators* and *maximum likelihood estimators* of θ and Λ. The basic picture is that the pseudo-likelihood estimators are computationally relatively straightforward and easy to implement, while the (full, semiparametric) maximum likelihood estimators are considerably more difficult, requiring an iterative algorithm in the computation of the profile likelihood. For other examples of the use of pseudo-likelihood to obtain computationally simple methods, see e.g. BETENSKY, RABINOWITZ, AND TSIATIS (2001) and RABINOWITZ, BETENSKY, AND TSIATIS (2000).

In section 3 we present information calculations for the semiparametric model described by the proportional mean function assumption (1) together with the non-homogeneous Poisson process assumption on N. This provides a baseline for comparisons of variances with the best possible asymptotic variance under the Poisson and proportional mean model assumptions. In section 4 we describe asymptotic normality results for the pseudo-likelihood and full maximum likelihood estimators $\widehat{\theta}_n^{ps}$ and $\widehat{\theta}_n$ of θ assuming only the proportional mean structure (1), but *not assuming* that N is a Poisson process. Proofs of these results will be presented in detail in WELLNER, ZHANG, AND LIU (2002). Finally, in section 4 we compare the pseudo-likelihood and full likelihood estimators of θ under three different scenarios with the goal of determining situations under which the pseudo-likelihood estimators will lose considerable efficiency relative to the full maximum likelihood estimators.

As will be seen, the rough upshot of the calculations here is that the efficiency of the pseudo-likelihood estimators relative to the full maximum likelihood estimators can be low when the distribution of K, the number of observation times per subject, is heavy-tailed.

2 Two Methods of Estimation

Maximum Pseudo-likelihood Estimation: The natural pseudo-likelihood estimators for this model use the marginal distributions of N, conditional on Z,

$$P(\mathbb{N}(t) = k|Z) = \frac{\Lambda(t|Z)^k}{k!} \exp(-\Lambda(t|Z))$$

and *ignore dependence* between $\mathbb{N}(t_1)$, $\mathbb{N}(t_2)$ to obtain the *pseudo-likelihood*:

$$l_n^{ps}(\theta, \Lambda) = \sum_{i=1}^n \sum_{j=1}^{K_i} \left\{ \mathbb{N}^{(i)}(T_{K_i,j}^{(i)}) \log \Lambda(T_{K_i,j}^{(i)}) \right.$$
$$\left. + \mathbb{N}^{(i)}(T_{K_i,j}^{(i)}) \theta' Z_i - e^{\theta' Z_i} \Lambda(T_{K_i,j}^{(i)}) \right\} .$$

Then the maximum pseudo-likelihood estimator $(\widehat{\theta}_n^{ps}, \widehat{\Lambda}_n^{ps})$ of (θ, Λ) is given by

$$(\widehat{\theta}_n^{ps}, \widehat{\Lambda}_n^{ps}) \equiv \operatorname{argmax}_{\theta, \Lambda} l_n^{ps}(\theta, \Lambda) .$$

This can be implemented in two steps via the usual (pseudo-) profile likelihood. For each fixed value of θ we set

$$\widehat{\Lambda}_n^{ps}(\cdot, \theta) \equiv \operatorname{argmax}_\Lambda l_n^{ps}(\theta, \Lambda) , \qquad (3)$$

and define

$$l_n^{ps,profile}(\theta) \equiv l_n^{ps}(\theta, \widehat{\Lambda}_n^{ps}(\cdot, \theta)).$$

Then

$$\widehat{\theta}_n^{ps} = \text{argmax}_\theta \, l_n^{ps,profile}(\theta), \qquad \text{and} \qquad \widehat{\Lambda}_n^{ps} = \widehat{\Lambda}_n^{ps}(\cdot, \widehat{\theta}_n^{ps}).$$

In fact, the optimization problem in (3) is easily solved as follows: Let $t_1 < \ldots < t_m$ denote the ordered distinct observation time points in the collection of all observations times, $\{T_{K_i,j}^{(i)}, \; j = 1, \ldots, K_i, \; i = 1, \ldots, n\}$, let $\mathbb{N}_{K_i,j}^{(i)} \equiv \mathbb{N}^{(i)}(T_{K_i,j}^{(i)})$, and set

$$w_l = \sum_{i=1}^{n} \sum_{j=1}^{K_i} 1_{[T_{K_i,j}^{(i)}=t_l]}, \quad \overline{N}_l = \frac{1}{w_l} \sum_{i=1}^{n} \sum_{j=1}^{K_i} \mathbb{N}_{K_i,j}^{(i)} 1_{[T_{K_i,j}^{(i)}=t_l]},$$

$$\overline{A}_l(\theta) = \frac{1}{w_l} \sum_{i=1}^{n} \sum_{j=1}^{K_i} \exp(\theta' Z^{(i)}) \, 1_{[T_{K_i,j}^{(i)}=t_l]}.$$

Then it is easily shown that

$$\widehat{\Lambda}_n^{ps}(\cdot, \theta) = \text{left-derivative of Greatest Convex Minorant of}$$

$$\{(\sum_{l \leq i} w_l \overline{A}_l(\theta), \sum_{l \leq i} w_l \overline{N}_l)\}_{i=1}^{m}$$

$$= \max_{i \leq l} \min_{j \geq l} \frac{\sum_{i \leq p} \leq w_p \overline{N}_p}{\sum_{i \leq p} \leq w_p \overline{A}_p(\theta)} \quad \text{at} \; t_l,$$

which is straightforward to compute.

Maximum Likelihood Estimation: Under the assumption that $\mathbb{N}$ is (conditionally, given Z) a non-homogeneous Poisson process, the likelihood can be calculated using the (conditional) independence of the increments of $\mathbb{N}$, $\Delta\mathbb{N}(s,t] \equiv \mathbb{N}(t) - \mathbb{N}(s)$, and the Poisson distribution of these increments:

$$P(\Delta\mathbb{N}(s,t] = k|Z) = \frac{[\Delta\Lambda((s,t]|Z)]^k}{k!} \exp(-\Delta\Lambda((s,t]|Z))$$

to obtain the *log-likelihood*:

$$l_n(\theta, \Lambda) = \sum_{i=1}^{n} \sum_{j=1}^{K_i} \left\{ \Delta\mathbb{N}_{K_i,j}^{(i)} \cdot \log \Delta\Lambda_{K_i,j} + \Delta\mathbb{N}_{K_i,j}^{(i)} \theta' Z_i - e^{\theta' Z_i} \Delta\Lambda_{K_i,j} \right\}$$

where

$$\Delta\mathbb{N}_{Kj} \equiv \mathbb{N}(T_{K,j}) - \mathbb{N}(T_{K,j-1}), \qquad j = 1, \ldots, K,$$
$$\Delta\Lambda_{Kj} \equiv \Lambda(T_{K,j}) - \Lambda(T_{K,j-1}), \qquad j = 1, \ldots, K,$$

with $\mathbb{N}(T_{K,0}) = 0$ and $\Lambda(T_{K,0}) = 0$. Then

$$(\widehat{\theta}_n, \widehat{\Lambda}_n) \equiv \text{argmax}_{\theta, \Lambda} \, l_n(\theta, \Lambda) \,.$$

This maximization can also be carried out in two steps via profile likelihood. For each fixed value of θ we set

$$\widehat{\Lambda}_n(\cdot, \theta) \equiv \text{argmax}_\Lambda \, l_n(\theta, \Lambda) \,,$$

and define

$$l_n^{profile}(\theta) \equiv l_n(\theta, \widehat{\Lambda}_n(\cdot, \theta)) \,.$$

Then

$$\widehat{\theta}_n = \text{argmax}_\theta \, l_n^{profile}(\theta) \,, \qquad \text{and} \qquad \widehat{\Lambda}_n = \widehat{\Lambda}_n(\cdot, \widehat{\theta}_n) \,.$$

Computation of the (profile) "estimator" $\widehat{\Lambda}_n(\cdot, \theta)$ is computationally involved, but possible via the iterative convex minorant algorithm; see e.g. JONGBLOED (1998). For more on computation without covariates see WELLNER AND ZHANG (2000).

3 Information bounds for θ under the Poisson model.

We first compute information bounds for estimation of θ under the proportional mean (non-homogeneous) Poisson process model.

Suppose that $(\mathbb{N}|Z) \sim \text{Poisson}(\Lambda(\cdot|Z))$, and $((K, T_K)|Z) \sim G(\cdot|Z)$ are conditionally independent given Z. We will assume here that $\mathbb{N}$ is conditionally a nonhomogeneous Poisson process with conditional mean function

$$E[\mathbb{N}(t)|Z] = \Lambda(t|Z) \equiv e^{\theta_0' Z} \Lambda_0(t) \,. \tag{4}$$

The second equality expresses the proportional mean regression model assumption.

The likelihood for one observation is, using the same notation introduced in Section 2,

$$p(X; \theta, \Lambda) = \prod_{j=1}^{K} \exp(-\Delta\Lambda_{Kj}) \frac{(\Delta\Lambda_{Kj})^{\Delta\mathbb{N}_{Kj}}}{(\Delta\mathbb{N}_{Kj})!} \,.$$

Thus the log-likelihood for (θ, Λ) for one observation is given by

$$\log p(X; \theta, \Lambda) = \sum_{j=1}^{K} \{\Delta\mathbb{N}_{Kj} \log \Delta\Lambda_{Kj} - \Delta\Lambda_{Kj} - \log(\Delta\mathbb{N}_{Kj}!)\} \,.$$

Differentiating this with respect to θ and Λ respectively, the scores for θ and Λ are easily seen to be

$$\dot{\mathbf{l}}_\theta(x) = \sum_{j=1}^{K} Z(\Delta N_{Kj} - e^{\theta_0' Z} \Delta \Lambda_{0Kj}), \tag{5}$$

while

$$\dot{\mathbf{l}}_\Lambda a(x) = \sum_{j=1}^{K} \left\{ \frac{\Delta N_{Kj}}{\Delta \Lambda_{0Kj}} - e^{\theta_0' Z} \right\} \Delta a_{Kj}$$

$$= \sum_{j=1}^{K} \left\{ \Delta N_{Kj} - e^{\theta_0' Z} \Delta \Lambda_{0Kj} \right\} \frac{\Delta a_{Kj}}{\Delta \Lambda_{0Kj}},$$

where

$$\Delta a_{Kj} = \int_{T_{K,j-1}}^{T_{K,j}} a \, d\Lambda_0, \qquad a \in L_2(\Lambda_0).$$

To compute the information bound for estimation of θ it follows from the results of BEGUN, HALL, HUANG, AND WELLNER (1983) and BICKEL, KLAASSEN, RITOV, AND WELLNER (1993) that we want to find a^* so that

$$\dot{\mathbf{l}}_\theta - \dot{\mathbf{l}}_\Lambda a^* \perp \dot{\mathbf{l}}_\Lambda a$$

for all $a \in L_2(\Lambda_0)$; i.e.

$$0 = E\left\{ (\dot{\mathbf{l}}_\theta - \dot{\mathbf{l}}_\Lambda a^*) \dot{\mathbf{l}}_\Lambda a \right\}$$

$$= E\left\{ \sum_{j=1}^{K} (\Delta N_{Kj} - e^{\theta_0' Z} \Delta \Lambda_{0Kj}) \left(Z - \frac{\Delta a_{Kj}^*}{\Delta \Lambda_{0Kj}} \right) \dot{\mathbf{l}}_\Lambda a \right\}$$

$$= E\left\{ \sum_{j=1}^{K} (\Delta N_{Kj} - e^{\theta_0' Z} \Delta \Lambda_{0Kj})^2 \left(Z - \frac{\Delta a_{Kj}^*}{\Delta \Lambda_{0Kj}} \right) \frac{\Delta a_{Kj}}{\Delta \Lambda_{0Kj}} \right\}$$

$$= E\left\{ \sum_{j=1}^{K} e^{\theta_0' Z} \Delta \Lambda_{0Kj} \left(Z - \frac{\Delta a_{Kj}^*}{\Delta \Lambda_{0Kj}} \right) \frac{\Delta a_{Kj}}{\Delta \Lambda_{0Kj}} \right\}$$

by conditioning on K, T_K, Z

$$= E_K\left\{ \sum_{j=1}^{K} E\left\{ e^{\theta_0' Z} \Delta \Lambda_{0Kj} \left(Z - \frac{\Delta a_{Kj}^*}{\Delta \Lambda_{0Kj}} \right) \frac{\Delta a_{Kj}}{\Delta \Lambda_{0Kj}} \Big| K \right\} \right\}$$

$$= E_K\left\{ \sum_{j=1}^{K} E\left\{ E\left\{ e^{\theta_0' Z} \Delta \Lambda_{0Kj} \right. \right. \right.$$

$$\left. \left. \left. \left(Z - \frac{\Delta a_{Kj}^*}{\Delta \Lambda_{0Kj}} \right) \frac{\Delta a_{Kj}}{\Delta \Lambda_{0Kj}} \Big| K, T_{K,j-1}, T_{K,j} \right\} \Big| K \right\} \right\}$$

$$= E_K \left\{ \sum_{j=1}^{K} E\left\{ \Delta\Lambda_{0Kj} \frac{\Delta a_{Kj}}{\Delta\Lambda_{0Kj}} \left(E\left\{ Ze^{\theta'_0 Z} | K, T_{K,j-1}, T_{K,j} \right\} \right. \right. \right.$$

$$\left. \left. \left. - \frac{\Delta a^*_{Kj}}{\Delta\Lambda_{0Kj}} E\left\{ e^{\theta'_0 Z} | K, T_{K,j-1}, T_{K,j} \right\} \right) \Big| K \right\} \right\}.$$

Thus we see that the desired orthogonality holds with

$$\frac{\Delta a^*_{Kj}}{\Delta\Lambda_{0Kj}} = \frac{E\left\{ Ze^{\theta'_0 Z} | K, T_{K,j-1}, T_{K,j} \right\}}{E\left\{ e^{\theta'_0 Z} | K, T_{K,j-1}, T_{K,j} \right\}}. \tag{6}$$

Hence the efficient score function for θ is given by

$$l^*_\theta(x) = \dot{l}_\theta(x) - \dot{l}_\Lambda a^*(x)$$

$$= \sum_{j=1}^{K} (\Delta\mathbb{N}_{Kj} - e^{\theta' Z} \Delta\Lambda_{0Kj}) \left(Z - \frac{E\left\{ Ze^{\theta' Z} | K, T_{K,j-1}, T_{K,j} \right\}}{E\left\{ e^{\theta' Z} | K, T_{K,j-1}, T_{K,j} \right\}} \right),$$

and the information for θ is, by computing conditionally on Z, K, T_K,

$$I(\theta) = E_0 \left\{ l^*_\theta(X)^{\otimes 2} \right\}$$

$$= E_0 \left\{ \sum_{j=1}^{K} e^{\theta'_0 Z} \Delta\Lambda_{0Kj} \left(Z - \frac{E\left\{ Ze^{\theta'_0 Z} | K, T_{K,j-1}, T_{K,j} \right\}}{E\left\{ e^{\theta'_0 Z} | K, T_{K,j-1}, T_{K,j} \right\}} \right)^{\otimes 2} \right\}.$$

In particular, we have the following corollary:

Corollary 1. (Current status data). If $P(K = 1) = 1$ (so that the only T_{Kj} of relevance is $T_{1,1} \equiv T$ while $T_{1,0} = 0$), then the efficient score function is

$$l^*_\theta(x) = \dot{l}_\theta(x) - \dot{l}_\Lambda a^*(x) = (\mathbb{N}(T) - e^{\theta'_0 Z} \Lambda_0(T)) \left(Z - \frac{E\left\{ Ze^{\theta'_0 Z} | T \right\}}{E\left\{ e^{\theta'_0 Z} | T \right\}} \right).$$

and the information for θ is given by

$$I(\theta) = E_0 \left\{ l^*_\theta(X)^{\otimes 2} \right\} = E_0 \left\{ e^{\theta'_0 Z} \Lambda_0(T) \left(Z - \frac{E\left\{ Ze^{\theta'_0 Z} | T \right\}}{E\left\{ e^{\theta'_0 Z} | T \right\}} \right)^{\otimes 2} \right\}.$$

This can be compared with the information for θ for the Cox proportional hazards model with current status data given by HUANG (1996), page 547 (with Huang's Y replaced by our present T for comparison):

$$I(\theta) = E\left\{ R(T, Z) \left\{ Z - \frac{E(ZR(T, Z) | T)}{E(R(T, Z) | T)} \right\}^{\otimes 2} \right\}$$

where $R(T, Z) = \Lambda^2(T, Z)O(T|Z)$ and

$$O(t|z) = \frac{\overline{F}(t|z)}{1 - \overline{F}(t|z)} = \frac{(1 - F_0(t))^{\exp(\theta_0' z)}}{1 - (1 - F_0(t))^{\exp(\theta_0' z)}}.$$

Corollary 2. (Case 2 Interval-censored data). If $P(K = 2) = 1$ (so that the only T_{Kj}'s of relevance are $T_{2,1} \equiv T_1$ and $T_{2,2} = T_2$, while $T_{2,0} = 0$), then the efficient score function is

$$l_\theta^*(x) = \dot{l}_\theta(x) - \dot{l}_\Lambda a^*(x)$$

$$= (\mathbb{N}(T_1) - e^{\theta_0' Z} \Lambda_0(T_1)) \left(Z - \frac{E\left\{ Z e^{\theta_0' Z} | T_1 \right\}}{E\left\{ e^{\theta_0' Z} | T_1 \right\}} \right)$$

$$+ \mathbb{N}(T_2) - \mathbb{N}(T_1)$$

$$- e^{\theta_0' Z} (\Lambda_0(T_2) - \Lambda_0(T_1))) \left(Z - \frac{E\left\{ Z e^{\theta_0' Z} | T_1, T_2 \right\}}{E\left\{ e^{\theta_0' Z} | T_1, T_2 \right\}} \right),$$

and the information for θ is given by

$$I(\theta) = E_0 \left\{ l_\theta^*(X)^{\otimes 2} \right\}$$

$$= E_0 \left\{ e^{\theta_0' Z} \Lambda_0(T_1) \left(Z - \frac{E\left\{ Z e^{\theta_0' Z} | T_1 \right\}}{E\left\{ e^{\theta_0' Z} | T_1 \right\}} \right)^{\otimes 2} \right\}$$

$$+ E_0 \left\{ e^{\theta_0' Z} (\Lambda_0(T_2) - \Lambda_0(T_2)) \left(Z - \frac{E\left\{ Z e^{\theta_0' Z} | T_1, T_2 \right\}}{E\left\{ e^{\theta_0' Z} | T_1, T_2 \right\}} \right)^{\otimes 2} \right\}.$$

This is much simpler than the information for θ for the Cox proportional hazards model with interval censored case II data given by HUANG AND WELLNER (1995). The calculations of Huang and Wellner resulted in an integral equation to be solved, analogously to the results for the mean functional considered by GESKUS AND GROENEBOOM (1996), GESKUS AND GROENEBOOM (1997), and GESKUS AND GROENEBOOM (1999).

4 Asymptotic normality of the two estimators of θ.

Here is the crucial theorem concerning the asymptotic behavior of the maximum pseudo-likelihood and maximum likelihood estimators of θ when the proportional mean model holds, but the Poisson assumption concerning $\mathbb{N}$ may fail.

Theorem 1. Under suitable regularity and integrability conditions, the estimators $\widehat{\theta}_n^{ps}$ and $\widehat{\theta}_n$ are asymptotically normal:

$$\sqrt{n}(\widehat{\theta}_n - \theta_0) \to_d Z \sim N_d\left(0, A^{-1}B\left(A^{-1}\right)'\right), \tag{7}$$

and

$$\sqrt{n}(\widehat{\theta}_n^{ps} - \theta_0) \to_d Z^{ps} \sim N_d\left(0, (A^{ps})^{-1}B^{ps}\left((A^{ps})^{-1}\right)'\right) \tag{8}$$

where

$$B \equiv Em^*(\theta_0, \Lambda_0; X)^{\otimes 2}$$

$$= E\left\{ \sum_{j,j'=1}^{K} C_{j,j'}(Z) \left[Z - \frac{E\left(Ze^{\theta_0'Z}|K, T_{K,j}, T_{K,j'}\right)}{E\left(e^{\theta_0'Z}|K, T_{K,j}, T_{K,j'}\right)} \right]^{\otimes 2} \right\},$$

$$A = E\left\{ \sum_{j=1}^{K} \Delta\Lambda_{0Kj} e^{\theta_0'Z} \left[Z - \frac{E\left(Ze^{\theta_0'Z}|K, T_{K,j-1}, T_{K,j}\right)}{E\left(e^{\theta_0'Z}|K, T_{K,j-1}, T_{K,j}\right)} \right]^{\otimes 2} \right\},$$

$$C_{j,j'}(Z) = \mathrm{Cov}\left[\Delta N_{Kj}, \Delta N_{Kj'}|Z, K, \underline{T}_K\right],$$

$$B^{ps} = Em^{*ps}(\theta_0, \Lambda_0; X)^{\otimes 2}$$

$$= E\left\{ \sum_{j,j'=1}^{K} C_{j,j'}^{ps}(Z) \left[Z - \frac{E\left(Ze^{\theta_0'Z}|K, T_{K,j}\right)}{E\left(e^{\theta_0'Z}|K, T_{K,j}\right)} \right] \right.$$

$$\left. \left[Z - \frac{E\left(Ze^{\theta_0'Z}|K, T_{K,j'}\right)}{E\left(e^{\theta_0'Z}|K, T_{K,j'}\right)} \right]' \right\},$$

$$A^{ps} = E\left\{ \sum_{j=1}^{K} \Lambda_{0Kj} e^{\theta_0'Z} \left[Z - \frac{E\left(Ze^{\theta_0'Z}|K, T_{K,j}\right)}{E\left(e^{\theta_0'Z}|K, T_{K,j}\right)} \right]^{\otimes 2} \right\},$$

$$C_{j,j'}^{ps}(Z) = \mathrm{Cov}\left[N_{Kj}, N_{Kj'}|Z, K, T_{K,j}, T_{K,j'}\right].$$

Our proof of this theorem is based on the results of ZHANG (1998). While we will not give the proof in detail, we will present here a sketch of the computation of the asymptotic variances given in (7) and (8).

Based on the Poisson model, the log-likelihood for (θ, Λ) with one observation is given by

$$m(\theta, \Lambda; X) = \log p(X; \theta, \Lambda) = \sum_{j=1}^{K} \{\Delta \mathbb{N}_{Kj} \log \Delta \Lambda_{Kj} - \Delta \Lambda_{Kj} - \log(\Delta \mathbb{N}_{Kj}!)\}$$

$$= \sum_{j=1}^{K} \{\Delta \mathbb{N}_{Kj} \log \Delta \Lambda_{Kj} + \Delta \mathbb{N}_{Kj} \theta' Z$$

$$- e^{\theta' Z} \Delta \Lambda_{0Kj} - \log(\Delta \mathbb{N}_{Kj}!)\} . \tag{9}$$

Thus the log-likelihood $l_n(\theta, \Lambda)$ for n i.i.d. observations is given by

$$l_n(\theta, \Lambda) = n \mathbb{P}_n m(\theta, \Lambda; \cdot) . \tag{10}$$

The maximum likelihood estimators $(\hat{\theta}, \hat{\Lambda})$ are obtained by maximizing (10).

A natural pseudo-likelihood is obtained by simply taking the product of the marginal distributions of the observed counts at the successive observation times. Thus a log-pseudo-likelihood for one observation is given by

$$m^{ps}(\theta, \Lambda; X) = \sum_{j=1}^{K} \left\{ \mathbb{N}_{Kj} \log \Lambda_{Kj} + \mathbb{N}_{Kj} \theta' Z - e^{\theta' Z} \Lambda_{Kj} - \log(\mathbb{N}_{Kj}!) \right\} \tag{11}$$

with $\Lambda_{K,j} = \Lambda(T_{K,j})$, and the log-pseudo-likelihood $l_n^{ps}(\theta, \Lambda)$ for n i.i.d. observations is given by

$$l_n^{ps}(\theta, \Lambda) = n \mathbb{P}_n m^{ps}(\theta, \Lambda; \cdot) , \tag{12}$$

and the corresponding pseudo-MLE's $(\hat{\theta}^{ps}, \hat{\Lambda}^{ps})$ are obtained by maximizing (12).

4.1 Asymptotic variance of the MLE

Based on the Poisson model, the log-likelihood for (θ, Λ) with one observation is given by (9). Using the notation of ZHANG (1998), page 29, we have

$$m_1(\theta, \Lambda; X) = \sum_{j=1}^{K} Z \left[\Delta \mathbb{N}_{Kj} - \Delta \Lambda_{Kj} e^{\theta' Z} \right],$$

$$m_2(\theta, \Lambda; X)[h] = \sum_{j=1}^{K} \left[\frac{\Delta \mathbb{N}_{Kj}}{\Delta \Lambda_{Kj}} - e^{\theta' Z} \right] \Delta h_{Kj},$$

$$m_{11}(\theta, \Lambda; X) = - \sum_{j=1}^{K} \Delta \Lambda_{Kj} Z Z' e^{\theta' Z},$$

$$m_{12}(\theta, \Lambda; X)[h] = m_{21}^T(\theta, \Lambda; X)[h] = - \sum_{j=1}^{K} Z e^{\theta' Z} \Delta h_{Kj},$$

$$m_{22}(\theta, \Lambda; X)[h, h] = - \sum_{j=1}^{K} \frac{\Delta \mathbb{N}_{Kj}}{(\Delta \Lambda_{Kj})^2} \Delta h_{Kj} \Delta h_{Kj},$$

where $\Delta h_{Kj} = \int_{T_{K,j-1}}^{T_{K,j}} h d\Lambda_0$ for $h \in L_2(\Lambda)$. By A2 of ZHANG (1998), page 30, we need to find a $\mathbf{h}^*$ such that

$$\dot{S}_{12}(\theta_0, \Lambda_0)[h] - \dot{S}_{22}(\theta_0, \Lambda_0)[\mathbf{h}^*, h]$$
$$= P\{m_{12}(\theta_0, \Lambda_0; X)[h] - m_{22}(\theta_0, \Lambda_0; X)[\mathbf{h}^*, h]\} = 0,$$

for all $h \in L_2(\Lambda_0)$. Note that

$$P\{m_{12}(\theta_0, \Lambda_0; X)[h] - m_{22}(\theta_0, \Lambda_0; X)[\mathbf{h}^*, h]\}$$

$$= -E\left\{\sum_{j=1}^{K}\left[Ze^{\theta_0'Z} - \frac{\Delta N_{Kj}}{(\Delta\Lambda_{0Kj})^2}\Delta\mathbf{h}^*_{Kj}\right]\Delta h_{Kj}\right\}$$

$$= -E_{(K,T_K,Z)}\left\{\sum_{j=1}^{K}\left[Ze^{\theta_0'Z} - \frac{e^{\theta_0'Z}\Delta\mathbf{h}^*_{Kj}}{\Delta\Lambda_{0Kj}}\right]\Delta h_{Kj}\right\}.$$

Therefore, an obvious choice of $\mathbf{h}^*$ is

$$\Delta\mathbf{h}^*_{Kj} = \Delta\Lambda_{0Kj}\frac{E\left(Ze^{\theta_0'Z}|K, T_{K,j-1}, T_{K,j}\right)}{E\left(e^{\theta_0'Z}|K, T_{K,j-1}, T_{K,j}\right)}.$$

Hence

$$m^*(\theta_0, \Lambda_0; X)$$
$$= m_1(\theta_0, \Lambda_0; X) - m_2(\theta_0, \Lambda_0; X)[\mathbf{h}^*]$$
$$= \sum_{j=1}^{K}\left\{Z\left(\Delta N_{Kj} - e^{\theta_0'Z}\Delta\Lambda_{0Kj}\right)\right.$$

$$\left. - \left(\frac{\Delta N_{Kj}}{\Delta\Lambda_{0Kj}} - e^{\theta_0'Z}\right)\Delta\Lambda_{0Kj}\frac{E\left(Ze^{\theta_0'Z}|K, T_{K,j-1}, T_{K,j}\right)}{E\left(e^{\theta_0'Z}|K, T_{K,j-1}, T_{K,j}\right)}\right\}$$

$$= \sum_{j=1}^{K}\left(\Delta N_{Kj} - e^{\theta_0'Z}\Delta\Lambda_{0Kj}\right)\left[Z - \frac{E\left(Ze^{\theta_0'Z}|K, T_{K,j-1}, T_{K,j}\right)}{E\left(e^{\theta_0'Z}|K, T_{K,j-1}, T_{K,j}\right)}\right].$$

By Theorem 2.3.5 of ZHANG (1998), page 32, the asymptotic variance will be $A^{-1}B\left(A^{-1}\right)'$, where

$$B = Em^*(\theta_0, \Lambda_0; X)^{\otimes 2}$$

$$= E_{(K,T_K,Z)}\left\{\sum_{j,j'=1}^{K} C(T_{K,j}, T_{K,j'}, T_{K,j-1}, T_{K,j'-1}; Z)\right.$$

$$\left[Z - \frac{E\left(Ze^{\theta_0'Z}|K, T_{K,j-1}, T_{K,j}\right)}{E\left(e^{\theta_0'Z}|K, T_{K,j-1}, T_{K,j}\right)}\right.$$

$$\left[Z - \frac{E\left(Ze^{\theta_0'Z}|K,T_{K,j'-1},T_{K,j'}\right)}{E\left(e^{\theta_0'Z}|K,T_{K,j'-1},T_{K,j'}\right)}\right]'\right\},$$

$$A = - \dot{S}_{11}(\theta_0,\Lambda_0) + \dot{S}_{21}(\theta_0,\Lambda_0)[\mathbf{h}^*]$$

$$= E\left\{\sum_{j=1}^{K}\left[\Delta\Lambda_{0Kj}e^{\theta_0'Z}ZZ'\right.\right.$$

$$\left.\left. - e^{\theta_0'Z}\Delta\Lambda_{0Kj}\frac{E\left(Ze^{\theta_0'Z}|K,T_{K,j'-1},T_{K,j'}\right)}{E\left(e^{\theta_0'Z}|K,T_{K,j'-1},T_{K,j'}\right)}Z'\right]\right\}$$

$$= E_{(K,T_K,Z)}\left\{\sum_{j=1}^{K}\Delta\Lambda_{0Kj}e^{\theta_0'Z}\left[Z - \frac{E\left(Ze^{\theta_0'Z}|K,T_{K,j-1},T_{K,j}\right)}{E\left(e^{\theta_0'Z}|K,T_{K,j-1},T_{K,j}\right)}\right]Z'\right\}$$

$$= E_{(K,T_K,Z)}\left\{\sum_{j=1}^{K}\Delta\Lambda_{0Kj}e^{\theta_0'Z}\left[Z - \frac{E\left(Ze^{\theta_0'Z}|K,T_{K,j-1},T_{K,j}\right)}{E\left(e^{\theta_0'Z}|K,T_{K,j-1},T_{K,j}\right)}\right]^{\otimes 2}\right\},$$

and

$$C(T_{K,j},T_{K,j'},T_{K,j-1},T_{K,j'-1};Z)$$
$$= E\left[\left(\Delta\mathbb{N}_{Kj} - e^{\theta_0'Z}\Delta\Lambda_{0Kj}\right)\right.$$
$$\left.\left(\Delta\mathbb{N}_{Kj'} - e^{\theta_0'Z}\Delta\Lambda_{0Kj'}\right)|Z,K,T_{K,j-1},T_{K,j},T_{K,j'-1},T_{K,j'}\right].$$

Note that if the counting process is indeed a conditional Poisson process with the mean function given as specified,

$$C(T_{K,j},T_{K,j'},T_{K,j-1},T_{K,j'-1};Z) = \begin{cases} \Delta\Lambda_{0Kj}e^{\theta_0'Z} &, \text{ if } j = j' \\ 0 &, \text{ if } j \neq j'. \end{cases}$$

This yields $B = A = I(\theta_0)$ and thus $A^{-1}B\left(A^{-1}\right)' = I^{-1}(\theta_0)$.

4.2 Asymptotic Variance of the Pseudo-MLE

Based on the Poisson model, the pseudo log-likelihood for (θ,Λ) with one observation is given by (11). Using the notation of Zhang (1998), page 29, we have

$$m_1^{ps}(\theta,\Lambda;X) = \sum_{j=1}^{K}Z\left[\mathbb{N}_{Kj} - \Lambda_{Kj}e^{\theta'Z}\right],$$

$$m_2^{ps}(\theta, \Lambda; X)[h] = \sum_{j=1}^{K} \left[\frac{\mathbb{N}_{Kj}}{\Lambda_{Kj}} - e^{\theta' Z} \right] h_{Kj},$$

$$m_{11}^{ps}(\theta, \Lambda; X) = -\sum_{j=1}^{K} \Lambda_{Kj} Z Z' e^{\theta' Z},$$

$$m_{12}^{ps}(\theta, \Lambda; X)[h] = m_{21}^{T}(\theta, \Lambda; X)[h] = -\sum_{j=1}^{K} Z e^{\theta' Z} h_{Kj},$$

$$m_{22}^{ps}(\theta, \Lambda; X)[\mathbf{h}, h] = -\sum_{j=1}^{K} \frac{\mathbb{N}_{Kj}}{(\Lambda_{Kj})^2} \mathbf{h}_{Kj} h_{Kj},$$

where $h_{Kj} = \int_0^{T_{K,j}} h \, d\Lambda$ for $h \in L_2(\Lambda)$. By A2 of ZHANG (1998), page 30, we need to find a $\mathbf{h}^*$ such that

$$\dot{S}_{12}^{ps}(\theta_0, \Lambda_0)[h] - \dot{S}_{22}^{ps}(\theta_0, \Lambda_0)[\mathbf{h}^*, h]$$
$$= P \{ m_{12}^{ps}(\theta_0, \Lambda_0; X)[h] - m_{22}^{ps}(\theta_0, \Lambda_0; X)[\mathbf{h}^*, h] \} = 0,$$

for all $h \in L_2(\Lambda_0)$. Note that

$$P \{ m_{12}^{ps}(\theta_0, \Lambda_0; X)[h] - m_{22}^{ps}(\theta_0, \Lambda_0; X)[\mathbf{h}^*, h] \}$$

$$= - E \left\{ \sum_{j=1}^{K} \left[Z e^{\theta_0' Z} - \frac{\mathbb{N}_{Kj}}{(\Lambda_{0Kj})^2} \mathbf{h}_{Kj}^* \right] h_{Kj} \right\}$$

$$= - E_{(K, T_K, Z)} \left\{ \sum_{j=1}^{K} \left[Z e^{\theta_0' Z} - \frac{e^{\theta_0' Z} \mathbf{h}_{Kj}^*}{\Lambda_{0Kj}} \right] h_{Kj} \right\}.$$

Therefore, an obvious choice of $\mathbf{h}^*$ is

$$\mathbf{h}_{Kj}^* = \Lambda_{0Kj} \frac{E \left(Z e^{\theta_0' Z} | K, T_{K,j} \right)}{E \left(e^{\theta_0' Z} | K, T_{K,j} \right)}.$$

Hence

$$m^{*ps}(\theta_0, \Lambda_0; X)$$
$$= m_1^{ps}(\theta_0, \Lambda_0; X) - m_2^{ps}(\theta_0, \Lambda_0; X)[\mathbf{h}^*]$$

$$= \sum_{j=1}^{K} \left\{ Z \left(\mathbb{N}_{Kj} - e^{\theta_0' Z} \Lambda_{0Kj} \right) - \left(\frac{\mathbb{N}_{Kj}}{\Lambda_{0Kj}} - e^{\theta_0' Z} \right) \Lambda_{0Kj} \frac{E \left(Z e^{\theta_0' Z} | K, T_{K,j} \right)}{E \left(e^{\theta_0' Z} | K, T_{K,j} \right)} \right\}$$

$$= \sum_{j=1}^{K} \left(\mathbb{N}_{Kj} - e^{\theta_0' Z} \Lambda_{0Kj} \right) \left[Z - \frac{E \left(Z e^{\theta_0' Z} | K, T_{K,j} \right)}{E \left(e^{\theta_0' Z} | K, T_{K,j} \right)} \right].$$

By Theorem 2.3.5 of ZHANG (1998), page 32, the asymptotic variance will be $(A^{ps})^{-1} B^{ps} \left((A^{ps})^{-1}\right)'$, where

$$B^{ps} = Em^{*ps}(\theta_0, \Lambda_0; X)^{\otimes 2}$$

$$= E_{(K,T_K,Z)} \left\{ \sum_{j,j'=1}^{K} C^{ps}(T_{K,j}, T_{K,j'}; Z) \left[Z - \frac{E\left(Ze^{\theta_0'Z}|K, T_{K,j}\right)}{E\left(e^{\theta_0'Z}|K, T_{K,j}\right)} \right] \right.$$

$$\left. \left[Z - \frac{E\left(Ze^{\theta_0'Z}|K, T_{K,j'}\right)}{E\left(e^{\theta_0'Z}|K, T_{K,j'}\right)} \right]' \right\},$$

$$A^{ps} = - \dot{S}_{11}^{ps}(\theta_0, \Lambda_0) + \dot{S}_{21}^{ps}(\theta_0, \Lambda_0)[h^*]$$

$$= E \left\{ \sum_{j=1}^{K} \left[\Lambda_{0Kj} e^{\theta_0'Z} ZZ' - e^{\theta_0'Z} \Lambda_{0Kj} \frac{E\left(Ze^{\theta_0'Z}|K, T_{K,j'}\right)}{E\left(e^{\theta_0'Z}|K, T_{K,j'}\right)} Z' \right] \right\}$$

$$= E_{(K,T_K,Z)} \left\{ \sum_{j=1}^{K} \Lambda_{0Kj} e^{\theta_0'Z} \left[Z - \frac{E\left(Ze^{\theta_0'Z}|K, T_{K,j}\right)}{E\left(e^{\theta_0'Z}|K, T_{K,j}\right)} \right] Z' \right\}$$

$$= E_{(K,T_K,Z)} \left\{ \sum_{j=1}^{K} \Lambda_{0Kj} e^{\theta_0'Z} \left[Z - \frac{E\left(Ze^{\theta_0'Z}|K, T_{K,j}\right)}{E\left(e^{\theta_0'Z}|K, T_{K,j}\right)} \right]^{\otimes 2} \right\},$$

and

$$C^{ps}(T_{K,j}, T_{K,j'}; Z)$$
$$= E\left[\left(\mathbb{N}_{Kj} - e^{\theta_0'Z}\Lambda_{0Kj}\right)\left(\mathbb{N}_{Kj'} - e^{\theta_0'Z}\Lambda_{0Kj'}\right)|Z, K, T_{K,j}, T_{K,j'}\right].$$

Note that if the counting process is indeed a conditional Poisson process with the mean function given as specified,

$$C^{ps}(T_{K,j}, T_{K,j'}; Z) = e^{\theta_0'Z}\Lambda_{0K(j\wedge j')}.$$

This yields

$$B^{ps} = A^{ps} + 2E_{(K,T_K,Z)} \left\{ \sum_{j<j'} e^{\theta_0 Z} \Lambda_{0Kj} \left[Z - \frac{E\left(Ze^{\theta_0'Z}|K, T_{K,j}\right)}{E\left(e^{\theta_0'Z}|K, T_{K,j}\right)} \right] \right.$$

$$\left. \left[Z - \frac{E\left(Ze^{\theta_0'Z}|K, T_{K,j'}\right)}{E\left(e^{\theta_0'Z}|K, T_{K,j'}\right)} \right]' \right\}$$

$$\neq A^{ps}.$$

5 Comparisons: MLE versus pseudo-MLE.

Scenario 1. We first suppose that the underlying counting process is in fact a standard homogeneous Poisson process conditionally given Z, with baseline mean function $\Lambda_0(t) = \lambda t$, We will also assume that the distribution of $(K, \underline{T}_K)$ is independent of Z. As a consequence, Z is independent of $(K, \underline{T}_K)$, and the formulas in the preceding section simplify considerably. Because of the Poisson process assumption, $A = B = I(\theta_0)$, and this matrix is given by

$$I(\theta_0) = E_{(K, T_K, Z)} \left\{ \sum_{j=1}^{K} \Delta \Lambda_{0Kj} e^{\theta_0' Z} \left[Z - \frac{E\left(Z e^{\theta_0' Z} | K, T_{K,j-1}, T_{K,j}\right)}{E\left(e^{\theta_0' Z} | K, T_{K,j-1}, T_{K,j}\right)} \right]^{\otimes 2} \right\}$$

$$= E_{(K, T_K)} \left\{ \Lambda_0(T_{K,K}) \right\} E_Z \left\{ e^{\theta_0' Z} \left[Z - \frac{E\left(Z e^{\theta_0' Z}\right)}{E\left(e^{\theta_0' Z}\right)} \right]^{\otimes 2} \right\}$$

$$\equiv E_{(K, T_K)} \left\{ \Lambda_0(T_{K,K}) \right\} C,$$

so that if C is nonsingular,

$$I(\theta_0)^{-1} = C^{-1} \frac{1}{E_{(K, T_K)} \left\{ \Lambda_0(T_{K,K}) \right\}}.$$

On the other hand,

$$A^{ps} = E_{(K, T_K, Z)} \left\{ \sum_{j=1}^{K} \Lambda_{0Kj} e^{\theta_0' Z} \left[Z - \frac{E\left(Z e^{\theta_0' Z} | K, T_{K,j}\right)}{E\left(e^{\theta_0' Z} | K, T_{K,j}\right)} \right]^{\otimes 2} \right\}$$

$$= E_{(K, T_K)} \left\{ \sum_{j=1}^{K} \Lambda_0(T_{Kj}) \right\} E \left\{ e^{\theta_0' Z} \left[Z - \frac{E\left(Z e^{\theta_0' Z}\right)}{E\left(e^{\theta_0' Z}\right)} \right]^{\otimes 2} \right\},$$

while

$$B^{ps} = E_{(K, T_K, Z)} \left\{ \sum_{j,j'=1}^{K} \Lambda_0(T_{K,j \wedge j'}) \right\} E_Z \left\{ e^{\theta_0' Z} \left[Z - \frac{E\left(Z e^{\theta_0' Z}\right)}{E\left(e^{\theta_0' Z}\right)} \right]^{\otimes 2} \right\},$$

so that

$$(A^{ps})^{-1} B^{ps} \left((A^{ps})^{-1}\right)' = C^{-1} \frac{E_{(K, T_K, Z)} \left\{ \sum_{j,j'=1}^{K} \Lambda_0(T_{K,j \wedge j'}) \right\}}{\left(E_{(K, T_K)} \left\{ \sum_{j=1}^{K} \Lambda_0(T_{Kj}) \right\}\right)^2}.$$

Thus it follows that the ARE of the pseudo-MLE of θ_0 relative to the MLE of θ_0 under the above scenario is given by

$$ARE(pseudo, mle) = \frac{A^{-1}B(A^{-1})^T}{(A^{ps})^{-1}B^{ps}((A^{ps})^{-1})^T}$$

$$= \frac{\left\{E\left\{\sum_{j=1}^{K}\Lambda_0(T_{K,j})\right\}\right\}^2}{E\left\{\Lambda_0(T_{K,K})\right\}E\left\{\sum_{j,j'=1}^{K}\Lambda_0(T_{K,j\wedge j'})\right\}}.$$

Note that this equals 1 if $P(K = 1) = 1$. Actually, we have not yet used the assumption about Λ_0. If we assume that $\Lambda_0(t) = \lambda t$, then

$$ARE(pseudo, mle) = \frac{\left\{E\left\{\sum_{j=1}^{K}T_{K,j}\right\}\right\}^2}{E\left\{T_{K,K}\right\}E\left\{\sum_{j,j'=1}^{K}T_{K,j\wedge j'}\right\}}$$

Scenario 1A. If we assume, further, that $P(K = k) = 1$ for a fixed integer $k \geq 2$, and $\underline{T}_K = (T_{K,1}, \ldots, T_{K,K})$ are the order statistics of a sample of k uniformly distributed random variables on an interval $[0, M]$, then

$$E\left\{\sum_{j=1}^{K}T_{K,j}\right\} = \sum_{j=1}^{k}\frac{j}{k+1}M = \frac{k}{2}M,$$

$$E\left\{T_{K,K}\right\} = \frac{k}{k+1}M,$$

and

$$E\left\{\sum_{j,j'=1}^{K}T_{K,j\wedge j'}\right\} = \sum_{j,j'=1}^{k}\frac{j\wedge j'}{k+1}M = \frac{k(2k+1)}{6}M.$$

Hence in this case

$$ARE(pseudo, mle) = \frac{(k/2)^2}{\frac{k}{k+1}\frac{k(2k+1)}{6}} = \frac{3(k+1)}{2(2k+1)} \to \frac{3}{4}$$

as $k \to \infty$.

k	1	2	3	4	5	6	7	8	9	10
$I(\theta)^{-1}(k)M\lambda$	2	3/2	4/3	5/4	6/5	7/6	8/7	9/8	10/9	11/10
$V^{ps}(k)M\lambda$	2	5/3	14/9	3/2	22/15	13/9	10/7	17/12	38/27	7/5
$ARE(k)$	1.00	.900	0.857	0.833	0.818	0.808	0.800	0.794	0.789	0.786

Scenario 1B. If we assume instead that K is random and for some $0 \leq c < 1/2$

$$T_{K,j} \sim \text{Uniform}[j - c, j + c], \qquad j = 1, \ldots, K,$$

and are independent (conditionally on K), then we calculate

$$E(T_{K,K}) = E(K),$$

$$E(\sum_{j=1}^{K} T_{K,j}) = E\left(\frac{K(K+1)}{2}\right),$$

$$E(\sum_{j,j'=1}^{K} T_{K,j \wedge j'}) = E\left(\frac{K(K+1)(2K+1)}{6}\right),$$

and hence

$$ARE(pseudo, mle) = \frac{\left\{E\left(\frac{K(K+1)}{2}\right)\right\}^2}{E(K)E\left(\frac{K(K+1)(2K+1)}{6}\right)}.$$

Note that this depends only on the first three moments of K, with the third moment appearing in the denominator. It does not depend on c, but only on $E(T_{K,j}|K) = j$, $j = 1, \ldots, K$. When $P(K = k) = 1$ we find that under this scenario

$$ARE(pseudo, mle) = \frac{3(k+1)}{2(2k+1)} \geq \frac{3}{4}.$$

It is clear that for random K the ARE in this scenario can be arbitrarily small if the distribution of K is heavy-tailed. This will be shown in more detail in Scenario 2.

Scenario 2. A variant on these calculations is to repeat all the assumptions about Z and $(K, \underline{T}_K)$, assume, conditionally on K, that $\underline{T}_K = (T_{K,1}, \ldots, T_{K,K})$ are the order statistics of a sample of K uniformly distributed random variables on an interval $[0, M]$, but now allow a distribution for K. Then

$$E\left\{\sum_{j=1}^{K} T_{K,j}\Big|K\right\} = \sum_{j=1}^{K} \frac{j}{K+1}M = \frac{K}{2}M,$$

$$E\left\{T_{K,K}\Big|K\right\} = \frac{K}{K+1}M,$$

and

$$E\left\{\sum_{j,j'=1}^{K} T_{K,j \wedge j'}\Big|K\right\} = \sum_{j,j'=1}^{K} \frac{j \wedge j'}{K+1}M = \frac{K(2K+1)}{6}M.$$

If we let K be distributed according to 1+Poisson(μ), then the ARE will be asymptotically 3/4 again as $\mu \to \infty$. A more interesting choice of the distribution of K is the Zeta(α) distribution given as follows: for $\alpha > 1$,

$$P(K = k) = \frac{1/k^\alpha}{\zeta(\alpha)}, \qquad k = 1, 2, \ldots,$$

where $\zeta(\alpha) = \sum_{j=1}^{\infty} j^{-\alpha}$ is the Riemann Zeta function. Then we can compute

$$E\left\{\sum_{j=1}^{K} T_{K,j}\right\} = E\left\{\sum_{j=1}^{K} \frac{j}{K+1}\right\} M = \frac{E_\alpha(K)}{2} M = \frac{M}{2}\frac{\zeta(\alpha-1)}{\zeta(\alpha)},$$

$$E\{T_{K,K}\} = E_\alpha\left(\frac{K}{K+1}\right) M,$$

and

$$E\left\{\sum_{j,j'=1}^{K} T_{K,j\wedge j'}\right\} = E_\alpha\left(\sum_{j,j'=1}^{K} \frac{j\wedge j'}{K+1}\right) M$$

$$= \frac{M}{6} E_\alpha(K(2K+1))$$

$$= \frac{M}{6}\left\{2E_\alpha(K^2) + E_\alpha(K)\right\}$$

$$= \frac{M}{6}\left\{\frac{2\zeta(\alpha-2) + \zeta(\alpha-1)}{\zeta(\alpha)}\right\}$$

Hence in this case

$$I(\theta)^{-1}(\alpha) = C^{-1}\frac{1}{M\lambda E_\alpha\left(\frac{K}{K+1}\right)},$$

$$V^{ps}(\alpha) = C^{-1}\frac{\left\{\frac{2\zeta(\alpha-2)+\zeta(\alpha-1)}{\zeta(\alpha)}\right\}}{6M\lambda\left(\frac{\zeta(\alpha-1)}{2\zeta(\alpha)}\right)^2},$$

and

$$ARE(pseudo, mle)(\alpha) \equiv ARE(\alpha)$$

$$= \frac{(E_\alpha(K)/2)^2}{E_\alpha\{\frac{K}{K+1}\}E_\alpha\frac{K(2K+1)}{6}}$$

$$= \frac{3}{2}\frac{\zeta(\alpha-1)/\zeta(\alpha)}{E_\alpha\{\frac{K}{K+1}\}\frac{2\zeta(\alpha-2)+\zeta(\alpha-1)}{\zeta(\alpha)}}$$

$$= \frac{3}{2}\frac{\zeta(\alpha-1)}{\{2\zeta(\alpha-2) + \zeta(\alpha-1)\}E_\alpha\{\frac{K}{K+1}\}},$$

and this varies between 0 and 1 as α varies from 3 to ∞; note that for $\alpha = 3$, $E(K^2) = \infty = \zeta(1)$, while $E(K) = \zeta(2)/\zeta(3) \doteq 10.5844\ldots$. See Figure 1.

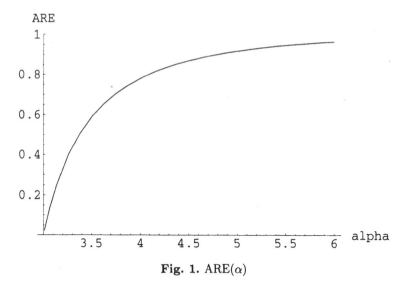

Fig. 1. ARE(α)

If we change the distribution of K to $K \sim \text{Unif}\{1,\ldots,k_0\}$, then

$$E\left\{\sum_{j=1}^{K} T_{K,j}\right\} = E\left\{\sum_{j=1}^{K} \frac{j}{K+1}\right\} M = \frac{E(K)}{2}M = \frac{k_0+1}{4}M,$$

$$\begin{aligned}
E\left\{\sum_{j,j'=1}^{K} T_{K,j\wedge j'}\right\} &= E_\alpha\left(\sum_{j,j'=1}^{K} \frac{j \wedge j'}{K+1}\right) M \\
&= \frac{M}{6}E(K(2K+1)) \\
&= \frac{M}{6}\{2E(K^2) + E(K)\} \\
&= \frac{M}{6}\left\{2\frac{(k_0+1)(2k_0+1)}{6} + \frac{k_0+1}{2}\right\}
\end{aligned}$$

while

$$E\{T_{K,K}\} = E\left(\frac{K}{K+1}\right) M,$$

Hence in this case

$$I(\theta)^{-1}(\alpha) = C^{-1}\frac{1}{M\lambda E\left(\frac{K}{K+1}\right)},$$

$$V^{ps}(k_0) = C^{-1}\frac{\frac{(k_0+1)(2k_0+1)/3+(k_0+1)/2}{6}}{M\lambda(k_0+1)^2/16},$$

and

$$ARE(pseudo, mle)(k_0) \equiv ARE(k_0)$$

$$= \frac{(E(K)/2)^2}{E\{\frac{K}{K+1}\}E\frac{K(2K+1)}{6}}$$

$$= \frac{(k_0+1)^2/16}{E\{\frac{K}{K+1}\}\frac{(k_0+1)(2k_0+1)/3+(k_0+1)/2}{6}},$$

and this varies between 1 and 9/16 as k_0 varies from 1 to ∞.

Scenario 3. We now suppose that the underlying counting process is *not* a Poisson process, conditionally given Z, but is, instead, defined as in terms of the "negative-binomialization" of an empirical counting process, as follows: suppose that $X_1, X_2, \ldots$ are i.i.d. with distribution function F on R, and define

$$\mathbb{N}_n(t) = \sum_{i=1}^{n} 1_{[X_i \leq t]} \qquad \text{for } t \geq 0.$$

Suppose that $(N|Z) \sim$ Negative Binomial$(r(Z, \gamma, \theta_0), p)$ where $r(Z, \gamma, \theta_0) = \gamma e^{\theta_0' Z}$, and define $\mathbb{N}$ by

$$\mathbb{N}(t) \equiv \mathbb{N}_N(t) = \sum_{i=1}^{N} 1_{[X_i \leq t]}.$$

Then, since

$$E(N|Z) = r(Z, \gamma, \theta_0)\frac{q}{p}, \qquad Var(N|Z) = r(Z, \gamma, \theta_0)\frac{q}{p^2},$$

it follows that

$$E\{\mathbb{N}(t)|Z\} = E\{E[\mathbb{N}(t)|Z, N]|Z\} = E\{NF(t)|Z\}$$
$$= \gamma e^{\theta_0' Z} F(t)\frac{q}{p} = e^{\theta_0' Z} \Lambda_0(t),$$

with $\Lambda_0(t) \equiv \gamma F(t)(q/p)$. Alternatively,

$$(\mathbb{N}(t)|Z) \sim \text{Negative Binomial}(r, \frac{p}{p+qF(t)})$$

by straightforward computation, and hence it follows that

$$E\{\mathbb{N}(t)|Z\} = r\frac{qF(t)/(p+qF(t))}{p/(p+qF(t))} = rF(t)\frac{q}{p} = \gamma e^{\theta_0' Z}\frac{q}{p}F(t) = e^{\theta_0' Z}\Lambda_0(t),$$

in agreement with the above calculation. Moreover

$$Var\{\mathbb{N}(t)|Z\} = r\frac{qF(t)/(p+qF(t))}{(p/(p+qF(t)))^2} = r\frac{q}{p}F(t)(1 + \frac{q}{p}F(t))$$

$$= r\frac{q}{p}F(t) + r\left(\frac{q}{p}\right)^2 F(t)^2.$$

Remark. It should be noted that this is somewhat different than the model obtained by supposing that the underlying counting process is a nonhomogeneous Poisson process conditionally given Z and an unobserved frailty $Y \sim \text{Gamma}(\gamma, \gamma)$ and conditional (on Y and Z) mean function

$$E\{\mathbb{N}(t)|Z, Y\} = Ye^{\theta_0' Z}\Lambda_0(t).$$

In this model we have

$$E\{\mathbb{N}(t)|Z\} = e^{\theta_0' Z}\Lambda_0(t),$$

but

$$Var\{\mathbb{N}(t)|Z\} = E\{Var[\mathbb{N}(t)|Y, Z]|Z\} + Var\{E[\mathbb{N}(t)|Y, Z]|Z\}$$
$$= e^{\theta_0' Z}\Lambda_0(t) + \gamma^{-1}e^{2\theta_0' Z}\Lambda_0^2(t).$$

Now we want to calculate

$$C(T_{K,j}, T_{K,j'}, T_{K,j-1}, T_{K,j'-1}; Z)$$
$$= E\left[\left(\Delta\mathbb{N}_{Kj} - e^{\theta_0' Z}\Delta\Lambda_{0Kj}\right)\right.$$
$$\left.\left(\Delta\mathbb{N}_{Kj'} - e^{\theta_0' Z}\Delta\Lambda_{0Kj'}\right)|Z, K, T_{K,j-1}, T_{K,j}, T_{K,j'-1}, T_{K,j'}\right].$$

By computing conditionally on N, and using the fact that conditionally on $Z, K, T_{K,j-1}, T_{K,j}, T_{K,j'-1}, T_{K,j'}$ and N, $\mathbb{N}$ has increments with a joint multinomial distribution, we find that

$$C(T_{K,j}, T_{K,j'}, T_{K,j-1}, T_{K,j'-1}; Z)$$
$$= E\left[\left(\Delta\mathbb{N}_{Kj} - e^{\theta_0' Z}\Delta\Lambda_{0Kj}\right)\right.$$
$$\left.\left(\Delta\mathbb{N}_{Kj'} - e^{\theta_0' Z}\Delta\Lambda_{0Kj'}\right)|Z, K, T_{K,j-1}, T_{K,j}, T_{K,j'-1}, T_{K,j'}\right]$$
$$= E\left\{E\left[\left(\Delta\mathbb{N}_{Kj} - E(\Delta\mathbb{N}_{Kj}|N) + E(\Delta\mathbb{N}_{Kj}|N) - e^{\theta_0' Z}\Delta\Lambda_{0Kj}\right)\right.\right.$$
$$\left.\cdot \left(\Delta\mathbb{N}_{Kj'} - E(\Delta\mathbb{N}_{Kj'}|N) + E(\Delta\mathbb{N}_{Kj'}|N) - e^{\theta_0' Z}\Delta\Lambda_{0Kj'}\right)\right.$$
$$\left.\left|N, Z, K, T_{K,j-1}, T_{K,j}, T_{K,j'-1}, T_{K,j'}\right.\right]$$
$$\left.\left|Z, K, T_{K,j-1}, T_{K,j}, T_{K,j'-1}, T_{K,j'}\right.\right\}$$

$$
= \begin{cases}
E\{N\Delta F_{Kj}(1 - \Delta F_{Kj})|Z, K, \underline{T}_K\} \\
\quad + E\{(N - rq/p)^2(\Delta F_{Kj})^2|Z, K, \underline{T}_K\}, & \text{if } j = j' \\
-E\{N\Delta F_{Kj}\Delta F_{Kj'}|Z, K, \underline{T}_K\} \\
\quad + E\{(N - rq/p)^2\Delta F_{Kj}\Delta F_{Kj'}|Z, K, \underline{T}_K\}, & \text{if } j \neq j'
\end{cases}
$$

$$
= \begin{cases}
r\frac{q}{p}\left(\Delta F_{K,j} - (\Delta F_{K,j})^2\right) + r\frac{q}{p^2}\Delta F_{K,j}^2, & \text{if } j = j' \\
\left\{r\frac{q}{p^2} - r\frac{q}{p}\right\}\Delta F_{Kj}\Delta F_{Kj'}, & \text{if } j \neq j'
\end{cases}
$$

$$
= \begin{cases}
r\frac{q}{p}\Delta F_{K,j} + r\frac{q^2}{p^2}(\Delta F_{K,j})^2, & \text{if } j = j' \\
r\frac{q^2}{p^2}\Delta F_{Kj}\Delta F_{Kj'}, & \text{if } j < j'
\end{cases}
$$

$$
= \begin{cases}
e^{\theta_0'Z}\Delta\Lambda_{0,K,j} + \gamma^{-1}e^{\theta_0'Z}\Delta(\Lambda_{0,K,j})^2, & \text{if } j = j', \\
\gamma e^{\theta_0'Z}\frac{q^2}{p^2}\Delta F_{Kj}\Delta F_{Kj'}, & \text{if } j \neq j',
\end{cases}
$$

$$
= \begin{cases}
e^{\theta_0'Z}\Delta\Lambda_{0,K,j} + \gamma^{-1}e^{\theta_0'Z}(\Delta\Lambda_{0,K,j})^2, & \text{if } j = j', \\
\gamma^{-1}e^{\theta_0'Z}\Delta\Lambda_{0Kj}\Delta\Lambda_{0Kj'}, & \text{if } j \neq j'.
\end{cases}
$$

Remark. Note that if $(N|Z) \sim \text{Poisson}(r(Z, \gamma, \theta_0))$, then the process $\mathbb{N} \equiv \mathbb{N}_N$ is conditionally, given Z, a non-homogeneous Poisson process with conditional mean function

$$
E\{\mathbb{N}(t)|Z\} = \gamma e^{\theta_0'Z}F(t) = e^{\theta_0'Z}\Lambda_0(t),
$$

and conditional variance function

$$
Var\{\mathbb{N}(t)|Z\} = \gamma e^{\theta_0'Z}F(t) = e^{\theta_0'Z}\Lambda_0(t)
$$

where $\Lambda_0(t) = \gamma F(t)$.

We will also assume, as in Scenarios 1 and 2, that the distribution of $(K, \underline{T}_K)$ is independent of Z. As a consequence, Z is independent of $(K, \underline{T}_K)$, and the formulas in the preceding section again simplify. By taking F uniform on $[0, M]$, $\Lambda_0(t) = \lambda t$ where $\lambda = (\gamma/M)(q/p)$, and we compute, using moments and covariances of uniform spacings, as found on page 721 of SHORACK AND WELLNER (1986),

$$
B = Em^*(\theta_0, \Lambda_0; X)^{\otimes 2}
$$

$$
= E_{(K,T_K,Z)}\left\{ \sum_{j,j'=1}^{K} C(T_{K,j}, T_{K,j'}, T_{K,j-1}, T_{K,j'-1}; Z) \right.
$$

$$
\left[Z - \frac{E\left(Ze^{\theta_0'Z}|K, T_{K,j-1}, T_{K,j}\right)}{E\left(e^{\theta_0'Z}|K, T_{K,j-1}, T_{K,j}\right)} \right]
$$

$$
\left. \left[Z - \frac{E\left(Ze^{\theta_0'Z}|K, T_{K,j'-1}, T_{K,j'}\right)}{E\left(e^{\theta_0'Z}|K, T_{K,j'-1}, T_{K,j'}\right)} \right]' \right\}
$$

$$= E_{(K,T_K,Z)} \left\{ \sum_{j=1}^{K} (e^{\theta_0' Z} \Delta\Lambda_{0Kj} \right.$$

$$\left. + \gamma^{-1} e^{\theta_0' Z} (\Delta\Lambda_{0Kj})^2) \left[Z - \frac{E\left(Z e^{\theta_0' Z}\right)}{E\left(e^{\theta_0' Z}\right)} \right]^{\otimes 2} \right\}$$

$$+ E_{(K,T_K,Z)} \left\{ \sum_{j \neq j'}^{K} \gamma^{-1} e^{\theta_0' Z} \Delta\Lambda_{0Kj} \Delta\Lambda_{0Kj'} \left[Z - \frac{E\left(Z e^{\theta_0' Z}\right)}{E\left(e^{\theta_0' Z}\right)} \right]^{\otimes 2} \right\}$$

$$= C \left\{ E_{K,T_K} \left\{ \sum_{j=1}^{K} (\Delta\Lambda_{0Kj} + \gamma^{-1}(\Delta\Lambda_{0Kj})^2) \right\} \right.$$

$$\left. + \gamma^{-1} E_{K,T_K} \left\{ \sum_{j \neq j'}^{K} \Delta\Lambda_{0Kj} \Delta\Lambda_{0Kj'} \right\} \right\}$$

$$= C \left\{ \lambda M E \left(\frac{K}{K+1} \right) + \gamma^{-1} \lambda^2 M^2 E \left(\frac{K}{K+2} \right) \right\}$$

$$= \lambda M C \left\{ E \left(\frac{K}{K+1} \right) + \gamma^{-1} \lambda M E \left(\frac{K}{K+2} \right) \right\}$$

where, as in scenario 1,

$$C \equiv E_Z \left\{ e^{\theta_0' Z} \left[Z - \frac{E\left(Z e^{\theta_0' Z}\right)}{E\left(e^{\theta_0' Z}\right)} \right]^{\otimes 2} \right\}.$$

On the other hand, we find that

$$A = E_{(K,T_K,Z)} \left\{ \sum_{j=1}^{K} \Delta\Lambda_{0Kj} e^{\theta_0' Z} \left[Z - \frac{E\left(Z e^{\theta_0' Z} | K, T_{K,j-1}, T_{K,j}\right)}{E\left(e^{\theta_0' Z} | K, T_{K,j-1}, T_{K,j}\right)} \right]^{\otimes 2} \right\}$$

$$= C \lambda M E \left\{ \frac{K}{K+1} \right\}.$$

Thus the asymptotic variance of the MLE for this scenario is

$$A^{-1} B (A^{-1})' = (\lambda M C)^{-1} \frac{E\left\{ \frac{K}{K+1} \right\} + \frac{\lambda M}{\gamma} E\left\{ \frac{K}{K+2} \right\}}{\left\{ E\left(\frac{K}{K+1} \right) \right\}^2}.$$

Now for the asymptotic variance of the pseudo-MLE under scenario 3. To calculate B^{ps} we first need to calculate

$$C^{ps}(T_{K,j}, T_{K,j'}; Z)$$

$$= E\left[\left(\mathbb{N}_{Kj} - e^{\theta_0' Z}\Lambda_{0Kj}\right)\left(\mathbb{N}_{Kj'} - e^{\theta_0' Z}\Lambda_{0Kj'}\right) | Z, K, T_{K,j}, T_{K,j'}\right]$$

$$= E\left\{E\left[\left(\mathbb{N}_{Kj} - e^{\theta_0' Z}\Lambda_{0Kj}\right)\left(\mathbb{N}_{Kj'} - e^{\theta_0' Z}\Lambda_{0Kj'}\right)\right.\right.$$
$$\left.\left.|N, Z, K, T_{K,j}, T_{K,j'}\right] \Big| Z, K, T_{K,j}, T_{K,j'}\right\}$$

$$= E\left\{N(F(T_{K,j} \wedge T_{K,j'}) - F(T_{K,j})F(T_{K,j'}))\right.$$
$$\left. + (N - rq/p)^2 F(T_{K,j})F(T_{K,j'}) \Big| Z, K, T_{K,j}, T_{K,j'}\right\}$$

$$= r\frac{q}{p}\{F(T_{K,j} \wedge T_{K,j'}) - F(T_{K,j})F(T_{K,j})\} + r\frac{q}{p^2}F(T_{K,j})F(T_{K,j'})$$

$$= e^{\theta_0' Z}\Lambda_0(T_{K,j} \wedge T_{K,j'}) + \gamma^{-1}e^{\theta_0' Z}\Lambda_0(T_{K,j})\Lambda_0(T_{K,j})$$

$$= e^{\theta_0' Z}\Lambda_0(T_{K,j})\left(1 + \gamma^{-1}\Lambda_0(T_{K,j'})\right) \qquad \text{if } j \le j'.$$

We can then calculate

$$B^{ps} = Em^{*ps}(\theta_0, \Lambda_0; X)^{\otimes 2}$$

$$= E_{(K,T_K,Z)}\left\{\sum_{j,j'=1}^{K} C^{ps}(T_{K,j}, T_{K,j'}; Z)\left[Z - \frac{E\left(Ze^{\theta_0' Z}|K, T_{K,j}\right)}{E\left(e^{\theta_0' Z}|K, T_{K,j}\right)}\right]\right.$$
$$\left.\left[Z - \frac{E\left(Ze^{\theta_0' Z}|K, T_{K,j'}\right)}{E\left(e^{\theta_0' Z}|K, T_{K,j'}\right)}\right]'\right\}$$

$$= E_{(K,T_K,Z)}\left\{\sum_{j,j'=1}^{K}\left(\Lambda_0(T_{K,j})\left(1 + \gamma^{-1}\Lambda_0(T_{K,j'})\right)\right)e^{\theta_0' Z}\right.$$
$$\left.\left[Z - \frac{E\left(Ze^{\theta_0' Z}\right)}{E\left(e^{\theta_0' Z}\right)}\right]^{\otimes 2}\right\}$$

$$= C\left\{\lambda M E\left(\sum_{j,j'=1}^{K}\frac{j \wedge j'}{k+1}\right) + \frac{\lambda^2 M^2}{\gamma}E\left(\sum_{j,j'}^{K} U_{K,j}U_{K,j'}\right)\right\}$$

$$= C\left\{\lambda M E\left(\frac{K(2K+1)}{6}\right) + \frac{\lambda^2 M^2}{\gamma}E\left(\sum_{j,j'}^{K} U_{K,j}U_{K,j'}\right)\right\}$$

$$= C\left\{\lambda M E\left(\frac{K(2K+1)}{6}\right) + \frac{\lambda^2 M^2}{\gamma}E\left(\frac{K(3K+1)}{12}\right)\right\}$$

$$= \lambda M C\left\{E\left(\frac{K(2K+1)}{6}\right) + \frac{\lambda M}{\gamma}E\left(\frac{K(3K+1)}{12}\right)\right\}$$

$$A^{ps} = E_{(K,T_K,Z)} \left\{ \sum_{j=1}^{K} \Lambda_{0Kj} e^{\theta_0' Z} \left[Z - \frac{E\left(Z e^{\theta_0' Z} | K, T_{K,j}\right)}{E\left(e^{\theta_0' Z} | K, T_{K,j}\right)} \right]^{\otimes 2} \right\}$$

$$= \lambda M C E\left(\frac{K}{2}\right).$$

Thus we find that the asymptotic variance of the pseudo-MLE $\widehat{\theta}_n^{ps}$ is given by

$$(A^{ps})^{-1} B^{ps} ((A^{ps})^{-1})' = (\lambda M C)^{-1} \frac{E\left(\frac{K(2K+1)}{6}\right) + \frac{\lambda M}{\gamma} E\left(\frac{K(3K+1)}{12}\right)}{\left\{E\left(\frac{K}{2}\right)\right\}^2},$$

and the asymptotic relative efficiency of the pseudo-mle to the mle is, under scenario 3,

$$ARE(pseudo, mle)(NegBin)$$

$$= \frac{\frac{E\left\{\frac{K}{K+1}\right\} + \frac{\lambda M}{\gamma} E\left\{\frac{K}{K+2}\right\}}{\left\{E\left(\frac{K}{K+1}\right)\right\}^2}}{\frac{E\left(\frac{K(2K+1)}{6}\right) + \frac{\lambda M}{\gamma} E\left(\frac{K(3K+1)}{12}\right)}{\left\{E\left(\frac{K}{2}\right)\right\}^2}}$$

$$= \frac{E\left\{\frac{K}{K+1}\right\} + \frac{\lambda M}{\gamma} E\left\{\frac{K}{K+2}\right\}}{E\left(\frac{K(2K+1)}{6}\right) + \frac{\lambda M}{\gamma} E\left(\frac{K(3K+1)}{12}\right)} \cdot \left(\frac{E\left(K/2\right)}{E\left(\frac{K}{K+1}\right)}\right)^2$$

$$= \frac{E\left\{\frac{K}{K+1}\right\} + \frac{\lambda M}{\gamma} E\left\{\frac{K}{K+2}\right\}}{E\left(\frac{K}{K+1}\right)} \cdot \frac{E\left(\frac{K(2K+1)}{6}\right)}{E\left(\frac{K(2K+1)}{6}\right) + \frac{\lambda M}{\gamma} E\left(\frac{K(3K+1)}{12}\right)}$$

$$\cdot ARE(pseudo, mle)(Poisson)$$

$$= \frac{\left(1 + \frac{\lambda M}{\gamma} \frac{E\left(\frac{K}{K+2}\right)}{E\left(\frac{K}{K+1}\right)}\right)}{\left(1 + \frac{\lambda M}{\gamma} \frac{E\left(\frac{K(3K+1)}{12}\right)}{E\left(\frac{K(2K+1)}{6}\right)}\right)} \cdot ARE(pseudo, mle)(Poisson).$$

Note that when factor $\lambda M/\gamma = q/p \to 0$, is zero then we recover our earlier result for the Poisson case. This is to be expected since $Poisson(\Lambda_0(t) \exp(\theta_0' Z))$ becomes the limiting distribution of Negative Binomial$(r, p/(p + qF(t)))$ as $p \to 1$.

6 Conclusions and Further Problems

Conclusions

As in the case of panel count data without covariates studied in SUN AND KALBFLEISCH (1995) and WELLNER AND ZHANG (2000), the pseudo likelihood estimation method for the semiparametric proportional mean model with panel count data proposed and studied in ZHANG (1998) and ZHANG (2002) also has advantages in terms of computational simplicity. The results of section 5 above show that the maximum pseudo-likelihood estimator of the regression parameters can be very inefficient relative to the maximum likelihood estimator, especially when the distribution of K is heavy - tailed. In such cases it is clear that we will want to avoid the pseudo-likelihood estimator, and the computational effort required by the "full" maximum likelihood estimators can be justified by the consequent gain in efficiency.

Our derivation of the asymptotic normality of the maximum likelihood estimator of the regression parameters results in a relatively complicated expression for the asymptotic variance which may be difficult to estimate directly. Hence it becomes important to develop efficient algorithms for computation of the maximum likelihood estimator in order to allow implementation, for example, of bootstrap inference procedures. Alternatively, profile likelihood inference may be quite feasible in this model; see e.g. MURPHY AND VAN DER VAART (1997), MURPHY AND VAN DER VAART (1999), MURPHY AND VAN DER VAART (2000) for likelihood ratio procedures in some related interval censoring models.

Further problems

The asymptotic normality results stated in section 4 will be developed and given in detail in WELLNER, ZHANG, AND LIU (2002). There are quite a large number of interesting problems still open concerning the semiparametric model for panel count data which has been studied here. Here is a short list:

• Find a fast and reliable *algorithm* for computation of the MLE $\hat{\theta}$ of θ. Although reasonable algorithms for computation of the maximum pseudo-likelihood estimators have been proposed in ZHANG (1998) and ZHANG (2002) based on the earlier work of SUN AND KALBFLEISCH (1995), good algorithms for computation of the maximum likelihood estimators have yet to be developed and implemented.

• Show that the natural semiparametric profile likelihood ratio procedures are valid for inference about the regression parameter θ via the theorems of MURPHY AND VAN DER VAART (1997), MURPHY AND VAN DER VAART (1999), and MURPHY AND VAN DER VAART (2000).

• Do the non-standard likelihood ratio procdures and methods of BANERJEE AND WELLNER (2001) extend to the present model to give tests and confidence intervals for $\Lambda_0(t)$?

• Are there compromise or hybrid estimators between the maximum pseudo-likelihood estimators and the full maximum likelihood estimators which have the computational advantages of the former and the efficiency advantages of the latter?

• Do similar results continue to hold for panel count data with covariates, but with other models for the mean function replacing the proportional mean model given by (1)?

• Are there computational or efficiency advantages to using the MLE's for one of the class of Mixed Poisson Process ($N|Z$), for example the Negative-Binomial model? Further comparisons with the work of DEAN AND BALSHAW (1997), HOUGAARD, LEE, AND WHITMORE (1997), and LAWLESS (1987A), LAWLESS (1987B) would be useful.

References

[Banerjee and Wellner (2001)] Banerjee, M. and Wellner, J. A. (2001). Likelihood ratio tests for monotone functions. *Ann. Statist.* **29**, 1699 - 1731.

[Begun, Hall, Huang, and Wellner (1983)] Begun, J. M., Hall, W. J., Huang, W.M., and Wellner, J. A. (1983). Information and asymptotic efficiency in parametric-nonparametric models. *Ann. Statist.* **11**, 432 - 452.

[Betensky, Rabinowitz, and Tsiatis (2001)] Betensky, R.A., Rabinowitz, D., and Tsiatis, A. A. (2001). Computationally simple accelerated failure time regression for interval censored data. *Biometrika 88*, 703-711.

[Bickel, Klaassen, Ritov, and Wellner (1993)] Bickel, P. J., Klaassen, C.A.J., Ritov, Y., and Wellner, J. A. (1993). *Efficient and Adaptive Estimation for Semiparametric Models.* Johns Hopkins University Press, Baltimore.

[Cook, Lawless, and Nadeau (1996)] Cook, R. J., Lawless, J. F., and Nadeau, C. (1996). Robust tests for treatment comparisons based on recurrent event responses. *Biometrics* **52**, 557 - 571.

[Dean and Balshaw (1997)] Dean, C. B. and Balshaw, R. (1997). Efficiency lost by analyzing counts rather than event times in Poisson and overdispersed Poisson regression models. *J. Amer. Statist. Assoc.* **92**, 1387-1398.

[Gaver and O'Muircheartaigh (1987)] Gaver, D. P., and O'Muircheartaigh, I. G. (1987). Robust Empirical Bayes analysis of event rates, *Technometrics,* **29**, 1-15.

[Geskus and Groeneboom (1996)] Geskus, R. and Groeneboom, P. (1996). Asymptotically optimal estimation of smooth functionals for interval censoring, part 1. *Statist. Neerlandica* **50**, 69 - 88.

[Geskus and Groeneboom (1997)] Geskus, R. and Groeneboom, P. (1997). Asymptotically optimal estimation of smooth functionals for interval censoring, part 2. *Statist. Neerlandica* **51**, 201-219.

[Geskus and Groeneboom (1999)] Geskus, R. and Groeneboom, P. (1999). Asymptotically optimal estimation of smooth functionals for interval censoring case 2. *Ann. Statist.* **27**, 626 - 674.

[Groeneboom (1991)] Groeneboom, P. (1991). Nonparametric maximum like-lihood estimators for interval censoring and deconvolution. *Technical Report 378*, Department of Statistics, Stanford University.

[Groeneboom (1996)] Groeneboom, P. (1996). Inverse problems in statistics. Proceedings of the St. Flour Summer School in Probability, 1994. *Lecture Notes in Math.* **1648**, 67 - 164. Springer Verlag, Berlin.

[Groeneboom and Wellner (1992)] Groeneboom, P. and Wellner, J. (1992). *Information Bounds and Nonparametric Maximum Likelihood Estimation*. Birkhäuser, Basel.

[Hougaard, Lee, and Whitmore (1997)] Hougaard, P., Lee, M.T., and Whitmore, G. A. (1997). Analysis of overdispersed count data by mixtures of Poisson variables and Poisson processes. *Biometrics* **53**, 1225 - 1238.

[Huang (1996)] Huang, J. (1996). Efficient estimation for the Cox model with interval censoring, *Annals of Statistics*, **24**, 540-568.

[Huang and Wellner (1995)] Huang, J., and Wellner, J. A. (1995). Efficient estimation for the Cox model with case 2 interval censoring, *Technical Report* **290**, University of Washington Department of Statistics, 35 pages.

[Jongbloed (1998)] Jongbloed, G. (1998). The iterative convex minorant algorithm for nonparametric estimation. *Journal of Computation and Graphical Statistics* **7**, 310-321.

[Kalbfleisch and Lawless (1981)] Kalbfleisch, J. D. and Lawless, J. F. (1981). Statistical inference for observational plans arising in the study of life history processes. In *Symposium on Statistical Inference and Applications In Honour of George Barnard's 65th Birthday*. University of Waterloo, August 5-8, 1981.

[Kalbfleisch and Lawless (1985)] Kalbfleisch, J. D. and Lawless, J. F. (1985). The analysis of panel count data under a Markov assumption. *Journal of the American Statistical Association* **80**, 863 - 871.

[Lawless (1987a)] Lawless, J. F. (1987a). Regression methods for Poisson process data. *J. Amer. Statist. Assoc.* **82**, 808-815.

[Lawless (1987b)] Lawless, J. F. (1987b). Negative binomial and mixed Poisson regression. *Canad. J. Statist.* **15**, 209-225.

[Lawless and Nadeau (1995)] Lawless, J. F. and Nadeau, C. (1995). Some simple robust methods for the analysis of recurrent events. *Technometrics* **37**, 158 - 168.

[Lin, Wei, Yang, and Ying (2000)] Lin, D. Y., Wei, L. J., Yang, I., and Ying, Z. (2000). Semiparametric regression for the mean and rate functions of recurrent events. *J. Roy. Statist. Soc. B*, 711-730.

[Murphy and Van der Vaart (1997)] Murphy, S. and Van der Vaart, A. W. (1997). Semiparametric likelihood ratio inference. *Ann. Statist.* **25**, 1471 - 1509.

[Murphy and Van der Vaart (1999)] Murphy, S. and Van der Vaart, A. W. (1999). Observed information in semi-parametric models. *Bernoulli* **5**, 381–412.

[Murphy and Van der Vaart (2000)] Murphy, S. and Van der Vaart, A. W. (2000). On profile likelihood. *J. Amer. Statist. Assoc.* **95**, 449 - 485.

[Rabinowitz, Betensky, and Tsiatis (2000)] Rabinowitz, D., Betensky, R. A., and Tsiatis, A. A. (2000). Using conditional logistic regression to fit proportional odds models to interval censored data. *Biometrics* **56**, 511-518.

[Shorack and Wellner (1986)] Shorack, G. R. and Wellner, J. A. (1986). *Empirical Processes with Applications to Statistics.* Wiley, New York.

[Sun and Kalbfleisch (1995)] Sun, J. and Kalbfleisch, J. D. (1995). Estimation of the mean function of point processes based on panel count data. *Statistica Sinica* **5**, 279 - 290.

[Sun and Wei (2000)] Sun, J. and Wei, L. J. (2000). Regression analysis of panel count data with covariate-dependent observation and censoring times. *J. R. Stat. Soc. Ser. B* **62**, 293 - 302.

[Thall and Lachin (1988)] Thall, P. F., and Lachin, J. M. (1988). Analysis of Recurrent Events: Nonparametric Methods for Random-Interval Count Data. *J. Amer. Statist. Assoc.* **83**, 339-347.

[Thall (1988)] Thall, P. F. (1988). Mixed Poisson likelihood regression models for longitudinal interval count data. *Biometrics* **44**, 197-209.

[Wellner and Zhang (2000)] Wellner, J. A. and Zhang, Y. (2000). Two estimators of the mean of a counting process with panel count data. *Ann. Statist.* **28**, 779 - 814.

[Wellner, Zhang, and Liu (2002)] Wellner, J. A., Zhang, Y., and Liu (2002). Large sample theory for two estimators in a semiparametric model for panel count data. Manuscript in progress.

[Zhang (1998)] Zhang, Y. (1998). Estimation for Counting Processes Based on Incomplete Data. Unpublished Ph.D. dissertation, University of Washington.

[Zhang (2002)] Zhang, Y. (2002). A semiparametric pseudo likelihood estimation method for panel count data. *Biometrika* **89**, 39 - 48.

UNIVERSITY OF WASHINGTON
STATISTICS
BOX 354322
SEATTLE, WASHINGTON 98195-4322
U.S.A.
e-mail: *jaw@stat.washington.edu*

DEPARTMENT OF STATISTICS
UNIVERSITY OF CENTRAL FLORIDA
P.O. BOX 162370
ORLANDO, FLORIDA 32816-2370
e-mail: *zhang@pegasus.cc.ucf.edu*

UNIVERSITY OF WASHINGTON
BIOSTATISTICS
BOX 357232
SEATTLE, WASHINGTON 98195-7232
U.S.A.
e-mail: hliu@u.washington.edu

Some Biases That May Affect Kin-Cohort Studies for Estimating the Risks from Identified Disease Genes

Mitchell Gail and Nilanjan Chatterjee

Division of Cancer Epidemiology and Genetics, National Cancer Institute, Rockville, MD 20852

ABSTRACT   The kin-cohort design can be used to estimate the absolute risk of disease (penetrance) associated with an identified mutation. In the kin-cohort design a volunteer (proband) is genotyped and provides information on the disease histories (phenotypes) of his or her first degree relatives. We review some of the strengths and weaknesses of this design before focusing on two types of bias. One bias can arise if the joint distribution of phenotypes of family members, conditional on their genotypes, is mis-specified. In particular, the assumption of conditional independence of phenotypes given genotypes can lead to overestimates of penetrance. If probands are sampled completely at random, a composite likelihood approach can be used that is robust to residual familial correlations, given genotypes. If the sample is enriched in probands with disease, however, one is forced into making some assumptions on the joint distribution of the phenotypes, given genotypes. For phenotypes characterized by age at disease onset, biases can result if no allowance is made for an influence of genotype on competing causes of mortality or on mortality rates following disease onset.

Key words: gene penetrance, absolute risk, genotyped proband design, Mendelian disease, autosomal dominant

1 Introduction

In the past twenty years, a number of major disease-producing genes have been identified, and it is now possible to test individuals to determine if they are carriers of disease-producing mutations. For counseling purposes it is important to estimate the absolute risk (penetrance) of disease associated with a given mutation. Initial estimates of the risk of breast cancer from mutations in the genes BRCA1 or BRCA2 were derived from families containing many women with breast cancer. For example, Ford et al. (1998) estimated that the cumulative risk to age 70 for carriers of mutations in BRCA1 was 84%. Because the risk in families with many affected members may not represent risk for women with mutations in the general population, there is a need for population-based studies to estimate risk. Data from such studies might be useful for estimating the burden of disease attributable to such mutations in the general population and for estimating risk for women whose families do not have many affected relatives.

Because the mutations in BRCA1 and BRCA2 can be measured, it is possible, in principle, to obtain population-based estimates of absolute risk from cohort or population-based case-control designs (Gail et al., 1999a). Another population-based approach, the "kin-cohort" design, was successfully used to estimate the age-specific cumulative risk of mutations in BRCA1 and BRCA2 (Struewing et al. 1997; Wacholder et al., 1998). In the kin-cohort design, volunteers (probands) agree to be genotyped, and they are interviewed to provide disease histories for their first-degree relatives. As showed by Struewing et al., this information can be used to estimate the penetrance of a rare dominant disease mutation, such as a mutation in BRCA1 or BRCA2. If the probands constitute a random sample from the general population, valid inference on penetrance can be obtained using a "marginal likelihood", even if the disease gene is not the only source of familial aggregation of disease (Chatterjee and Wacholder, 2001). Often probands will tend to have a higher prevalence of disease than in the general population, as was the case in the study of Struewing et al. Moreover, it may be efficient to design a study to have a high proportion of probands with disease (Gail et al., 1999a). We use the term "case-enriched ascertainment" to describe such studies, and we show that correction for such ascertainment requires assumptions on the joint distributions of disease status (phenotypes) of family members, conditional on their genotypes. In particular, residual correlation of phenotypes, conditional on genotypes, must be taken into account in order to avoid bias.

In this paper we review the definition of the kin-cohort design and mention some strengths and weaknesses of the design before focusing on two types of bias and their remedies: bias that arises from residual familial correlation of phenotypes, conditional on genotype; and certain biases that can result when the phenotype is age at disease onset and when competing causes of death, ascertainment probabilities, or survival following disease onset depend on the disease gene under study. Most of our examples concern rare autosomal dominant disease alleles, but many of the formulae and ideas apply more generally. We will refer to the disease of interest as cancer or breast cancer.

2 Notation and Analytic Approaches for the Kin-Cohort Design

Let Y_0 be the disease status (phenotype) of a proband, and let g_0 be that volunteer's genotype. Let $\mathbf{Y} = (Y_1, Y_2, \ldots, Y_r)'$ be the vector of phenotypes of first-degree relatives of the proband, and let $\mathbf{g} = (g_1, g_2, \ldots, g_r)'$ be their genotypes. The object of inference is the penetrance of the genotype g. If disease status is a dichotomous variable with values $Y = 1$ or 0 according as an individual is diseased or not, then $P(Y = 1|g)$ is the penetrance for genotype g. If disease status is time to onset of cancer, then $Y = (t, \delta)$, where t is the age of the earlier of cancer onset or end of follow-up, and $\delta = 1$ or 0 according as cancer was observed or not. We are interested in the "pure" cumulative distributions $F_g(a)$ that give the probability of cancer onset at or before age a in a person with genotype g, in the absence of competing causes of mortality. For an autosomal dominant disease gene, we let $g = 1$ if the individual carries one or two copies of the disease-producing allele and $g = 0$ if the individual has no copies of this allele. Otherwise, the previous notation is unchanged. Thus, for autosomal dominant genes, g indicates carrier status.

Before discussing likelihood-based inference, it is instructive to recall how Struewing et al. (1997) estimated $F_g(a)$, $g = 0, 1$ for autosomal dominant mutations in BRCA1 or BRCA2. First they used survival methods to estimate the cumulative risk function for breast cancer in first-degree relatives of non-carrier probands. Because the disease-producing alleles are rare, this provides an estimate of $F_0(a)$. Next they considered the cumulative risk function of breast cancer in first-degree relatives of carrier probands. Because first-degree relatives have nearly a $50 : 50$ chance of being carriers, their cumulative risk has expectation approximately $0.5F_1(a) + 0.5F_0(a)$. Thus, Struewing et al. were able to solve these two equations at each age a for $F_1(a)$, the cumulative risk in carriers. Their important finding was that the cumulative risk of breast cancer to age 70 was 56%, which is substantially lower than the 84% found from studies of highly affected families (Ford et al., 1998).

Likelihood-based methods can also be used to estimate penetrance (Gail et al., 1999a; Chatterjee and Wacholder, 2001). If probands are sampled at random, the likelihood can be based on $P(\mathbf{Y}, Y_0, g_0)$. If case-enriched ascertainment is used by design or suspected to have occurred, a conditional likelihood based on $P(\mathbf{Y}, g_0|Y_0)$ is more appropriate. Before we discuss assumptions needed to carry out such analyses, we briefly review other strengths and weaknesses of the kin-cohort design.

3 Some Strengths and Weaknesses of the Kin-Cohort Design

Compared to other population-based designs, the kin-cohort design enjoys several advantages (Wacholder et al.,1998; Gail et al., 1999a, 1999b). Struewing et al. (1997) were able to plan, conduct and publish their study in about one year, which is astonishingly rapid. The kin-cohort study can be completed quickly because probands are sampled cross-sectionally and disease history information on the relatives are collected retrospectively. It would take several years to accrue incident cases needed for a population-based case-control study with comparable precision. A second advantage of the kin-cohort design is the ability to estimate the penetrances for several disease outcomes from a single study. For example, Struewing et al. interviewed probands concerning their relatives' histories of prostate and ovarian cancer at the same time they inquired about breast cancer. They were able to produce valuable information on the risk of ovarian and prostate cancers in women and men with BRCA1 and BRCA2 mutations. A third advantage of the kin-cohort design is that the penetrance information reflects the period before the study. The penetrance estimates may therefore reflect the natural history of disease better than would a prospective study conducted during a period when high-risk women might take tamoxifen or other measures to prevent breast cancer. Finally, the kin-cohort design requires slightly smaller samples than cohort or case-control designs when disease history of both probands and relatives are used as in equations (6) and (7) (Gail et al., 1999a).

There are, however, some disadvantages to be considered. If subjects volunteer to be probands more readily if they have affected relatives, the estimates of penetrance will be upwardly biased, both for mutation carriers and non-carriers (Struewing et al., 1997; Wacholder et al., 1998; Gail et al., 1999a, 1999b). This potential upward bias suggests that the estimated cumulative risk of breast cancer to age 70 of 0.56 in the study of Struewing et al. may be too high; thus the force of the conclusions of Struewing et al., is, if anything, strengthened, because the principal result of the study was that risks were lower than previously thought. In general, however, one would need to be concerned about this upward ascertainment bias. Cohort and case-control designs are much more robust to such selection bias and are completely robust to it if the probability of disease depends only on gene carrier status and not on other factors that might be shared by family members (Gail et al., 1999a).

A second concern about kin-cohort data is that probands may err in describing the disease history of their relatives. If probands tend to report disease that is not present (imperfect specificity), penetrance can be seriously overestimated, whereas if probands fail to report extant disease (imperfect sensitivity), penetrance will be underestimated (Gail et al., 1999a,1999b, 2001).

Another potential difficulty concerns the statistical behavior of estimates of penetrance obtained from the kin-cohort design. For rare disease alleles with high penetrance, very large sample sizes are needed before Wald type confidence intervals have the correct coverage (Gail et al., 1999b, 2001). Test-based confidence intervals derived from the likelihood ratio statistic performed better in limited simulations.

We now turn to two other potential problems with analysis of kin-cohort data. To analyze studies with "case-enriched ascertainment", there is a need for joint modeling of phenotypes, that may need to allow for residual familial correlation of phenotypes, conditional on genotypes (Section 4). In studies of the effects of genotype on time to cancer onset, one may need to take into account the possibilities that genotype may affect competing causes of mortality and survival after cancer onset (Section 5).

4 Likelihood Analyses and the Need for Joint Modeling of Phenotypes, Conditional on Genotypes

4.1 Randomly Selected Probands

Suppose probands are selected completely at random from the population. Then the likelihood is the product over families of

$$P(\mathbf{Y}, Y_0, g_0) = P(g_0)P(Y_0|g_0)P(\mathbf{Y}|Y_0, g_0). \tag{1}$$

Here $P(g_0)$ depends on the allele frequency q and can be computed assuming Hardy-Weinberg equilibrium. If genotype is the only determinant of disease risk so that phenotypes are conditionally independent given genotypes, equation (1) can be written as

$$P(g_0)P(Y_0|g_0) \int \prod_{i=1}^{r} P(Y_i|g_i)dP(\mathbf{g}|g_0). \tag{2}$$

The term $P(\mathbf{Y}|g_0)$ is computed assuming no residual familial correlations among phenotypes given genotypes. The quantity $P(\mathbf{g}|g_0)$ is based on standard Mendelian calculations. Suppose, however, that family members share a random familial effect, b (Gail et al., 1999a). Then the object of interest $P(Y|g) = \int P(Y|b, g)dF(b)$, if b is independent of genotype and has distribution F. Under this model

$$P(\mathbf{Y}, Y_0, g_0) = P(g_0) \int P(Y_0|b, g_0) \int \prod_{i=1}^{r} P(Y_i|b, g_i)dP(\mathbf{g}|g_0)dF(b). \tag{3}$$

Thus assuming conditional independence leads to model mis-specification. In particular, using equation (2) when equation (3) is correct leads to exaggerated estimates of genetic effects. In the case of an autosomal dominant gene, $P(Y = 1|g = 1)$ tends to be overestimated, $P(Y = 1|g = 0)$ tends to be underestimated, and q tends to be overestimated. These biases result because model (2) attempts to account for both genetic and random familial sources of familial aggregation of phenotypes using only genetic parameters (Gail et al.,1999b, Chatterjee and Wacholder, 2001). Similar results are found for survival data (Gail et al., 1999b).

Chatterjee and Wacholder (2001) observed that for randomly sampled probands, each of the proband-relative doublets can be treated as a random sample from the population of such doublets, even though doublets from the same family are correlated. Also, for each doublet, given the genotype of the proband, g_0, the phenotype of a relative, Y_i, is representative of the distribution $P(Y_i|g_0)$. Under the random effect model described above,

$$P(Y_i|g_0) = \int \int P(Y_i|b, g_i)dP(g_i|g_0)dF(b) \tag{4}$$

$$= \int P(Y_i|g_i)dP(g_i|g_0).$$

Under random sampling, given g_0, Y_0 is also representative of the distribution $P(Y_0|g_0)$. Hence we can replace equation (1) with a composite likelihood (Lindsay, 1988) that is product over families of

$$P(g_0)P(Y_0|g_0) \prod_{i=1}^{r} \int P(Y_i|g_i) dP(g_i|g_0). \tag{5}$$

Chatterjee and Wacholder (2001) used the term "marginal likelihood" instead of "composite likelihood", but the latter term is more accurate, as pointed out by the editor. Even though we start with the random effect model, we note that, the composite likelihood depends on the parameters of interest $P(Y|g)$ and q and no assumption is needed about the distribution of the random effects. The key feature, however, is reproducibility (Whittemore, 1995), $P(Y_i|g_i, g_0) = P(Y_i|g_i)$, so that the second expression for $P(Y_i|g_0)$ in equation (4) holds more generally. The random effect model described above automatically implies reproducibility. Figure 1A depicts the causal relationships in this model.

Chatterjee and Wacholder give "sandwich" estimators of variance for the composite likelihood estimates that take into account correlations among scores from doublets in the same family. Computationally, the composite likelihood also enjoys certain advantages. Since all the computation in the composite likelihood is done at an individual level, the method is relatively easy to implement irrespective of family sizes. Furthermore, the composite likelihood approach has been found to be much faster than joint likelihood based approaches for non-parametric or weakly parametric estimation of the age-at-onset distribution from kin-cohort survival data (Moore et al., 2001). When the conditional independence assumption is true, however, full maximum likelihood based on (2) can be more efficient (Chatterjee and Wacholder, 2001; Moore et al., 2001).

Even the composite likelihood approach can yield biased results if the models are not reproducible. Two scenarios come to mind. Suppose the disease allele under study is in linkage disequilibrium with another nearby disease-producing allele at a separate locus (i.e. the two alleles are correlated in samples of chromosomes). This situation could arise if there are disease-producing mutations at two loci on the same gene or if the polymorphism under study is a marker that is in linkage disequilibrium with a disease-producing allele at another locus. If Y_i, g_i and Y_0, g_0 correspond to two siblings, for example, then $P(Y_i|g_i, g_0) \neq P(Y_i|g_i)$, because knowing g_0 gives information on the unmeasured linked disease-allele in sib 0, and because sibs i and 0 are related, g_0 thus also gives indirect information on the status of that allele in sib i (see figure 1B). In another scenario, suppose sib i is a smoker at risk of lung cancer. Because a high risk genotype g_0 is present in sib 0, sib 0 develops lung cancer at an early age. This causes sib i to stop smoking, reducing his risk. Thus $P(Y_i|g_i, g_0) \neq P(Y_i|g_i)$.

4.2 Case-Enriched Ascertainment

The sample may be enriched in probands with disease either because such probands have a higher tendency to volunteer to be genotyped or by design (Gail et al., 1999a). The appropriate conditional likelihood for such data is the product over families of

$$P(\mathbf{Y}, g_0|Y_0) = P(g_0|Y_0)P(\mathbf{Y}|g_0, Y_0). \tag{6}$$

The first term in the product above can be computed by Bayes Theorem as a function of the disease allele frequency and the penetrance parameters (Gail et al., 1999a). If $\mathbf{Y}$ is conditionally independent of Y_0 given g_0, the second term can be simplified to $P(\mathbf{Y}|g_0)$. Under the additional assumption that $Y_1, \ldots, Y_r$ are conditionally independent given $g_1, \ldots, g_r$, equation (6) can be written as

$$P(\mathbf{Y}, g_0|Y_0) = P(g_0|Y_0) \int \prod_{i=1}^{r} P(Y_i|g_i) dP(\mathbf{g}|g_0). \tag{7}$$

Gail et al. (1999b, 2001) and Chatterjee and Wacholder (2001) found that equation (7) led to overestimates of the penetrance associated with an autosomal dominant gene, underestimates of the penetrance associated with the wild type, and overestimates of the allele frequency of the disease-producing allele when a random effect model held (Figure 1A). The model (7) tries to accommodate the residual familial aggregation associated with the random familial effect by exaggerating the genetic effects. Chatterjee and Wacholder (2001) replaced the second term in equation (7) to obtain

$$P(g_0|Y_0) \prod_{i=1}^{r} \int P(Y_i|g_i) dP(g_i|g_0). \tag{8}$$

The composite likelihood approach in (8) yields similarly biased results in the presence of residual aggregation, but the magnitudes of the biases are less than in analyses based on equation (7). This is because equation (8) only requires that Y_i be conditionally independent of Y_0 given g_i for each i, whereas (7) requires that Y_i be conditionally independent of Y_0 and of all other $Y_j, j \neq i$, given g_i.

Two approaches seem worth exploring to eliminate these biases. One can attempt to model the joint distribution $P(\mathbf{Y}, Y_0|\mathbf{g}, g_0)$ in order to compute the required conditional distribution $P(\mathbf{Y}|g_0, Y_0)$ in equation (6). For example, one might assume a random effects model to allow for residual familial correlations given genotypes. It is an open question how robust such a procedure would be to mis-specification of the random effects distribution. Another approach might be to regard the triplets $(Y_i, g_0|Y_0)$ as a random sample of values Y_i, g_0 given Y_0. Then, by analogy to equation (7), one could use the composite likelihood (Chatterjee and Wacholder, 2001)

$$P(g_0|Y_0) \prod_{i=1}^{r} P(Y_i|g_0, Y_0). \tag{9}$$

Even this composite likelihood would require joint modeling of Y_i and Y_0 conditional on g_i and g_0. Indeed, $P(Y_i|g_0, Y_0) = P(Y_i, Y_0|g_0)/P(Y_0|g_0)$, and, $P(Y_i, Y_0|g_0) = \int P(Y_i, Y_0|g_i, g_0) dP(g_i|g_0)$. This approach requires less elaborate joint modeling than for the full conditional likelihood $P(\mathbf{Y}|g_0, Y_0)$ in equation (6).

Thus the analysis of data with case-enriched ascertainment requires assumptions on the joint distribution of phenotypes conditional on genotypes. It is not uncommon to assume that phenotypes are conditionally independent given genotypes, as in equation (7), but this assumption can lead to overestimates of the penetrance among carriers when residual correlations are present. It seems prudent to conduct some analyses using random effects models to determine how sensitive the results are to the conditional independence assumptions required in equations equation (7) or (8). Unfortunately, the comparatively assumption-free approach of composite likelihood used in equation (5) is not unbiased for case-enriched ascertainment.

5 Analysis of Time to Cancer Onset, and Biases that Arise When the Gene Under Study Affects Competing Risks or Survival Following Cancer Onset

Age at disease onset is an important feature of disease history (phenotype) for cancer and other chronic diseases. Because probands who volunteer for kin-cohort studies must be alive at the time of the kin-cohort study, certain biases can arise if g affects not only the pure cumulative risk of cancer to age a, $F_g(a)$, but also the distribution $H_g(a)$ of mortality from competing non-cancer causes of death, or the distribution $J_g(d)$ of duration of survival after cancer onset. Figure 2 depicts four potential study probands. The date of birth corresponds to the left end of each time line. The first (topmost) subject died before developing cancer and before the study and therefore could not serve as a proband. The second subject developed cancer at age a but died before the additional time interval d to age $t = a + d$ at the time of the study; thus this subject is also not available for study. The third subject developed cancer at age a and survived to age $t = a + d$ at the date of the study; this person is thus available to be a "case proband". The fourth subject was cancer-free and alive at age t when the study took place and is therefore available to be a "control proband". Even assuming conditional independence of phenotypes given genotypes, as in equation (7), there is a need to account for sampling in Figure 2 in computing $P(g_0|Y_0)$. Under conditional independence, the second term in (7) is unaffected, because sampling influences only the selection of probands and not the disease histories of relatives. In the presence of residual familial correlation, the second term in equation (6) would also need to take the sampling into account, but we assume conditional independence in what follows. For a case-proband, the term corresponding to $P(g_0|Y_0)$ in equation (7) becomes

$$P(g_0|Y_0 = (a, \delta = 1), \text{sampled}) = \frac{P(g_0)h_{g_0}(a)S_{g_0}(a)H_{g_0}(a)J_{g_0}(t-a)\chi_{g_0}(t,a)}{\sum_g P(g)h_g(a)S_g(a)H_g(a)J_g(t-a)\chi_g(t,a)},$$
(10)

where the survival curve and hazard corresponding to $F_g(a)$ are $S_g(a) = 1 - F_g(a)$ and $h_g(a) = -\partial \log S_g(a)/\partial a$, respectively, and, where $\chi_g(t,a)$ is the probability that a subject with genotype g who developed cancer at age a and survived to age t at the date of the study would be sampled for the study. If H, J and χ are independent of g, equation (10) reduces to

$$P(g_0|Y_0 = (a, \delta = 1), \text{sampled}) = \frac{P(g_0)h_{g_0}(a)S_{g_0}(a)}{\sum_g P(g)h_g(a)S_g(a)}$$
(11)

as discussed by Gail et al. (1999a).

For control probands, with $Y_0 = (t, \delta = 0)$ the analogue of equation (10) is

$$P(g_0|Y_0 = (t, \delta = 0), \text{sampled}) = \frac{P(g_0)S_{g_0}(t)H_{g_0}(t)\psi_{g_0}(t)}{\sum_g P(g)S_g(t)H_g(t)\psi_g(t)},$$
(12)

where $\psi_g(t)$ is the probability that a subject with genotype g who remained cancer-free to age t at the date of the study would be sampled. If H and ψ are independent of g, equation (12) reduces to

$$P(g_0|Y_0 = (t, \delta = 0), \text{sampled}) = \frac{P(g_0)S_{g_0}(t)}{\sum_g P(g)S_g(t)}.$$
(13)

Under conditional independence, terms $P(Y_j|g_j)$ in equation (7) and (8) are $\{h_{g_j}(t_j)\}^{\delta_j} S_{g_j}(t_j)$, where t_j is the minimum of the age at cancer onset or end of follow-up. To examine the possibility that older cohorts have different penetrance than younger cohorts, one may need to analyze the disease history data of parents alone. Because parents can be part of the study only if they have offspring who are available to volunteer as probands, the disease incidence data of the parents are left-truncated. This problem, however, can be handled by excluding the person-year contributions of the parents before their age at first birth.

We studied the biases that can result by ignoring the dependence of H or J on g and using the simple expressions (11) and (13). We used the improper Weibull distributions described in Gail et al. (1999a) to match the means and variances of the estimates of $F_1(a)$ and $F_0(a)$ given by Claus et al. (1991) for autosomal dominant breast cancer mutations such as those in BRCA1 and BRCA2. In particular, we used $F_0(t) = 0.10 \left[1 - \exp\left\{-(0.0133t)^{5.148}\right\}\right]$ and $F_1(t) = 0.92 \left[1 - \exp\left\{-(0.0164t)^{4.047}\right\}\right]$. These distributions have means 69.0 and 55.4 years respectively. The allele frequency $q = 0.0033$ was based on Claus et al. (1991). The distribution of ages at the time of study were obtained as described in Gail et al. (1999a).

The bottom curve in Figure 3 depicts $S_1(a) = 1 - F_1(a)$ for carriers. We created 1000 simulated data sets each containing 5000 families consisting of a daughter-proband and mother. We averaged the resulting estimated survival curves to produce each of the other loci in Figure 3. First, we assumed equal competing risks in carriers ($g = 1$) and non-carriers ($g = 0$). These hazards of competing risks were obtained from national U.S. death rates, 1973-1979, for non-breast cancer causes of death. We also assumed a constant mortality hazard of 1/50 per year following breast cancer onset, both in carriers and non-carriers. Finally, we let $\chi = \psi = 1$. Under these conditions estimates based on equations (11) and (13) should yield asymptotically unbiased estimates of $S_1(a)$, but we notice some slight upward bias (solid squares) in samples of this size.

If the hazard of competing risks is doubled in carriers, but not in non-carriers, the upward bias in the estimate of $S_1(a)$ (crosses in Figure 3) is substantial. A possible explanation is that fewer case-probands who are carriers will enter the study than in the previous scenario, because they have a higher rate of competing mortality. Thus, the empirical estimate of $P(g_0 = 1 | Y_0 = (t, \delta = 1), \text{sampled})$ will be reduced, and the estimate of $F_g(a)$ will be reduced. The most severe upward bias in $S_1(a)$, results when the hazard of mortality following breast cancer onset is 1/10 in carriers compared to 1/50 in non-carriers (open circles in Figure 3). Again the proportion of sampled carriers among case probands will be reduced, resulting in an underestimate of $F_1(a)$ and an overestimate of $S_1(a)$. Similarly, there is a potential for bias if χ or ψ depend on g. For example, suppose cases who are carriers tend to volunteer for study more readily than cases who are not carriers, namely, $\chi_1 > \chi_0$. This can induce an upward bias in $F_1(a)$.

In view of the possibilities of these various biases associated with the use of the simple expressions (11) and (13), one may consider use of the original but more complex expressions of (10) and (12). This, however, will require extensive modeling of various components of the sources of different biases, namely, J_g, H_g, χ_g and ψ_g. Moreover, this may be computationally intractable, since fitting the full maximum likelihood with large number of hazard parameters even with the simple expressions (11) and (13) has been found to be numerically challenging (Moore et al., 2001). A simple yet robust approach to avoid these biases could be to use the relatives' disease incidence data alone to estimate the penetrance parameters. Since the disease history data of the relatives are collected through the probands, the survival of the relatives after disease onset does not affect their disease incidence data. The sampling probabilities for the probands also do not affect the disease incidence data of the relatives as long as there is no residual familial correlation. But dependence of competing causes of death on genotype can still cause bias with this approach. We are currently examining how such biases can be eliminated by simultaneously estimating the penetrances for the disease of interest and competing causes of death from the relatives' disease histories and data on vital status. This approach is also being used to examine the effect of BRCA1 and BRCA2 mutations on overall mortality of men and women after adjusting for the known effect of these genes on breast, ovary and prostate cancer.

6 Discussion

We have reviewed some of the strengths and weakness of the kin-cohort design and concentrated on biases that can result when one incorrectly models the joint distribution of phenotypes, conditional on genotypes (Section 4), or when competing risks, mortality rates after cancer onset, or study selection probabilities can depend in genotype (Section 5). The latter issues can affect cohort or case-control designs, but the need to model joint distributions correctly seems to be a special requirement of the kin-cohort design, at least for case-enriched sampling. We are currently exploring use of multivariate survival analysis methods to adjust for case-enrichment sampling in kin-cohort estimation of penetrance.

Despite potential biases, the kin-cohort design has proven to be a powerful and useful design for estimating the risks associated with identified genes. Some recent papers using the design are discussed by Begg (2002).

Acknowledgements
We wish to thank Mr. David Pee for the simulations and graphics leading to Figure 3 and the editor and referees for helpful suggestions.

References

Begg, C.B. (2002). On the use of familial aggregation in population-based case probands for calculating penetrance. *Journal of the National Cancer Institute* **94**, 1221-1226.

Chatterjee, N., and Wacholder, S. (2001). A marginal likelihood approach for estimating penetrance from kin-cohort designs. *Biometrics* **57**, 245-262.

Ford, D., Easton, D.F., Stratton, M., et al. (1998). Genetic heterogeneity and penetrance analysis of the BRCA1 and BRCA2 genes in breast cancer families. *American Journal of Human Genetics* **62**, 676-689.

Gail, M..H., Pee, D., Benichou, J., and Carroll, R. (1999a).Designing studies to estimate the penetrance of an identified autosomal dominant mutation: cohort, case-control and genotyped-proband designs. *Genetic Epidemiology* **16**, 15-39.

Gail, M.H., Pee, D., and Carroll, R.(1999b). Kin-cohort designs for gene characterization. *Monographs of the National Cancer Institute* **26**, 55-60.

Gail, M.H., Pee, D., and Carroll, R. (2001) Effects of violation of assumptions on likelihood methods for estimating the penetrance of an autosomal dominant mutation from kin-cohort studies. *Journal of Statistical Planning and Inference, Special Issue* **96** 167-177.

Lindsay, B. (1998). Composite likelihood methods. *Contemporary Mathematics* **80**, 221-239.

Moore, D.F., Chatterjee, N., Pee, D., and Gail, M.H. (2001). Pseudo-likelihood estimates of the cumulative risk of an autosomal dominant disease from a kin-cohort study. *Genetic Epidemiology* **20** 210-227.

Struewing, J.P., Hartge, P., Wacholder, S., Baker, S.M., Berlin, M., McAdams, M., Timmerman, M.M., Brody, L.C. and Tucker M.A. (1997). The risk of cancer associated with specific mutations of BRCA1 and BRCA2 among Ashkenazi Jews. *The New England Journal of Medicine* **336**, 1401-1408.

Wacholder, S., Hartge, P., Struewing, J.P., Pee, D., McAdams, M., Brody, L.C. and Tucker M.A.(1998). The kin-cohort study for estimating penetrance. *American Journal of Epidemiology* **148**, 623-630.

Whittemore, A. (1995). Logistic Regression of family data from case-control studies. *Biometrika* **82**, 57-67.

- **Legend to figure 1:** The random effect model in Figure 1A is reproducible, because as shown in text, $P(Y_i|g_i, g_0) = P(Y_i|g_i)$. In this figure b is the random effect and g_i and g_0 are genotypes. In Figure 1B, the unmeasured disease genes a_i and a_0 are associated with g_i and g_0, respectively and with each other because subject i and 0 are related. In this figure, the model is not reproducible because $P(Y_i|g_i, g_0) \neq P(Y_i|g_i)$.
- **Legend to figure 2:** Sampling probands in a kin-cohort study. The date of birth is represented by the left terminus of each line and the date of death by a plus (+) mark, if any. The symbol a is the age at cancer incidence and d is the duration of time from cancer incidence to the date of the study. Dashed lines represent unobserved survival after the study.
- **Legend to figure 3:** Biases in estimates of survival functions $S_1(a) = 1 - F_1(a)$ induced by genetic effects on competing risks or on the mortality rate following cancer incidence. The true survival curve ($\bullet$) and estimates ($\blacksquare$) obtained from equations (6), (11) and (13), when genotype does not affect competing risks or mortality are shown. Substantial upward biases in estimates of $S_1(a)$ result when mutation carriers have twice the competing risk hazards as non-carriers (+) and, especially, when the mortality rate after cancer incidence is 5 times greater in carriers than in non-carriers (o).

Optimal Structural Nested Models for Optimal Sequential Decisions

James M. Robins

Departments of Epidemiology and Biostatistics, Harvard School of Public Health, 677 Huntington Avenue, Boston, MA 02115, email: robins@hsph.harvard.edu

ABSTRACT: I describe two new methods for estimating the optimal treatment regime (equivalently, protocol, plan or strategy) from very high dimesional observational and experimental data: (i) g-estimation of an *optimal* double-regime structural nested mean model (drSNMM) and (ii) g-estimation of a standard single regime SNMM combined with sequential dynamic-programming (DP) regression. These methods are compared to certain regression methods found in the sequential decision and reinforcement learning literatures and to the regret modelling methods of Murphy (2003). I consider both Bayesian and frequentist inference. In particular, I propose a novel "Bayes-frequentist compromise" that combines honest subjective non- or semiparametric Bayesian inference with good frequentist behavior, even in cases where the model is so large and the likelihood function so complex that standard (uncompromised) Bayes procedures have poor frequentist performance.

1 Introduction

The goal of this paper is to describe several methods for estimating the optimal treatment regime (equivalently, protocol, plan or strategy) from observational (i.e. nonexperimental) and randomized studies when a data on high dimensional time-dependent response (i.e. covariate) processes are available. The first method is based on doubly robust locally semiparametric efficient (dr-lse) g-estimation of the so-called blip (i.e. treatment effect) function of an *optimal* double-regime structural nested mean model (drSNMM). The second method is based on a dynamic-programming (DP) -like regression model applied to g-estimates of the blip (treatment effect) function of a standard single regime SNMM. I shall refer to the models required by this method as DP-regression SNMMs.

I introduced *standard* single-regime structural nested mean model (srSNMMs) and proposed dr-lse g-estimation of their blip function in Robins

(1994,1997,2000). *Standard* srSNMMs model the effect of a final blip of active treatment (versus zero treatment) at time m before following the zero treatment regime from time $m+1$ to end of follow-up. Here "zero" treatment refers to a substantively meaningful baseline level of treatment such as "no treatment". Double-regime SNMMs and optimal drSNMMs are introduced here. A drSNMM models the effect of a final blip of active treatment (versus zero treatment) at time m before following a given prespecified regime from *time* $m+1$ to end of follow-up. An optimal drSNMM is a drSNMM in which the regime followed from time $m+1$ onwards is the optimal treatment regime. In Sections 3 and 4 I show drSNMMs and optimal drSNMMs are but a minor technical generalization of the standard srSNMMs of Robins (1994).

My methods were motivated by but differ from but those proposed by Susan Murphy in her seminal paper on this topic. Section 6 compares and contrasts Murphy's methods with mine. I show that Murphy's semiparametric regret model is a particular *nonstandard* single-regime SNMM, not only in terms of the observed data likelihood, but also as a counterfactual model. A *nonstandard* srSNMM differs from a standard srSNMM only in that the data analyst's definition of the "zero" level of treatment at any time m may vary both with time and with past treatment and covariate history, and thus may have little or no consistent substantive meaning. From a mathematical and statistical point of view, standard and non-standard srSNMMs are identical; they only differ in the substantive meaning of the treatment effect encoded in their blip functions. It follows, as conjectured by Murphy, that my prior work on SNMMs indicates how to extend her results to include (i) sensitivity analysis and instrumental variable methodologies that allow for unmeasured confounders (Robins, Rotnitzky, Sharfstein, 1999a, Sec 8.1b,8.2b; Robins, Greenland, Hu 1999d, Sec.2d.5; Section 7 below) (ii) continuous time treatments (Robins,1998ab; Section 8 below), (iii) locally semiparametric efficient doubly- robust (lse-dr) estimation (Robins,1994, 2000a; Sections 3-4 below), and (iv) an asymptotic distribution-free test of the g-null hypothesis that the mean response is the same for all regimes (Robins, 1994,1997; Sections 3-4 below) [provided the treatment probabilities are known (as in a randomized study) or can be correctly modelled.].

In addition I show in Section 6.1 that the proposed optimal drSNMMs have two advantages over the semiparametric regret models proposed by Murphy (2003). First, when the time interval between treatment innovations is not too short, they admit closed formed estimators of the optimal treatment regime for non-continuous (e.g. dichotomous) treatments without requiring smoothing or (differentiable) approximation of indicator functions. Second, and more importantly, I believe it is easier to specify substantively meaningful (e.g. biologically meaningful) optimal drSNMMs than semiparametric regret models, because regrets are not effect measures about which scientists have clear substantive opinions amenable to easy modelling. I believe this last statement to be true not only for the sequential decision problem that is the subject of this paper but also for the simpler single time decision problem.

Section 6.2 compares and contrasts optimal regime SNMMs with DP-regression SNMMs. Optimal drSNMMs enjoy a certain robustness property not shared by the DP-regression SNMMs. Specifically, when the treatment probabilities are known (as in a randomized study) or can be correctly modelled, optimal drSNMMs quite generally allow consistent estimation of the optimal treatment regime without restricting or modelling the joint distribution of the time -dependent covariate processes. In contrast, the DP-regression component of a DP-regression SNMM model is a model for aspects of the joint distribution of this covariate process. I show that misspecification of the DP-regression model results in inconsistent estimation of the optimal treatment regime, except when the g-null hypothesis of no treatment effect holds. However, I do not consider this lack of robustness to be a shortcoming of the DP-regression SNMM compared to the optimal drSNMM methodology for the following reason. To obtain a consistent estimate of the optimal regime $\bar{d}_{op}$ under an optimal drSNMM, the optimal drSNMM must be correct. But, due to the high dimension of the covariate processes, this is not possible whenever the g-null hypothesis is false. Indeed, no method can provide a consistent estimator for $\bar{d}_{op}$ under such a high dimensional alternative, even when the treatment probabilities are known. The relevant question then is whether, based on our substantive subject specific knowledge, do we expect to obtain less biased estimates of $\bar{d}_{op}$ by specifying a DP-regression SNMM or by specifying an optimal drSNMM? Even when we possess a great deal of accurate substantive knowledge, this is often a very difficult question to answer. As a consequence I would recommend estimation of the optimal regime based on both models and then either (i) checking whether the optimal regimes and estimated expected utilities (or confidence sets for the optimal regime and for their expected utility) computed under the two different models agree at least qualitatively or (ii) choosing among the estimated optimal regimes by comparing independent estimates of their expected utilities by employing the cross-validation methods described in Section 9.

Overview: To fix ideas consider the HIV infected patients receiving their health care at a large HMO. Suppose that each patient is seen weekly beginning shortly after their time of infection with the virus. At each visit clinical and laboratory data are obtained. On the basis of a patient's treatment, clinical, and laboratory history, the patient's physician decides whether to treat with anti-virals in the next week, and, if so, the particular drugs and dosages to prescribe. Physicians wish to maximize the quality-adjusted survival time of their patients. Because there is no single agreed upon treatment protocol, different physicians make different treatment decisions in the face of the same patient history. Suppose that, after several years, the HMO wishes to estimate from data collected to date an optimal treatment protocol that, when implemented uniformly by all HMO-physicians, will maximize quality adjusted survival time. A treatment protocol or regime is a rule (function) that at the beginning of each week m takes as input a patients treatment, laboratory, and clinical history up to m and deterministically prescribes the dosage of each available antiviral drug to be taken during the week. Our goal is to develop methods for estimating the optimal treatment protocol by utilizing the variability in treatment found in the HMO data. This variability exists because different physicians have made different treatment decisions in the face of similar patient histories.

A key identifying assumption that we shall assume until Section 7 is the assumption of no unmeasured confounders, which is also referred to as the assumption of sequential randomization. It says that, in the HMO data, among patients with a common measured (i.e. recorded for data analysis) treatment, laboratory, and clinical history up to any time m, those receiving a particular dose of treatment in week m do not differ on unmeasured (unrecorded) determinants of quality-adjusted survival. This assumption will be true if all determinants of quality-adjusted survival that are used by physicians to determine the dosage of treatment at m have been recorded in the data base. For example, since physicians tend to withhold anti-viral treatment from subjects with very low white blood count (WBC), and in untreated subjects, low white blood count is a predictor of survival, the assumption of no unmeasured confounders would be false if data on WBC history was not recorded. It is a primary goal of the HMO epidemiologists to record data on a sufficient number of covariates to ensure that the assumption of no unmeasured confounders will be at least approximately true.

The assumption of no unmeasured confounders is the fundamental condition that will allow us to draw causal inferences and to estimate the effect of interventions from observational data. It is precisely because it cannot be guaranteed to hold in an observational study and is not empirically testable that it is so very hazardous to draw causal inferences from observational data. On the other hand, the assumption of no unmeasured confounders is guaranteed to be true in a sequential randomized trial. A sequential randomized trial is a trial in which, at each time m, the dose of treatment is chosen at random by the flip of a (possibly multi-sided) coin, with the coin probabilities depending on past measured laboratory, clinical and treatment-history . It is because physical randomization guarantees the assumption of sequential randomization that most people accept that valid causal inferences can be obtained from a randomized trial. In Section 7, we discuss how the consequences of violations of the assumption of no unmeasured confounders can be explored through sensitivity analysis.

The problem of determining an optimal treatment strategy is a sequential decision problem in that the treatment to be prescribed at each week m is decided based on updated information. As discussed by Murphy (2003), Sutton and Barto (1998), Cowell et. al. (1999), and Bertsekas and Tsitsiklis (1996), this same problem is of concern in many other disciplines and subdisciplines including the disciplines of Markov Decision Processes, Multi-stage or Sequential Decision Analysis, Influence Diagrams, Decision Trees, Dynamic Programming, Partially Observed Markov Decision Processes, and Reinforcement Learning. Susan Murphy (2003) showed that under the assumption of no unmeasured confounders, the mathematical problem we are attempting to solve is identical to that treated in these other disciplines. Thus the estimation methods developed in these disciplines could be used in place of the proposed methodologies to estimate the optimal treatment regime. However, we argue that in principle for many, if not most, of the very high dimensional sequential decision problems faced in clinical medicine, the estimation methods of Murphy and myself are better than any previous approach for the following reason. In biomedical studies, it is often the case that the treatment being evaluated has no effect on survival but may cause mild to moderately severe side effects. If so, the treatment regime that maximizes the quality-adjusted survival is to withhold all treatment. In section 2, I argue that in this setting, previous methods, other than Murphy's and my own, can, with probability near 1, estimate an optimal treatment regime that inappropriately recommends treatment for certain patients. The advantage of Murphy and my methods is intimately connected with recent work on the foundations of statistics in very high dimensional models (Robins and Ritov, 1997; Robins Rotnitzky, van der Laan, 2000, Robins and Rotnitzky,2001). This work shows that in high dimensional, sequential randomized trials with known randomization probabilities (i.e. known conditional probabilities of treatment at each time m), any method, whether Bayesian or frequentist, that satisfies the likelihood principle must ignore the known randomization probabilities. However any method of estimation that ignores these probabilities will, with high probability, incorrectly estimate, as optimal, regimes that prescribe active drug, even under the null hypothesis of no drug effect. In contrast, methods such as Murphy's and mine, that violate the likelihood principle by using these probabilities, will correctly estimate as optimal the regime that withholds all drug. In this paper the question of optimal experimental design is not adressed. Rather we take the data as given and develop analytic methods for estimation of optimal or near optimal decision rules.

Organization of the Paper: In Section 2, we formalize our problem and describe its relation with the problem treated in the sequential decision literature. In Section 3, we define drSNMMs and srSNMMs. and construct dr-lse estimators of the model parameters. In Section 4, we define optimal drSNMMs and construct dr-lse estimators. In Section 5 , we consider how to use our estimates of an optimal drSNMM to make optimal decisions. We consider both frequentist and Bayesian approaches. Because, for an optimal drSNMM, the expectation of our dr-lse estimating functions may not be differentiable with respect to the model parameters, standard methods of confidence interval construction can fail. In Section 5 we describe a novel method for the construction of frequentist confidence intervals in this setting. Furthermore, in Section 5, we show that, due to the curse of dimesionality, standard Bayesian methods fail when analyzing high dimensional data arising from either a sequential randomized trial or an observational study data. We therefore propose a new type of Bayes-Frequentist compromise procedure that allows a valid Bayesian analysis of high dimensional data by reducing the data to the locally efficient doubly robust frequentist estimating function for the data, which is then viewed as a stochastic process whose index is the parameter vector of our optimal drSNMM. In Section 6 we compare and contrast drSNMMs with Murphy's regret models and DP-regression SNMMs. In Section 7, we allow for unmeasured confounding variables and propose sensitivity analysis and instrumental variable methodologies. Section 8 briefly considers extensions to the continuous time setting in which the treatment and covariate processes can jump at random times. Results in Sections 1-8 rely on two assumptions that will never be strictly correct: the first that our optimal drSNMM is correct and the second that either (but not necessarily both) a low dimensional model for the conditional law of treatment or a low dimensional model for the mean of the counterfactual utility given the past is correct. In section 9, we relax both assumptions, although not simultaneously. To accomplish this, we use recent results of van der Laan and Dudoit (2003) on model selection via cross-validation and of Robins and van der Vaart (2003,2004) on adaptive non-parametric confidence intervals and inference based on higher order influence functions. [Robins and van der Vaart (2004) consider relaxing both assumptions simultaneously.] In Appendix 1, we provide detailed calculations for a specific example in order to clarify the inferential consequences of using estimating functions with the non- differentiable expectations. Finally, Appendix 2 and 3 contain the deferred proofs of several theorems.

2 The Data and Analysis Goals

2.1 Observational Studies and Sequential Randomized Trials:

In an observational study or sequential randomized trial we assume that we observe n i.i.d. copies O_i, $i = 1, ..n$, of the random vector $O = (\overline{L}_{K+1}, \overline{A}_{K+1})$ where $\overline{A}_{K+1} = \{A_0, \ldots, A_{K+1}\}$ are temporally ordered treatment variables given at non-random times $t_0, \ldots, t_{K+1}$, $\overline{L}_{K+1} = \{L_0, L_1, \ldots, L_{K+1}\}$ are responses (i.e. covariates) with L_m temporally subsequent to A_{m-1} but prior to A_m, and we have represented random variables by capital letters. Both A_m and L_m may be multivariate. For example in a study of HIV infected subjects, $A_m = (A_{m1}, A_{m2}, A_{m3})^T$ might be the three vector of doses of protease inhibitor, nonnucleoside reverse transcriptase inhibitor (RTI) and nucleoside RTI received in the interval $(t_m, t_{m+1}]$, while L_m might be a vector with components of white count, red count, CD4 count, level of serum HIV RNA, indicators for each HIV associated opportunistic infection, weight, height, blood pressure, etc. recorded at time t_m. [In particular L_m would include the indicator D_m of survival to t_m.] In typical applications, the number of time steps K would be in the range of 10 to 500. If the time subscript is absent, we take the history indicated by the overbar through the end of the study. For example, $\overline{L} = \overline{L}_{K+1}$. Without loss of generality, we will take $A_{K+1} = 0$ with probability one, as A_{K+1} cannot causally influence $\overline{L}_{K+1}$. Thus, in a mild abuse of notation, we can write $\overline{A} = \overline{A}_K$. For any random vector Z_k, we use the corresponding lower case letter z_k to denote a realization of Z_k and the corresponding calligraphic letter $\mathcal{Z}_k$ to denote the support set (i.e. possible values of) of Z_k. We write $\overline{Z}_k = \{Z_0, Z_1, \ldots, Z_k\}$ and, by convention, set $\overline{Z}_{-1} \equiv Z_{-1} \equiv \overline{z}_{-1} \equiv z_{-1} \equiv 0$ with probability one.

We assume there is a known function $y(\cdot)$ of the observed data O whose expectation $E[y(O)]$ we would like to maximize. That is $Y = y(O)$ can be thought of as a utility and our goal is to maximize expected utility. For example, $y(O) = \sum_{m=1}^{K+1} D_m w_m (\overline{L}_m, \overline{A}_m)$ is quality-adjusted years of life where $D_m = 1$ if alive at t_m, 0 otherwise and $w_m(\cdot, \cdot)$ is an agreed upon function of past treatment and covariate history quantifying the quality of life at t_m. If $w_m(\cdot, \cdot) \equiv 1$, $y(O)$ is total years of life during the study period. [Note that a subject who survived until end of follow-up at time t_{K+1}, will presumably survive a considerable time past end of follow-up. This implies that the weight function $w_{K+1}(\cdot, \cdot)$ should dominate the function $w_m(\cdot, \cdot)$, $m < K + 1$, especially for values of $\overline{L}_{K+1}, \overline{A}_K$ that suggest the subject is healthy and is expected to live a long time after the study comes to an end.]

A treatment regime or strategy $\overline{p} = (p_0, \ldots, p_K)$ is a collection of conditional densities $p_m = p_m(a_m | \overline{l}_m, \overline{a}_{m-1})$ for the density of treatment at t_m given past treatment and covariate history. A given treatment strategy $\overline{p}$ is a deterministic strategy, say $\overline{d} = (d_0, \ldots, d_K)$, if for all m, a_m is a deterministic function $d_m = d_m(\overline{l}_m, \overline{a}_{m-1})$ of $(\overline{l}_m, \overline{a}_{m-1})$. That is $\overline{p} = \overline{d}$ means $p_m(a_m | \overline{l}_m, \overline{a}_{m-1}) = 1$ if $a_m = d_m(\overline{l}_m, \overline{a}_{m-1})$. Let $\overline{p}_{obs} = (p_{0,obs}, \ldots, p_{K,obs})$ be the set of conditional treatment densities that generated the observed data. Then we can write the density $f_{obs} = f_{obs}(o)$ of the law that generated the observed data with respect to a dominating measure $\mu(\cdot)$ as the product of the conditional response densities f_{res} and the conditional treatment densities $f_{tr,\overline{p}_{obs}}$. Specifically we write, $f_{obs} \equiv f_{\overline{p}_{obs}} \equiv f_{res} f_{tr,\overline{p}_{obs}}$ where for any $\overline{p}$

$$f_{\overline{p}}(o) = f_{res}(o) f_{tr,\overline{p}}(o), \tag{2.1}$$

$$f_{res} = f_{res}(o) = \prod_{m=0}^{K+1} f\left[l_m \mid \overline{l}_{m-1}, \overline{a}_{m-1}\right],$$

$$f_{tr,\overline{p}} = f_{tr,\overline{p}}(o) = \prod_{m=0}^{K} p_m\left(a_m | \overline{l}_m, \overline{a}_{m-1}\right)$$

Note that knowing $f_{res}(o)$ is the same as knowing each $f\left[l_m \mid \overline{l}_{m-1}, \overline{a}_{m-1}\right]$, $m = 0, \ldots, K + 1$, since the $f\left[l_m | \overline{l}_{m-1}, \overline{a}_{m-1}\right]$ are densities; for example $f(l_0) = f\left[l_0 | \overline{l}_{0-1}, \overline{a}_{0-1}\right] = \int \cdots \int f_{res}(o) \prod_{m=1}^{K+1} d\mu(l_m)$. In an observational study neither f_{res} nor $f_{tr,\overline{p}_{obs}}$ are known and must therefore be estimated from the observed data $O_i, i = 1, \ldots, n$. In a sequential randomized trial f_{res} is unknown but $f_{tr,\overline{p}_{obs}}$ is known by design since the randomization probabilities $p_{m,obs}(a_m | \overline{l}_m, \overline{a}_{m-1})$ are chosen by the investigators .

Note $f_{\bar{p}}(o) = f_{\bar{p}} = f_{res}f_{tr,\bar{p}}$ is a law in which the treatment regime $\bar{p}$ replaces the observed regime $\bar{p}_{obs}$. Actually $f_{\bar{p}}$ is not well-defined unless $\bar{p}$ is a feasible regime defined as follows.

Definition: A regime $\bar{p}$ is feasible if $f_{\bar{p}}(\bar{l}_m, \bar{a}_{m-1}) > 0$ implies the support of A_m under the conditional law $p_m(\cdot|\bar{l}_m, \bar{a}_{m-1})$ is contained in the support of $p_{m,obs}(\cdot|\bar{l}_m, \bar{a}_{m-1})$. We let $\overline{\mathcal{P}}$ be the set of all feasible regimes and let $\overline{\mathcal{D}}$ be the set of all deterministic feasible regimes.

If $\bar{p}$ is not feasible, then there must exist $(\bar{l}_m, \bar{a}_m)$ such that $f_{\bar{p}}(\bar{l}_m, \bar{a}_m) > 0$ but $f_{\bar{p}_{obs}}(\bar{l}_m, \bar{a}_m) = 0$. Thus $f_{\bar{p}}(l_{m+1}|\bar{l}_m, \bar{a}_m)$ is not a function of $f_{obs} \equiv f_{\bar{p}_{obs}}$ and thus is not non-parametrically identified. For any given $\bar{p} \in \overline{\mathcal{P}}$, $f_{\bar{p}}$ is identified from the observed data, since $f_{\bar{p}}$ is a function of f_{res} and f_{res} is a functional of the joint density $f_{\bar{p}_{obs}}$ of the observed data. Until Section 3.2, we restrict attention to feasible regimes. In Section 3.2, we make additional modelling assumptions that allow borrowing of information across regimes. As a consequence, the restriction to feasible regimes becomes unnecessary.

Let $f_{int}^{\bar{p}}(o)$ be the density of O that would have been observed if, contrary to fact, all subjects had followed regime $\bar{p}$. The subscript "int" denotes that $f_{int}^{\bar{p}}$ is the density of the data that would have been observed under an intervention that forced all subjects to follow regime $\bar{p}$. Our interest in $f_{\bar{p}}$ derives from the fact that, as formally discussed in section 3, under a sequential randomization assumption, $f_{int}^{\bar{p}}(o) = f_{\bar{p}}(o)$ for all $\bar{p} \in \overline{\mathcal{P}}$, which implies $f_{int}^{\bar{p}}(o)$ is identified from the observed data. Let $J_{int}^{\bar{p}} = E_{int,\bar{p}}[Y]$ and $J^{\bar{p}} = E_{\bar{p}}[Y]$ be the expectation of $Y = y(O)$ under $f_{int}^{\bar{p}}$ and $f_{\bar{p}}$, respectively. Also for a deterministic strategy $\bar{d}$, define $J^{\bar{d}}$ to be $J^{\bar{p}}$ for $\bar{p} = \bar{d}$. Note $J^{\bar{p}_{obs}}$ is the mean of Y in the observed study. If our goal is to treat a new patient, exchangeable with the n patients in the study, with the regime that maximizes expected utility, we wish to treat with a (possibly nonunique) regime $\bar{p}_{op}$ that maximizes $J_{int}^{\bar{p}}$ over $\bar{p} \in \overline{\mathcal{P}}$. Under sequential randomization, this is equivalent to maximizing $J^{\bar{p}}$. It is clear that we can always take $\bar{p}_{op}$ to be a deterministic strategy $\bar{d}_{op}$, because one can always match a random strategy with a deterministic one. That is, $\sup_{\bar{p} \in \overline{\mathcal{P}}} J^{\bar{p}} = \sup_{\bar{d} \in \overline{\mathcal{D}}} J^{\bar{d}}$. Thus, under sequential randomization, our goal is to find $\bar{d}_{op}$ maximizing $J^{\bar{d}}$.

2.2 The Sequential Decision Literature:

The standard sequential decision literature with a finite time horizon $K + 1$ deals with the following problem. A set $\overline{\mathcal{P}}$ of strategies and a product of conditional densities $f_{res}(o) = \prod_{m=0}^{K+1} f[l_m \mid \bar{l}_{m-1}, \bar{a}_{m-1}]$ are given such that $f_{\bar{p}} = f_{res}f_{tr,\bar{p}}$ is well defined for all $\bar{p} \in \overline{\mathcal{P}}$. The goal is again to find $\bar{d}_{op} \in \overline{\mathcal{D}} \subset \overline{\mathcal{P}}$ maximizing $J^{\bar{d}}$ over $\bar{d} \in \overline{\mathcal{D}}$. See Sutton and Barto (1998) and Bertsekas and Tsitsiklis (1996). Thus the problem treated in this literature is exactly as above except now (i) f_{res} is known rather than estimated from the data and (ii) there is no data. Thus the problem is purely computational rather than statistical. The dynamic programming algorithm of Bellman (1957) is the classic method of computing $\bar{d}_{op}$. However in high dimensional problems the classical dynamic programming algorithm cannot be implemented because it depends on the calculation of conditional expectations that require the evaluation of very high dimensional integrals and thus only approximate solutions are available. These approximate solutions are often based on choosing a known regime $\bar{p}_{obs}$ and simulating data O_i, $i = 1, ..., n$, from $f_{\overline{p_{obs}}}$. The needed conditional expectations are then evaluated by fitting linear or non-linear (e.g. neural network) regression models by least squares. These models are meant to roughly approximate the true functional form of the conditional expectations determined by $f_{res}(o)$ (Bertekas and Tsilikis,1996). We will call this fitting method the *regression method*. Thus in the recent sequential decision literature, the analysts actually create sequential randomized trials to approximately solve an intractable computational problem by simulation. However we will argue that, for the high dimensional problems typically occurring in biomedical studies, the regression method is inferior to dr-lse g-estimation of optimal double-regime SNMMs. Indeed the difficulty with the regression approach is already evident in high dimensional single decision problems.

Difficulty with the regression-method: We will consider the special case where $K = 1$ so the observed data is $o = (l_0, a_0, l_1, a_1, l_2)$. Further, to simplify matters, we suppose A_1 is the constant 0 with probability 1 so we can only consider treating with $a_1 = 0$ at t_1 and so A_1 can be ignored. For convenience we suppress the subscript 0 so $d_0 = d, l_0 = l, a_0 = a$. Our goal is then to find the function $d_{op}(\cdot)$ of l that maximizes $J^{\bar{d}} = \int y(l_2, l_1, l, a) \, dF(l_2 \mid a, l, l_1) \, dF(l) \, dF(l_1 \mid a, l)$. Thus $d_{op}(l) = \arg\max_{a \in \mathcal{A}} E[Y \mid A = a, L = l] = \int y(l_2, l_1, l, a) \, dF(l_2 \mid a, l, l_1) dF(l_1 \mid a, l)$. Now if l_1 and/or l_2 is very high dimensional the integral is intractable even if as in the sequential decision literature $f(l_1 \mid a, l)$ and $f(l_2 \mid a, l, l_1)$ are known . In that case we choose a known density $p_{obs}(a \mid l)$ and simulate n iid copies $O_i = (L_{2i}, L_{1i}, A_i, L_i)$ from $f_{res} f_{tr,p_{obs}}(o) = f(l_2 \mid a, l, l_1) f(l_1 \mid a, l) f(l) p_{obs}(a \mid l)$. In the regression method we obtain the OLS estimate $\hat{\eta}$ of η from the fit of a regression model $E(Y \mid A, L) = \eta^T w(A, L)$ to the data $Y_i = y(L_{2i}, L_{1i}, L_i, A_i), A_i, L_i$, $i = 1, ..., n$, where $w(A, L)$ is an investigator chosen vector of regressors selected to have $\eta^T w(a, l)$ approximate the true regression function $E(Y \mid A = a, L = l) = \int y(l_2, l_1, l, a) \, dF(l_2 \mid a, l, l_1) dF(l_1 \mid a, l)$. The regression-estimate of $d_{op}(l)$ is $\hat{d}_{op}(l) = \arg\max_{a \in \mathcal{A}} \hat{\eta}^T w(a, l)$. Suppose, for the moment, the utility $y(l_2, l_1, l, a) = l_2$ where L_2 is the biological outcome of interest. In biomedical studies, it is often the case that the treatment being evaluated has no effect on the biological outcome L_2. In that case all treatment regimes d result in the same utility, so the true regression function $E(Y \mid A = a, L = l)$ does not depend on a. However when l is very high dimensional, the regression model $\eta^T w(A, L)$ is almost guaranteed to be misspecified and, as discussed further below, because of this misspecification, even in large samples $\hat{\eta}^T w(a, l)$

will nearly always depend on a . It follows that if for some non-zero dose a, $\hat{\eta}^T w(a, l)$ exceeds $\hat{\eta}^T w(0, l)$, treatment will be unneccessarily recommended.

Remark : Of course, when $y(l_2, l_1, l, a)$ does not depend on a and both $f(l_1 | a, l)$ and $f(l_2 \mid a, l, l_1)$ are known then a sufficient condition for the null hypothesis to hold is that both the known densities $f(l_1 | a, l)$ and $f(l_2 \mid a, l, l_1)$ do not depend on a, which can be checked by inspection. However, surprisingly, as discussed by Robins and Wasserman (1997), it often happens in realistic biomedical settings that both densities depend on a and yet the null hypothesis that the integral $J^{\bar{d}}$ is the same for all $\bar{d} \in \bar{\mathcal{D}}$ is true. Thus whether this null hypothesis holds cannot be checked without evaluation of the integral $J^{\bar{d}}$ but, in high dimensions, this is not possible. Robins and Wasserman (1997) refer to this as the null paradox since the factors in the integral $J^{\bar{d}}$ depend on a but the integral does not. Although such a cancellation may appear miraculous it is quite common in many realistic biomedical settings. Specifically it will occur whenever (i) neither A nor L_1 affects L_2 (ii) treatment A affects L_1 and (iii), as will nearly always be the case, pre-treatment unmeasured health status, say U, is a causal determinant of both L_1 and L_2. As a specific example in HIV patients infected with AZT-resistant HIV, A being treatment with AZT, L_1 being red blood count (RBC) and L_2 being HIV RNA, (i) and (ii) will hold as (i) *neither* AZT nor RBC will influence HIV RNA but (ii) AZT is a direct red blood cell toxin.

Now if the null hypothesis of no treatment effect is false and thus $E(Y|A = a, L = l)$ depends on a, then, because of the high dimension of l and logistical limits to the number of observations n we can obtain or simulate, we cannot hope to correctly estimate $d_{op}(l)$. Thus some approximation is necessary. But we would like to use a statistical method to do this approximation that, in contrast to the regression method, does not lead us to falsely conclude that $E(Y|A = a, L = l)$ depends on a when in fact the null hypothesis is true. We now describe such a method after first giving a more precise treatment of the failings of the regression method.

Let $\gamma(l, a) = E(Y|A = a, L = l) - E(Y|A = 0, L = l)$ and $b(l) = E(Y|A = 0, L = l)$, where 0 is a substantively meaningful baseline level of a (e.g. no treatment). Then $E(Y|A = a, L = l) = \gamma(l, a) + b(l)$. Note $\gamma(l, 0) = 0$. The optimal strategy depends solely on the function $\gamma(l, a)$ since $d_{op}(l) = \arg\max_{a \in \mathcal{A}} \gamma(l, a)$. Suppose, as an example, we model $\gamma(l, a)$ by $\gamma(l, a, \psi) = \sum_{j=1}^{s} \psi_j h_j(a) w_{1j}(l)$ and $E(Y|A = 0, L = l)$ by $b(l, \theta) = \sum_{j=1}^{r} \theta_j w_{2j}(l)$ where h_j, w_{1j} and w_{2j} are functions chosen by the analyst with $h_j(0) = 0$, so $\gamma(l, 0, \psi) = 0$ as it must. The model $\gamma(l, a, \psi)$ for $\gamma(l, a)$ is a simple special case of an optimal drSNMM of Section 4. Thus our model is

$$E(Y|A = a, L = l) = \eta^T w(a, l) = \gamma(l, a, \psi) + b(l, \theta) \tag{2.2}$$

Consider also the larger semiparametric partially linear model

$$E(Y|A = a, L = l) = \gamma(l, a, \psi) + b(l) \tag{2.3}$$

where $b(l)$ is a completely unknown function of l. Note, under the null hypothesis $E(Y|A = a, L = l) = E(Y|L = l)$, model (2.3) is guaranteed to be correctly specified with $\psi = 0$ since $E(Y|A = a, L = l)$ does not depend on a if and only if $\psi = (\psi_1, ..., \psi_s)^T = 0$. In contrast, under the null, the model $\gamma(l, a, \psi) + b(l, \theta)$ is correctly specified only if $b(l, \theta)$ equals $E(Y|A = 0, L = l)$ for some θ, which is almost certainly false when L is high dimensional. Because of this model misspecification, the regression method will fail. Specifically the OLS estimate $\widehat{\psi}$ from the fit of the model $\gamma(l, a, \psi) + b(l, \theta)$ will , except for certain exceptional data generating processes, be biased with confidence intervals that in large samples will fail to include zero, even though the null $\psi = 0$ is true. [In exceptional cases the OLS estimate $\widehat{\psi}$ of $\psi = 0$ remains unbiased under the null ($\psi = 0$) even though the model $b(l, \theta)$ for $E(Y|A = 0, L = l)$ is misspecified. An example of such an exception is the special case in which, in the definitions of $\gamma(l, a, \psi)$ and $b(l, \theta)$, we have $r = s$, $w_{1j}(l) = w_{2j}(l)$ for each j, and A is independent of L under $p_{obs}(a|l) = p_{obs}(a)$.]

If we could obtain a consistent estimator of ψ in the semiparametric model (2.3) we would be guaranteed to not be led astray under the null as, then, (2.3) is a correctly specified model with $\psi = 0$. The key to doing so is to use the fact that $p_{obs}(a|l)$ is determined by the simulator or randomizer and thus is known. For example, consider the so-called g-estimator $\widehat{\psi}(s)$ solving $0 = \sum_i U_i(\psi, s)$ with $U(\psi, s) = H(\psi)\{s(A, L) - E[s(A, L)|L]\}, H(\psi) = Y - \gamma(L, A, \psi)$, $s(A, L)$ is a vector function of the dimension of ψ chosen by the analyst, and $E[\cdot|L]$ is computed under the known $p_{obs}(a|l)$. Because under the model (2.3), $U(\psi, s)$ has mean zero at the true ψ, it follows that under standard regularity conditions $\widehat{\psi}(s)$ is a consistent asymptotically normal estimate of ψ, i.e., as $n \to \infty$, $n^{1/2}\left(\widehat{\psi}(s) - \psi\right)$ converges in law to a normal with mean zero and variance that depends on the particular choice of $s(A, L)$. Efficient choices for $s(A, L)$ are discussed in Section 3. However a goal that may be more important than efficiency is to choose $s(A, L)$ and $p_{obs}(a|l)$ such that $E[s(A, L)|L]$ can be computed in closed form. For example if we choose $s(A, L) = As^*(L)$ and $p_{obs}(a|l)$ to have mean $v(L)$ then $E[s(A, L)|L] = v(L)s^*(L)$. In section 3, we extend this approach to the sequential decision setting.

Remark 2.1: Dimension Reduction and Estimation of ψ Using A Deterministic Design: Suppose A and L are discrete with card($\mathcal{A}$) and card($\mathcal{L}$) levels respectively. It would not be unusual to have the vector L have card($\mathcal{L}$) = 10^8 in a biomedical application. Then in a saturated model $\gamma(l, a, \psi)$ for $\gamma(l, a)$, ψ is $\{card(\mathcal{A}) - 1\}$card($\mathcal{L}$) dimensional and its value determines which of the card($\mathcal{A}$)$^{card(\mathcal{L})}$ treatment regimes is optimal. Our use of an unsaturated model $\gamma(l, a, \psi)$ with ψ of dimension much less than $\{card(\mathcal{A}) - 1\}$card($\mathcal{L}$) makes the problem tractable at the cost of possible misspecification bias when the null hypothesis is false. If ψ is sufficiently low dimensional and, as in the sequential decision literature, the design parameters of a simulation study are under the analyst's control, it is computationally feasible to estimate ψ without bias under the null hypothesis and without using g-estimation by employing a deterministic design. We describe 2 such methods. Suppose $\gamma(l, a, \psi) = a\left(\psi_0 + \sum_{j=1}^{s}\psi_j l_j\right)$. where $l = (l_1, ..., l_s)^T$. Then we can estimate ψ_0 by simulating O_i $i = 1, ..., n$ as above but with $L_i = 0$ for all i and with $A_i = a_{\max} = \max\{a; a \in \mathcal{A}\}$ for $i \leq n/2$ and with $A_i = a_{\min} = \min\{a; a \in \mathcal{A}\}$ for $i > n/2$, and estimating the mean of ψ_0 by $\{a_{\max} - a_{\min}\}^{-1}$ times the difference between the averages of Y_i in the first and second half of the sample. We can then estimate $\psi_0 + \psi_j$ and thus ψ_j for each j by repeating the above with L_i the vector that has a 1 in entry j and 0 elsewhere. This approach is unbiased under the null hypothesis. Alternatively we could use a L−matched design to control confounding wherein we first take a random sample $O_{1i} = (L_{1i}, A_{1i}, Y_{1i})$ $i = 1, ..., n$ of size n and then create a second sample O_{2i} $i = 1, ..., n$ where $O_{2i} = (L_{2i} = L_{1i}, A_{2i} = 1 - A_{1i}, Y_{2i})$ with Y_{2i} drawn from the conditional law of Y given (L_{2i}, A_{2i}) and then minimize $\sum_{i=1}^{n}\left\{Y_{2i} - Y_{1i} - (A_{2i} - A_{1i})\left(\psi_0 + \sum_{j=1}^{s}\psi_j L_{ji}\right)\right\}^2$ over ψ.

2.3 A Counterfactual Formulation:

Following Murphy (2002), we will find it useful to have a counterfactual formulation of the problem. We adopt the model of Robins (1986). In this model associated with each treatment history $\bar{a} = \bar{a}_K \in \bar{A} = \bar{A}_K$ and each m we have a counterfactual response vector $\bar{L}_{\bar{a},m} = \bar{L}_{\bar{a}_{m-1},m} = (L_{\bar{a},0,}, L_{\bar{a},1}, ..., L_{\bar{a},m}) = \left(L_0,, L_{\bar{a}_0,1}, ..., L_{\bar{a}_{m-1},m}\right)$ where $L_{\bar{a},j} = L_{\bar{a}_{j-1},j}$ records a subjects outcome at t_j if, possibly contrary to fact, the subject had followed treatment history $\bar{a}_{j-1}$. This notation includes the assumption that the future does not determine the past, since for any two treatment histories $\bar{a}$ and $\bar{a}^*$ that agree through t_{j-1}, $L_{\bar{a},j} = L_{\bar{a}^*,j}$. The counterfactual data is linked to the observed data by the consistency assumption that if a subject's observed treatment history $\bar{A}$ agrees with a treatment history $\bar{a}$ through t_{j-1} then a subject's observed response L_j equals the counterfactual response $L_{\bar{a},j}$ at time t_j. That is,

$$If\ \bar{A}_{j-1} = \bar{a}_{j-1},\ then\ L_j = L_{\bar{a}_{j-1},j} \tag{2.4}$$

In particular, $L_{\bar{a},0}$ equals L_0.

Let D_m be the set of all functions d_m that are the mth component of some $\bar{d} \in \bar{\mathcal{D}}$. Let $\bar{\mathcal{D}}_m$ and $\underline{\mathcal{D}}_m$ be the set of $\bar{d}_m = (d_0, ..., d_m)$ and $\underline{d}_m = (d_m, ..., d_K)$ respectively, each of whose components is in some D_k. We define the counterfactual outcome and treatment histories $\bar{L}_{\bar{d},m} = \bar{L}_{\bar{d}_{m-1},m} = \left(L_{\bar{d},0,}, ..., L_{\bar{d},m}\right) = \left(L_0, L_{\bar{d}_0,1}, ..., L_{\bar{d}_{m-1},m}\right)$ and $\bar{A}_{\bar{d},m} = \bar{A}_{\bar{d}_m,m} = \left(A_{\bar{d},0,}, ..., A_{\bar{d},m}\right) = \left(A_{\bar{d}_0,0}, ..., A_{\bar{d}_m,m}\right)$ associated with following regime $\bar{d}$ in terms of the $L_{\bar{a},j}$ recursively as follows: $L_{\bar{d},0} = L_0$ and, for $m = 0, ..., K+1$, $A_{\bar{d}_j,j} = d_j\left(\bar{L}_{\bar{d}_{j-1},j}, \bar{A}_{\bar{d}_{j-1},j-1}\right)$, where $L_{\bar{d}_{j-1},j} = L_{\bar{a}_{j-1},j}$ with $\bar{a}_{j-1} = \bar{A}_{\bar{d}_{j-1},j-1}$. That is ones counterfactual treatment $A_{\bar{d},j} = A_{\bar{d}_j,j}$

under $\bar{d}$ at time t_j is the treatment assignment function $d_j(\cdot,\cdot)$ applied to the past counterfactual history $\left(\bar{L}_{\bar{d}_{j-1},j}, \bar{A}_{\bar{d}_{j-1},j-1}\right)$. Similarly, ones counterfactual outcome $L_{\bar{d},j} = L_{\bar{d}_{j-1},j}$ under $\bar{d}$ at time t_j is ones counterfactual outcome $L_{\bar{a}_{j-1},j}$ associated with the treatment $\bar{a}_{j-1}$ equal to one's counterfactual treatment history $\bar{A}_{\bar{d}_{j-1},j-1}$ through t_{j-1} under $\bar{d}$. This notation incorporates the assumption that the response of a given subject under regime $\bar{d}$ does not depend on the treatments received by any other subject. By definition, the distribution of these counterfactuals are linked to the previously introduced intervention distributions $f_{int}^{\bar{d}}$ by $f_{int}^{\bar{d}}(\bar{l},\bar{a}) = f_{\bar{L}_{\bar{d}},\bar{A}_{\bar{d}}}(\bar{l},\bar{a})$ where, for any random variable X, $f_X(x)$ is the density of X at x and $F_X(x)$ is the distribution function of X at x.

The distribution $F_{int}^{\bar{d}}(\bar{l}) = F_{\bar{L}_{\bar{d}}}(\bar{l})$ of the counterfactual data $\bar{L}_{\bar{d}} = \bar{L}_{\bar{d},K+1}$ for $\bar{d} \in \bar{\mathcal{D}}$ is identified from the distribution of the observables under the following sequential randomization assumption.

$$\text{Sequential Randomization:} \{\bar{L}_{\bar{a}}; \bar{a} \in \bar{A}\} \coprod A_k \mid \bar{L}_k, \bar{A}_{k-1} \text{ w.p.1,} \qquad (2.5)$$
$$\text{for } k = 0, 1, \ldots, K \text{ and } \bar{a} \in \bar{A}$$

We also refer to (2.5) as the assumption of no unmeasured confounders. Eq. (2.5) states that among subjects with covariate history $\bar{L}_k$ through t_k, and treatment history $\bar{A}_{k-1}$ through t_{k-1}, treatment A_k at time t_k is independent of the set of counterfactual outcomes $\bar{L}_{\bar{a}}$. It can be shown that if (2.5) holds, it also holds with $\{\bar{L}_{\bar{d}}, \bar{d} \in \bar{\mathcal{D}}\}$ substituted for $\{\bar{L}_{\bar{a}}; \bar{a} \in \bar{A}\}$ (Robins, 1986). A sequential randomized trial is a designed study in which treatment level is randomly assigned at each time t_k with the known randomization probabilities $p_k\left(a_k|\bar{L}_k, \bar{A}_{k-1}\right)$, possibly depending on past outcome and treatment history $\left(\bar{L}_k, \bar{A}_{k-1}\right)$. Eq. (2.5) will be true in a sequential randomized trial because $\bar{L}_{\bar{a}}$, like gender or age at enrollment, is a fixed characteristic of a subject unaffected by the randomized treatments A_k actually received and thus is independent of A_k given the determinants $\left(\bar{L}_k, \bar{A}_{k-1}\right)$ of A_k. As stated in the following theorem of Robins (1986), Eqs. (2.5) implies that the density of $f_{int}^{\bar{d}}\left(\bar{l}_{K+1}\right)$ of $\bar{L}_{\bar{d}}$ is a functional (termed the g-computational algorithm functional or g-functional) of the distribution of the observables O and thus is identified.

Theorem 2.1 : Under (2.5), for all $\bar{d} \in \bar{\mathcal{D}}, (i)$ $f_{int}^{\bar{d}}\left(\bar{l}_{K+1}\right)$ is equal to

$$f_{\bar{d}}\left(\bar{l}_{K+1}\right) = \prod_{m=0}^{K+1} f\left[l_m \mid \bar{l}_{m-1}, \bar{a}_{m-1}\right], \text{ where, recursively, } a_m = d_m\left(\bar{l}_m, \bar{a}_{m-1}\right),$$

for $m = 0, 1, ..., K$, and

$$(ii) f_{int}^{\bar{d}}(y) = \int \cdots \int y\left(\bar{l}_{K+1}, \bar{a}_K\right) \prod_{m=0}^{K} dF\left[l_m \mid \bar{l}_{m-1}, \bar{a}_{m-1}\right]$$

with $a_m = d_m\left(\bar{l}_m, \bar{a}_{m-1}\right)$

Note: The expression for $f_{\overline{d}}(\overline{l}_{K+1})$ given in the theorem is equivalent to the previous definition of $f_{\overline{d}}(\overline{l}_{K+1})$, because the treatment density at each m is degenerate, taking the value $a_m = d_m(\overline{l}_m, \overline{a}_{m-1})$ with probability 1.

We have two goals. The first goal is to develop useful models for estimating the mean $E\left[Y_{\overline{d}}\right] \equiv E_{int}^{\overline{d}}[Y] \equiv J_{int}^{\overline{d}}$ of Y under a given regime $\overline{d}$ and to derive easily computed locally-efficient doubly-robust estimators of the model parameters. Note, by Theorem 2.1, under (2.5), $E\left[Y_{\overline{d}}\right]$ equals the identifiable quantity $J^{\overline{d}}$. The second goal is to find the optimal regime(s) maximizing $E\left[Y_{\overline{d}}\right] = J^{\overline{d}}$ over $\overline{d} \in \mathcal{D}$ and to estimate $E\left[Y_{\overline{d}}\right]$ for the optimal regime. We turn next to goal one.

3 Regime-Specific Additive Structural Nested Mean Models

3.1 Definition and Characterization:

In this section we show that regime-specific additive structural nested mean models can be used to estimate the mean of $Y_{\overline{d}}$ for a given regime $\overline{d}$.

We begin with some definitions. For any z_k, let $\underline{z}_k = (z_k, ..., z_{K+1})$. Given regimes $\overline{d} = (d_0, ..., d_K)$ and $\overline{d}^*$ and a treatment history $\overline{a}_{k-1}$, we write $Y_{\overline{a}_{k-1}, d_k^*, \underline{d}_{k+1}}$, as the response (utility) Y under the regime $\left(\overline{a}_{k-1}, d_k^*, \underline{d}_{k+1}\right)$, assumed to be $\overline{\mathcal{D}}$, in which the nondynamic regime $\overline{a}_{k-1}$ is followed through t_{k-1}, $\overline{d}^*$ is followed at t_k and the regime $\overline{d}$ is followed from t_{k+1} onwards. Let the "blip" function

$$\gamma^{\overline{d},\overline{d}^*}(\overline{l}_m, \overline{a}_m) \equiv \gamma^{\underline{d}_{m+1}, d_m^*}(\overline{l}_m, \overline{a}_m) =$$
$$E\left[Y_{\overline{a}_m, \underline{d}_{m+1}} - Y_{\overline{a}_{m-1}, d_m^*, \underline{d}_{m+1}} | \overline{L}_m = \overline{l}_m, \overline{A}_m = \overline{a}_m\right]$$

be the causal effect on the mean of Y among those with history $\overline{L}_m = \overline{l}_m, \overline{A}_m = \overline{a}_m$ of taking one's observed treatment a_m versus treatment $d_m^*(\overline{l}_m, \overline{a}_{m-1})$ at time t_m and then following the regime $\overline{d}$ from t_{m+1} onwards. Note that from its definition $\gamma^{\overline{d},\overline{d}^*}(\overline{l}_K, \overline{a}_K)$ is the same for all $\overline{d} \in \mathcal{D}$ at the final treatment time t_K (since $\underline{d}_{K+1}$ is empty). The functions $\gamma^{\overline{d},\overline{d}^*}(\overline{l}_m, \overline{a}_m)$ will be useful for estimating $E\left[Y_{\overline{d}}\right]$. The regime $\overline{d}^*$ functions only as a baseline level of treatment and will commonly be chosen to be the regime in which treatment is always withheld. It is for this reason that we give $\overline{d}$ pride of place before $\overline{d}^*$ when writing $\gamma^{\overline{d},\overline{d}^*}$.

Remark 3.1: The preceding definition includes a minor abuse of notation: Technically we should have written $\gamma^{\overline{d},\overline{d}^*}(\overline{l}_m, \overline{a}_m)$ as $\gamma_m^{\overline{d},\overline{d}^*}(\overline{l}_m, \overline{a}_m)$ because, for $k \neq m$, $\gamma^{\overline{d},\overline{d}^*}(\overline{l}_m, \overline{a}_m)$ and $\gamma^{\overline{d},\overline{d}^*}(\overline{l}_k, \overline{a}_k)$ have different domains and are different functions .

Remark 3.2: If for $k \geq m$, $d_{k+1}\left(\bar{l}_{k+1}, \bar{a}_k\right)$ only depends on the variables $\left(\bar{l}_m, \bar{a}_{m-1}\right)$ prior to a_m, then $\gamma^{\bar{d}, \bar{d}^*}\left(\bar{l}_m, \bar{a}_m\right)$ represents the effect of one last blip of treatment a_m (versus $d_m^*(\bar{l}_m, \bar{a}_{m-1})$) at time t_m. However when, for some $k > m$, $d_{k+1}\left(\bar{l}_{k+1}, \bar{a}_k\right)$ depends on $\left(\underline{l}_{m+1}, \underline{a}_m\right)$, the actual treatment of subjects following regime $\left(\bar{a}_m, \underline{d}_{m+1}\right)$ may differ from those following regime $\left(\bar{a}_{m-1}, d_m^*, \underline{d}_{m+1}\right)$ at times subsequent to t_m and thus $\gamma^{\bar{d}, \bar{d}^*}\left(\bar{l}_m, \bar{a}_m\right)$ may depend on the effect of treatments at times subsequent to t_m.

The following lemma that is a consequence of Theorem 2.1 states that under sequential randomization $\gamma^{\underline{d}_{m+1}, d_m^*}\left(\bar{l}_m, \bar{a}_m\right)$ is also equal to the above counterfactual contrast among all subjects who would have history $\bar{l}_m$ under the counterfactual treatment history $\bar{a}_{m-1}$.

Lemma 3.1: Under the sequential randomization assumption (2.5),

$$\gamma^{\bar{d}, \bar{d}^*}\left(\bar{l}_m, \bar{a}_m\right) = \gamma^{\underline{d}_{m+1}, d_m^*}\left(\bar{l}_m, \bar{a}_m\right)$$

$$= E\left[Y_{\bar{a}_m, \underline{d}_{m+1}} - Y_{\bar{a}_{m-1}, d_m^*, \underline{d}_{m+1}} \middle| \bar{L}_{\bar{a}_{m-1}, m} = \bar{l}_m\right].$$

Note that sequential randomization in the hypothesis of Lemma 3.1 guarantees that the conditional means of $Y_{\bar{a}_m, \underline{d}_{m+1}}$ and $Y_{\bar{a}_{m-1}, d_m^*, \underline{d}_{m+1}}$ among the subset of the population with observed history $\left(\bar{l}_m, \bar{a}_m\right)$ is equal to the means among the larger subset who would have had history $\bar{l}_m$ upon receiving the (possibly counterfactual) treatment $\bar{a}_{m-1}$ through t_{m-1}. It follows from Theorem 2.1 and Lemma 3.1 that the function $\gamma^{\bar{d}, \bar{d}^*}\left(\bar{l}_m, \bar{a}_m\right)$ is nonparametrically identified under sequential randomization. The following theorem below states that under sequential randomization the function $\gamma^{\bar{d}, \bar{d}^*}\left(\bar{l}_m, \bar{a}_m\right)$ being identically zero for a single regime pair $\left(\bar{d}, \bar{d}^*\right)$ is equivalent to the $g - null$ hypothesis

$$E\left[Y_{\bar{d}^{***}}\right] = E\left[Y_{\bar{d}^{**}}\right] \quad \text{for all } \bar{d}^{***}, \bar{d}^{**} \in \mathcal{D} \tag{3.1}$$

of no effect of any feasible treatment regime on the mean of Y. Further the theorem provides formulae for $E\left[Y_{\bar{d}}\right]$ when $\gamma^{\bar{d}, \bar{d}^*}\left(\bar{l}_m, \bar{a}_m\right)$ is non-zero. Below we use the notational convention $h\left(x\right) \equiv 0$ to denote that the range of the function $h\left(x\right)$ is zero. Parts (i)-(ii) are special cases of Theorem 7.1 below. Part (iii) is a special case of Theorem 7.6.

Theorem 3.1: Given sequential randomization (2.5), and regimes $\bar{d}$ and $\bar{d}^* \in \mathcal{D}$,

(i) $\gamma^{\bar{d}, \bar{d}^*}\left(\bar{L}_m, \bar{A}_m\right) \equiv 0$ w.p.1 for $m = 0, ..., K$ if and only if the g-null mean hypothesis (3.1) holds.

(ii)

$$E\left[Y_{\bar{d}}\right] = E\left[H^{\bar{d}}\right] \tag{3.2}$$

where $H^{\bar{d}} = Y + \sum_{m=0}^K \varrho^{\bar{d}}\left(\bar{L}_m, \bar{A}_m\right)$ and

$$\varrho^{\bar{d}}\left(\bar{L}_m, \bar{A}_m\right) = \gamma^{\bar{d}, \bar{d}^*}\left(\bar{L}_m, \bar{A}_{m-1}, d_m\left(\bar{L}_m, \bar{A}_{m-1}\right)\right) - \gamma^{\bar{d}, \bar{d}^*}\left(\bar{L}_m, \bar{A}_m\right)$$

$$= E\left[Y_{\bar{A}_{m-1}, \underline{d}_m} - Y_{\bar{A}_m, \underline{d}_{m+1}} \middle| \bar{L}_m, \bar{A}_m\right] = -\gamma^{\bar{d}, \bar{d}}(\bar{L}_m, \bar{A}_m)$$

More generally,

$$E\left[Y_{\overline{a}_{k-1},\underline{d}_k}|\overline{L}_k = \overline{l}_k, \overline{A}_k = \overline{a}_k\right] = E\left[H_k^{\overline{d}}|\overline{L}_k = \overline{l}_k, \overline{A}_k = \overline{a}_k\right] \qquad (3.3)$$

where $H_k^{\overline{d}} = Y + \sum_{m=k}^{K} \varrho^{\overline{d}}\left(\overline{L}_m, \overline{A}_m\right)$.

(iii) For any other $\overline{d}^{**} \in \overline{\mathcal{D}}$,

$$E\left[Y_{\overline{d}^{**}}\right] =$$

$$E\left[Y_{\overline{d}}\right] + \int \cdots \int \left[\sum_{m=0}^{K}\left\{\gamma^{\overline{d},\overline{d}^*}\left(\overline{l}_m, \overline{a}_m\right) - \gamma^{\overline{d},\overline{d}^*}\left(\overline{l}_m, \overline{a}_{m-1}, d_m\left(\overline{l}_m, \overline{a}_{m-1}\right)\right)\right\}\right]$$

$$\times \prod_{m=0}^{K} dF\left[l_m \mid \overline{l}_{m-1}, \overline{a}_{m-1}\right]$$

where, for $m = 0, 1, ..., K, a_m = d_m^{**}\left(\overline{l}_m, \overline{a}_{m-1}\right)$.

Note that neither $H^{\overline{d}}, H_k^{\overline{d}}$ nor $\varrho^{\overline{d}}(\overline{l}_m, \overline{a}_m)$ depend on $\overline{d}^*$. It follows from Theorem 3.1(ii) that if the identifiable function $\gamma^{\overline{d},\overline{d}^*}\left(\overline{l}_m, \overline{a}_m\right)$ were known, a $n^{1/2}$- consistent estimate of $E\left[Y_{\overline{d}}\right]$ would be the sample average of the observable random variable $H^{\overline{d}}$. Intuitively at each time t_m, $H^{\overline{d}}$ removes the effect of observed treatment A_m (compared to treatment $d_m^*\left(\overline{L}_m, \overline{A}_{m-1}\right)$) from Y by subtracting $\gamma^{\overline{d},\overline{d}^*}\left(\overline{L}_m, \overline{A}_m\right)$ and then adds back the effect $\gamma^{\overline{d},\overline{d}^*}\left(\overline{L}_m, \overline{A}_{m-1}, d_m\left(\overline{L}_m, \overline{A}_{m-1}\right)\right)$ of the treatment $d_m\left(\overline{L}_m, \overline{A}_{m-1}\right)$ specified by the regime $\overline{d}$ (again compared to treatment $d_m^*(\overline{L}_m, \overline{A}_{m-1})$)

Why Eq. (3.2) and (3.3) should be expected to hold is particularly transparent under *additive local rank preservation*, which we now define.

Definition: Let $\gamma^{\overline{d},\overline{d}^*}\left(y, \overline{L}_m, \overline{A}_m\right)$ be the counterfactual conditional quantile-quantile function $F_{Y_{\overline{A}_{m-1},d_m^*,\underline{d}_{m+1}}}^{-1}\left[\left\{F_{Y_{\overline{A}_m,\underline{d}_{m+1}}}\left(y|\overline{L}_m, \overline{A}_m\right)\right\}|\overline{L}_m, \overline{A}_m\right]$. We say we have local rank preservation w.r.t. $\left(\overline{d}, \overline{d}^*\right)$ if $\gamma^{\overline{d},\overline{d}^*}\left(Y_{\overline{A}_m,\underline{d}_{m+1}}, \overline{L}_m, \overline{A}_m\right) = Y_{\overline{A}_{m-1},d_m^*,\underline{d}_{m+1}}$ w.p.1. for all m.

Definition: If $\gamma^{\overline{d},\overline{d}^*}\left(y, \overline{L}_m, \overline{A}_m\right) = y - \gamma^{\overline{d},\overline{d}^*}\left(\overline{L}_m, \overline{A}_m\right)$ w.p.1. and we have local rank preservation w.r.t. $\left(\overline{d}, \overline{d}^*\right)$, we say we have additive local rank preservation w.r.t. $\left(\overline{d}, \overline{d}^*\right)$.

The existence of local rank preservation is non-identifiable (i.e. untestable) since we never observe both $Y_{\overline{A}_m,\underline{d}_{m+1}}$ and $Y_{\overline{A}_{m-1},d_m^*,\underline{d}_{m+1}}$ on any subject with $A_m \neq d_m^*\left(\overline{L}_m, \overline{A}_{m-1}\right)$. However, we can rule out additive local rank preservation under sequential randomization as both $\gamma^{\overline{d},\overline{d}^*}\left(y, \overline{L}_m, \overline{A}_m\right)$ and $\gamma^{\overline{d},\overline{d}^*}\left(\overline{L}_m, \overline{A}_m\right)$ are identifiable so the truth of $\gamma^{\overline{d},\overline{d}^*}\left(y, \overline{L}_m, \overline{A}_m\right) = y - \gamma^{\overline{d},\overline{d}^*}\left(\overline{L}_m, \overline{A}_m\right)$ is subject to empirical test.

Lemma: Suppose additive local rank preservation w.r.t. $\left(\bar{d}, \bar{d}^*\right)$ holds. Then, with probability 1,

$$Y = Y_{\bar{A}_K},$$

$$Y - \gamma^{\underline{d}_{K+1}, d_K^*}\left(\bar{L}_K, \bar{A}_K\right) = Y_{\bar{A}_{K-1}, d_K^*},$$

$$H_K^{\bar{d}} = Y - \gamma^{\underline{d}_{K+1}, d_K^*}\left(\bar{L}_K, \bar{A}_K\right) +$$

$$\gamma^{\underline{d}_{K+1}, d_K^*}\left(\bar{L}_K, \bar{A}_{K-1}, d_K\left(\bar{L}_K, \bar{A}_{K-1}\right)\right) = Y_{\bar{A}_{K-1}, d_K}$$

$$H_k^{\bar{d}} = Y + \sum_{m=k}^{K} \varrho^{\bar{d}}\left(\bar{L}_m, \bar{A}_m\right) = Y_{\bar{A}_{k-1}, \underline{d}_k}$$

$$H_k^{\bar{d}} - \gamma^{\bar{d}, \bar{d}^*}\left(\bar{L}_{k-1}, \bar{A}_{k-1}\right) = Y + \sum_{m=k}^{K} \varrho^{\bar{d}}\left(\bar{L}_m, \bar{A}_m\right) - \gamma^{\bar{d}, \bar{d}^*}\left(\bar{L}_{k-1}, \bar{A}_{k-1}\right)$$

$$= Y_{\bar{A}_{k-2}, d_{k-1}^*, \underline{d}_k},$$

$$H_{k-1}^{\bar{d}} = H_k^{\bar{d}} - \gamma^{\bar{d}, \bar{d}^*}\left(\bar{L}_{k-1}, \bar{A}_{k-1}\right) +$$

$$\gamma^{\bar{d}, \bar{d}^*}\left(\bar{L}_{k-1}, \bar{A}_{k-2}, d_{k-1}\left(\bar{L}_{k-1}, \bar{A}_{k-2}\right)\right) = Y_{\bar{A}_{k-2}, \underline{d}_{k-1}}$$

In particular, (3.2) and (3.3) hold.

Proof: All results follow directly from the definitions and the assumption of additive local rank preservation w.r.t. $\left(\bar{d}, \bar{d}^*\right)$.

It follows that (3.2) and (3.3) hold under additive local rank preservation w.r.t. $\left(\bar{d}, \bar{d}^*\right)$ even without the assumption of sequential randomization. In fact, Theorem 7.1 below implies the following more general result.

Lemma 3.2 : Eqs. (3.2) and (3.3) hold if

$$\gamma^{\bar{d}, \bar{d}^*}\left(\bar{L}_m, \bar{A}_{m-1}, d_m\left(\bar{L}_m, \bar{A}_{m-1}\right)\right)$$

$$= E\left[Y_{\bar{A}_{m-1}, d_m, \underline{d}_{m+1}} - Y_{\bar{A}_{m-1}, d_m^*, \underline{d}_{m+1}} \middle| \bar{L}_m, \bar{A}_{m-1}, A_m \neq d_m\left(\bar{L}_m, \bar{A}_{m-1}\right)\right].$$

The left hand side of the above equation is, by definition,

$$E\left[Y_{\bar{A}_{m-1}, d_m, \underline{d}_{m+1}} - Y_{\bar{A}_{m-1}, d_m^*, \underline{d}_{m+1}} \middle| \bar{L}_m, \bar{A}_{m-1}, A_m = d_m\left(\bar{L}_m, \bar{A}_{m-1}\right)\right]$$

The previous equation will be true if any one of the following are true: the assumption of sequential randomization, the assumption of additive local rank preservation w.r.t. $\left(\bar{d}, \bar{d}^*\right)$, or the regime $\bar{d}$ is the same as the regime $\bar{d}^*$ (since in this latter case the left hand side and right hand side of the equation are both zero).

Since $\gamma^{\bar{d}, \bar{d}^*}\left(\bar{l}_m, \bar{a}_m\right)$ has a high dimensional argument $\left(\bar{l}_m, \bar{a}_m\right)$, nonparametric estimation is not feasible. Therefore we shall consider parametric models for $\gamma^{\bar{d}, \bar{d}^*}\left(\bar{l}_m, \bar{a}_m\right)$.

Definition: A $\bar{d},\bar{d}^*$ double-regime additive SNMM for the outcome Y specifies that

$$\gamma^{\bar{d},\bar{d}^*}\left(\bar{l}_m,\bar{a}_m\right) = \gamma^{\bar{d}^*}\left(\bar{l}_m,\bar{a}_m;\psi^\dagger\right) \tag{3.4}$$

where $\gamma^{\bar{d}^*}\left(\bar{l}_m,\bar{a}_m;\psi\right)$ is a known function depending on a finite dimensional parameter $\psi \in \Psi \subset R^p$ that (i) satisfies $\gamma^{\bar{d}^*}\left(\bar{l}_m,\bar{a}_m;\psi\right) = 0$ if $a_m = d_m^*\left(\bar{l}_m,\bar{a}_{m-1}\right)$ and (ii) $\gamma^{\bar{d}^*}\left(\bar{l}_m,\bar{a}_m;\psi\right) \equiv 0$ for all m if and only if $\psi = 0$, so under sequential randomization, $\psi^\dagger = 0$ is equivalent to the g-null mean hypothesis (3.1).

An example of such a function is $\gamma^{\bar{d}^*}\left(\bar{l}_m,\bar{a}_m;\psi\right) = a_m\left(1,l_m,a_{m-1}\right)\psi_m = a_m\left(\psi_{1m} + \psi_{2m}l_m + \psi_{3m}a_{m-1}\right)$. Note it is comprised of a main effect term for a_m plus terms representing interactions of a_m with past treatment and covariates. In this example the dimension of $\psi = (\psi_1^T,...,\psi_K^T)^T$ is $3K$.

Notational Conventions: The function $\gamma^{\bar{d}^*}\left(\bar{l}_m,\bar{a}_m;\psi\right)$ is indexed by $\bar{d}^*$ to indicate that condition (i) in the definition below Equation (3.4) holds. Sometimes to help the reader recall the $\bar{d},\bar{d}^*$ regime that we are modelling, we will write the function $\gamma^{\bar{d}^*}\left(\bar{l}_m,\bar{a}_m;\psi\right)$ as $\gamma^{\bar{d},\bar{d}^*}\left(\bar{l}_m,\bar{a}_m;\psi\right)$. Similarly we will sometimes write the parameter ψ as $\psi^{\bar{d},\bar{d}^*}$ to indicate it is the parameter of a drSNMM for $\gamma^{\bar{d},\bar{d}^*}\left(\bar{l}_m,\bar{a}_m\right)$. Occasionally we will write $\gamma^{\bar{d}^*}\left(\bar{l}_m,\bar{a}_m;\psi\right)$ simply as $\gamma\left(\bar{l}_m,\bar{a}_m;\psi\right)$ to indicate a generic drSNMM model.

Remark: Robins (1994,1997) proved Theorem 3.1 and then studied estimation of the parameters $\psi^\dagger$ for $(\bar{d},\bar{d}^*)$-double-regime additive SNMMs in the special cases in which $\bar{d}$ and $\bar{d}^*$ are (i) the same treatment regime and (ii) this common regime $\bar{d}$ is the identically "zero" regime- that is $d_m(\bar{l}_m,\bar{a}_{m-1}) \equiv 0$ for all m where 0 is a baseline level of treatment selected by the data analyst. Because, as discussed in Robins (1986), we are free to define the "zero" level of treatment a_m for subjects with history $(\bar{l}_m,\bar{a}_{m-1})$ to be $d_m\left(\bar{l}_m,\bar{a}_{m-1}\right)$ (even though the substantive meaning of $a_m = 0$ now depends on the $(\bar{l}_m,\bar{a}_{m-1})$), it follows that Robins' (1994) additive SNMM model applies whenever property (i) of this remark holds, with (ii) simply a notational convention. When $\bar{d}$ equals $\bar{d}^*$, we refer to our model as a $\bar{d}$-regime additive srSNMM where sr stands for single-regime. If, in addition, $\bar{d}$ is the zero regime and the treatment level 0 has a natural substantive meaning (such as no treatment), we shall refer to the $\bar{0}$-regime srSNMM as a standard srSNMM.

Remark: From the fact that, by definition,

$$\gamma^{\bar{d},\bar{d}^*}\left(\bar{L}_m,\bar{A}_{m-1},d_m\left(\bar{L}_m,\bar{A}_{m-1}\right)\right) - \gamma^{\bar{d},\bar{d}^*}\left(\bar{L}_m,\bar{A}_m\right)$$
$$= E\left[Y_{\bar{A}_{m-1},\underline{d}_m} - Y_{\bar{A}_m,\underline{d}_{m+1}}|\bar{L}_m,\bar{A}_m\right]$$

it follows that if $\gamma^{\bar{d}^*}\left(\bar{L}_m,\bar{A}_m,\psi\right)$ is a correctly specified $\bar{d},\bar{d}^*$ drSNMM for $\gamma^{\bar{d},\bar{d}^*}\left(\bar{L}_m,\bar{A}_m\right)$, then

$$\varrho^{\bar{d}}\left(\bar{L}_m,\bar{A}_m,\psi\right) = \gamma^{\bar{d}^*}\left(\bar{L}_m,\bar{A}_m,\psi\right) - \gamma^{\bar{d}^*}\left(\bar{L}_m,\bar{A}_{m-1},d_m\left(\bar{L}_m,\bar{A}_{m-1}\right),\psi\right)$$

is a correctly specified $\bar{d}$–regime srSNMM for $\gamma^{\bar{d},\bar{d}}\left(\bar{l}_m,\bar{a}_m\right)$.

3.2 Inefficient Estimation

We now discuss (inefficient) estimation of the parameter $\psi^\dagger$ of a $\left(\bar{d},\bar{d}^*\right)$ - double-regime additive SNMM when, as in a sequential randomized trial, $p_m\left[a_m\mid\overline{A}_{m-1},\overline{L}_m\right]$ is known by design. Efficient estimation and estimation in observational studies with unknown $p_m\left[a_m\mid\overline{A}_{m-1},\overline{L}_m\right]$ is considered in Section 3.3. Our fundamental tool is the characterization of the true blip function $\gamma^{\bar{d},\bar{d}^*}\left(\bar{l}_m,\bar{a}_m\right)$ given in Theorem 3.2. Let $\gamma^{\bar{d}^**}\left(\bar{l}_m,\bar{a}_m\right)$ denote an arbitrary function of $\left(\bar{l}_m,\bar{a}_m\right)$ satisfying (3.6) below, where the second "$*$" denotes that this is a particular, but arbitrary, function. Let

$$H_m^{\bar{d}}\left(\gamma^{\bar{d}^**}\right) = H_m^{\bar{d}_m}\left(\gamma^{\bar{d}^**}\right) \tag{3.5}$$

$$= Y + \sum_{j=m}^{K}\left\{\gamma^{\bar{d}^**}\left(\overline{L}_j,\overline{A}_{j-1},d_j\left(\overline{L}_j,\overline{A}_{j-1}\right)\right) - \gamma^{\bar{d}^**}\left(\overline{L}_j,\overline{A}_j\right)\right\}$$

The following is a special case of Theorems 7.1 and 7.2.

Theorem 3.2: Given a regime $\bar{d}$, sequential randomization (2.5), and any function $\gamma^{\bar{d}^**}\left(\overline{L}_m,\overline{A}_m\right)$ satisfying for all m

$$\gamma^{\bar{d}^**}\left(\overline{L}_m,\overline{A}_m\right) = 0 \text{ if } A_m = d_m^*\left(\overline{L}_m,\overline{A}_{m-1}\right) \tag{3.6}$$

the following three conditions are equivalent.

(i) $\gamma^{\bar{d}^**}\left(\overline{L}_m,\overline{A}_m\right) = \gamma^{\bar{d},\bar{d}^*}\left(\overline{L}_m,\overline{A}_m\right)$ w.p. 1,

i.e., $\gamma^{\bar{d}^**}\left(\overline{L}_m,\overline{A}_m\right)$ is the true blip function $\gamma^{\bar{d},\bar{d}^*}\left(\overline{L}_m,\overline{A}_m\right)$

(ii) For $m = 0,\ldots,K$,

$$E\left[H_m^{\bar{d}_m}\left(\gamma^{\bar{d}^**}\right)\mid\overline{A}_m,\overline{L}_m\right] \tag{3.7}$$

does not depend on A_m w.p. 1.

(iii) For each function $S_m\left(A_m\right) \equiv s_m\left(A_m,\overline{A}_{m-1},\overline{L}_m\right)$

$$E\left[H_m^{\bar{d}_m}\left(\gamma^{\bar{d}^**}\right)\left\{S_m\left(A_m\right) - E\left[S_m\left(A_m\right)\mid\overline{A}_{m-1},\overline{L}_m\right]\right\}\right] \tag{3.8}$$

$$= 0.$$

provided the expectation exists.

Remark: In contrast with theorem 3.1, neither the assumption of additive local rank preservation w.r.t. $\left(\bar{d},\bar{d}^*\right)$ nor having the regime $\bar{d}$ be the same as the regime $\bar{d}^*$ can substitute for the assumption of sequential randomization in theorem 3.2.

We now show how to use the Theorem 3.2 to estimate the parameters of a drSNMM. Given a dr SNMM, define

$$H_m^{\overline{d},\overline{d}^*}(\psi) = H_m^{\underline{d}_m,\underline{d}_m^*}(\psi)$$

$$= Y + \sum_{j=m}^{K}\left\{\gamma^{\overline{d}^*}\left(\overline{L}_j,\overline{A}_{j-1},d_j\left(\overline{L}_j,\overline{A}_{j-1}\right),\psi\right) - \gamma^{\overline{d}^*}\left(\overline{L}_j,\overline{A}_j,\psi\right)\right\}$$

and

$$U^{\overline{d},\overline{d}^*}(\psi,s) = \sum_{m=0}^{K} U_m^{\overline{d},\overline{d}^*}(\psi,s) \text{ with} \tag{3.9}$$

$$U_m^{\overline{d},\overline{d}^*}(\psi,s) = H_m^{\underline{d}_m,\underline{d}_m^*}(\psi)\left\{S_m\left(A_m\right) - E\left[S_m\left(A_m\right) \mid \overline{A}_{m-1},\overline{L}_m\right]\right\}$$

where $s = (s_0,...,s_K)$ and $S_m\left(A_m\right) \equiv s_m\left(A_m,\overline{A}_{m-1},\overline{L}_m\right)$ is a vector valued function with range the dimension of ψ, chosen by the analyst. Note $U^{\overline{d},\overline{d}^*}(\psi,s)$ can be explicitly computed from the data when $p\left[a_m \mid \overline{A}_{m-1},\overline{L}_m\right]$ is known, since then the expectation in (3.9) can be calculated. It follows from (3.8) that $U^{\overline{d},\overline{d}}(\psi,s)$ is an unbiased estimating function, i.e., $E\left[U^{\overline{d},\overline{d}^*}(\psi^\dagger,s)\right] = 0$. Define P_n to be the expectation operator with respect to the empirical distribution so $P_n[Z] = n^{-1}\sum_i Z_i$. Then, by the central limit theorem, $n^{1/2}P_n[U^{\overline{d},\overline{d}^*}(\psi^\dagger,s)]$ is asymptotically normal with mean 0 and covariance $\Sigma(\psi^\dagger,s)$ which can be consistently estimated by $\hat{\Sigma}(\psi^\dagger,s) = P_n[U^{\overline{d},\overline{d}^*}(\psi^\dagger,s)^{\otimes 2}]$. Thus the set of ψ for which $nP_n[U^{\overline{d}\overline{d}^*}(\psi,s)]^T\hat{\Sigma}(\psi,s)^{-1}P_n[U^{\overline{d}\overline{d}^*}(\psi,s)]$ is less than the α upper quantile of a χ^2 distribution on the dimension of ψ degrees of freedom is a large sample $1 - \alpha$ confidence interval for $\psi^\dagger$. Further $U^{\overline{d},\overline{d}}(\psi,s)$ is smooth in ψ when $\gamma\left(\overline{L}_m,\overline{A}_m,\psi\right)$ is smooth in ψ and is linear in ψ when $\gamma\left(\overline{L}_m,\overline{A}_m,\psi\right)$ is linear. Suppose $E\left[\partial U^{\overline{d},\overline{d}*}(\psi^\dagger,s)/\partial\psi\right]$ exists and is invertible. Then under standard regularity conditions there will be a consistent asymptotically normal (CAN) root $\hat{\psi} = \hat{\psi}(s)$ of the estimating function $P_n\left[U^{\overline{d},\overline{d}^*}(\psi,s)\right] = 0$ under (2.5). That is $n^{1/2}\left(\hat{\psi} - \psi^\dagger\right)$ will converge to a normal distribution with zero mean and finite variance; further $P_n\left[H_0^{\underline{d}_0\underline{d}_0^*}\left(\hat{\psi}\right)\right]$ is a CAN estimator of $E\left[Y_{\overline{d}}\right]$ that does not require knowing or modelling $f\left[l_m \mid \overline{l}_{m-1},\overline{a}_{m-1}\right]$.

Remark: In fact $P_n\left[H_0^{\underline{d}_0\underline{d}_0^*}\left(\hat{\psi}\right)\right]$ is a CAN estimator of $E\left[Y_{\overline{d}}\right]$ even if $\overline{d}$ is not a feasible regime, because, by assuming the parametric model (3.4) is correct, the estimator $P_n\left[H_0^{\underline{d}_0\underline{d}_0^*}\left(\hat{\psi}\right)\right]$ succeeds in borrowing sufficient information from subject's following other regimes to estimate $E\left[Y_{\overline{d}}\right]$ at an $n^{1/2}$-rate.

When $\gamma^{\bar{d}^*}\left(\bar{L}_m, \bar{A}_m, \psi\right)$ is a linear function of ψ, $P_n\left[U^{\bar{d},\bar{d}^*}(\psi, s)\right] = 0$ will, with probability approaching 1, have a unique root. However when $\gamma^{\bar{d}^*}\left(\bar{L}_m, \bar{A}_m, \psi\right)$ is a nonlinear function of ψ, $E\left[U^{\bar{d},\bar{d}^*}(\psi, s)\right] = 0$ may have roots in addition to $\psi^\dagger$, in which case even asymptotically $P_n\left[U^{\bar{d},\bar{d}}(\psi, s)\right] = 0$ will have additional inconsistent roots. In that case it can help to choose functions s_m whose range is of greater dimension than ψ and find the minimizer $\widehat{\psi}(s)$ of the smooth function $\left\{P_n\left[U^{\bar{d},\bar{d}^*}(\psi, s)\right]\right\}^T \times$ $B\{P_n\left[U^{\bar{d},\bar{d}^*}(\psi, s)\right]\}$ for some positive definite matrix B (e.g. the identity matrix) [as $P_n\left[U^{\bar{d},\bar{d}^*}(\psi, s)\right] = 0$ will no longer have a solution.] It follows from Theorem 3.2(iii) that in sufficiently large samples, this should solve the multiple root problem provided that one can solve the computational problem of minimizing $\left\{P_n\left[U^{\bar{d},\bar{d}^*}(\psi, s)\right]\right\}^T B\{P_n\left[U^{\bar{d},\bar{d}^*}(\psi, s)\right]\}$.

Remark: The approach based on choosing functions s_m whose range is of greater dimension than ψ will fail when the model (3.4) is even slightly misspecified as then there will in general be no ψ for which $E[U^{\bar{d},\bar{d}^*}(\psi, s)] = 0$. Unfortunately, in practice, the drSNMM (3.4) would never be expected to be precisely correct (unless saturated) [even though it might well be close enough to being correct that the bias of $P_n\left[H_0^{\underline{d}_0\underline{d}_0^*}\left(\widehat{\psi}\right)\right]$ as an estimator of $E\left[Y_{\bar{d}}\right]$ is of little substantive importance.] Nonetheless we will continue to assume (3.4) is precisely correct until Section 9. In Section 9 we explore the consequences of dropping this assumption.

3.3 Locally Efficient Doubly-Robust Estimation:

We now consider how to obtain a locally semiparametric efficient estimator of the parameter ψ^* of a drSNMM. To do so we introduce a generalization of the estimating function $U(\psi, s)$.

Again let $S_m(A_m) \equiv s_m\left(A_m, \bar{A}_{m-1}, \bar{L}_m\right)$ have range the dimension of ψ. Now given $dim\ \psi$ vector-valued functions $C_m = c_m\left(\bar{A}_m, \bar{L}_m\right)$ chosen by the investigator, define $C = c\left(\bar{L}_K, \bar{A}_K\right) = \sum_{m=0}^{K}\left\{C_m - E\left[C_m|\bar{A}_{m-1}, \bar{L}_m\right]\right\}$ and

$$U^\dagger(\psi, s, c) = U(\psi, s) - C$$

where for notational convenience we have suppressed the $\bar{d}$ and $\bar{d}^*$ superscripts denoting the regimes under consideration. We will now consider estimators of ψ under three different semiparametric models which we denote by (a.1), (a.2), and (a.3). The three models differ only in the a priori knowledge about the conditional treatment laws $p\left[A_m\mid\bar{L}_m, \bar{A}_{m-1}\right]$. Specifically, they are characterized by an $\bar{d}, \bar{d}^*-$regime specific additive SNMM model $\gamma\left(\bar{l}_m, \bar{a}_m, \psi\right)$, the sequential randomization assumption (2.5), and a model $\left\{p_m\left(a_m \mid \bar{l}_m, \bar{a}_{m-1}; \alpha\right); \alpha \in \alpha\right\}$ for $p_m\left(a_m \mid \bar{l}_m, \bar{a}_{m-1}\right)$ with true parameter $\alpha^\dagger$ where $p_m\left(a_m \mid \bar{l}_m, \bar{a}_{m-1}; \alpha\right)$ is a conditional density known up to α. In model (a.1), $\alpha = \left\{\alpha^\dagger\right\}$ is a singleton, so $p_m\left(a_m \mid \bar{l}_m, \bar{a}_{m-1}\right) = p_m\left(a_m \mid \bar{l}_m, \bar{a}_{m-1}; \alpha^\dagger\right)$ is known as in a sequential randomized trial. In model (a.2), $\alpha \subset R^p$ is a finite-dimensional parameter. In model (a.3), α is an infinite-dimensional set indexing all conditional densities possibly restricted by the requirement that they belong to some prespecified smoothness class.

To avoid misspecification bias we would like to use model (a.3) in analyzing observational data. Due to the high dimension of $\left(\bar{L}_m, \bar{A}_{m-1}\right)$ this is often not possible, and thus in practice, model (a.2) would often be used for dimension reduction. Let $U^\dagger\left(\psi, \alpha, s, c\right)$ be $U^\dagger\left(\psi, s, c\right)$ with $p_m\left[A_m \mid \bar{L}_m, \bar{A}_{m-1}\right]$ replaced by $p\left[A_m \mid \bar{L}_m, \bar{A}_{m-1}; \alpha\right]$ in the expectation in (3.9) and let $\widehat{\psi}\left(s, c; \alpha\right)$ denote a solution to

$$P_n\left[U^\dagger\left(\psi, \alpha, s, c\right)\right] = 0.$$

Finally, in model (a.2), let $\widehat{\alpha}$ solve the parametric partial likelihood score equation

$$P_n\left[S_{part}\left(\alpha\right)\right] = 0$$

with $S_{part}\left(\alpha\right) = \partial \log \prod_{m=0}^{K} p_m\left[A_m \mid \bar{L}_m, \bar{A}_{m-1}; \alpha\right] / \partial \alpha$, and in model (a.3) let $p_m\left[A_m \mid \bar{L}_m, \bar{A}_{m-1}; \widehat{\alpha}_{smooth}\right]$ denote a high-dimensional non-parametric estimate of $p_m\left[A_m \mid \bar{L}_m, \bar{A}_{m-1}\right]$ possibly obtained by smoothing.

The following theorem 3.3 states results related to the asymptotic properties of estimators of the form $\widehat{\psi}\left(s, c; \alpha^\dagger\right), \widehat{\psi}\left(s, c; \widehat{\alpha}\right)$ and $\widehat{\psi}\left(s, c; \widehat{\alpha}_{smooth}\right)$. Theorem 3.3 and 3.4 below are special cases of Theorem 4.3 in Robins and Rotnitzky (2003). We stress that when, as will usually be the case, $\left(\bar{L}_m, \bar{A}_{m-1}\right)$ is high dimensional, $p_m\left[A_m \mid \bar{L}_m, \bar{A}_{m-1}; \widehat{\alpha}_{smooth}\right]$ will be a poor estimate of $p_m\left[A_m \mid \bar{L}_m, \bar{A}_{m-1}\right]$ in the moderate sized samples occurring in practice and thus the asymptotic results for model (a.3) described in the theorem will not be a useful guide to finite sample properties. However knowledge of the asymptotic results for model (a.3) will be useful in understanding the mathematical structure of the problem.

We shall need the following definitions. An estimator $\widehat{\psi}$ of $\psi^\dagger$ is asymptotically linear if $n^{1/2}\left(\widehat{\psi} - \psi^\dagger\right) = n^{1/2} P_n\left[D\right] + o_p\left(1\right)$ with $E\left[D\right] = 0, E\left[D^T D\right] < \infty$, and $o_p(1)$ denotes a random variable converging to zero in probability. D is to referred to as the influence function of $\widehat{\psi}$. If an estimator is asymptotically linear then $n^{1/2}\left(\widehat{\psi} - \psi^\dagger\right)$ is asymptotically normal with mean 0 and variance $E\left[DD^T\right]$. An estimator $\widehat{\psi}$ is regular if its convergence to its limiting distribution is locally uniform in $n^{-1/2}$ neighborhoods of the truth.

Theorem 3.3: Suppose that the sequential randomization assumption (2.5) holds and we have a correctly specified dr SNMM $\gamma\left(\bar{l}_m, \bar{a}_m, \psi\right)$. Suppose that for all c and for all s such that $\partial E\{U(\psi, s)\}/\partial \psi_{|\psi=\psi^\dagger}$ exists and is non-singular, $\widehat{\psi}(s, c; \widehat{\alpha}_{smooth})$ is a regular asymptotically linear (RAL) estimator in model (a.3) and thus in models (a.2) and (a.1), $\widehat{\psi}(s, c; \widehat{\alpha})$ is a RAL estimator in model (a.2) and thus in model (a.1), and $\widehat{\psi}(s, c; \alpha^\dagger)$ is a RAL estimator in model (a.1). Then

(i) The influence function of any RAL estimator of ψ in models (a.1), (a.2) and (a.3) is equal to that of $\widehat{\psi}(s, c; \alpha^\dagger)$, $\widehat{\psi}(s, c; \widehat{\alpha})$, and $\widehat{\psi}(s, c; \widehat{\alpha}_{smooth})$, respectively for some (s, c).

(ii) For a given s, the asymptotic variance of any RAL estimator of the form $\widehat{\psi}(s, c; \alpha^\dagger)$, $\widehat{\psi}(s, c; \widehat{\alpha})$, or $\widehat{\psi}(s, c; \widehat{\alpha}_{smooth})$ is minimized at $c^s(\overline{L}_K, \overline{A}_K) =$
$$\sum_{m=0}^{K}\left\{C_m^s - E\left[C_m^s|\overline{A}_{m-1}, \overline{L}_m\right]\right\} \text{ with}$$

$$C_m^s \equiv E\left[U\left(\psi^\dagger, s\right) \mid \overline{A}_m, \overline{L}_m\right]$$

Further, under (2.5), $E\left[H_m(\psi) \mid \overline{A}_j, \overline{L}_j\right] = E\left[H_m(\psi) \mid \overline{A}_{j-1}, \overline{L}_j\right]$ for $j \geq m$. Thus

$$C_m^s - E\left[C_m^s|\overline{A}_{m-1}, \overline{L}_m\right]$$
$$= E\left[U_m\left(\psi^\dagger, s\right) \mid \overline{A}_m, \overline{L}_m\right] - E\left[U_m\left(\psi^\dagger, s\right)|\overline{A}_{m-1}, \overline{L}_m\right]$$
$$= E\left[H_m\left(\psi^{\dagger}\right)\left\{S_m(A_m) - E\left[S_m(A_m) \mid \overline{A}_m, \overline{L}_m\right]\right\} \mid \overline{A}_m, \overline{L}_m\right]$$
$$= E\left[H_m\left(\psi^{\dagger}\right)|\overline{A}_{m-1}, \overline{L}_m\right]\left\{S_m(A_m) - E\left[S_m(A_m) \mid \overline{A}_{m-1}, \overline{L}_m\right]\right\}.$$

Hence

$$U^\dagger(\psi, s, c^s) = \qquad\qquad (3.10)$$

$$\sum_{m=0}^{K}\left\{H_m(\psi) - E\left[H_m(\psi)|\overline{A}_{m-1}, \overline{L}_m\right]\right\}\left\{S_m(A_m) - E\left[S_m(A_m) \mid \overline{A}_{m-1}, \overline{L}_m\right]\right\}.$$

Further, in model (a.3) the RAL estimators $\widehat{\psi}(s, c; \widehat{\alpha}_{smooth})$ have the same influence function for all c.

(iii) The influence functions of $\widehat{\psi}(s, c; \alpha^\dagger)$, $\widehat{\psi}(s, c; \widehat{\alpha})$, and $\widehat{\psi}(s, c; \widehat{\alpha}_{smooth})$ are respectively equal to $I^{-1}U^\dagger(s, c)$,
$I^{-1}\left\{U^\dagger(s, c) - E\left[U^\dagger(s, c) S_{part}^T\right]\left\{E\left[S_{part}^{\otimes 2}\right]\right\}^{-1} S_{part}\right\}$, and $I^{-1}U^\dagger(s, c^s)$ where $U^\dagger(s, c) = U^\dagger(\psi^\dagger, s, c)$, $S_{part} = S_{part}(\alpha^\dagger)$, and $I = -E\left[\partial U(\psi^\dagger, s)/\partial \psi\right]$. The asymptotic variance of $\widehat{\psi}(s, c; \widehat{\alpha}_{smooth})$ is always less than or equal to that of $\widehat{\psi}(s, c; \widehat{\alpha})$, which is always less than or equal to that of $\widehat{\psi}(s, c; \alpha^\dagger)$. However, when $c = c^s$, all three estimators have the same asymptotic variance.

(iv) The semiparametric variance bound is the same in models (a.1), (a.2) and (a.3) and is equal to the asymptotic variance of $\widehat{\psi}(s_{eff}, c^{s_{eff}})$. An explicit closed form expression for s_{eff} is given in Robins (1994). The expression is very complex except in the special case in which

$$var\left(H_m\left(\psi^\dagger\right)|\overline{L}_m,\overline{A}_m\right) = var\left(H_m\left(\psi^\dagger\right)|\overline{L}_m,\overline{A}_{m-1}\right) \qquad (3.11)$$

does not depend on A_m for all m. In that case

$$s_{eff,m}\left(\overline{L}_m,\overline{A}_m\right) \equiv S_{eff,m}\left(A_m,\psi^\dagger\right) \text{ with} \qquad (3.12)$$
$$S_{eff,m}\left(A_m,\psi\right) = \left\{E\left[\partial H_m\left(\psi\right)/\partial\psi|\overline{L}_m,\overline{A}_m\right]\right\}\left\{var\left(H_m\left(\psi\right)|\overline{L}_m,\overline{A}_{m-1}\right)\right\}^{-1}.$$

Double Robustness: Surprisingly, given (2.5) and a correct drSNMM, the estimator $\widehat{\psi}\left(s,c^s;\widehat{\alpha}\right)$ is a CAN estimator of $\psi^\dagger$ even if the model $p_m\left[A_m\mid\overline{L}_m,\overline{A}_{m-1};\alpha\right]$ for $p_m\left[A_m\mid\overline{L}_m,\overline{A}_{m-1}\right]$ is misspecified because $E\left[U^\dagger\left(\psi^\dagger,s,c^s;\widehat{\alpha}\right)\right] = 0$ under misspecification of $p_m\left[A_m\mid\overline{L}_m,\overline{A}_{m-1};\alpha\right]$. However this is of no direct use because $E\left[H_m\left(\psi\right)|\overline{A}_{m-1},\overline{L}_m\right]$ is unknown and thus $U^\dagger\left(\psi^\dagger,s,c^s;\widehat{\alpha}\right)$ is not computable. Therefore we consider a model $\varsigma^T W_m$ for $E\left[H_m\left(\psi^\dagger\right)|\overline{L}_m,\overline{A}_{m-1}\right]$ where $W_m = w_m\left(\overline{A}_{m-1},\overline{L}_m\right)$ is a known vector function of $\left(\overline{A}_{m-1},\overline{L}_m\right)$ and ς is an unknown parameter. Define $\widehat{\psi}\left(s,c^s;\widehat{\alpha},\widehat{\varsigma}\right)$ to be a solution to $P_n\left[U^\dagger\left(\psi,s,c^s;\widehat{\alpha},\widehat{\varsigma}\right)\right] = 0$ where

$$U^\dagger\left(\psi,s,c^s;\widehat{\alpha},\widehat{\varsigma}\right) \qquad (3.13)$$
$$= \sum_{m=0}^{K}\left\{H_m\left(\psi\right)-\widehat{\varsigma}^T\left(\psi\right)W_m\right\}\left\{S_m\left(A_m\right)-E_{\widehat{\alpha}}\left[S_m\left(A_m\right)\mid\overline{A}_{m-1},\overline{L}_m\right]\right\}$$

is Equation (3.10) with $-E_{\widehat{\alpha}}\left[S_m\left(A_m\right)\mid\overline{A}_{m-1},\overline{L}_m\right]\}$ substituted for $-E\left[S_m\left(A_m\right)\mid\overline{A}_{m-1},\overline{L}_m\right]$ and with $\widehat{\varsigma}^T\left(\psi\right)W_m$ substituted for $E\left[H_m\left(\psi\right)|\overline{A}_{m-1},\overline{L}_m\right]$. Here $\widehat{\varsigma}^T\left(\psi\right)$ solves the OLS estimating equation $P_n\left[\sum_{m=0}^{K}\left(H_m\left(\psi\right)-\varsigma^T W_m\right)W_m\right] = 0$. The following theorem and Remark 3.1 below describe the so called "double-robustness" properties of $\widehat{\psi}\left(s,c^s;\widehat{\alpha},\widehat{\varsigma}\right)$ and $U^\dagger\left(\psi^\dagger,s,c^s;\widehat{\alpha},\widehat{\varsigma}\right)$.

Theorem 3.4: Consider the $\overline{d},\overline{d}^*$"union" model characterized by (i) the sequential randomization assumption (2.5), (ii) a correctly specified $(\overline{d},\overline{d}^*)$-double-regime-specific SNMM $\gamma\left(\overline{l}_m,\overline{a}_m,\psi\right)$ and that either (but not necessarily both) the parametric model $p_m\left[A_m\mid\overline{L}_m,\overline{A}_{m-1};\alpha\right]$ for $p_m\left[A_m\mid\overline{L}_m,\overline{A}_{m-1}\right]$ is correct or the regression model $\varsigma^T W_m$ for $E\left[H_m\left(\psi^\dagger\right)|\overline{L}_m,\overline{A}_{m-1}\right]$ is correct. Then, under standard regularity conditions, (i) $n^{-1/2}P_n\left[U^\dagger\left(\psi^\dagger,s,c^s;\widehat{\alpha},\widehat{\varsigma}\right)\right] = n^{-1/2}P_n\left[U_{adj}^\dagger\left(\psi^\dagger,s,c^s;\alpha^*,\varsigma^*\right)\right]+o_p\left(1\right)$, where

$$U^\dagger_{adj}\left(\psi^\dagger, s, c^s; \alpha^*, \varsigma^*\right) =$$
$$U^\dagger\left(\psi^\dagger, s, c^s; \alpha^*, \varsigma^*\right) -$$
$$E\left[\partial U^\dagger\left(\psi^\dagger, s, c^s; \alpha^*, \varsigma^*\right)/\partial \alpha^T\right] E\left[\partial S_{part}\left(\alpha^*\right)/\partial \alpha^T\right]^{-1} S_{part}\left(\alpha^*\right) +$$
$$E\left[\partial U^\dagger\left(\psi^\dagger, s, c^s; \alpha^*, \varsigma^*\right)/\partial \varsigma\left(\psi^\dagger\right)^T\right] \times$$
$$E\left[\sum_{m=0}^{K} W_m^{\otimes 2}\right]^{-1} \sum_{m=0}^{K}\left(H_m\left(\psi^\dagger\right) - \varsigma^*\left(\psi^\dagger\right) W_m\right) W_m$$

(3.14)

and $\left(\alpha^*, \varsigma^*\right)$ is the probability limit of $(\widehat{\alpha}, \widehat{\varsigma})$. Since $S_{part}\left(\alpha^*\right)$, $\sum_{m=0}^{K}\left(H_m\left(\psi^\dagger\right) - \varsigma^*\left(\psi^\dagger\right) W_m\right) W_m$ and, under the union model, $U^\dagger\left(\psi^\dagger, s, c^s; \alpha^*, \varsigma^*\right)$ all have mean 0, it follows that, by Slutsky's theorem, (i) $n^{-1/2} P_n\left[U^\dagger\left(\psi^\dagger, s, c^s; \widehat{\alpha}, \widehat{\varsigma}\right)\right]$ is asymptotically normal with mean zero and co-variance $E\left[U^\dagger_{adj}\left(\psi^\dagger, s, c^s; \alpha^*, \varsigma^*\right)^{\otimes 2}\right]$, (ii) $\widehat{\psi}\left(s, c^s; \widehat{\alpha}, \widehat{\varsigma}\right)$ is asymptotically linear with influence function

$$-E\left[\partial U^\dagger_{adj}\left(\psi^\dagger, s, c^s; \alpha^*, \varsigma^*\right)/\partial \psi\right]^{-1} U^\dagger_{adj}\left(\psi^\dagger, s, c^s; \alpha^*, \varsigma^*\right)$$

provided $E\left[\partial U^\dagger_{adj}\left(\psi^\dagger, s, c^s; \alpha^*, \varsigma^*\right)/\partial \psi\right]$ exists and is invertible and (iii) $\widehat{\psi}\left(s_{eff}, c^{s_{eff}}; \widehat{\alpha}, \widehat{\varsigma}\right)$ attains the semiparametric efficiency bound for the "union" model at the submodel in which (3.11) holds and both the model $p_m\left[A_m \mid \overline{L}_m, \overline{A}_{m-1}; \alpha\right]$ and the model $\varsigma^T W_m$ for $E\left[H_m\left(\psi^\dagger\right) | \overline{L}_m, \overline{A}_{m-1}\right]$ are correct. Theorem 3.4 suggests an analysis based on the following algorithm.

Algorithm:

Step 1: Specify regimes of interest $\overline{d}$ and $\overline{d}^*$.

Step 2: Specify a drSNMM model $\gamma\left(\overline{L}_m, \overline{A}_m, \psi\right)$ for $\gamma^{\overline{d}, \overline{d}^*}\left(\overline{L}_m, \overline{A}_m\right)$

Step 3: For each subject calculate $H_m\left(\psi\right)$, $m = 0, ..., K$ for each possible value of ψ. (Obviously this is not computationally feasible since ψ can take values in $R^{\dim(\psi)}$. Below we discuss how one can reduce the number of ψ for which $H_m\left(\psi\right)$ must be evaluated in order to make the algorithm feasible).

Step 4: For each subject estimate $E\left[H_m\left(\psi\right) | \overline{L}_m, \overline{A}_{m-1}\right]$ under a model $\varsigma^T W_m$ by $\widehat{\varsigma}^T\left(\psi\right) W_m$ where $\widehat{\varsigma}^T\left(\psi\right)$ solves the OLS estimating equation $P_n\left[\sum_{m=0}^{K}\left(H_m\left(\psi\right) - \varsigma W_m\right) W_m\right] = 0$ and $W_m = w_m\left(\overline{A}_{m-1}, \overline{L}_m\right)$ is known vector function of $\left(\overline{A}_{m-1}, \overline{L}_m\right)$.

Step 5. For each subject estimate $var\left(H_m\left(\psi^\dagger\right) | \overline{A}_{m-1}, \overline{L}_m\right)$ by the fitted value $exp\left(\widehat{\varkappa}\left(\psi\right)^T B_m\right)$ from the nonlinear least squares fit of the regression of the estimated squared residual $\{H_m\left(\psi\right) - \widehat{\varsigma}\left(\psi\right) W_m\}^2$ on the regression function $exp\left(\varkappa B_m\right)$ where $B_m = b_m\left(\overline{L}_m, \overline{A}_{m-1}\right)$ is a known vector function.

Step 6. For each subject estimate $E\left[\partial H_m\left(\psi\right)/\partial \psi | \overline{L}_m, \overline{A}_m\right]$ under a multivariate regression model ζR_m by the fitted value $\widehat{\zeta}\left(\psi\right) R_m$ from the multivariate OLS regression of $\partial H_m\left(\psi\right)/\partial \psi$ on R_m where $R_m = r_m\left(\overline{A}_m, \overline{L}_m\right)$ is a known vector function and ζ is a matrix of regression coefficients.

Step 7: Specify a parametric model $p_m \left[A_m \mid \overline{L}_m, \overline{A}_{m-1}; \alpha \right]$ and find $\widehat{\alpha}$ solving $P_n \left[S_{part} \left(\alpha \right) \right] = 0$

Step 8: For each subject compute

$$\widehat{S}_{eff,m} \left(A_m \right) = \widehat{\zeta} \left(\psi \right) R_m \left\{ exp \left(\widehat{\varkappa} \left(\psi \right)^T B_m \right) \right\}^{-1} \text{ and}$$

$$U^{\dagger} \left(\psi, \widehat{s}_{eff}, c^{\widehat{s}_{eff}}, \widehat{\alpha}, \widehat{\varsigma}, \widehat{\varkappa}, \widehat{\zeta} \right) \tag{3.15}$$

$$= \sum_{m=0}^{K} \left\{ H_m \left(\psi \right) - \widehat{\varsigma} \left(\psi \right) W_m \right\} \left\{ \widehat{S}_{eff,m} \left(A_m \right) - E_{\widehat{\alpha}} \left[\widehat{S}_{eff,m} \left(A_m \right) \mid \overline{A}_{m-1}, \overline{L}_m \right] \right\}$$

Step 9: Compute

$$P_n \left[\partial U^{\dagger} \left(\psi, \widehat{s}_{eff}, c^{\widehat{s}_{eff}}, \widehat{\alpha}, \widehat{\varsigma}, \widehat{\varkappa}, \widehat{\zeta} \right) / \partial \widehat{\varsigma} \left(\psi \right)^T \right],$$

$$P_n \left[\partial U^{\dagger} \left(\psi, \widehat{s}_{eff}, c^{\widehat{s}_{eff}}, \widehat{\alpha}, \widehat{\varsigma}, \widehat{\varkappa}, \widehat{\zeta} \right) / \partial \widehat{\alpha}^T \right],$$

$$P_n \left[\sum_{m=0}^{K} W_m^{\otimes 2} \right],$$

$$P_n \left[\partial S_{part} \left(\widehat{\alpha} \right) / \partial \alpha^T \right],$$

$$P_n \left[\partial U^{\dagger} \left(\psi, \widehat{s}_{eff}, c^{\widehat{s}_{eff}}, \widehat{\alpha}, \widehat{\varsigma}, \widehat{\varkappa}, \widehat{\zeta} \right) / \partial \psi^T \right]$$

Step 10: For each subject compute $U^{\dagger}_{adj} \left(\psi, \widehat{s}_{eff}, c^{\widehat{s}_{eff}}, \widehat{\alpha}, \widehat{\varsigma}, \widehat{\varkappa}, \widehat{\zeta} \right)$

$$= U^{\dagger} \left(\psi, \widehat{s}_{eff}, c^{\widehat{s}_{eff}}, \widehat{\alpha}, \widehat{\varsigma}, \widehat{\varkappa}, \widehat{\zeta} \right) - \tag{3.16}$$

$$P_n \left[\partial U^{\dagger} \left(\psi, \widehat{s}_{eff}, c^{\widehat{s}_{eff}}, \widehat{\alpha}, \widehat{\varsigma}, \widehat{\varkappa}, \widehat{\zeta} \right) / \partial \widehat{\alpha}^T \right] P_n \left[\partial S_{part} \left(\widehat{\alpha} \right) / \partial \alpha^T \right] S_{part} \left(\widehat{\alpha} \right) +$$

$$P_n \left[\partial U^{\dagger} \left(\psi, \widehat{s}_{eff}, c^{\widehat{s}_{eff}}, \widehat{\alpha}, \widehat{\varsigma}, \widehat{\varkappa}, \widehat{\zeta} \right) / \partial \widehat{\varsigma} \left(\psi \right)^T \right] P_n \left[\sum_{m=0}^{K} W_m^{\otimes 2} \right]^{-1} \times$$

$$\sum_{m=0}^{K} \left(H_m \left(\psi \right) - \widehat{\varsigma} \left(\psi \right) W_m \right) W_m$$

Step 11: Declare the set ψ for which

$$\chi^2_{score} \left(\psi \right) = n P_n [U^{\dagger}_{adj} \left(\psi, \widehat{s}_{eff}, c^{\widehat{s}_{eff}}, \widehat{\alpha}, \widehat{\varsigma}, \widehat{\varkappa}, \widehat{\zeta} \right)^T] \times \tag{3.17}$$

$$\widehat{\Sigma}_{adj} \left(\psi, \widehat{s}_{eff}, c^{\widehat{s}_{eff}}, \widehat{\alpha}, \widehat{\varsigma}, \widehat{\varkappa}, \widehat{\zeta} \right)^{-1} P_n [U^{\dagger}_{adj} \left(\psi, \widehat{s}_{eff}, c^{\widehat{s}_{eff}}, \widehat{\alpha}, \widehat{\varsigma}, \widehat{\varkappa}, \widehat{\zeta} \right)]$$

is less than the α upper quantile of a χ^2 distribution on the dimension of ψ degrees of freedom to be a locally efficient large sample $1 - \alpha$ score confidence interval for $\psi^\dagger$ where

$$\hat{\Sigma}_{adj}\left(\psi,\hat{s}_{eff},c^{\hat{s}_{eff}},\hat{\alpha},\hat{\varsigma},\hat{\varkappa},\hat{\zeta}\right) = P_n\left[U_{adj}^\dagger\left(\psi,\hat{s}_{eff},c^{\hat{s}_{eff}},\hat{\alpha},\hat{\varsigma},\hat{\varkappa},\hat{\zeta}\right)^{\otimes 2}\right].$$

Step 12: Solve $P_n\left[U_{adj}^\dagger\left(\psi,\hat{s}_{eff},c^{\hat{s}_{eff}},\hat{\alpha},\hat{\varsigma},\hat{\varkappa},\hat{\zeta}\right)\right] = 0$ to obtain the estimator $\hat{\psi}\left(\hat{s}_{eff},c^{\hat{s}_{eff}},\hat{\alpha},\hat{\varsigma},\hat{\varkappa},\hat{\zeta}\right)$.

Estimate $J^{\bar{d}} = E\left[Y^{\bar{d}}\right]$ by $P_n\left[H_0\left(\hat{\psi}\left(\hat{s}_{eff},c^{\hat{s}_{eff}},\hat{\alpha},\hat{\varsigma},\hat{\varkappa},\hat{\zeta}\right)\right)\right].$

Step13: Declare the set ψ for which $\chi^2_{wald}(\psi) =$

$$n\left(\hat{\psi}\left(\hat{s}_{eff},c^{\hat{s}_{eff}},\hat{\alpha},\hat{\varsigma},\hat{\varkappa},\hat{\zeta}\right)^T - \psi^T\right) \times$$

$$P_n\left[\partial U_{adj}^\dagger\left(\hat{\psi},\hat{s}_{eff},c^{\hat{s}_{eff}},\hat{\alpha},\hat{\varsigma},\hat{\varkappa},\hat{\zeta}\right)/\partial\psi^T\right] \times$$

$$\hat{\Sigma}_{adj}\left(\hat{\psi},\hat{s}_{eff},c^{\hat{s}_{eff}},\hat{\alpha},\hat{\varsigma},\hat{\varkappa},\hat{\zeta}\right)^{-1}P_n\left[\partial U_{adj}^\dagger\left(\hat{\psi},\hat{s}_{eff},c^{\hat{s}_{eff}},\hat{\alpha},\hat{\varsigma},\hat{\varkappa},\hat{\zeta}\right)/\partial\psi\right] \times$$

$$\left(\hat{\psi}\left(\hat{s}_{eff},c^{\hat{s}_{eff}},\hat{\alpha},\hat{\varsigma},\hat{\varkappa},\hat{\zeta}\right) - \psi\right) \tag{3.18}$$

is less than the α upper quantile of a χ^2 distribution on the dimension of ψ degrees of freedom to be a locally efficient large sample $1 - \alpha$ Wald confidence interval for $\psi^\dagger$. Here $\hat{\psi} = \hat{\psi}\left(\hat{s}_{eff},c^{\hat{s}_{eff}},\hat{\alpha},\hat{\varsigma},\hat{\varkappa},\hat{\zeta}\right)$

Remark: If inference is to be based on Steps 12 and 13 then we can use Newton-Raphson to obtain the solution in Step 12 and we only need to run the algorithm for the values of ψ required by the Newton-Raphson updates. If Step 11 is to be used for inference then we might use a finite search procedure and run the algorithm for the values of ψ on a finite lattice. Other computational approaches are also possible. It follows from Theorems 3.3 and 3.4 above that the estimator $\hat{\psi}\left(\hat{s}_{eff},c^{\hat{s}_{eff}},\hat{\alpha},\hat{\varsigma},\hat{\varkappa},\hat{\zeta}\right)$ is, under the union model, RAL and locally efficient at the submodel in which (3.11) holds and the model $p_m\left[A_m \mid \bar{L}_m,\bar{A}_{m-1};\alpha\right]$, the model $\varsigma^T W_m$ for $E\left[H_m\left(\psi^\dagger\right)|\bar{L}_m,\bar{A}_{m-1}\right]$, the model $exp(\varkappa B_m)$ for $var\left(H_m\left(\psi^\dagger\right)|\bar{L}_{m-1},\bar{A}_m\right)$, and the model ζR_m for $E\left[\partial H_m\left(\psi^\dagger\right)/\partial\psi|\bar{L}_m,\bar{A}_m\right]$ are all correct. Analogously the estimator $P_n\left[H_0\left(\hat{\psi}\left(\hat{s}_{eff},c^{\hat{s}_{eff}},\hat{\alpha},\hat{\varsigma},\hat{\varkappa},\hat{\zeta}\right)\right)\right]$ is a RAL estimator of $J^{\bar{d}} = E\left[Y^{\bar{d}}\right]$ in the union model that is efficient at the above submodel. We therefore refer to these estimators as locally semiparametric efficient in the union model at the above submodel. These estimators are also locally semiparametric efficient (at the same submodel) in the more restrictive models (a.1) and (a.2) which, in addition to the assumptions of the union model, respectively assume that $p_m\left[A_m \mid \bar{L}_m,\bar{A}_{m-1}\right]$ is known and the model $p_m\left[A_m \mid \bar{L}_m,\bar{A}_{m-1};\alpha\right]$ is correct.

Remark: We henceforth refer to $\hat{\psi}\left(\hat{s}_{eff},c^{\hat{s}_{eff}},\hat{\alpha},\hat{\varsigma},\hat{\varkappa},\hat{\zeta}\right)$ as a doubly-robust locally semiparametric efficient (dr-lse) estimator. It is doubly robust because it is a RAL estimator in the union model that assumes either a model for $p_m \left[A_m \mid \overline{L}_m, \overline{A}_{m-1} \right]$ or a model for $E \left[H_m \left(\psi^\dagger \right) \mid \overline{L}_m, \overline{A}_{m-1} \right]$ be correct. It is locally semiparametric efficient because it is efficient in the union model at the submodel described above.

All the results obtained in the this and the previous section in regards to point and interval estimates of $\psi^\dagger$ (but not of $E[Y_{\overline{d}}]$) remain true when we replace $H_m^{\underline{d}_m, \underline{d}_m^*} (\psi)$ by the modified version

$$H_{\text{mod},m}^{\underline{d}_m, \underline{d}_m^*} (\psi) = H_m^{\underline{d}_m, \underline{d}_m^*} (\psi) - \gamma^{\overline{d}^*} \left(\overline{L}_m, \overline{A}_{m-1}, d_m \left(\overline{L}_m, \overline{A}_{m-1} \right), \psi \right) \quad (3.19)$$

$$= Y - \gamma^{\overline{d}^*} \left(\overline{L}_m, \overline{A}_m, \psi \right) +$$

$$\sum_{j=m+1}^{K} \left\{ \gamma^{\overline{d}^*} \left(\overline{L}_j, \overline{A}_{j-1}, d_j \left(\overline{L}_j, \overline{A}_{j-1} \right), \psi \right) - \gamma^{\overline{d}^*} \left(\overline{L}_j, \overline{A}_j, \psi \right) \right\}$$

to obtain modified estimating functions $U_{\text{mod}}^{\overline{d}, \overline{d}^*}$ and $U_{\text{mod}}^{\overline{d}, \overline{d}^*, \dagger}$. This follows from the fact that the difference between $H_{\text{mod},m}^{\underline{d}_m, \underline{d}_m^*} (\psi)$ and $H_m^{\underline{d}_m, \underline{d}_m^*} (\psi)$ is fixed when we condition on $\overline{L}_m, \overline{A}_{m-1}$. Futher the efficient choice s_{eff} is exactly the same function of the data whether we use $H_{\text{mod},m}^{\underline{d}_m, \underline{d}_m^*} (\psi)$ or $H_m^{\underline{d}_m, \underline{d}_m^*} (\psi)$. The usefulness of this modification will become clear in Section 4.1.1 below.

4 Optimal drSNMM

4.1 Estimation

We now turn attention to estimation of the optimal treatment regime when, as in a sequential RCT , sequential randomization (2.5) holds and $p_m \left[A_m \mid \overline{L}_m, \overline{A}_{m-1} \right]$ is known. We first characterize the optimal regime. Define

$$d_{op,K} \left(\overline{L}_K, \overline{A}_{K-1} \right) = \arg \max_{a_K \in \mathcal{A}_K} E \left[Y_{\overline{A}_{K-1}, a_K} \mid \overline{L}_K, \overline{A}_{K-1} \right], \quad (4.1)$$

so $d_{op,K} \left(\overline{L}_K, \overline{A}_{K-1} \right)$ is the optimal treatment at time t_K for someone with observed history $\left(\overline{L}_K, \overline{A}_{K-1} \right)$. If there is more than one value of $a_K \in \mathcal{A}_K$ at which $E \left[Y_{\overline{A}_{K-1}, a_K} \mid \overline{L}_K, \overline{A}_{K-1} \right]$ is maximized, $d_{op,K} \left(\overline{L}_K, \overline{A}_{K-1} \right)$ can be arbitrarily chosen to be any one of the maximizers.

For $m = K - 1, \dots 0$, recursively define

$$d_{op,m} \left(\overline{L}_m, \overline{A}_{m-1} \right) = \arg \max_{a_m \in \mathcal{A}_m} E \left[Y_{\overline{A}_{m-1}, a_m, \underline{d}_{op,m+1}} \mid \overline{L}_m, \overline{A}_{m-1} \right] \quad (4.2)$$

where $\underline{d}_{op,m+1} = (d_{op,m+1}, \dots, d_{op,K})$ with ties again broken arbitrarily. Thus $d_{op,m} \left(\overline{L}_m, \overline{A}_{m-1} \right)$ is the optimal treatment at time t_m for someone with observed history $\left(\overline{L}_m, \overline{A}_{m-1} \right)$ who is planning to follow regime $\underline{d}_{op,m+1}$ beginning at time t_{m+1}. The following trivial Lemma follows directly from the definitions.

Lemma 4.1:
$$d_{op,m} = d_{op,m}\left(\overline{L}_m, \overline{A}_{m-1}\right) = \arg\max_{a_m \in \mathcal{A}_m} \gamma^{\overline{d}_{op}, \overline{d}^*}\left(\overline{L}_m, \overline{A}_{m-1}, a_m\right).$$
We then have the following which is a special case of Theorem 7.4 below.

Theorem 4.1: Under the sequential randomization assumption (2.5), the regime $\underline{d}_{op,m}$ maximizes

$E\left[Y_{\overline{A}_{m-1},\underline{d}_m} | \overline{L}_m, \overline{A}_{m-1}\right]$ over all regimes $\underline{d}_m \in \mathcal{D}_m$ where $\mathcal{D}_m$ is the set of all feasible regimes beginning at time t_m. Further $\overline{d}_{op} = \underline{d}_{op,0}$ maximizes $E\left[Y_{\overline{d}}\right]$ over all $\overline{d} \in \overline{\mathcal{D}}$. In addition Theorems 3.1 and 3.2 still hold with $\overline{d}_{op}$ substituted for $\overline{d}$ and with $H_m^{\underline{d}_m}\left(\gamma^{\overline{d}^*}\right) = H_m^{\underline{d}_{op,m}}\left(\gamma^{\overline{d}^*}\right)$ redefined to be

$$H_m^{\underline{d}_{op,m}}\left(\gamma^{\overline{d}^*}\right) = Y + \sum_{j=m}^{K} \left\{\gamma^{\overline{d}^*}\left(\overline{L}_j, \overline{A}_{j-1}, d_j^{**}\left(\overline{L}_j, \overline{A}_{j-1}\right)\right) - \gamma^{\overline{d}^*}\left(\overline{L}_j, \overline{A}_j\right)\right\}$$

with $d_m^{**}\left(\overline{L}_m, \overline{A}_{m-1}\right) = \arg\max_{a_m \in \mathcal{A}_m} \gamma^{\overline{d}^*}\left(\overline{L}_m, \overline{A}_{m-1}, a_m\right)$.

Suppose for a given subject we are unable to intervene prior to time t_m although data on $\overline{L}_m, \overline{A}_{m-1}$ is available. Theorem 4.1 implies that $\underline{d}_{op,m}$ is the optimal treatment plan beginning at time t_m.

Remark: Note that without sequential randomization Theorem 4.1 will not hold, because then, for example, $\underline{d}_{op,K-1} = (d_{op,K-1}, d_{op,K})$ may not maximize $E\left[Y_{\overline{A}_{K-2}, \underline{d}_{K-1}} | \overline{L}_{K-1}, \overline{A}_{K-2}\right]$. To see this consider the subset of subjects with observed history $\left(\overline{l}_{K-1}, \overline{a}_{K-2}\right)$. Note, without sequential randomization, the mean of $Y_{\overline{a}_{K-2}, d_{op,K-1}\left(\overline{l}_{K-1}, \overline{a}_{K-2}\right), a_K}$ among the subgroup with observed history $\left(\overline{l}_K, \overline{a}_{K-2}, a_{K-1} = d_{op,K-1}\left(\overline{l}_{K-1}, \overline{a}_{K-2}\right)\right)$ need not equal the mean among the larger subgroup who would have had history $\left(\overline{l}_K, \overline{a}_{K-2}, a_{K-1} = d_{op,K-1}\left(\overline{l}_{K-1}, \overline{a}_{K-2}\right)\right)$ if, contrary to fact, the entire subset with observed history $\left(\overline{l}_{K-1}, \overline{a}_{K-2}\right)$ had followed following regime $d_{op,K-1}$ and thus received treatment $d_{op,K-1}\left(\overline{l}_{K-1}, \overline{a}_{K-2}\right)$ at t_{K-1}. In that case one cannot use the basic method of backward induction (i.e. dynamic programming) to solve the sequential decision problem. See section 7.2 below for a more complete discussion.

Definition: Given a regime $\overline{d}^*$, an optimal drSNMM model $\gamma^{\overline{d}_{op}, \overline{d}^*}\left(\overline{l}_m, \overline{a}_m\right) \equiv \gamma^{\overline{d}^*}\left(\overline{l}_m, \overline{a}_m; \psi\right)$ is a drSNMM model for $\gamma^{\overline{d}_{op}, \overline{d}^*}\left(\overline{l}_m, \overline{a}_m\right)$.

Definition: Define

$$d_{op,m}\left(\overline{L}_m, \overline{A}_{m-1}, \psi\right) = \arg\max_{a_m \in \mathcal{A}_m} \gamma^{\overline{d}^*}\left(\overline{L}_m, \overline{A}_{m-1}, a_m, \psi\right)$$

Note we shall model $\gamma^{\overline{d}_{op}, \overline{d}^*}\left(\overline{l}_m, \overline{a}_m\right)$ even though $\overline{d}_{op}$ is unknown. However the model itself determines $\overline{d}_{op}$ as a function of the parameter $\psi^\dagger$ via $d_{op,m}\left(\overline{l}_m, \overline{a}_{m-1}\right) = \arg\max_{a_m \in \mathcal{A}_m} \gamma^{\overline{d}^*}\left(\overline{l}_m, \overline{a}_m; \psi^\dagger\right)$. We shall see that under sequential randomization the parameter $\psi^\dagger$ can be estimated at a $n^{1/2}-$rate.

Without loss of generality, we shall usually take the regime $\overline{d}^*$ to be the zero-regime $\overline{0}$.

Example (1): Suppose $\gamma^{\overline{0}}\left(\overline{l}_m,\overline{a}_m,\psi\right) = a_m r\left(m,\overline{l}_m,\overline{a}_{m-1},\psi_m\right)$ with a the common maximum and 0 the common minimum element in each $\mathcal{A}_m$, r a known function of ψ_m, and $\psi^T = (\psi_0,...,\psi_K)$. Then $d_{op,m}\left(\overline{l}_m,\overline{a}_{m-1},\psi\right) = a\left[I\left\{r\left(m,\overline{l}_m,\overline{a}_{m-1},\psi_m\right) > 0\right\}\right]$. We consider the explicit choice $r\left(m,\overline{l}_m,\overline{a}_{m-1},\psi_m\right) = (1,l_m,a_{m-1})\psi_m = \psi_{1m} + \psi_{2m}l_m + \psi_{3m}a_{m-1}$ in much of the ensuing discussion.

Example (2): Suppose now

$$\gamma^{\overline{0}}\left(\overline{l}_m,\overline{a}_m,\psi\right) = a_m\left[r_1\left(m,\overline{l}_m,\overline{a}_{m-1},\psi_1\right)\right] + a_m^2\left[r_2\left(m,\overline{l}_m,\overline{a}_{m-1},\psi_2\right)\right]$$

with each $\mathcal{A}_m$ being the interval $[0,a]$ on the real line and r_1 and r_2 are known functions of ψ_1 and ψ_2. Then

$$d_{op,m}\left(\overline{l}_m,\overline{a}_{m-1},\psi\right) =$$
$$\left\{I\left[r_2\left(m,\overline{l}_m,\overline{a}_{m-1},\psi_2\right) < 0\right]\right\}I\left(0 \le g\left(m,\overline{l}_m,\overline{a}_{m-1},\psi\right) \le a\right)g\left(m,\overline{l}_m,\overline{a}_{m-1},\psi\right)$$
$$+a\left\{I\left[r_2\left(m,\overline{l}_m,\overline{a}_{m-1},\psi_2\right) \ge 0\right]\right\}\left\{I\left[\begin{array}{c}ar_2\left(m,\overline{l}_m,\overline{a}_{m-1},\psi_2\right)\\+r_1\left(m,\overline{l}_m,\overline{a}_{m-1},\psi_1\right)\end{array}\right] > 0\right\}$$

where $g\left(m,\overline{l}_m,\overline{a}_{m-1},\psi\right) = -r_1\left(m,\overline{l}_m,\overline{a}_{m-1},\psi_1\right)/2r_2\left(m,\overline{l}_m,\overline{a}_{m-1},\psi_2\right)$ and the first term corresponds to a maximum in the interior of $[0,a]$ and the second term corresponds to a maximum at the boundary point a. Here $I[B]$ is the indicator function that takes the value 1 if B is true and 0 otherwise.

Under sequential randomization (2.5) and $p_m\left(a_m|\overline{L}_m,\overline{A}_{m-1}\right)$ known, we now consider the properties of approximate minimizers of $\left\{P_n\left[U\left(\psi,s\right)\right]\right\}^T B\left\{P_n\left[U\left(\psi,s\right)\right]\right\}$ with $U\left(\psi,s\right) = U^{\overline{d}_{op},\overline{0}}\left(\psi,s\right)$ as defined in Equation (3.9), each function s_m having range the dimension of ψ, B a positive definite square matrix, and $H_m^{\overline{d}_{op},\overline{0}}\left(\psi\right)$ defined by

$$H_m^{\overline{d}_{op},\overline{0}}\left(\psi\right) = Y + \sum_{j=m}^{K}\left\{\gamma^{\overline{0}}\left(\overline{L}_j,\overline{A}_{j-1},d_{op,j}\left(\overline{L}_j,\overline{A}_{j-1},\psi\right),\psi\right) - \gamma^{\overline{0}}\left(\overline{L}_j,\overline{A}_j,\psi\right)\right\}.$$

Note that even when as in examples 1 and 2, $\gamma^{\overline{0}}\left(\overline{l}_m,\overline{a}_m,\psi\right)$ is smooth (or even linear) in ψ, $H^{\overline{d}_{op},\overline{0}}\left(\psi\right)$ and $U^{\overline{d}_{op},\overline{0}}\left(\psi,s\right)$ will not be everywhere differentiable in ψ (because ψ appears within indicator functions), although both remain continuous in ψ. Because $U^{\overline{d}_{op},\overline{0}}\left(\psi,s\right)$ is a nonlinear function of ψ, $E\left[U^{\overline{d}_{op},\overline{0}}\left(\psi,s\right)\right] = 0$ may have roots in addition to $\psi^\dagger$ in which case $\left\{P_n\left[U\left(\psi,s\right)\right]\right\}^T B\left\{P_n\left[U\left(\psi,s\right)\right]\right\}$ will have an inconsistent minimizer even asymptotically. As before if we increase the dimension of the s, then in sufficiently large samples the problem of multiple minimizers should disappear under correct specification, but not if the model $\gamma^{\overline{0}}\left(\overline{l}_m,\overline{a}_m,\psi\right)$ is misspecified.

Define $U^{\dagger \overline{d}_{op}, \overline{0}} \left(\psi, \widehat{s}_{eff}, c^{\widehat{s}_{eff}}, \widehat{\alpha}, \widehat{\varsigma}, \widehat{\varkappa}, \widehat{\zeta} \right)$ as above but restricted to the set of ψ at which the required ψ−derivatives exist. Refer to this set as the admissible set. [In example 1, these ψ−derivatives will fail to exist only for values of ψ satisfying $(1, L_{m,i}, A_{m-1,i}) \psi_m = 0$ for some study subject i as it is only at these values of ψ for which the contribution of subject i is nondifferentiable. Specifically in that case $d_{op,j} \left(\overline{L}_{j,i}, \overline{A}_{j-1,i}, \psi \right)$ and $H_{j,i}^{\overline{d}_{op}, \overline{0}} (\psi), j \leq m$ are non differentiable for that subject.] A unique $n^{1/2} -$ consistent member $\widehat{\psi} \left(\widehat{s}_{eff}, c^{\widehat{s}_{eff}}, \widehat{\alpha}, \widehat{\varsigma}, \widehat{\varkappa}, \widehat{\zeta} \right)$ of the admissible set solving $P_n \left[U^{\dagger \overline{d}_{op}, \overline{0}} \left(\psi, \widehat{s}_{eff}, c^{\widehat{s}_{eff}}, \widehat{\alpha}, \widehat{\varsigma}, \widehat{\varkappa}, \widehat{\zeta} \right) \right] = 0$ will exist with probability approaching one. It is a dr-lse estimator (i.e. it is RAL and lse not only in model (a.1) with $p_m \left(a_m | \overline{L}_m, \overline{A}_{m-1} \right)$ known but also in the larger $\overline{d}_{op}, \overline{0}$ "union" model of Theorem 3.4 in which $p_m \left(a_m | \overline{L}_m, \overline{A}_{m-1} \right)$ is not known), except under the exceptional laws F_O defined as those laws at which, for some m, $\arg \max_{a_m \in \mathcal{A}_m} \gamma^{\overline{0}} \left(\overline{L}_m, \overline{A}_{m-1}, a_m, \psi^{\dagger} \right)$ is not unique with positive probability. In example 1, these exceptional laws are the laws under which $(1, \overline{L}_m, \overline{A}_{m-1}) \psi_m^{\dagger} = 0$ with positive probability. Even at these laws this estimator remains $n^{1/2} - consistent$ for $\psi^{\dagger}$ although not CAN and thus not RAL. These exceptional laws are discussed in detail in Section 5.1 and Appendix 1.

A Closed-Form Estimator of an Optimal drSNMM

We now show that, if, as in our examples, $\gamma^{\overline{0}} \left(\overline{l}_m, \overline{a}_m, \psi \right)$ is linear in ψ, we can obtain a closed -form $n^{1/2}$-consistent estimator $\widetilde{\psi}$ under the union model of Theorem 3.4 based on solving a sequence of linear estimating functions. Then $P_n \left[H_0^{\overline{d}_{op}, \overline{0}} \left(\widetilde{\psi} \right) \right]$ is a closed-form $n^{1/2}$-consistent estimator of $E \left[Y_{\overline{d}_{op}} \right]$ that does not require modelling $f \left[l_m \mid \overline{l}_{m-1}, \overline{a}_{m-1} \right]$. The importance of having a closed-form $n^{1/2}$-consistent estimator of $\psi^{\dagger}$ is that it avoids the problem with our earlier estimating functions. That is they could have multiple roots, an unknown one of which is consistent. Although the closed-form estimator $\widetilde{\psi}$ is not locally efficient, the one-step update

$$\widetilde{\psi}^{(1)} = \widetilde{\psi} + P_n \left[EIF \left(\widetilde{\psi} \right) \right] \text{ where}$$

$$EIF \left(\widetilde{\psi} \right) = P_n \left[\partial U_{adj}^{\dagger} \left(\widetilde{\psi}, \widehat{s}_{eff}, c^{\widehat{s}_{eff}}, \widehat{\alpha}, \widehat{\varsigma}, \widehat{\varkappa}, \widehat{\zeta} \right) / \partial \psi^T \right]^{-1} \times$$
$$P_n \left[U_{adj}^{\dagger} \left(\widetilde{\psi}, \widehat{s}_{eff}, c^{\widehat{s}_{eff}}, \widehat{\alpha}, \widehat{\varsigma}, \widehat{\varkappa}, \widehat{\zeta} \right) \right]$$

is locally efficient in the union model of Theorem 3.4. Note $EIF \left(\widetilde{\psi} \right)$ is an estimator of the efficient influence function for ψ in the union model at a particular submodel. The key to obtaining $\widetilde{\psi}$ is to use $U_{mod}^{\overline{d}_{op}, \overline{0}} (\psi, s) =$

$\sum_{m=0}^{K} U_{\text{mod},m}^{\overline{d}_{op},\overline{0}}(\psi, s_m)$ defined just before Section 4 as a basis for estimation rather than $U^{\overline{d}_{op},\overline{0}}(\psi, s)$.

We first show how to construct $\widetilde{\psi}$ in the case in which $p_m\left(a_m | \overline{L}_m, \overline{A}_{m-1}\right)$ is known, $\psi = (\psi_0, ..., \psi_K)$ and $\gamma^{\overline{0}}\left(\overline{l}_m, \overline{a}_m, \psi\right) = \gamma^{\overline{0}}\left(\overline{l}_m, \overline{a}_m, \underline{\psi}_m\right)$ with $\gamma^{\overline{0}}\left(\overline{l}_m, \overline{a}_m, \underline{\psi}_m\right)$ linear and/or smooth in ψ_m but not necessarily in $\underline{\psi}_{m+1}$. It is crucial that at time t_m, our model $\gamma^{\overline{0}}\left(\overline{l}_m, \overline{a}_m, \psi\right)$ depends on ψ only through $\underline{\psi}_m$. We estimate the ψ_m recursively beginning with ψ_K so that at the step in which we estimate ψ_m, we have already estimated the vector $\underline{\psi}_{m+1}$. Specifically let $\widetilde{\psi}_K$ solve $P_n\left[U_{\text{mod},K}^{\overline{d}_{op},\overline{0}}(\psi_K, s_K)\right] = 0$ where $U_{\text{mod},K}^{\overline{d}_{op},\overline{0}}(\psi_K, s_K) = H_{\text{mod},K}^{\overline{d}_{op},\overline{0}}(\psi_K)\left\{S_K(A_K) - E\left[S_K(A_K) | \overline{A}_{K-1}, \overline{L}_K\right]\right\}$, and $H_{\text{mod},K}^{\overline{d}_{op},\overline{0}}(\psi_K) = Y - \gamma^{\overline{0}}\left(\overline{L}_K, \overline{A}_K, \psi_K\right)$. Then, for $m = K - 1, ..., 0$, let $\widetilde{\psi}_m$ recursively solve, $P_n\left[U_{\text{mod},m}^{\overline{d}_{op},\overline{0}}\left(\psi_m, \underline{\widetilde{\psi}}_{m+1}, s_m\right)\right] = 0$, where

$$U_{\text{mod},m}^{\overline{d}_{op},\overline{0}}\left(\psi_m, \underline{\widetilde{\psi}}_{m+1}, s_m\right)$$
$$= H_{\text{mod},m}^{d_{op},m,\overline{0}}\left(\psi_m, \underline{\widetilde{\psi}}_{m+1}\right)\left\{S_m(A_m) - E\left[S_m(A_m) | \overline{A}_{m-1}, \overline{L}_m\right]\right\},$$

$$H_{\text{mod},m}^{d_{op},m,\overline{0}}\left(\psi_m, \underline{\widetilde{\psi}}_{m+1}\right) = Y - \gamma^{\overline{0}}\left(\overline{L}_m, \overline{A}_m, \psi_m, \underline{\widetilde{\psi}}_{m+1}\right)$$
$$+ \sum_{j=m+1}^{K}\left\{\gamma^{\overline{0}}\left(\overline{L}_j, \overline{A}_{j-1}, d_{op,j}\left(\overline{L}_j, \overline{A}_{j-1}, \underline{\widetilde{\psi}}_j\right), \underline{\widetilde{\psi}}_j\right) - \gamma^{\overline{0}}\left(\overline{L}_j, \overline{A}_j, \underline{\widetilde{\psi}}_j\right)\right\},$$

and $S_m(a_m) = s_m\left(\overline{L}_m, \overline{A}_{m-1}, a_m\right)$ has range the dimension of ψ_m. Note $E\left[U_{\text{mod},m}^{\overline{d}_{op},\overline{0}}\left(\psi_m^{\dagger}, \underline{\psi}_{m+1}^{\dagger}, s_m\right)\right] = 0$. Further each of these estimating functions are smooth in ψ_m when $\gamma^{\overline{0}}\left(\overline{l}_m, \overline{a}_m, \underline{\psi}_m\right)$ is smooth in ψ_m and will be linear in ψ_m when $\gamma^{\overline{0}}\left(\overline{l}_m, \overline{a}_m, \underline{\psi}_m\right)$ is linear in ψ_m. In the linear case $\widetilde{\psi}(s) = \widetilde{\psi}_0(s) = \widetilde{\psi}_0 = \left(\widetilde{\psi}_0, .., \widetilde{\psi}_K\right)^T$ is unique and exists in closed form. In the following, we suppress the dependence on s and write $\widetilde{\psi}_0(s) = \widetilde{\psi}_0 = \left(\widetilde{\psi}_0, .., \widetilde{\psi}_K\right)^T$. With $\gamma^{\overline{0}}\left(\overline{l}_m, \overline{a}_m, \psi\right) = (1, l_m, a_{m-1})\psi_m$ of Example 1,

$$\widetilde{\psi}_m = \widetilde{I_m}^{-1} \times P_n$$
$$\left[\left\{Y + \sum_{j=m+1}^{K}\left\{\gamma^{\overline{0}}\left(\overline{L}_j, \overline{A}_{j-1}, d_{op,j}\left(\overline{L}_j, \overline{A}_{j-1}, \widetilde{\psi}_j\right), \widetilde{\psi}_j\right) - \gamma^{\overline{0}}\left(\overline{L}_j, \overline{A}_j, \widetilde{\psi}_j\right)\right\}\right\}\right]$$
$$\left\{S_m(A_m) - E[S_m(A_m) | \overline{A}_{m-1}, \overline{L}_m]\right\} \times$$

whenever the three by three derivative matrix $\tilde{I}_m =$
$P_n\left[\{S_m(A_m) - E[S_m(A_m)|\overline{A}_{m-1}, \overline{L}_m]\}A_m(1, L_m, A_{m-1})\right]$ is invertible. Further, when $\gamma^{\overline{0}}\left(\overline{L}_m, \overline{A}_m, \psi_m, \underline{\tilde{\psi}}_{m+1}\right)$ is linear in ψ_m, $\tilde{\psi}_m\left(\hat{s}_{eff}, c^{\hat{s}_{eff}}, \hat{\alpha}, \hat{\varsigma}, \hat{\varkappa}, \hat{\zeta}\right)$
solving $P_n\left[U_{mod,adj,m}^{\dagger, \overline{d}_{op}, \overline{0}}\left(\psi_m, \underline{\tilde{\psi}}_{m+1}, \hat{s}_{eff}, c^{\hat{s}_{eff}}, \hat{\alpha}, \hat{\varsigma}, \hat{\varkappa}, \hat{\zeta}\right)\right] = 0$ is a closed form
dr-lse estimator (i.e. it is lse not only in model a.1 with $p_m\left(a_m|\overline{L}_m, \overline{A}_{m-1}\right)$
known but also in the larger $\overline{d}_{op}, \overline{0}$ "union" model of Theorem 3.4 in which
$p_m\left(a_m|\overline{L}_m, \overline{A}_{m-1}\right)$ is not known) except at the exceptional laws mentioned
above where it remains $n^{1/2}-$ consistent.

Remark on Estimation Under A Deterministic Design: When
ψ_m is of sufficiently low dimension and, as in the sequential decision literature, the design parameters of the simulation generating the data under
analysis are in the analyst's control, it is computationally feasible to accurately estimate the ψ_m without using the above estimation methods by
recursively employing time-specific deterministic designs to obtain estimators $\hat{\psi}_m, m = K, ..., 0$ as described in Section 2.2. For example at time t_m
we can estimate ψ_{1m} by fixing $\left(\overline{L}_{m,i}, \overline{A}_{m-1,i}\right) = 0$ for all i, $i = 1, ..., n$,
and simulating Y_i under the subsequent regime $\left\{a_{\max, m}, \underline{d}_{op, m+1}\left(\underline{\hat{\psi}}_{m+1}\right)\right\}$ for
$i \leq n/2$ and $\left\{a_{\min, m}, \underline{d}_{op, m+1}\left(\underline{\hat{\psi}}_{m+1}\right)\right\}$ for $i > n/2$, and taking $\hat{\psi}_{1m}$ to be
$\{a_{\max, m} - a_{\min, m}\}^{-1}$ times the difference between the averages of Y_i in the
first and second half of the sample of size n. One can gain computational
efficiency by reusing relevant simulations from times greater than t_m. Alternatively one could use a matched design as described in Remark 2.1 of Section
2.2.

Now suppose that, as in example 1, ψ_m is the same for each m so
$\gamma^{\overline{0}}\left(\overline{l}_m, \overline{a}_m, \psi_m\right) = (1, l_m, a_{m-1})\psi$. One can still artificially regard the common ψ as $K + 1$ separate time-specific parameter vectors ψ_m. We can obtain the $K + 1$ estimates $\tilde{\psi}_m(s)$ and their (estimated) covariance matrix and
combine them by inverse covariance weighting to give a final more efficient
estimate $\tilde{\psi}(s)$. Indeed if we let $\tilde{\psi}_m\left(\hat{s}_{eff}, c^{\hat{s}_{eff}}, \hat{\alpha}, \hat{\varsigma}, \hat{\varkappa}, \hat{\zeta}\right)$ be as above, the
inverse covariance weighted estimator will be a dr-lse of the time-independent
parameter ψ, except at the exceptional laws. This efficiency result requires
that $\hat{s}_{eff}$ estimate the optimal choice s_{eff} for the model that does not impose equality of the different ψ_m. Alternatively the estimator $\tilde{\psi}^{(1)}$ is a dr-lse,
but here $\hat{s}_{eff}$ must estimate s_{eff} for the model that does impose equality of
the different ψ_m

Suppose the time $\Delta t = t_{m+1} - t_m$ between treatments is so short that
very few subjects have A_{m+1} different from A_m. Then, $\tilde{\psi}_m, m < K$, can have
unacceptable small sample bias, even though it is asymptotically unbiased if
Δt stays fixed as $n \to \infty$. To see why note that $\tilde{\psi}_K$ will then be excessively
variable because its variance is an increasing function of the inverse of the
conditional variance of A_K given $\left(\overline{A}_{K-1}, \overline{L}_K\right)$ that increases to infinity as the

conditional variance of A_{K+1} decreases to zero. The excessive variability in $\widetilde{\psi}_K$ will then lead to severe small sample bias in $\widetilde{\psi}_{K-1}$ because $\widetilde{\psi}_K$ enters the estimating function $U_{\text{mod},K-1}^{\overline{d}_{op}}\left(\psi_{K-1}, \widetilde{\psi}_K, s_{K-1}^*\right)$ in a highly non-linear manner through it's inclusion within an indicator function. Thus even when all the $\psi_m = \psi$ are known to be equal and K is large so there is plenty of information available to estimate ψ, our locally efficient one-step estimator $\widetilde{\psi}^{(1)}$ can be very biased. Thus we have no choice but to solve the non-differentiable vector of estimating functions $U_{\text{mod}}^{\overline{d}_{op}}(\psi, s)$ non-sequentially, which can be computationally difficult and may suffer from the problem of multiple roots . In Section 8 we consider the extreme case of treatment innovations in continuous time, where Δt can be arbitrarily small.

Uniform Asymptotic Confidence Intervals For ψ and $\overline{d}_{op}$ By Inverting Tests

Although the estimators $\widetilde{\psi}$ and $\widehat{\psi}$ of the previous subsections will be $n^{1/2}$-consistent (i.e., $n^{1/2}\left(\widehat{\psi} - \psi^\dagger\right)$ and $n^{1/2}\left(\widetilde{\psi} - \psi^\dagger\right)$ are bounded in probability) at all laws allowed by our model , they will be neither asymptotically unbiased nor asymptotically normal under "exceptional" laws F_O satisfying, for some m, $\arg\max_{a_m \in A_m} \gamma^{\overline{0}}\left(\overline{L}_m, \overline{A}_{m-1}, a_m, \psi^\dagger\right)$ is not unique with positive probability. Specifically, as discussed in Appendix 1.1, the limiting distributions of $n^{1/2}\left(\widehat{\psi} - \psi^\dagger\right)$ and $n^{1/2}\left(\widetilde{\psi} - \psi^\dagger\right)$ will be non-normal with a non zero mean (and thus will not be CAN) at such exceptional laws. Indeed, as shown in Appendix 1.1, $\psi^\dagger$ is not a regular parameter at these laws in the sense that it is not a differentiable function of a smooth finite dimensional parameterization of the law of O. It follows that, because of their unknown asymptotic bias, we cannot obtain uniformly asymptotically unbiased estimators of $\psi^\dagger$ and thus cannot construct valid (i.e. uniform over the entire model) asymptotic Wald-type confidence intervals for $\psi^\dagger$ centered on any estimator including $\widehat{\psi}$ or $\widetilde{\psi}$ of the previous subsections.

However one can obtain valid uniform confidence intervals for such non-regular parameters by inverting tests. For example, uniformly over all laws F_O allowed by the model with $p_m\left(a_m | \overline{L}_m, \overline{A}_{m-1}\right)$ known the sets $C\left(1 - \alpha\right)$ and $C_{\text{mod}}\left(1 - \alpha\right)$ of ψ for which $nP_n[U^{\overline{d}_{op},\overline{0}}(\psi, s)]^T \widehat{\Sigma}(\psi, s)^{-1} P_n[U^{\overline{d}_{op},\overline{0}}(\psi, s)]$ and $nP_n[U_{\text{mod}}^{\overline{d}_{op},\overline{0}}(\psi, s)]^T \widehat{\Sigma}_{\text{mod}}(\psi, s)^{-1} P_n[U_{\text{mod}}^{\overline{d}_{op},\overline{0}}(\psi, s)]$, respectively, are less than the α upper quantile, say, $\chi_{\alpha,\dim(\psi)}$, of a χ^2 distribution on the dimension of ψ degrees of freedom are uniform large sample $1 - \alpha$ confidence interval for $\psi^{\dagger\cdot}$. [The set $C\left(1 - \alpha\right)$ has no relation to the random variable C defined in Section 3.3.] Further under the $\overline{d}_{op},\overline{0}$ union model of Theorem 3.4 or the more restrictive models (a.1) and (a.2), the interval $C_{op}\left(1 - \alpha\right)$ based on $\chi_{score}^{2,\overline{d}_{op},\overline{0}}(\psi)$ of Eq (3.17) will be a uniform asymptotic confidence interval over all laws allowed by the model.

One can also obtain conservative uniform large sample (i.e. asymptotic) $1 - \alpha$ confidence intervals for functions of $\psi^\dagger$, even discrete functions such as $\bar{d}_{op}$. The set

$$D_{op}(1 - \alpha) = \tag{4.3}$$

$$\left\{ \bar{d}_{op}(\psi) ; d_{op,m}(\psi) = \arg \max_{a_m \in \mathcal{A}_m} \gamma^{\bar{d}_{op}\bar{0}} \left(\bar{l}_m, \bar{a}_m ; \psi \right), \ \psi \in C_{op}(1 - \alpha) \right\}$$

is an example. That is, writing $\bar{d}_{op}(\psi^\dagger)$ as $\bar{d}_{op}(F_O)$ and $D_{op}(1 - \alpha)$ as $D_{op,n}(1 - \alpha)$ to emphasize the dependence on sample size n, by the definition of an conservative uniform asymptotic confidence interval in Appendix 1.1, we have that given any $\delta > 0$, there exists a $N(\delta)$ such that

for all $n > N(\delta)$ and all sequences $F_{O,1}, F_{O,2}, ...$ in the union model

$$(1 - \alpha) - \Pr_{F_{O,n}} \left[\bar{d}_{op}(F_{O,n}) \in D_{op,n}(1 - \alpha) \right] < \delta. \tag{4.4}$$

In contrast, by definition, a non-uniform conservative asymptotic $(1 - \alpha)$ confidence interval $D_n^*(1 - \alpha)$ satisfies: given any $\delta > 0$ and any F_O in the union model, there exists a $N(\delta, F_O)$ depending on F_O, such that

for all $n > N(\delta, F_O)$ \qquad\qquad (4.5)

$$(1 - \alpha) - \Pr_{F_O} \left[\bar{d}_{op}(F_O) \in D_n^*(1 - \alpha) \right] < \delta$$

Thus only the conservative uniform asymptotic confidence interval has the property that there exists some finite sample size $N(\delta)$ such that for $n > N(\delta)$, the interval $D_{op,n}(1 - \alpha)$ contains the true optimal regime $\bar{d}_{op}$ with probability greater than $(1 - \alpha - \delta)$. In contrast a conservative non-uniform asymptotic $(1 - \alpha)$ confidence interval is not guaranteed to contain the true $\bar{d}_{op}$ with probability greater than $(1 - \alpha - \delta)$ at any sample size. For this reason we are only interested in uniform asymptotic confidence intervals. Now because the volume of $C_{op}(1 - \alpha)$ is asymptotically equivalent to the volume of the Wald intervals based on the dr-lse estimator. $\hat{\psi} \left(\hat{s}_{eff}, c^{\hat{s}_{eff}}, \hat{\alpha}, \hat{\varsigma}, \hat{\varkappa}, \hat{\zeta} \right)$ at the unexceptional laws, we doubt it will be possible to obtain an interval for $\bar{d}_{op}(\psi^\dagger)$ that is substantially narrower (say by a factor of more than 2 under any law in the union model) than $D_{op,n}(1 - \alpha)$. However the confidence interval $D_{op,n}(1 - \alpha)$ for the optimal regime $\bar{d}_{op}$ may at a given sample size n be too wide (i.e., contain too many candidate regimes $\bar{d}_{op}(\psi)$) to provide reliable optimal decisions. In that case we must make a choice among these $\bar{d}_{op}(\psi)$. We discuss this issue further below and in particular discuss a Bayesian solution based on informative priors for the unknown parameters.

It is useful to understand when $D_{op,n}(1 - \alpha)$ may contain many candidate regimes $\bar{d}_{op}(\psi)$. In a slight abuse of notation we say the confidence interval $C_{op,n}(1 - \alpha)$ contains a law F_O if $C_{op,n}(1 - \alpha)$ contains a value ψ such that

$\gamma^{\overline{0}}\left(\overline{L}_m, \overline{A}_{m-1}, a_m, \psi\right)$ equals the blip function $\gamma^{\overline{d}_{op}\overline{0}}\left(\overline{L}_m, \overline{A}_{m-1}, a_m\right)$ associated with F_O. At a fixed sample size n, even if the data were generated under a (unknown) nonexceptional law $F_{ne,O}$ and n is very large, the confidence interval $C_{op,n}(1-\alpha)$ may contain one or more exceptional laws (i.e a law $F_{e,O}$ under which $\arg\max_{a_m \in A_m} \gamma^{\overline{d}_{op}\overline{0}}\left(\overline{L}_m, \overline{A}_{m-1}, a_m\right)$ is not unique with positive probability). It then follows that the interval $C_{op,n}(1-\alpha)$ will (generally) also contain another non-exceptional law $F^*_{ne,O}$ such that $\overline{d}_{op}(F_{ne,O})$ differs from $\overline{d}_{op}\left(F^*_{ne,O}\right)$, *as the exceptional laws form the boundary separating non-exceptional laws corresponding to different optimal treatment regimes.*

Thus $C_{op,n}(1-\alpha)$ may often contain both $F_{ne,O}$ and $F^*_{ne,O}$ and thus $D_{op,n}(1-\alpha)$ will often contain both $\overline{d}_{op}(F_{ne,O})$ and $\overline{d}_{op}\left(F^*_{ne,O}\right)$. Because both $F_{ne,O}$ and $F^*_{ne,O}$ are non-exceptional laws, we know that under $F_{ne,O}$, the maximal expected utility $E[Y_{\overline{d}_{op}(F_{ne,O})}]$ is strictly greater than $E[Y_{\overline{d}_{op}\left(F^*_{nc,O}\right)}]$ while under $F^*_{ne,O}$, $E[Y_{\overline{d}_{op}\left(F^*_{nc,O}\right)}]$ is strictly greater than $E[Y_{\overline{d}_{op}(F_{ne,O})}]$. Now since, without further information we remain uncertain whether $F_{ne,O}$ or $F^*_{ne,O}$ or neither generated the data, we do not know whether to choose $\overline{d}_{op}(F_{ne,O})$ or $\overline{d}_{op}\left(F^*_{ne,O}\right)$ or neither. Such further information may be available as informative priors for unknown parameters.

Note that because (i) the data were generated under $F_{ne,O}$ and (ii) $\overline{d}_{op}(F_{ne,O})$ differs from $\overline{d}_{op}\left(F^*_{ne,O}\right)$, it is true that our non-uniform asymptotics guarantees that there exists some sample size $\tilde{n} = \tilde{n}\left(F_{ne,O}, F^*_{ne,O}\right), \tilde{n} > n$, such that $D_{op,n}(1-\alpha)$ will exclude $\overline{d}_{op}\left(F^*_{ne,O}\right)$ with very high probability. But of course this fact is of no use when the actual sample size is n. Thus, we see that a "uniform asymptotics" in contrast to a "non-uniform asymptotics" correctly recognizes that even when data is generated under an unknown non-exceptional law $F_{ne,O}$, at (even a large) fixed sample size n, we often cannot rule out the hypothesis that the data were generated either under an exceptional law $F_{e,O}$ or under a non-exceptional law $F^*_{ne,O}$ with $\overline{d}_{op}\left(F^*_{ne,O}\right)$ different from $\overline{d}_{op}(F_{ne,O})$.

5 Locally Efficient Optimal Treatment Decisions For Individual Patients

In this section we will restrict attention to dichotomous $(0,1)$ treatments, so that any model for $\gamma^{\overline{d}_{op},\overline{0}}\left(\overline{l}_m, \overline{a}_m\right)$ takes the form $\gamma^{\overline{0}}\left(\overline{l}_m, \overline{a}_m, \psi\right) = a_m r\left(m, \overline{l}_m, \overline{a}_{m-1}, \psi\right)$ of example 1 of Section 4.1 with $a_m \in \{0,1\}$. Thus $d_{op,m}\left(\overline{l}_m, \overline{a}_{m-1}, \psi\right) = I\left\{r\left(m, \overline{l}_m, \overline{a}_{m-1}, \psi\right) > 0\right\}$. Suppose, after the study is completed, a new patient appears in his physicians office at time t_m since diagnosis with past data $\left(\overline{l}_m, \overline{a}_{m-1}\right)$. One might suppose that for this patient on day t_m, the parameter of immediate interest is $\psi_{int} = r\left(m, \overline{l}_m, \overline{a}_{m-1}, \psi\right)$, as the patient should be treated if $\psi^\dagger_{int} = r\left(m, \overline{l}_m, \overline{a}_{m-1}, \psi^\dagger\right)$ is positive and not treated if negative. [Here 'int' abbreviates 'interest' and not 'intervention']. If this supposition were correct we might wish to obtain locally efficient tests of the single null hypothesis $H_0 : \psi_{int}^\dagger \leq 0$ versus the alternative $H_1 : \psi_{int}^\dagger > 0$ without any consideration given to simultaneous inference or the multiple testing problem that results from testing similar hypotheses at many times and for many patients with different $\left(\overline{l}_m, \overline{a}_{m-1}\right)$ histories. However the sign of $\psi_{int}^\dagger$ only determines the optimal treatment decision on day t_m for this patient if in fact the patient follows the optimal regime from t_{m+1} onwards. But because of uncertainty we cannot be assured that the subject will follow the optimal regime subsequent to time t_m unless $m = K$, as t_K is the final treatment time (even if we assume, as we shall do for the time being, that all uncertainty is attributable to sampling variability and not also to model misspecification, to unmeasured confounding, or to lack of compliance.) Nonetheless we shall study the interesting mathematical issue of how to obtain locally efficient tests of the single null hypothesis $H_0 : \psi_{int}^\dagger \leq 0$ versus the alternative $H_1 : \psi_{int}^\dagger > 0$, in the prescence of exceptional laws, as the results will be useful later.

5.1   A Frequentist Approach to Locally Efficient Tests of $H_0 : \psi_{int}^\dagger \leq 0$

It follows from Equation (3.19) that we can rewrite $H_{mod,m}^{\overline{d}_{op},\overline{0}}\left(\psi\right) =$

$$Y - A_m r\left(m, \overline{L}_m, \overline{A}_{m-1}, \psi\right) +$$
$$\sum_{j=m+1}^{K} \left\{I\left\{r\left(j, \overline{L}_j, \overline{A}_{j-1}, \psi_j\right) > 0\right\} - A_j\right\} r\left(j, \overline{L}_j, \overline{A}_{j-1}, \psi\right),$$

and from Equation (3.9) and (3.10) that we can rewrite $U_{mod}^{\dagger, \overline{d}_{op}, \overline{0}}\left(\psi, s_{eff}, c_{eff}^s\right) =$

$$\sum_{m=0}^{K} \left\{H_{mod,m}^{\overline{d}_{op}, \overline{0}}\left(\psi\right) - E\left[H_{mod,m}^{\overline{d}_{op}, \overline{0}}\left(\psi\right) | \overline{A}_{m-1}, \overline{L}_m\right]\right\} \times$$
$$\left\{S_{eff,m}\left(1, \psi\right) - S_{eff,m}\left(0, \psi\right)\right\} \left\{A_m - E\left[A_m \mid \overline{A}_{m-1}, \overline{L}_m\right]\right\}$$

In the remainder of this section we suppress the $\overline{d}_{op}, \overline{0}$ superscript and assume $r\left(m, \overline{L}_m, \overline{A}_{m-1}, \psi\right)$ is twice continuously differentiable with respect to ψ with probability one. Differentiability of $U_{mod}^\dagger\left(\psi^\dagger, s_{eff}, c_{eff}^s\right)$ at $\psi^\dagger$ with probability one will turn out to be of crucial concern. We now show that $U_{mod}^\dagger\left(\psi^\dagger, s_{eff}, c_{eff}^s\right)$ and (indeed $U_{mod}^\dagger\left(\psi^\dagger, s, c^s\right)$ for any s) is differentiable at $\psi^\dagger$ w.p.1 except for laws F_O under which for some (j, m), with non-zero probability all of the following hold, (i) $r\left(j, \overline{L}_j, \overline{A}_{j-1}, \psi^\dagger\right) = 0$ (ii) $m < j$ and (iii) $B_{mj}\left(\psi^\dagger\right) = 1$. Here $B_{mj}\left(\psi^\dagger\right)$ is the indicator of the event that $r\left(j, \overline{L}_j, \overline{A}_{j-1}, \psi\right)$ depends on at least one component of $\left(\underline{A}_m, \underline{L}_{m+1}\right)$ for some ψ in every open neighborhood of $\psi^\dagger$. To obtain this result note (i) $H_{\text{mod},m}(\psi) - E\left[H_{\text{mod},m}(\psi)|\overline{A}_{m-1}, \overline{L}_m\right]$ will be a function of $I\left\{r\left(j, \overline{L}_j, \overline{A}_{j-1}, \psi\right) > 0\right\}$ unless $B_{mj}(\psi) = 0$ for all $j > m$ and (ii) if, for all ψ in a neighborhood of $\psi^\dagger$, $B_{mj}(\psi) = 0$ w.p1. for all $(m, j), j > m$, then $U^\dagger_{\text{mod}}\left(\psi, s_{eff}, c^s_{eff}\right)$ does not have ψ occurring within an indicator function and is thus smooth at $\psi^\dagger$. A law F_O satisfying (i)-(iii) is said to be an exceptional law. In general any law F_O under which the g-null hypothesis $\psi^\dagger = 0$ holds will be an exceptional law, except if the model $r\left(m, \overline{l}_m, \overline{a}_{m-1}, \psi\right)$ rules out all treatment interactions apriori by specifying that $r\left(m, \overline{l}_m, \overline{a}_{m-1}, \psi\right) = r(m, \psi)$ does not depend on $\overline{l}_m, \overline{a}_{m-1}$ for all ψ, in which case $U^\dagger_{\text{mod}}\left(\psi, s_{eff}, c^s_{eff}\right)$ is smooth in ψ.

Remark: The non-doubly robust statistic $U_{\text{mod}}(\psi, s)$, in contrast to $U^\dagger_{\text{mod}}(\psi, s, c^s)$, will be nondifferentiable at $\psi^\dagger$ with positive probability when, for some m, $r\left(m, \overline{L}_m, \overline{A}_{m-1}, \psi^\dagger\right) = 0$ with non-zero probability. This is equivalent to saying that $\arg_{a_m \in \mathcal{A}_m} \gamma^{\overline{0}}\left(\overline{L}_m, \overline{A}_{m-1}, a_m, \psi^\dagger\right)$ is not unique with positive probability. Thus, when earlier, we were considering tests and estimators based on $U_{\text{mod}}(\psi, s)$, we referred to any law F_O satisfying only condition (i) as an exceptional law.

We now reparametrize so that the parameter ψ_{int} is substituted for some component of ψ on which $r\left(m, \overline{l}_m, \overline{a}_{m-1}, \psi\right)$ functionally depends, so now, in a slight abuse of notation,

$$\psi = \left(\psi_{int}, \psi^T_{-int}\right)^T \text{ where } \psi_{-int} \text{ are the unchanged components of the}$$
original ψ.

Write $U^\dagger_{\text{mod}\,adj}\left(\psi, \widehat{s}_{eff}, c^{\widehat{s}_{eff}}, \widehat{\alpha}, \widehat{\varsigma}, \widehat{\varkappa}, \widehat{\zeta}\right)$ as

$$\left(U^\dagger_{\text{mod}\,adj,int}\left(\psi, \widehat{s}_{eff}, c^{\widehat{s}_{eff}}, \widehat{\alpha}, \widehat{\varsigma}, \widehat{\varkappa}, \widehat{\zeta}\right), U^\dagger_{\text{mod}\,adj,-int}\left(\psi, \widehat{s}_{eff}, c^{\widehat{s}_{eff}}, \widehat{\alpha}, \widehat{\varsigma}, \widehat{\varkappa}, \widehat{\zeta}\right)^T\right)^T$$

Define $S_{int,eff}\left(\psi, \widehat{\alpha}, \widehat{\varsigma}, \widehat{\varkappa}, \widehat{\zeta}\right) =$

$$U^\dagger_{\text{mod}\,adj,int}\left(\psi, \widehat{s}_{eff}, c^{\widehat{s}_{eff}}, \widehat{\alpha}, \widehat{\varsigma}, \widehat{\varkappa}, \widehat{\zeta}\right) -$$
$$E[\partial U^\dagger_{\text{mod}\,adj,int}\left(\psi, \widehat{s}_{eff}, c^{\widehat{s}_{eff}}, \widehat{\alpha}, \widehat{\varsigma}, \widehat{\varkappa}, \widehat{\zeta}\right)/\partial \psi^T_{-int}]\times$$
$$E[\partial U^\dagger_{\text{mod}\,adj,-int}\left(\psi, \widehat{s}_{eff}, c^{\widehat{s}_{eff}}, \widehat{\alpha}, \widehat{\varsigma}, \widehat{\varkappa}, \widehat{\zeta}\right)/\partial \psi^T_{-int}]^{-1}\times$$
$$U^\dagger_{\text{mod}\,adj,-int}\left(\psi, \widehat{s}_{eff}, c^{\widehat{s}_{eff}}, \widehat{\alpha}, \widehat{\varsigma}, \widehat{\varkappa}, \widehat{\zeta}\right)$$

The (locally) efficient score $S_{int,eff}\left(\psi^\dagger, \alpha^*, \varsigma^*, \varkappa^*, \zeta^*\right)$ for ψ_{int} with the other components of ψ_{-int} treated as nuisance parameters is the probability limit of $S_{int,eff}\left(\psi^\dagger, \widehat{\alpha}, \widehat{\varsigma}, \widehat{\varkappa}, \widehat{\zeta}\right)$ in the $\overline{d}_{op}, \overline{0}$ union model of Theorem 3.4, provided F_O is not an exceptional law. The locally efficient score for ψ_{int} is undefined at exceptional laws, because ψ_{int} is a non-regular parameter under these laws. See appendix A1.1.

We now construct a conservative $1 - \alpha$ uniform asymptotic confidence interval for $\psi_{int}^\dagger$ that quite generally will be narrower than the so-called $1 - \alpha$ projection interval $\{\psi_{int}; \psi_{int} = \psi_{int}(\psi)$ for some $\psi \in C_{op}(1 - \alpha)\}$ based on the interval $C_{op}(1 - \alpha)$ for the vector ψ. In the following $\varnothing$ denotes the null set and $C_{-int,}(1 - \varepsilon, \psi_{int})$ is a uniform large sample $1 - \varepsilon$ joint confidence interval for ψ_{-int} when assuming that $\psi_{int}^\dagger$ is known apriori to be equal to ψ_{int}. For example, $C_{-int,}(1 - \varepsilon, \psi_{int})$ could be the interval $C_{mod}(1 - \varepsilon)$ of the last subsection given by $U_{mod}^{\overline{d}_{op}, \overline{0}}(\psi, s)^T \hat{\Sigma}_{mod}(\psi, s)^{-1} U_{mod}^{\overline{d}_{op}, \overline{0}}(\psi, s)$ is less than the ε upper quantile of a χ^2 distribtion on $\dim(\psi_{-int}) = \dim(\psi) - 1$ d.f. except that one component (say the last) of $U_{mod}^{\overline{d}_{op}, \overline{0}}(\psi, s)$ has been eliminated so $U_{mod}^{\overline{d}_{op}, \overline{0}}(\psi, s)$ is now of $\dim(\psi) - 1$ to reflect the fact that ψ_{int} is regarded as known.

Theorem 5.1: . Let the interval $C_{-int,}(1 - \varepsilon, \psi_{int})$ be a uniform large sample $1 - \varepsilon$ joint confidence interval for ψ_{-int}, when assuming that $\psi_{int}^\dagger$ is known apriori to be equal to ψ_{int}. Under regularity conditions sketched in the proof below, the region

$$\left\{ \inf_{\psi_{-int} \in C_{-int,}(1-\varepsilon,\psi_{int})} \left| \frac{n^{1/2} P_n\left[S_{int,eff}\left((\psi_{int},\psi_{-int}),\hat{\alpha},\hat{\varsigma},\hat{\varkappa},\hat{\zeta}\right)\right]}{P_n\left[S_{int,eff}\left((\psi_{int},\psi_{-int}),\hat{\alpha},\hat{\varsigma},\hat{\varkappa},\hat{\zeta}\right)^2\right]^{1/2}} \right| < z_{\alpha/2} \right\}$$
(5.1)

is a conservative $1 - \alpha - \varepsilon$ uniform asymptotic confidence region for $\psi_{int}^\dagger$ over all laws allowed by the model. The interval's coverage and length are asymptotically equivalent to the asymptotic coverage of $(1 - \alpha)$ and the length of the locally optimal interval $\left\{ \psi_{int}; \left| \frac{n^{1/2} P_n\left[S_{int,eff}\left((\psi_{int},\psi_{-int}^\dagger),\alpha^*,\varsigma^*,\varkappa^*,\zeta^*\right)\right]}{E\left[S_{int,eff}\left((\psi_{int},\psi_{-int}^\dagger),\alpha^*,\varsigma^*,\varkappa^*,\zeta^*\right)^2\right]^{1/2}} \right| < z_{\alpha/2} \right\}$
at all laws but the exceptional laws. Similarly for $z_\alpha > 1$, the test that rejects when

$$I\left\{ \inf_{\psi_{-int} \in C_{-int,}(1-\varepsilon,\psi_{int})} \frac{n^{1/2} P_n\left[S_{int,eff}\left((0,\psi_{-int}),\hat{\alpha},\hat{\varsigma},\hat{\varkappa},\hat{\zeta}\right)\right]}{P_n\left[S_{int,eff}\left((0,\psi_{-int}),\hat{\alpha},\hat{\varsigma},\hat{\varkappa},\hat{\zeta}\right)^2\right]^{1/2}} > z_\alpha \right\}$$

is a conservative uniform asymptotic $\alpha + \varepsilon - level$ test of $H_0 : \psi_{int}^\dagger \leq 0$ versus $H_1 : \psi_{int}^\dagger > 0$ whose asymptotic level will be α and whose asymptotic local power will be equal to that of the locally optimal test

$$I\left\{ \frac{n^{1/2} P_n\left[S_{int,eff}\left((0,\psi_{-int}^\dagger),\alpha^*,\varsigma^*,\varkappa^*,\zeta^*\right)\right]}{P_n\left[S_{int,eff}\left((0,\psi_{-int}^\dagger),\alpha^*,\varsigma^*,\varkappa^*,\zeta^*\right)^2\right]^{1/2}} > z_\alpha \right\} \text{ under all laws but the excep-}$$

tional laws.

Remark: When a conservative uniform asymptotic confidence interval for a vector ψ is available, the method given in Theorem 5.1 is a quite general method of obtaining a conservative uniform asymptotic confidence interval for a subvector ψ_{int} of ψ that will in general be narrower than the projection interval. The narrowness of the interval and the power of the associated test depend critically on the fact that, when $\psi_{int} = \psi_{int}^\dagger$, the statistic's numerator, here $n^{1/2}P_n\left[S_{int,eff}\left((\psi_{int},\psi_{-int}),\widehat{\alpha},\widehat{\varsigma},\widehat{\varkappa},\widehat{\zeta}\right)\right]$, has an expectation that, for n sufficiently large, varies less (to a smaller order) as ψ_{-int} varies over a $1-\varepsilon$ confidence interval $C_{-int}\left(1-\varepsilon,\psi_{int}^\dagger\right)$ than as ψ_{int} varies around $\psi_{int}^\dagger$ over an interval of length $O\left(n^{-1/2}\right)$. This general approach would allow us to construct confidence intervals for ψ_{int} that can do better than projection intervals even when ψ_{-int} is infinite dimensional and/or ψ_{int} is only estimable at non square-root n rates.

Proof: At any law that is not an exceptional law, ψ_{int} and ψ_{-int} are regular parameters. At any such law we assume that, with probability one, $U_{\text{mod }adj}^\dagger\left(\psi,\widehat{s}_{eff},c^{\widehat{s}_{eff}},\widehat{\alpha},\widehat{\varsigma},\widehat{\varkappa},\widehat{\zeta}\right)$ has bounded second derivatives with respect to ψ_{-int}. [Note this assumption cannot hold at an exceptional law since at these laws $U_{\text{mod }adj}^\dagger\left(\psi,\widehat{s}_{eff},c^{\widehat{s}_{eff}},\widehat{\alpha},\widehat{\varsigma},\widehat{\varkappa},\widehat{\zeta}\right)$, although continuous, will not be even once differentiable.] Further, when $\psi_{int} = \psi_{int}^\dagger$, the value $\widehat{\psi}_{\inf,-int}$ where the infimum is attained will be uniformly $n^{1/2}-consistent$ for $\psi_{-int}^\dagger$ as all members of the set $C_{-int},(1-\varepsilon,\psi_{int})$ are uniformly $n^{1/2}-consistent$ over all laws in the model. It then follows from the following lemma 5.1 and some standard limit arguments using contiguity theory that

$$\frac{n^{1/2}P_n\left[S_{int,eff}((\psi_{int},\widehat{\psi}_{\inf,-int}),\widehat{\alpha},\widehat{\varsigma},\widehat{\varkappa},\widehat{\zeta})\right]}{P_n\left[S_{int,eff}((\psi_{int},\widehat{\psi}_{\inf,-int}),\widehat{\alpha},\widehat{\varsigma},\widehat{\varkappa},\widehat{\zeta})^2\right]^{1/2}} = \frac{n^{1/2}P_n\left[S_{int,eff}((\psi_{int},\psi_{-int}^\dagger),\alpha^*,\varsigma^*,\varkappa^*,\zeta^*)\right]}{E\left[S_{int,eff}((\psi_{int},\psi_{-int}^\dagger),\alpha^*,\varsigma^*,\varkappa^*,\zeta^*)^2\right]^{1/2}} +$$

$o_p(1)$ when $\psi_{int} = \psi_{int}^\dagger + kn^{-1/2}$ for any constant k.

Suppose now we are at an exceptional law and $\psi_{int} = \psi_{int}^\dagger$. Let $\widehat{\psi}_{\inf,-int}$ be the minimizer of (5.1). We know with probability $1-\varepsilon$ that $C_{-int},(1-\varepsilon,\psi_{int})$ contains $\psi_{-int}^\dagger$. Thus with uniform probability $1-\varepsilon$,

$$\left|\frac{n^{1/2}P_n\left[S_{int,eff}((\psi_{int},\widehat{\psi}_{\inf,-int}),\widehat{\alpha},\widehat{\varsigma},\widehat{\varkappa},\widehat{\zeta})\right]}{P_n\left[S_{int,eff}((\psi_{int},\widehat{\psi}_{\inf,-int}),\widehat{\alpha},\widehat{\varsigma},\widehat{\varkappa},\widehat{\zeta})^2\right]^{1/2}}\right| \leq \left|\frac{n^{1/2}P_n\left[S_{int,eff}((\psi_{int},\psi_{-int}^\dagger),\widehat{\alpha},\widehat{\varsigma},\widehat{\varkappa},\widehat{\zeta})\right]}{P_n\left[S_{int,eff}((\psi_{int},\psi_{-int}^\dagger),\widehat{\alpha},\widehat{\varsigma},\widehat{\varkappa},\widehat{\zeta})^2\right]^{1/2}}\right|.$$

But $\left|\dfrac{n^{1/2}P_n\left[S_{int,eff}((\psi_{int},\psi_{-int}^\dagger),\widehat{\alpha},\widehat{\varsigma},\widehat{\varkappa},\widehat{\zeta})\right]}{P_n\left[S_{int,eff}((\psi_{int},\psi_{-int}^\dagger),\widehat{\alpha},\widehat{\varsigma},\widehat{\varkappa},\widehat{\zeta})^2\right]^{1/2}}\right| < z_{\alpha/2}$ with uniform probability $1-\alpha$ as $n\to\infty$. Thus as $n\to\infty$, $\left|\dfrac{n^{1/2}P_n\left[S_{int,eff}((\psi_{int},\widehat{\psi}_{\inf,-int}),\widehat{\alpha},\widehat{\varsigma},\widehat{\varkappa},\widehat{\zeta})\right]}{P_n\left[S_{int,eff}((\psi_{int},\widehat{\psi}_{\inf,-int}),\widehat{\alpha},\widehat{\varsigma},\widehat{\varkappa},\widehat{\zeta})^2\right]^{1/2}}\right| < z_{\alpha/2}$ with uniform probability at least $1-\varepsilon-\alpha$.

Lemma 5.1: Suppose $E_{\psi_1,\psi_2}\left[U_a\left(\psi_1,\psi_2\right)\right] = E_{\psi_1,\psi_2}\left[U_b\left(\psi_1,\psi_2\right)\right]$ and $\partial^2 U_a\left(\psi_1,\psi_2\right)/\partial^2\psi_2$ and $\partial^2 U_b\left(\psi_1,\psi_2\right)/\partial^2\psi_2$ are continuous and bounded with probability 1. Define

$U_1 (\psi_1, \psi_2)$

$= U_a (\psi_1, \psi_2) - P_n [\partial U_a (\psi_1, \psi_2) / \partial \psi_2] \{P_n [\partial U_b (\psi_1, \psi_2) / \partial \psi_2]\}^{-1} U_b (\psi_1, \psi_2)$

Then under mild regularity conditions $P_{\psi_1, \psi_2}, n^{1/2} P_n \left[U_1 \left(\psi_1, \widehat{\psi}_2 \right) \right]$

$= n^{1/2} P_n [U_1 (\psi_1, \psi_2)] + o_p (1)$ whenever $n^{1/2} \left(\widehat{\psi}_2 - \psi_2 \right)$ is uniformly bounded in probability.

Proof: see Appendix 2

Remark: Note that, even if $U_a (\psi_1, \psi_2)$ and $U_b (\psi_1, \psi_2)$ are non differentiable, Lemma 5.1 remains true under weak regularity conditions if the derivatives $m_a (\psi_1, \psi_2) = \partial E_{\psi_1, \psi_2} [U_a (\psi_1, \psi_2^*)] / \partial \psi_2^*|_{\psi_2^* = \psi_2}$ and $m_b (\psi_1, \psi_2) = \partial E_{\psi_1, \psi_2} [U_b (\psi_1, \psi_2^*)] / \partial \psi_2^*|_{\psi_2^* = \psi_2}$ exist and $U_1 (\psi_1, \psi_2)$ is redefined to be

$U_1 (\psi_1, \psi_2)$

$= U_a (\psi_1, \psi_2) - \widetilde{m}_a (\psi_1, \psi_2) \{\widetilde{m}_b (\psi_1, \psi_2)\}^{-1} U_b (\psi_1, \psi_2)$

where $\widetilde{m}_a (\psi_1, \psi_2)$ and $\widetilde{m}_b (\psi_1, \psi_2)$ are based on "numerical derivatives" of $P_n [U_a (\psi_1, \psi_2)]$ and $P_n [U_b (\psi_1, \psi_2)]$ with step sizes of $O \left(n^{-1/2} \right)$ whenever $U_a (\psi_1, \psi_2)$ and $U_b (\psi_1, \psi_2)$ are non differentiable. This still does not help at exceptional laws since, under exceptional laws, the derivative of $E \left[S_{int, eff} \left(\left(\psi_{int}, \psi_{-int}^\dagger \right), \alpha^*, \varsigma^*, \varkappa^*, \zeta^* \right) \right]$ with respect to $\psi_{-int}^\dagger$ does not exist.

Remark 5.1: $\left\{ \psi_{int}; \left| \dfrac{n^{1/2} P_n \left[S_{int, eff} \left((\psi_{int}, \widehat{\psi}_{-int}), \widehat{\alpha}, \widehat{\varsigma}, \widehat{\varkappa}, \widehat{\zeta} \right) \right]}{P_n \left[S_{int, eff} \left((\psi_{int}, \widehat{\psi}_{-int}), \widehat{\alpha}, \widehat{\varsigma}, \widehat{\varkappa}, \widehat{\zeta} \right)^{\times 2} \right]^{1/2}} \right| < z_{\alpha/2} \right\}$ for

$\widehat{\psi}_{-int}$ an arbitrary $n^{1/2}$-consistent estimator of $\psi_{-int}^\dagger$ need not be a $1 - \alpha - \varepsilon$ uniform asymptotic confidence interval for $\psi_{int}^\dagger$ for any given ε because, at the exceptional laws, we do not obtain guaranteed coverage of $1 - \alpha - \varepsilon$ unless we use the minimizer $\widehat{\psi}_{\inf, -int}$ of (5.1). Similarly

$I \left\{ \dfrac{n^{1/2} P_n \left[S_{int, eff} \left((0, \widehat{\psi}_{-int}), \widehat{\alpha}, \widehat{\varsigma}, \widehat{\varkappa}, \widehat{\zeta} \right) \right]}{P_n \left[S_{int, eff} \left((0, \widehat{\psi}_{-int}), \widehat{\alpha}, \widehat{\varsigma}, \widehat{\varkappa}, \widehat{\zeta} \right)^{\times 2} \right]^{1/2}} > z_\alpha \right\}$ need not be a conservative asymp-

totic $\alpha + \varepsilon - level$ test under an exceptional law. Furthermore had we taken the infimum over all ψ_{-int} (rather than just over ψ_{-int} in $C_{-int}, (1 - \varepsilon, \psi_{int})$), the resulting test

$$I \left\{ \inf_{\psi_{-int}} \dfrac{n^{1/2} P_n \left[S_{int, eff} \left((0, \psi_{-int}), \widehat{\alpha}, \widehat{\varsigma}, \widehat{\varkappa}, \widehat{\zeta} \right) \right]}{P_n \left[S_{int, eff} \left((0, \psi_{-int}), \widehat{\alpha}, \widehat{\varsigma}, \widehat{\varkappa}, \widehat{\zeta} \right)^{\times 2} \right]^{1/2}} > z_\alpha \right\}$$

with $z_\alpha > 1$, though conservative, may have power zero, as it is possible that *the* test statistic may equal zero with probability one, at both local and global alternatives to $\psi_{int}^\dagger. < 0$ whether the data were generated under an exceptional or nonexceptional law. To see why the power can be poor if we take the infimum over all ψ_{-int}, consider the following simple example of a model with an exceptional law.

Example: Suppose we observe n iid copies of $X \sim N(\beta, 1), Y \sim N(\psi - I(\beta > 0)\beta, 1)$, X and Y independent. Then ψ is in the role of ψ_{int}, β is in the role of ψ_{-int} and ψ is a regular parameter except at the exceptional laws that have $\beta = 0$. If $\beta \neq 0$, the efficient score based on one observation for ψ at $\psi = 0$ is $I(\beta \le 0)Y + I(\beta > 0)(Y + X)$. Thus our .05 level test of $\psi > 0$ that takes the infimum over all β rejects only if $I\{min(n^{1/2}Y_{av}, n^{1/2}(Y_{av} + X_{av})/\sqrt{2}) > 1.64\} = 1$. Suppose the law generating the data has $\beta = -100n^{-1/2}$, $\psi = 10n^{-1/2}$ so Y has mean $10n^{-1/2}$, X has mean $-100n^{-1/2}$ and $Y + X$ has mean $-90n^{-1/2}$, and $X - Y$ has mean $-110n^{-1/2}$. Then the test will fail to accept the true alternative $\psi > 0$ with probability essentially one (i.e it has power zero). On the other hand the efficient score for β with $\psi = 0$ is $I(\beta \le 0)(X - \beta) + I(\beta > 0)(X - Y - 2\beta)$ so $C_\beta(1 - \varepsilon, \psi = 0) =$

$$\left\{ \begin{array}{c} \beta; \beta \le 0 \text{ and } X_{av} - n^{-1/2}z_\varepsilon < \beta < X_{av} + n^{-1/2}z_\varepsilon, \text{ or} \\ \beta > 0 \text{ and } \left[\frac{(X_{av} - Y_{av}) - n^{-1/2}z_\varepsilon\sqrt{2}}{2}\right] < \beta < \left[\frac{(X_{av} - Y_{av}) + n^{-1/2}z_\varepsilon\sqrt{2}}{2}\right] \end{array} \right\}.$$

Now, if we choose ε large enough that $z_\varepsilon < 100/\sqrt{2}$, then $C_\beta(1 - \varepsilon, \psi = 0)$ is, with probability essentially one, the set $\{\beta; \beta \le 0 \text{ and } X_{av} - n^{-1/2}z_\varepsilon < \beta < X_{av} + n^{-1/2}z_\varepsilon \}$. Thus the test of $\psi > 0$ that takes the infimum only over all $\beta \in C_\beta(1 - \varepsilon, \psi = 0)$ rejects whenever $I\{n^{1/2}Y_{av} > 1.64\} = 1$ and thus has power essentially 1. If we take the infimum over all β, the power of zero is not only against local alternatives or near exceptional laws as can be seen by noting that again we have power zero if $\beta = -100$, $\psi = 10$ or $\beta = -100$, $\psi = 10n^{-1/2}$.

We can also use this example to understand why we needed to add the condition $C_{-int}(1 - \varepsilon, \psi_{int}) \neq \emptyset$ to our interval and testing procedures. Suppose the true data generating process has $\beta = 100n^{-1/2}$ and $\psi = 300n^{-1/2}$. Then with probability essentially one, the interval $C_\beta(1 - \varepsilon, \psi = 0)$ will be empty for any reasonably small ε since X has mean $100n^{-1/2}$ and $X - Y$ has mean $100n^{-1/2} - 200n^{-1/2} = -100n^{-1/2}$. The emptiness of the confidence interval for β can be taken as evidence of model misspecification due to assuming, for the purpose of hypothesis testing, that ψ is known apriori to be equal to 0. Thus $\psi = 0$ should, as is appropriate, not be included in the confidence interval and also be rejected when doing two-sided testing. For a one sided test we may not wish to reject as we may not know which side of $\psi = 0$ we are on.

The above results leave open the question of what $\alpha - level$ or more precisely $\alpha + \varepsilon - level$ to choose to make the best treatment decision. We shall see there is no easy answer. Suppose we choose ε to be much smaller than α so we can ignore the distinction between α and $\alpha + \varepsilon$. The classical thoughtless frequentist tradition is to choose $\alpha = .05$, but there is really no justification for this convention. Further as patients are seen at many different times t_m

from diagnosis with different histories $(\bar{l}_m, \bar{a}_{m-1})$, we will be testing the null hypothesis $\psi_{int} \leq 0$ about many time-history-specific parameters ψ_{int}. How should we adjust the $\alpha-level$ of our tests to account for the multiple hypotheses being tested? How should we account for the fact that with the exception of the last treatment occasion K, we cannot be certain we shall succeed in following the optimal regime in the future? Perhaps a Bayesian approach is best. We next explore such an approach.

5.2 Approximate Bayesian Inference:

To begin we will study the following two decision rules (i) and (ii) in which we treat a patient with past data $(\bar{l}_m, \bar{a}_{m-1})$ on day t_m if (i) the posterior probability that $\psi_{int} = r\left(m, \bar{l}_m, \bar{a}_{m-1}, \psi\right)$ is positive exceeds $1/2$ (i.e. the posterior median is positive) or (ii) the posterior mean of $\psi_{int} = r\left(m, \bar{l}_m, \bar{a}_{m-1}, \psi\right)$ is positive. In our complex high-dimensional model, exact Bayesian inference that respects the semiparametric nature of the problem is not computationally feasible nor, as we shall argue, would it be desirable even if computationally feasible. Therefore, we consider an approximate (i.e. asymptotic) Bayesian analysis. Our analysis will face 2 separate problems. First how do we obtain an approximate posterior for the model parameter $\psi^\dagger$ and thus for $r\left(m, \bar{l}_m, \bar{a}_{m-1}, \psi^\dagger\right)$. Our second problem will be to consider whether either of the two decision rules (i) and (ii) is the optimal Bayes decision rule and, if not, how might we approximate the optimal Bayes rule. The first problem we shall consider now. As for the second, we shall later show that neither decision rule may be the Bayes rule.

Let $\mathbf{t}$ be the $dim(\psi)$ vector with each component equal to t. For any $dim(\psi)$ random variable V, define the the $t - truncated$ version

$$V_t = VI\left[V^T V < dim\left(\psi\right) t^2\right] + \mathbf{t}I\left[V^T V > dim\left(\psi\right) t^2\right]$$

of V to the variable that takes the value $\mathbf{t}$ whenever the norm of V exceeds $dim\left(\psi\right)^{1/2} t$. In this section, our approach will be to pretend that rather than observing the data O_i, $i = 1, ..., n$, we *only* observed the $t - truncated$ version $\widehat{Z}_t\left(\cdot\right) = Z_t\left(\cdot, \widehat{s}_{eff}, c^{\widehat{s}_{eff}}, \widehat{\alpha}, \widehat{\varsigma}, \widehat{\varkappa}, \widehat{\zeta}\right)$ of the multivariate stochastic process $\widehat{Z}\left(\cdot\right)$ indexed by ψ

where

$$\widehat{Z}\left(\cdot\right) = Z\left(\cdot, \widehat{s}_{eff}, c^{\widehat{s}_{eff}}, \widehat{\alpha}, \widehat{\varsigma}, \widehat{\varkappa}, \widehat{\zeta}\right)$$

$$= \widehat{\Sigma}^{-1/2}\left(\cdot, \widehat{s}_{eff}, c^{\widehat{s}_{eff}}, \widehat{\alpha}, \widehat{\varsigma}, \widehat{\varkappa}, \widehat{\zeta}\right) n^{1/2} P_n\left[U_{adj}^\dagger\left(\cdot, \widehat{s}_{eff}, c^{\widehat{s}_{eff}}, \widehat{\alpha}, \widehat{\varsigma}, \widehat{\varkappa}, \widehat{\zeta}\right)\right].$$

We now argue that for large n and for $t = t(n)$ going to infinity slowly enough with n, the distribution associated with the stochastic process $\widehat{Z}_t\left(\cdot\right)$ under a law F_O with parameter $\psi^\dagger = \psi^\dagger\left(F_O\right)$ depends on F_O only through $\psi^\dagger$ with a "density" proportional to that of the t-truncated version of a dim

(ψ) $MVN(0, I)$ random variable evaluated at the argument $\widehat{Z}_t\left(\psi^\dagger\right)$. That is $f\left(\widehat{Z}_t\left(\cdot\right)|F_O\right)$ is proportional to $\phi_{t-Normal}\left(\widehat{Z}_t\left(\psi^\dagger\right)\right)$ where $\phi_{t-Normal}\left(u\right)$ is the density of a t-truncated MVN$(0,1)$ random variable. Thus with p the dimension of $\psi^\dagger$ we can approximate the likelihood $f\left(\widehat{Z}_t\left(\cdot\right)|F_O\right)$ with $(2\pi)^{-p/2}\exp\left(-\widehat{Z}_t\left(\psi^\dagger\right)^T\widehat{Z}_t\left(\psi^\dagger\right)/2\right)$ uniformly in F_O, whenever $\widehat{Z}_t\left(\psi^\dagger\right)^T\widehat{Z}_t\left(\psi^\dagger\right) < \dim\left(\psi\right)t^2$. To see why, write Z_t as $Z_{n,t(n)}$ and $\widehat{Z}_t$ as $\widehat{Z}_{n,t(n)}$. Then, the approximation follows from the fact that, under regularity conditions, it can be shown that (i) $\widehat{Z}_{n,t(n)}\left(\cdot\right)$ is uniformly asymptotically degenerate, i.e. given any $\epsilon > 0$, there exists $N\left(\epsilon\right)$ such that for $n > N\left(\epsilon\right)$

$$\sup_{F_O} pr_{F_O}\left[\left|\frac{f\left(\widehat{Z}_{n,t(n)}\left(\cdot\right)|F_O\right)}{f\left(\widehat{Z}_{n,t(n)}\left(\psi^\dagger\right)|F_O\right)}-1\right|>\epsilon\right]<\epsilon$$

where $\psi^\dagger = \psi^\dagger\left(F_O\right)$, (ii) $\widehat{Z}_{n,t(n)}\left(\psi^\dagger\right)$ can be approximated by the t-truncated version $Z_{n,t(n)}\left(\psi^\dagger, F_O\right)$ of the limit random variable $Z_n\left(\psi^\dagger, F_O\right)$, where $Z_n\left(\psi, F_O\right) = Z\left(\psi\right) =$

$$Z\left(\psi, s^*_{eff}, c^{s^*}_{eff}, \alpha^*, \varsigma^*, \varkappa^*, \zeta^*\right)$$
$$=\widehat{\Sigma}^{-1/2}\left(\psi, s^*_{eff}, c^{s^*}_{eff}, \alpha^*, \varsigma^*, \varkappa^*, \zeta^*\right)n^{+1/2}\times$$
$$P_n\left[U^\dagger_{\text{mod} adj}\left(\psi, s^*_{eff}, c^{s^*}_{eff}, \alpha^*, \varsigma^*, \varkappa^*, \zeta^*\right)\right]$$

with the * limits evaluated under F_O; that is, for any $\epsilon > 0$, there exists $N^*\left(\epsilon\right)$ such that for $n > N^*\left(\epsilon\right)$

$$\sup_{F_O} pr_{F_O}\left\{\left|\widehat{Z}_{n,t(n)}\left(\psi^\dagger\right)-Z_{n,t(n)}\left(\psi^\dagger\left(F_O\right), F_O\right)\right|>\epsilon\right\}<\epsilon$$

and (iii) the limit variable $Z_{n,t(n)}\left(\psi^\dagger\left(F_O\right), F_O\right)$ is uniformly asymptotically t-truncated normal i.e., given u, for any $\epsilon > 0$, there exists $N^{**}\left(\epsilon\right)$ such that for $n > N^{**}\left(\epsilon\right)$

$$\sup_{F_O}\left|pr_{F_O}\left[Z_{n,t(n)}\left(\psi^\dagger\left(F_O\right), F_O\right)>u\right]-\Phi_{t(n),normal}\left(u\right)\right|<\epsilon$$

where $\phi_{t-Normal}\left(u\right)$ is the distribution function of a t-truncated MVN$(0, I)$ random variable. In each case the sup is over the F_O in the union model of Theorem 3.4. Thus we have a uniform large sample approximation to the likelihood function based on observing $Z_t\left(\cdot, \widehat{s}_{eff}, c^{\widehat{s}_{eff}}, \widehat{\alpha}, \widehat{\varsigma}, \widehat{\varkappa}, \widehat{\zeta}\right)$.

We give a rough sketch of the proof. The key idea is to show that Theorem 3.4 implies that under the $\overline{d}_{op}, \overline{0}$ union model, for $\left(\psi - \psi^\dagger\right)$ of $O\left(n^{-1/2}\right)$,

$$n^{+1/2} P_n \left[U^\dagger_{mod\,adj} \left(\psi, \widehat{s}_{eff}, c^{\widehat{s}_{eff}}, \widehat{\alpha}, \widehat{\varsigma}, \widehat{\varkappa}, \widehat{\zeta} \right) \right] \tag{5.2}$$

$$= n^{+1/2} P_n \left[U^\dagger_{mod\,adj} \left(\psi^\dagger, s^*_{eff}, c^{s^*_{eff}}, \alpha^*, \varsigma^*, \varkappa^*, \zeta^* \right) \right] + \kappa \left(\psi, \psi^\dagger, F_O \right) + o_P (1)$$

where $\psi^\dagger = \psi^\dagger (F_O)$, the $o_P (1)$ is uniform over the model, and $\kappa (\cdot, \cdot, \cdot)$ is a non-random function that equals 0 at $\psi = \psi^\dagger$, is everywhere continuous in ψ, and differentiable when F_O is a non-exceptional law. Note if it were not for exceptional laws, where $E \left[U^\dagger_{mod\,adj} \left(\psi, s^*_{eff}, c^{s^*_{eff}}, \alpha^*, \varsigma^*, \varkappa^*, \zeta^* \right) \right]$ may be non-differentiable in ψ (although continuous), standard arguments could be used to show that Eq.(5.2) was true with $\kappa \left(\psi, \psi^\dagger, F_O \right)$ equal to

$$\partial E \left[U^\dagger_{mod\,adj} \left(\psi, s^*_{eff}, c^{s^*_{eff}}, \alpha^*, \varsigma^*, \varkappa^*, \zeta^* \right) \right] / \partial \psi^T_{|\psi = \psi^\dagger} \, n^{1/2} \left(\psi - \psi^\dagger \right)$$

Because it would be notationally complex and thereby obscure the essential idea, we do not provide a general proof of (5.2); rather in appendix $A1.2$, we provide, with essentially no loss of generality, an explicit proof for a simple paradigmatic example.

Remark 5.2: Under an exceptional law F_O, for all ψ (except $\psi^\dagger$) in a neighborhood of $\psi^\dagger$ $DER (\psi) = DER (\psi, F_O)$
$= \partial E \left[U^\dagger_{mod\,adj} \left(\psi, s^*_{eff}, c^{s^*_{eff}}, \alpha^*, \varsigma^*, \varkappa^*, \zeta^* \right) \right] / \partial \psi^T$ exists and $\kappa \left(\psi, \psi^\dagger (F_O), F_O \right) = DER (\psi) n^{1/2} \left(\psi - \psi^\dagger \right)$; however, $DER (\psi^\dagger)$ is undefined because for different sequences $seq_m = \{ \psi_{mj}; j = 1, 2, ... \}$ all converging to $\psi^\dagger$, $\{ DER (\psi_{mj}); j = 1, 2, ... \}$ may converge to different limits depending on the particular seq_m. Nonetheless since the set of limits is bounded, $\kappa \left(\psi, \psi^\dagger (F_O), F_O \right)$ converges to 0 as $\psi \to \psi^\dagger$. See Appendix A1.2 for an example. One can view the lack of existence of the derivative of $DER (\psi^\dagger)$ at $\psi^\dagger$ under an exceptional law as the reason that $\widehat{\psi}$ solving $n^{-1/2} P_n \left[U^\dagger_{mod\,adj} \left(\psi, \widehat{s}_{eff}, c^{\widehat{s}_{eff}}, \widehat{\alpha}, \widehat{\varsigma}, \widehat{\varkappa}, \widehat{\zeta} \right) \right] = 0$ is asymptotically biased since, plugging $\widehat{\psi}$ in place of ψ in (5.2) with $\kappa \left(\psi, \psi^\dagger, F_O \right) = DER (\psi) n^{1/2} \left(\psi - \psi^\dagger \right)$, we have

$$n^{+1/2} P_n \left[U^\dagger_{mod\,adj} \left(\widehat{\psi}, \widehat{s}_{eff}, c^{\widehat{s}_{eff}}, \widehat{\alpha}, \widehat{\varsigma}, \widehat{\varkappa}, \widehat{\zeta} \right) \right] \tag{5.3}$$

$$= n^{+1/2} P_n \left[U^\dagger_{mod\,adj} \left(\psi^\dagger, s^*_{eff}, c^{s^*_{eff}}, \alpha^*, \varsigma^*, \varkappa^*, \zeta^* \right) \right] +$$

$$DER \left(\widehat{\psi}, F_O \right) n^{1/2} \left(\widehat{\psi} - \psi^\dagger \right) + o_P (1)$$

so $n^{1/2} \left(\widehat{\psi} - \psi^\dagger \right) =$

$$- \left\{ DER \left(\widehat{\psi} \right) \right\}^{-1} n^{-1/2} P_n \left[U^\dagger_{mod\,adj} \left(\psi^\dagger, s^*_{eff}, c^{s^*_{eff}}, \alpha^*, \varsigma^*, \varkappa^*, \zeta^* \right) \right] + o_P (1).$$

The bias results from the fact that $DER \left(\widehat{\psi} \right)$ is not converging in probability but rather, due to the lack of continuity of the derivative $DER (\psi)$ at $\psi^\dagger$,

$DER\left(\widehat{\psi}\right)$ has variance $O\left(1\right)$. Eq (5.2) implies that, uniformly, for $\left(\psi - \psi^\dagger\right)$ in a ball of radius $O\left(n^{-1/2}\right)$,

$$\widehat{Z}\left(\psi\right) = Z\left(\psi^\dagger\right) + \kappa^*\left(\psi, \psi^\dagger, F_O\right) + o_P\left(1\right) \qquad (5.4)$$

where $\kappa^*\left(\psi, \psi^\dagger, F_O\right)$ is a non-random function that is continuous in ψ, differentiable at non-exceptional laws, equal to 0 at $\psi = \psi^\dagger$, and, for $\psi \neq \psi^\dagger$, equal to

$$\kappa^*\left(\psi, \psi^\dagger, F_O\right) = \left[\partial E_{F_O}\left[Z\left(\psi\right)\right]/\partial\psi\right] n^{1/2}\left(\psi - \psi^\dagger\right) \qquad (5.5)$$

in a neighborhood of $\psi^\dagger$.

It follows from Eqs. (5.4) and (5.5) that if, as we assume, $n^{1/2} E\left[U^\dagger_{\text{mod adj}}\left(\psi, s^*_{eff}, c^{s^*_{eff}}, \alpha^*, \varsigma^*, \varkappa^*, \zeta^*\right)\right]$ is greater than $O\left(1\right)$ whenever $\left(\psi - \psi^\dagger\right)$ is greater than $O\left(n^{-1/2}\right)$, the stochastic process $\widehat{Z}_t\left(\cdot\right)$ (with t going to infinity slowly enough with n) is asymptotically degenerate under F_O, because (i) the local process $\left\{\widehat{Z}\left(\psi\right); \left(\psi - \psi^\dagger\right) \text{ in a ball of radius } O\left(n^{-1/2}\right)\right\}$ is, to order $o_p\left(1\right)$, a deterministic function of $Z\left(\psi^\dagger\right)$ and (ii) for $\left(\psi - \psi^\dagger\right)$ greater than $O\left(n^{-1/2}\right)$, $\widehat{Z}\left(\psi\right)$ is greater than $O\left(1\right)$ so $\widehat{Z}_t\left(\psi\right) = t$ with probability going to one. Finally, the limiting distribution of $Z\left(\psi^\dagger\right)$ under F_O is $MVN(0, I)$.

We can use the approximation $(2\pi)^{-p/2}\exp\left(-\widehat{Z}_t\left(\psi^\dagger\right)^T \widehat{Z}_t\left(\psi^\dagger\right)/2\right)$ to the likelihood $f\left(Z_t\left(\cdot, \widehat{s}_{eff}, c^{\widehat{s}_{eff}}, \widehat{\alpha}, \widehat{\varsigma}, \widehat{\varkappa}, \widehat{\zeta}\right)|F_O\right)$ to compute an asymptotic approximation

$$\pi_{post}\left(\psi^\dagger\right)$$
$$= \frac{I\left\{\psi^\dagger; \left\|\widehat{Z}_t\left(\psi^\dagger\right)\right\| < t\dim\left(\psi^\dagger\right)^{1/2}\right\}\exp\left(-\widehat{Z}_t\left(\psi^\dagger\right)^T \widehat{Z}_t\left(\psi^\dagger\right)/2\right)\pi\left(\psi^\dagger\right)}{\int_{\left\{\psi^\dagger; \|\widehat{Z}_t(\psi^\dagger)\| < t\dim(\psi^\dagger)^{1/2}\right\}}\exp\left(-\widehat{Z}_t\left(\psi^\dagger\right)^T \widehat{Z}_t\left(\psi^\dagger\right)/2\right)\pi\left(\psi^\dagger\right)d\psi^\dagger}$$

to the posterior $\pi\left(\psi^\dagger|Z_t\left(\cdot, \widehat{s}_{eff}, c^{\widehat{s}_{eff}}, \widehat{\alpha}, \widehat{\varsigma}, \widehat{\varkappa}, \widehat{\zeta}\right)\right)$ given $Z_t\left(\cdot, \widehat{s}_{eff}, c^{\widehat{s}_{eff}}, \widehat{\alpha}, \widehat{\varsigma}, \widehat{\varkappa}, \widehat{\zeta}\right)$ for $t = t\left(n\right)$, n sufficiently large, with $t\left(n\right)$ going slowly to ∞ with n, so we can ignore the set where $\left\|\widehat{Z}_t\left(\psi^\dagger\right)\right\| > t\dim\left(\psi\right)^{1/2}$. Consider a prior $\pi\left(\psi^\dagger\right)$ that is absolutely continuous wrt Lesbegue measure, and charges $\psi^\dagger$ in a volume of radius $O\left(1\right)$ (that includes the true parameter value). Such a prior is effectively uniform on a volume with radius $O\left(n^{-1/2}\right)$ around the truth. Since the likelihood is highly peaked on a volume of $O\left(n^{-1/2}\right)$, it follows that the approximate posterior based on a prior $\pi\left(\psi^\dagger\right)$ is just the rescaled likelihood i.e. set the prior $\pi\left(\psi^\dagger\right)$ to be 1 in the previous display.

Thus for sufficiently large t and n, an approximate highest posterior $(1 - \alpha)$ credible regions $C_{cred}(1 - \alpha)$ for, $\psi^\dagger$ is

$C_{cred}(1 - \alpha) = \left\{ \psi; \widehat{Z}_t(\psi)^T \widehat{Z}_t(\psi) < c_\alpha^2 \right\}$ where c_α^2 satisfies

$$1 - \alpha$$

$$= \frac{\int_{\left\{\psi^\dagger; \widehat{Z}_t(\psi^\dagger)^T \widehat{Z}_t(\psi^\dagger) < c_\alpha^2\right\}} \exp\left(-\widehat{Z}_t(\psi^\dagger)^T \widehat{Z}_t(\psi^\dagger)/2\right) d\psi^\dagger}{\int_{\left\{\psi^\dagger; \|\widehat{Z}_t(\psi^\dagger)\| < t\, \dim(\psi^\dagger)^{1/2}\right\}} \exp\left(-\widehat{Z}_t(\psi^\dagger)^T \widehat{Z}_t(\psi^\dagger)/2\right) d\psi^\dagger}$$

$$\approx \frac{\int_0^{c_\alpha} \exp\left(-u^2/2\right) area\,(u)\, du}{\int_0^\infty \exp\left(-u^2/2\right) area\,(u)\, du}$$

and

$$area\,(u)\, du = \int_{\left\{\psi^\dagger; \widehat{Z}_t(\psi^\dagger)^T \widehat{Z}_t(\psi^\dagger) = (u+du)^2\right\}} d\psi^\dagger - \int_{\left\{\psi^\dagger; \widehat{Z}_t(\psi^\dagger)^T \widehat{Z}_t(\psi^\dagger) = u^2\right\}} d\psi^\dagger$$

is the volume of the infinitesmal annulus between $\left\{\psi^\dagger; \widehat{Z}_t(\psi^\dagger)^T \widehat{Z}_t(\psi^\dagger) = (u + du)^2\right\}$ and $\left\{\psi^\dagger; \widehat{Z}_t(\psi^\dagger)^T \widehat{Z}_t(\psi^\dagger) = u^2\right\}$. Thus $area\,(u)$ is the (surface) area of the set $\left\{\psi^\dagger; \widehat{Z}_t(\psi^\dagger)^T \widehat{Z}_t(\psi^\dagger) = u^2\right\}$ of dimesion $R^{\dim(\psi^\dagger)-1}$ imbedded in $R^{\dim(\psi^\dagger)}$. The surface area of this set is well-defined with probability one since, under any law including an exceptional law, $\widehat{Z}_t(\psi^\dagger)$ is almost surely a continuous function of $\psi^\dagger$ and smooth except on a set of $\psi^{\dagger\cdot}$ of Lesbegue measure 0. We have used the fact that $\int_t^\infty \exp\left(-u^2/2\right) area\,(u)\, du$ goes to zero as $t = t\,(n) \to \infty$

Henceforth, it will be convenient to index the likelihood approximation $\exp\left(-\widehat{Z}_t(\psi)^T \widehat{Z}_t(\psi)/2\right)$ by ψ and again only use $\psi^\dagger$ to denote the true value of ψ. Upon inserting the expansion (5.4) − (5.5) into the approximate likelihood $(2\pi)^{-p/2} \exp\left(-\widehat{Z}_t(\psi)^T \widehat{Z}_t(\psi)/2\right)$, we see that with probability going to one, the posterior for ψ is asymptotically quadratic in $E\left[\partial Z(\psi)/\partial\psi^T\right](\psi - \psi^\dagger)$ for $(\psi - \psi^\dagger)$ of $O\left(n^{-1/2}\right)$. Thus the posterior will be asymptotically quadratic in $(\psi - \psi^\dagger)$ (and indeed asymptotically normal with mean $\widehat{\psi}$) if $E\left[\partial U_{mod\,adj}^\dagger(\psi)/\partial\psi^T\right] = E\left[\partial U_{mod\,adj}^\dagger(\psi^\dagger)/\partial\psi^T\right] + o\,(1)$ and thus $E\left[\partial Z(\psi)/\partial\psi^T\right] = E\left[\partial Z(\psi^\dagger)/\partial\psi^T\right] + o\,(1)$ does not depend on ψ to this order. Here $\widehat{\psi}$ is our locally efficient doubly robust estimator solving $\widehat{Z}_t(\psi) = \widehat{Z}(\psi) = 0$. This lack of dependence on ψ will be true, when, as we are assuming, $r\left(m, \bar{l}_m, \bar{a}_{m-1}, \psi\right)$ is smooth in ψ, except for the case where the data were generated under an exceptional law. Thus, in large samples, under non-exceptional laws, the posterior distribution of ψ will be normal. It follows that under non-exceptional laws we can substitute for $area\,(u)$ the suface area of the $\dim(\psi)$ ball of radius u in $R^{\dim(\psi)}$. Thus, for example, if $\dim(\psi) = 3$, then $area\,(u) = 4\pi u^2$. In that case c_α is equal to the upper

α quantile $\chi_{\alpha,\dim(\psi)}$ of a χ^2 random variable on $\dim(\psi)$-d.o.f. and thus our highest posterior credible interval $C_{cred}(1-\alpha)$ for ψ is exactly the same as the frequentist confidence interval $C_{op}(1-\alpha)$ based on the pivotal statistic $\widehat{Z}(\psi)$. Thus a result which is well known for regular parametric models continues to hold for our semiparametric model at non-exceptional laws.

However, under the exceptional laws, the posterior distribution for $\psi^\dagger$ will be non-quadratic and the surface $\left\{\psi; \widehat{Z}_t(\psi)^T \widehat{Z}_t(\psi) = u^2\right\}$ will not be a sphere of radius u. Thus area(u) will not be proportional to the suface area of the $\dim(\psi)$ ball of radius u in $R^{\dim(\psi)}$. Nonetheless, the frequentist interval $C_{op}(1-\alpha)$ will remain a highest posterior credible interval $C_{cred}(1-\alpha^*)$ with the 'frequency-calibrated' α^* given by

$$\alpha^* = \alpha^*(\alpha) \approx \frac{\int_0^{\chi_{\alpha,\dim(\psi)}} \exp\left(-u^2/2\right) area\,(u)\,du}{\int_0^\infty \exp\left(-u^2/2\right) area\,(u)\,du}$$

where $\chi_{\alpha,\dim(\psi)}$ is again the upper α quantile $\chi_{\alpha,\dim(\psi)}$ of a χ^2 random variable on $\dim(\psi)$ d.o.f.

Indeed even when the data are not generated under an exceptional law, for $(\psi - \psi^\dagger)$ of $O\left(n^{-1/2}\right)$, the $o(1)$ in the equation $E\left[\partial U^\dagger_{\mathrm{mod}\,adj}(\psi)/\partial \psi^T\right] - E\left[\partial U^\dagger_{\mathrm{mod}\,adj}(\psi^\dagger)/\partial \psi^T\right] = o(1)$ is non-uniform in $\psi^\dagger$ because $\psi^\dagger$ may still be close to an exceptional law (see Appendix A1.2 for additional discussion). However the Lebesgue measure of the set of $\psi^\dagger$ for which this $o(1)$ difference will not be small will decrease as n increases so that posterior associated with a prior absolutely continuous wrt Lesbegue measure that charges $\psi^\dagger$ in a volume of radius $O(1)$ will eventually be quadratic.

Nonetheless, in practice, if frequentist interval $C_{op}(1-\alpha)$ includes exceptional laws (or laws very close to exceptional laws) and thus the set where the likelihood is relatively large contains an exceptional law, it is best not to use a normal approximation, but rather to use either Markov chain Monte Carlo or rejection sampling techniques to generate a sample $\psi^{(v)}$, $v = 1, ..., V$ from a density proportional to $\exp\left(-\widehat{Z}(\psi)^T \widehat{Z}(\psi)/2\right)$ to construct a highest posterior credible intervals, even if one had a prior mass of zero on the exceptional laws. Informally, this recommendation represents the possibility that one may be in asymptopia in regards to using the uniform approximation $\exp\left(-\widehat{Z}(\psi)^T \widehat{Z}(\psi)/2\right)$ to the likelihood of $Z\left(\cdot, \widehat{s}_{eff}, c^{\widehat{s}_{eff}}, \widehat{\alpha}, \widehat{\varsigma}, \widehat{\varkappa}, \widehat{\zeta}\right)$, but may not be in asymptopia as far as the non-uniform approximation $E\left[\partial U^\dagger_{\mathrm{mod}\,adj}(\psi)/\partial \psi^T\right] - E\left[\partial U^\dagger_{\mathrm{mod}\,adj}(\psi^\dagger)/\partial \psi^T\right] = o(1)$ is concerned.

A way to formalize this approach to approximate Bayes inference when the set where the likelihood is relatively large contains an exceptional law is to assume that our prior $\pi(\psi)$, although still absolutely continuous, only charges a volume with radius $O\left(n^{-1/2}\right)$ but that volume includes the set where the likelihood is relatively large. [Robins, Scheines, Spirtes, and Wasserman (2003) also discuss the fact that Bayesian inference can be made to qualitatively agree with uniform asymptotic frequentist inference by letting the support of the prior vary with the sample size.] When the support of the prior only charges a volume with radius $O\left(n^{-1/2}\right)$, the posterior may be non-normal even under non-exceptional laws and even if the prior $\pi\left(\psi\right)$ is uniform on its support. In finite samples, one's substantive priors in high dimensional semiparametric problems are often not 'washed out' by the data and thus an asymptotics that assumes the prior charges a volume with radius $O\left(n^{-1/2}\right)$ may be more relevant to finite sample inference than an asymptotics that takes priors as being $O\left(1\right)$ since the latter priors are not sensitive to the fact that, due to non-uniform convergence, even at a reasonably large sample size n, the uniform asymptotic frequentist interval $C_{op}\left(1-\alpha\right)$ may contain several subsets with nearly equal measure such that the subset-specific typical values of $E\left[\partial U^{\dagger}_{\text{mod adj}}\left(\psi\right)/\partial\psi^{T}\right]$ and thus $\bar{d}_{op}\left(\psi\right)$, differ between subsets by $O\left(1\right)$. Indeed, as discussed in the introduction, in many biomedical studies, one may wish not to use an absolutely continuous prior but rather to give a positive prior mass to $\psi=0$ representing laws (essentially always exceptional) satisfying the g-null hypothesis. In that case, the posterior can often be far from normal.

Failure of the Bernstein–Von Mises Theorem Based on all the Data: It is natural to inquire how a highest posterior $(1-\alpha)$ credible region based on a posterior $\pi\left(\psi|O_{i},i=1,...,n\right)$ that conditions on all the data compares to that based on observing only $Z_{t}\left(\cdot,\widehat{s}_{eff},c^{\widehat{s}_{eff}},\widehat{\alpha},\widehat{\varsigma},\widehat{\varkappa},\widehat{\zeta}\right)$. In regular parametric models, the standardized estimated efficient score process for a subset of the model parameters is asymptotically sufficient so the intervals should be asymptotically equivalent. A formal proof relies on the Bernstein–Von Mises theorem that shows that $\pi\left(\psi|O_{i},i=1,...,n\right)$ is asymptotically normal centered on an efficient estimator of $\psi^{\dagger}$ with variance converging to the Cramer Rao variance bound for $\psi^{\dagger}$. In particular it implies that the posterior median is $n^{1/2}-consistent$ under the true data generating process F_{O}. In semiparametric models, a general proof of the Bernstein–Von Mises theorem does not yet exist. However we can prove that, if L_{m} has continuous components, then in model (a.1) with the $p_{m}\left(a_{m}|\overline{L}_{m},\overline{A}_{m-1}\right)$ known (and thus in the larger $\bar{d}_{op},\bar{0}$ union model of Theorem 3.4 as well), the Bernstein Von Mises theorem cannot hold for any Bayesian who would use the same prior $\pi\left(f_{res}\right)$ for the response densities f_{res}, whatever be the known treatment probabilities $p_{m}\left(a_{m}|\overline{L}_{m},\overline{A}_{m-1}\right)$. This follows from the fact that, under such an 'independence' prior, the posterior $\pi\left(\psi^{\dagger}|O_{i},i=1,...,n\right)$ and thus the posterior median is not a function of $p_{m}\left(a_{m}|\overline{L}_{m},\overline{A}_{m-1}\right)$. But Robins and Ritov (1997) showed that any estimator of $\psi^{\dagger}$ that does not depend on the $p_{m}\left(a_{m}|\overline{L}_{m},\overline{A}_{m-1}\right)$ must converge at rate no greater than $\log\left(\log n\right)$ under some treatment process $p_{m}\left(a_{m}|\overline{L}_{m},\overline{A}_{m-1}\right)$ and response law f_{res}, contradicting the conclusion of the Bernstein–Von Mises theorem. Indeed Robins and Ritov (1997) prove that under an 'independence' prior, the highest posterior $(1 - \alpha)$ credible regions based on posterior $\pi(\psi|O_i, i = 1, ..., n)$ cannot both have asymptotic frequentist coverage of $1 - \alpha$ and volume converging to zero as $n \to \infty$. Since both these desirable properties are true of the intervals based on $\pi\left(\psi|Z_t\left(\cdot, \widehat{s}_{eff}, c^{\widehat{s}_{eff}}, \widehat{\alpha}, \widehat{\varsigma}, \widehat{\varkappa}, \widehat{\zeta}\right)\right)$, it follows that intervals based on $\pi(\psi|O_i, i = 1, ..., n)$ and $\pi\left(\psi|Z_t\left(\cdot, \widehat{s}_{eff}, c^{\widehat{s}_{eff}}, \widehat{\alpha}, \widehat{\varsigma}, \widehat{\varkappa}, \widehat{\zeta}\right)\right)$ are not asymptotically equivalent and from a frequentist point of view those based on $\pi\left(\psi|Z_t\left(\cdot, \widehat{s}_{eff}, c^{\widehat{s}_{eff}}, \widehat{\alpha}, \widehat{\varsigma}, \widehat{\varkappa}, \widehat{\zeta}\right)\right)$ are preferable. The good performance of intervals based on $\pi\left(\psi|Z_t\left(\cdot, \widehat{s}_{eff}, c^{\widehat{s}_{eff}}, \widehat{\alpha}, \widehat{\varsigma}, \widehat{\varkappa}, \widehat{\zeta}\right)\right)$ in our union model depends critically on the fact that $Z_t\left(\cdot, \widehat{s}_{eff}, c^{\widehat{s}_{eff}}, \widehat{\alpha}, \widehat{\varsigma}, \widehat{\varkappa}, \widehat{\zeta}\right)$ is a function of either the true $p_m\left(a_m|\overline{L}_m, \overline{A}_{m-1}\right)$ (when the latter is known) or of a model-based estimate of $p_m\left(a_m|\overline{L}_m, \overline{A}_{m-1}\right)$ (when the true function is unknown). It can be argued from general decision theoretic results that there exists a particular prior for $f_O = f_{res} f_{tr,obs}$ with f_{res} and the $f_{tr,obs} = \prod_m p_m\left(a_m|\overline{L}_m, \overline{A}_{m-1}\right)$ apriori dependent such that $\pi(\psi|O_i, i = 1, ..., n)$ is an accurate large sample approximation to $\pi\left(\psi|Z_t\left(\cdot, \widehat{s}_{eff}, c^{\widehat{s}_{eff}}, \widehat{\alpha}, \widehat{\varsigma}, \widehat{\varkappa}, \widehat{\zeta}\right)\right)$ when the treatment probabilities are known. However the prior may be hard to derive and will essentially never represent the analyst's subjective beliefs.

Marginal Bayesian inference: Bayesian inference concerning the marginal ψ_{int} is based on integration of $\pi\left(\psi|Z_t\left(\cdot, \widehat{s}_{eff}, c^{\widehat{s}_{eff}}, \widehat{\alpha}, \widehat{\varsigma}, \widehat{\varkappa}, \widehat{\zeta}\right)\right) \propto$ $(2\pi)^{-p/2} \exp\left(-\widehat{Z}_t(\psi)^T \widehat{Z}_t(\psi)/2\right) \pi(\psi)$ over ψ_{-int}. Thus, if $\pi(\psi)$ is smooth and charges $\psi^\dagger$ in a volume of $O(1)$, then, in large samples, under non-exceptional laws, the posterior distribution of ψ_{int} will be normal if, as we have assumed, $r\left(m, \bar{l}_m, \bar{a}_{m-1}, \psi\right)$ is smooth in ψ and and thus (a) the posterior median and posterior mean of ψ_{int} will agree in sign and (b) furthermore the highest $(1 - \alpha)$ posterior credible region for ψ_{int} will be asymptotically equivalent to the univariate (non-simultaneous) $(1 - \alpha)$ confidence interval for ψ_{int} considered in the last subsection. However because of the possibility that the data were generated under an exceptional law or because we are not in asymptopia in regards to the non-uniform approximation $E\left[\partial U_{mod\,adj}^\dagger(\psi)/\partial \psi^T\right] - E\left[\partial U_{mod\,adj}^\dagger(\psi^\dagger)/\partial \psi^T\right] = o(1)$, it is again best not to use a normal approximation but rather to use either Markov chain Monte Carlo or rejection sampling techniques to generate a sample $\psi^{(v)}$, $v = 1, ..., V$ from a density proportional to $\exp\left(-\widehat{Z}_t(\psi)^T \widehat{Z}_t(\psi)/2\right)$ or $\exp\left(-\widehat{Z}_t(\psi)^T \widehat{Z}_t(\psi)/2\right) \pi(\psi)$ and then report whether the sample mean or median of the $\psi_{int}^{(v)}$ exceeds zero as an estimate of the posterior mean $E\left(\psi_{int}|Z_t\left(\cdot, \widehat{s}_{eff}, c^{\widehat{s}_{eff}}, \widehat{\alpha}, \widehat{\varsigma}, \widehat{\varkappa}, \widehat{\zeta}\right)\right)$ or median of ψ_{int}. In this setting, the posterior mean and median may fail to agree in sign, leading to different decisions under our two different decision rules. Further, the highest $(1 - \alpha^*)$ posterior credible region for ψ_{int}, in contrast to the credible interval $C_{cred}(1 - \alpha^*)$ for the entire vector ψ, (i) may have frequentist coverage less than $(1 - \alpha)$ when we choose α^* equal to $\alpha^*(\alpha)$ and (ii) may not be asymptotically equivalent (in terms of shape and volume) to the univariate (non-simultaneous) $(1 - \alpha)$ confidence interval for ψ_{int} considered in the last subsection for any value of α^*.

Optimal Bayes Decison Rules: The actual fact is that the optimal Bayes decision rule (i.e. the rule that maximizes posterior expected utility) that a Bayesian should use in deciding whether to treat a patient with past data $(\bar{l}_m, \bar{a}_{m-1})$ on day t_m may be captured by neither of our decision rules. Thus, in principle, we should not choose between them but calculate the optimal Bayes rule. First suppose we have a correctly specified model $\gamma^{\bar{0}}(\bar{l}_m, \bar{a}_m, \psi) = a_m r(m, \bar{l}_m, \bar{a}_{m-1}, \psi)$ for $\gamma^{\bar{d}_{op}, \bar{0}}(\bar{l}_m, \bar{a}_m)$ so the true optimal regime $d_{op} = d_{op}(\psi^\dagger)$ is a deterministic function of the true value $\psi^\dagger$. Let Ψ be a set that contains ψ with posterior probability one so $D_{op}(\Psi) = \{d_{op}(\psi) ; \psi \in \Psi\}$ contains the optimal regime with posterior probability one. Further we can assume the true $\psi^\dagger$ that actually generated the data is in Ψ. Nonetheless the optimal Bayes decision rule (i.e. treatment regime) need not be an element of $D_{op}(\Psi)$. Here is a specific simple example. Suppose the data is $A_0, A_1,$ and $Y = L_2$ with no L_0 or L_1. Suppose we have a saturated model $\gamma^{\bar{0}}(\bar{l}_m, \bar{a}_m, \psi) = \gamma^{\bar{0}}(\bar{a}_m, \psi)$, $\psi = (\psi_{m=0}, \psi_{m=1, a_0=1}, \psi_{m=1, a_0=0})$ for $\gamma^{\bar{d}_{op}, \bar{0}}(\bar{l}_m, \bar{a}_m)$ and the posterior distribution is discrete with 2 support points: $\psi_{m=0} = -100, \psi_{m=1, a_0=1} = 0, \psi_{m=1, a_0=0} = 10$ with posterior probability .4 and $\psi_{m=0} = 50, \psi_{m=1, a_0=1} = 1, \psi_{m=1, a_0=0} = -20$ with posterior probability .6. Then, with posterior probability .4, the optimal treatment regime is $d_0^{op} = 0, d_1^{op} = 1$ and with posterior probability .6, $d_0^{op} = 1,$ $d_1^{op} = 1$. So the set Ψ consists of two vectors ψ and $D_{op}(\Psi)$ contains only the two regimes $d_0^{op} = 0, d_1^{op} = 1$ and $d_0^{op} = 1, d_1^{op} = 1$. But the optimal Bayes decision rule is $d_0^{op} = 0, d_1^{op} = 0$ as it has posterior expected utility of $.4 \times (-10 + c_1) + .6 \times (-50 + c_2)$ while the posterior expected utility of $d_0^{op} = 0, d_1^{op} = 1$ is $.4 \times c_1 + .6 \times (-50 - 20 + c_2)$, of $d_0^{op} = 1, d_1^{op} = 1$ is $.4 \times (-100 + c_1) + .6 \times (c_2)$ and of $d_0^{op} = 1, d_1^{op} = 0$ is $.4 \times (-100 + c_1) + .6 \times (-1 + c_2)$, where c_1 is the posterior utility of $d_0^{op} = 0,$ $d_1^{op} = 1$ conditional on the first support point and c_2 is the posterior utility of $d_0^{op} = 1, d_1^{op} = 1$ conditional on the second support point.

Note in this simple example, the optimal Bayes decision rule was a function of the marginal posterior distribution of ψ. In the next paragraph we will see that, when the sample size is large, this remains true even when data on covariates L_m are available, provided the data is generated under a nonexceptional law and the prior for ψ charges a volume with radius $O(1)$. However, we show in the next paragraph but one that, even in large samples, if either the prior for ψ only charges a volume of radius $O(n^{-1/2})$ or the data were generated under an exceptional law, the optimal Bayes decision rule will generally be a complex function of the posterior distribution of the infinite-dimensional nuisance parameters.

Suppose the data were generated under an unexceptional law and the prior $\pi(\psi)$ is absolutely continuous and charges a volume with radius $O(1)$. We therefore approximate the posterior $\pi\left(\psi|Z_t\left(\cdot,\widehat{s}_{eff},c^{\widehat{s}_{eff}},\widehat{\alpha},\widehat{\varsigma},\widehat{\varkappa},\widehat{\zeta}\right)\right)$ by the approximate posterior

$$\pi_{post}(\psi) = \frac{I\left\{\psi;\left\|\widehat{Z}_t(\psi)\right\| < t\dim(\psi)^{1/2}\right\}\exp\left(-\widehat{Z}_t(\psi)^T\widehat{Z}_t(\psi)/2\right)}{\int_{\left\{\psi;\|\widehat{Z}_t(\psi)\|<t\dim(\psi)^{1/2}\right\}}\exp\left(-\widehat{Z}_t(\psi)^T\widehat{Z}_t(\psi)/2\right)d\psi}.$$

Then, for sufficiently large n and t, the posterior mean $\int a_K r\left(K,\bar{l}_K,\bar{a}_{K-1},\psi\right)\pi_{post}(\psi)d\psi$ of $\gamma^{\bar{d}_{op},\bar{0}}\left(\bar{l}_K,\bar{a}_K\right)$ based on a correct smooth model $\gamma^{\bar{0}}\left(\bar{l}_m,\bar{a}_m,\psi\right) = a_m r\left(m,\bar{l}_m,\bar{a}_{m-1},\psi\right)$ will to $o(1)$ be $a_K r\left(K,\bar{l}_K,\bar{a}_{K-1},\widehat{\psi}\right)$ because $\pi_{post}(\psi)$ is normal with mean equal to the locally efficient doubly robust estimator $\widehat{\psi}$ solving $\widehat{Z}_t(\psi) = \widehat{Z}(\psi) = 0$, the variance of $\widehat{\psi}$ is $O(1/n)$, and $\widehat{\psi}$ is greater than $O(n^{-1/2})$ away from any ψ for which $\arg\max_{a_m \in A_m}\gamma^{\bar{0}}\left(\bar{L}_m,\bar{A}_{m-1},a_m,\psi\right)$ is not unique with positive probability (by our assumption the data were generated under a nonexceptional law.) The optimal Bayes decison $d_{bayes,K}\left(\bar{l}_K,\bar{a}_{K-1}\right)$ for a subject known to have history $\bar{l}_K,\bar{a}_{K-1}$ is $\arg\max_{a_k \in A_k}$ of the posterior mean, which under our assumptions is equal to $\arg\max_{a_k \in A_k} a_K r\left(K,\bar{l}_K,\bar{a}_{K-1},\widehat{\psi}\right)$ with probability going to 1. Further because $\widehat{\psi}$ is $n^{1/2}-consistent$ for $\psi^\dagger$, results described in the following paragraph imply that, with probability going to one, the optimal Bayes decison $d_{bayes,K-1}\left(\bar{l}_{K-1},\bar{a}_{K-2}\right)$ for a subject known to have history $\bar{l}_{K-1},\bar{a}_{K-2}$ is $\arg\max_{a_{k-1}\in A_{k-1}}$ of the posterior mean $\int a_{K-1} r\left(K-1,\bar{l}_{K-1},\bar{a}_{K-2},\psi\right)\pi_{post}(\psi)d\psi$ of $\gamma^{\bar{d}_{op},\bar{0}}\left(\bar{l}_{K-1},\bar{a}_{K-1}\right) = a_{K-1} r\left(K-1,\bar{l}_{K-1},\bar{a}_{K-2},\psi^\dagger\right)$ which, under our assumptions is equal, with probability approaching 1, to $\arg\max_{a_{k-1}\in A_{k-1}} a_{K-1} r\left(K-1,\bar{l}_{K-1},\bar{a}_{K-2},\widehat{\psi}\right)$. Continuing in this manner we see that the optimal bayes decision rule $d_{bayes,m}\left(\bar{l}_m,\bar{a}_{m-1}\right)$ is $d_{op,m}\left(\bar{l}_m,\bar{a}_{m-1},\widehat{\psi}\right)$ for each m.

Suppose next the data were generated under an exceptional law and/or the prior $\pi(\psi)$ only charges a volume with radius $O\left(n^{-1/2}\right)$. Although we still approximate the posterior by $\pi_{post}(\psi)$, now $\pi_{post}(\psi)$ may neither have mean $\widehat{\psi}$ nor be normal, and thus

$$d_{bayes,K}\left(\bar{l}_K,\bar{a}_{K-1}\right) = \arg\max_{a_k \in A_k}\int a_K r\left(K,\bar{l}_K,\bar{a}_{K-1},\psi\right)\pi_{post}(\psi)d\psi$$

may differ from $d_{op,K}\left(\bar{l}_K,\bar{a}_{K-1},\widehat{\psi}\right)$. Now, by definition, $d_{bayes,K-1}\left(\bar{l}_{K-1},\bar{a}_{K-2}\right)$ is the optimal Bayes choice for a_{K-1} given that a_K will equal $d_{bayes,K}\left(\bar{l}_K,\bar{a}_{K-1}\right)$.

That is $d_{bayes,K-1}\left(\bar{l}_{K-1},\bar{a}_{K-2}\right)$ equals $\arg\max_{a_{k-1}\in\mathcal{A}_{k-1}}$ of the posterior mean of $E\left[Y_{\bar{a}_{K-2},a_{K-1},d_{bayes,K}}|\bar{A}_{K-2}=\bar{a}_{K-2},\bar{L}_{K-1}=\bar{l}_{K-1}\right]$ and, thus, of

$$E\left[Y_{\bar{a}_{K-2},a_{K-1},d_{bayes,K}} - Y_{\bar{a}_{K-2},0,d_{op,K-1}}|\bar{A}_{K-2}=\bar{a}_{K-2},\bar{L}_{K-1}=\bar{l}_{K-1}\right].$$

At $\psi=\psi^{\dagger}$, this contrast can be written as

$$E\left[Y_{\bar{a}_{K-2},a_{K-1},d_{bayes,K}} - Y_{\bar{a}_{K-2},a_{K-1},d_{op,K-1}}|\bar{A}_{K-2}=\bar{a}_{K-2},\bar{L}_{K-1}=\bar{l}_{K-1}\right] +$$
$$\gamma^{\bar{d}_{op},\bar{0}}\left(\bar{l}_{K-1},\bar{a}_{K-1},\psi\right)$$
$$= E\left\{\begin{array}{l}E\left[Y_{\bar{a}_{K-2},a_{K-1},d_{bayes,K}} - Y_{\bar{a}_{K-2},a_{K-1},d_{op,K}}|\bar{A}_{K-1}=\bar{a}_{K-1},\bar{L}_K\right]\\|\bar{A}_{K-1}=\bar{a}_{K-1},\bar{L}_{K-1}=\bar{l}_{K-1}\end{array}\right\} +$$
$$+ \gamma^{\bar{d}_{op},\bar{0}}\left(\bar{l}_{K-1},\bar{a}_{K-1},\psi\right)$$
$$= E\left[j_{Bayes}\left(\bar{L}_K,\bar{A}_{K-1}\right)|\bar{A}_{K-1}=\bar{a}_{K-1},\bar{L}_{K-1}=\bar{l}_{K-1}\right] + \gamma^{\bar{d}_{op},\bar{0}}\left(\bar{l}_{K-1},\bar{a}_{K-1},\psi\right)$$

where

$$j_{Bayes}\left(\bar{l}_K,\bar{a}_{K-1}\right)$$
$$= \gamma^{\bar{d}_{op},\bar{0}}\left(\bar{l}_K,\bar{a}_{K-1},d_{bayes,K}\left(\bar{l}_K,\bar{a}_{K-1}\right),\psi\right) -$$
$$\gamma^{\bar{d}_{op},\bar{0}}\left(\bar{l}_K,\bar{a}_{K-1},d_{op,K}\left(\bar{l}_K,\bar{a}_{K-1},\psi\right),\psi\right)$$
$$= \left\{d_{bayes,K}\left(\bar{l}_K,\bar{a}_{K-1}\right) - d_{op,K}\left(\bar{l}_K,\bar{a}_{K-1},\psi\right)\right\}r\left(K,\bar{l}_K,\bar{a}_{K-1},\psi\right)$$

Hence

$$d_{bayes,K-1}\left(\bar{l}_{K-1},\bar{a}_{K-2}\right)$$
$$= \arg\max_{a_{k-1}\in\mathcal{A}_{k-1}}$$
$$\left[\int\left\{d_{bayes,K}\left(\bar{l}_K,\bar{a}_{K-1}\right) - d_{op,K}\left(\bar{l}_K,\bar{a}_{K-1},\psi\right)\right\}\times\right.$$
$$r\left(K,\bar{l}_K,\bar{a}_{K-1},\psi\right)dF\left(l_K|\bar{l}_{K-1},\bar{a}_{K-1};\eta\right)\pi_{post}\left(\eta|\psi\right)\pi_{post}\left(\psi\right)d\psi d\mu\left(\eta\right) +$$
$$\left.\int a_{K-1}r\left(K-1,\bar{l}_{K-1},\bar{a}_{K-2},\psi\right)\pi_{post}\left(\psi\right)d\psi\right]$$

where η denotes the parameter governing the density $f\left(l_K|\bar{l}_{K-1},\bar{a}_{K-1}\right)$ and $\pi_{post}\left(\eta|\psi\right)$ is the conditonal posterior of η with respect to the measure $\mu\left(\cdot\right)$. One possible approach to obtaining $d_{bayes,K-1}\left(\bar{l}_{K-1},\bar{a}_{K-2}\right)$ would be to specify a parametric model $f\left(l_m|\bar{l}_{m-1},\bar{a}_{m-1};\eta\right)$, estimate η by the MLE $\hat{\eta}$ and take $\pi_{post}\left(\eta|\psi\right)=\pi_{post}\left(\eta\right)$ to be normal with mean $\hat{\eta}$ and variance given by the inverse Hessian matrix for $\hat{\eta}$. A second approach, analogous to that taken in Section 6.2 and (more specifically) Section 7.2 below, is to assume the law of $j\left(\bar{L}_K,\bar{A}_{K-1}\right)|\bar{A}_{K-1}=\bar{a}_{K-1},\bar{L}_{K-1}=\bar{l}_{K-1}$ is normal with mean $\nu\left(\bar{a}_{K-1},\bar{l}_{K-1};\beta_K\right)$ and, say, variance σ_K^2 where $\nu\left(\bar{a}_{K-1},\bar{l}_{K-1};\beta_K\right)$ is a known function and β_K and σ_K^2 are unknown parameters. We might take the posterior of β_K given ψ to be normal with mean equal to the (possibly nonlinear) least squares regression estimator $\hat{\beta}_K(\psi)$ from the regression of $j\left(\overline{L}_K, \overline{A}_{K-1}\right) = j\left(\overline{L}_K, \overline{A}_{K-1}, \psi\right)$ on $\left(\overline{L}_{K-1}, \overline{A}_{K-1}\right)$ with regression function $\nu\left(\overline{a}_{K-1}, \overline{l}_{K-1}; \beta_K\right)$. Then take $d_{bayes,K-1}\left(\overline{l}_{K-1}, \overline{a}_{K-2}\right) =$

$\arg\max_{a_{k-1}\in\mathcal{A}_{k-1}} \int\int \left\{\nu\left(\overline{a}_{K-1}, \overline{l}_{K-1}; \beta_K\right) + a_{K-1} r\left(K-1, \overline{l}_{K-1}, \overline{a}_{K-2}, \psi\right)\right\} \times$
$\pi_{post}\left(\beta_K|\psi\right)\pi_{post}\left(\psi\right) d\psi d\mu\left(\beta_K\right)$.. More generally, under this second approach, it follows from results in Section 6.2 and 7.2 that $d_{bayes,m}\left(\overline{l}_m, \overline{a}_{m-1}\right)$ is

$$\arg\max_{a_m\in\mathcal{A}_m} \left[\int \left\{\nu\left(\overline{a}_m, \overline{l}_m; \beta_{m+1}\right) + a_m r\left(m, \overline{l}_m, \overline{a}_{m-1}, \psi\right)\right\} \times\right.$$
$$\pi_{post}\left(\beta_{m+1}|\psi, \underline{\beta}_{m+2}\right) \times$$
$$\left.\pi_{post}\left(\psi, \underline{\beta}_{m+2}\right) d\psi d\mu\left(\psi, \underline{\beta}_{m+2}, \beta_{m+1}\right)\right]$$

where $\nu\left(\overline{a}_m, \overline{l}_m; \beta_{m+1}\right)$ is a parametric model for $E\left[j\left(\overline{L}_{m+1}, \overline{A}_m\right)|\overline{L}_m = \overline{l}_m, \overline{A}_m = \overline{a}_m\right]$ with
$j\left(\overline{L}_m, \overline{A}_{m-1}\right) = E\left[Y_{\overline{A}_{m-1}, \underline{d}_{bayes,m}} - Y_{\overline{A}_{m-1}, \underline{d}_{op,m}} | \overline{L}_m, \overline{A}_{m-1}\right].$

Under either of the 2 approaches, the principal benefit of specifying a optimal drSNMM $\gamma^{\overline{d}_{op}, \overline{0}}\left(\overline{l}_m, \overline{a}_m, \psi\right)$ is lost when computing the optimal Bayes decision, in the sense that, even when the treatment probabilities are known, we must model, in addition to $\gamma^{\overline{d}_{op}, \overline{0}}\left(\overline{l}_m, \overline{a}_m\right)$, other aspects of the joint distribution of the observed data. Further the second approach may result in incompatible models in the sense that there is no joint distribution for the observed data satisfying all the functional form restrictions imposed by the models $\nu\left(\overline{a}_m, \overline{l}_m; \beta_{m+1}\right)$ and $\gamma^{\overline{d}_{op}, \overline{0}}\left(\overline{l}_m, \overline{a}_m, \psi\right)$. Indeed, Robins (1994) shows that even the first approach may suffer from model incompatibility. At the cost of a complex reparametrization of the joint distribution of the observed data described in the Appendix of Robins (1994), the possibility of model incompatibility when using the first approach can be resolved.

To overcome the need to model other aspects of the joint distribution of the observed data we might specify a drSNMM $\gamma^{\overline{d}_{Bayes}, \overline{0}}\left(\overline{l}_m, \overline{a}_m, \psi\right)$ for

$E\left[Y_{\overline{A}_{m-1}, a_m, \underline{d}_{bayes,m+1}} - Y_{\overline{A}_{m-1}, 0, \underline{d}_{bayes,m+1}} | \overline{L}_m = \overline{l}_m, \overline{A}_{m-1} = \overline{a}_{m-1}\right]$
$= \gamma^{\overline{d}_{Bayes}, \overline{0}}\left(\overline{l}_m, \overline{a}_m\right)$ so that $d_{bayes,m}\left(\overline{l}_m, \overline{a}_{m-1}, \psi\right)$
$= \arg\max_{a_m\in\mathcal{A}_m} \int \gamma^{\overline{d}_{Bayes}, \overline{0}}\left(\overline{l}_m, \overline{a}_m, \psi\right) \pi_{post}\left(\psi\right) d\psi$. This idea raises all sorts of interesting and unresolved philosophical and statistical questions because of course $d_{bayes,m}\left(\overline{l}_m, \overline{a}_{m-1}, \psi\right)$ is a function of the data through the posterior $\pi_{post}\left(\psi\right)$. [However the above expectation is to be computed treating $\underline{d}_{bayes,m+1}$ as a given fixed regime rather than as a random regime that depends on the data.] This idea will be further pursued elsewhere.

6 Comparison of Optimal drSNMMs with Alternative Approaches

6.1 Susan Murphy's semiparametric regret model are SNMMS

I now show that, under sequential randomization Murphy's semiparametric regret model is a particular parametrization of an additive $\bar{d}-regime$ srSNMM with $\bar{d}$ the optimal regime $\bar{d}_{op}$. Specifically, Murphy's semiparametric regret model specifies that the regret $E\left[Y_{\bar{a}_{m-1},\underline{d}_{op,m}} - Y_{\bar{a}_m,\underline{d}_{op,m+1}}|\overline{L}_{\bar{a}_{m-1},m} = \bar{l}_m\right]$ equals $u_m\left(\bar{l}_m,\bar{a}_m,\beta^\dagger\right)$ where $u_m\left(\bar{l}_m,\bar{a}_m,\beta\right) = \eta_m\left(\bar{l}_m,\bar{a}_{m-1},\beta_{scale}\right) \times$
$f\left(a_m - d_{op,m}\left(\bar{l}_m,\bar{a}_{m-1},\beta_{regime}\right)\right), \beta = \left(\beta_{scale},\beta_{regime}\right)$ is a finite dimensional parameter vector, $f\left(\cdot\right)$ is a known non-negative function satisfying $f\left(0\right) = 0, \eta_m\left(\bar{l}_m,\bar{a}_{m-1},\beta_{scale}\right)$ is a known non-negative scale function, and $d_{op,m}\left(\bar{l}_m,\bar{a}_{m-1},\beta^\dagger_{regime}\right)$ is the optimal regime $d_{op,m}\left(\bar{l}_m,\bar{a}_{m-1}\right)$. In all her examples $\beta = \left(\beta_{scale},\beta_{regime}\right)$ had (i) β_{scale} and β_{regime} as variation independent and (ii) $\eta_m\left(\bar{l}_m,\bar{a}_{m-1},\beta_{scale}\right) = 0$ if and only if $\beta_{scale} = 0$. [Murphy also allows the possibility that $u_m\left(\bar{l}_m,\bar{a}_m,\beta\right)$ is a sum of J_m terms indexed by j of the form $\eta_{j,m}\left(\bar{l}_m,\bar{a}_{m-1},\beta_{j,scale}\right) \times f_j\left(a_m - d_{j,op,m}\left(\bar{l}_m,\bar{a}_{m-1},\beta_{j,regime}\right)\right)$]. It follows that Murphy's model is a $\bar{d}_{op}-regime$ srSNMM with $-u_m\left(\bar{l}_m,\bar{a}_m,\beta\right)$ equal to $\gamma^{\bar{d}_{op}}\left(\bar{l}_m,\bar{a}_m;\beta\right)$ in my notation. Note that Murphy uses a particular parametrization, similar to one suggested by Robins (1999, p.125), under which the "scale" components β_{scale} of β being zero implies both the g-null hypothesis and that the other components of β_{regime} are undefined. That is her parametrization is such that the parameters β_{regime} are only defined under the alternative $\beta_{scale} \neq 0$. (This parametrization can result in certain additional inferential difficulties that have been discussed frequently in the statistical literature; however, as discussed by Robins (1999) the parametrization has a certain conceptual justification.)

Comparisons

Limitations of Murphy's regret model include a) estimation of $\beta^\dagger$ based on smooth function optimization methods requires (differentiable) approximations (e.g., with sigmoid functions) of indicator functions and b) regrets are not effect measures about which scientists have clear substantive opinions amenable to easy modelling. Optimal drSNMMs do not suffer as severely from these limitations. We will consider these two limitations within the context of one specific example offered by Murphy. She considers the model for dichotomous A_m and univariate positive L_m given by $u_m\left(\bar{l}_m,\bar{a}_m,\beta\right) = \beta_{scale}\left\{a_m - d_{op,m}\left(\bar{l}_m,\bar{a}_{m-1},\beta_{regime}\right)\right\}^2$ with $d_{op,m}\left(\bar{l}_m,\bar{a}_{m-1},\beta_{regime}\right) = I\left(l_m > \beta_{regime}\right)$, so that treatment is preferred whenever L_m exceeds $\beta^\dagger_{regime}$. Because β_{regime} lies inside an indicator function, Murphy's criterion function is not differentiable with respect to β_{regime}. In order to use

smooth function optimization methods, she uses a differentiable approxima-
tion $e^{30(l_m - \beta_{regime})} / \left\{ 1 + e^{30(l_m - \beta_{regime})} \right\}$ for $I\left(l_m > \beta_{regime} \right)$. The performance of this approximation in her simulations was rather poor (in the sense
that estimates of the model parameters were biased).

Murphy's model also has substantive limitations: it assumes apriori that
the dose response as a function of L_m is positive in the sense that if treatment
is preferred at a given level of L_m, it is preferred at all higher levels; if the
data may imply a negative dose response this cannot be detected using this
model. Further the model implies that the regret β_{scale} of taking treatment
when one should not $\left(L_m < \beta_{regime}^{\dagger} \right)$ is exactly equal to the regret of not
taking treatment when one should $\left(L_m > \beta_{regime}^{\dagger} \right)$. Further it assumes that
the advantage β_{scale} of taking treatment once $L_m > \beta_{regime}^{\dagger}$ is independent
of the value of L_m and the advantage β_{scale} of not taking treatment once
$L_m < \beta_{regime}^{\dagger}$ also does not depend on L_m. It is substantively hard to imagine
such a sharp cut-point $\beta_{regime}^{\dagger}$. Now Murphy clearly did not intend this regret
model to be substantively realistic and one could clearly elaborate the model ,
perhaps by including additional parameters, in order to make it substantively
realistic. I will argue that precisely how to do so requires quite a bit of thought,
tedious calculation, and some mathematical ability.

The substantive difficulty in specifying Murphy's regret model is already
evident in the simplest of all settings : the setting in which we have a single
time-independent treatment $(K = 0)$. Thus assume the data are $L = L_0, A =
A_0, Y = L_1$ with A dichotomous, L univariate and positive and Y continuous.
Then under sequential randomization any $(\bar{d}, \bar{0}) - drSNMM$ $\gamma^{\bar{0}}\left(\bar{l}_0, \bar{a}_0; \psi \right)$ for
$\gamma^{\bar{d},\bar{0}}\left(\bar{l}_0, \bar{a}_0 \right) = \gamma^{\bar{0}}\left(l, a \right)$ does not depend on $\bar{d}$ as our only treatment decision
is the final one; in particular $\gamma^{\bar{d}_{op},\bar{0}}\left(\bar{l}_m, \bar{a}_m \right)$ equals $\gamma^{\bar{d},\bar{0}}\left(\bar{l}_m, \bar{a}_m \right) = \gamma^{0}\left(l, a \right) =
E\left[Y | L = l, A = a \right] - E\left[Y | L = l, A = 0 \right]$ under sequential randomization. Thus
an optimal drSNMM model is just a model $\gamma^{0}\left(l, a, \psi \right)$ for $E\left[Y | L = l, A = a \right] -
E\left[Y | L = l, A = 0 \right]$. The simplest such model that includes the possibility
that optimal treatment may change at some value of L is the simple (semi-
parametric) linear regression model $\gamma^{0}\left(l, a, \psi \right) = a\left(\psi_0 + \psi_1 l \right)$ [i.e. the model
$E\left[Y | L = l, A = a \right] = a\left(\psi_0 + \psi_1 l \right) + b(l)$ with $b(l)$ unrestricted.] It is trivial to derive the optimal regime and the regret from this linear regression
model. Specifically, $d_{op}\left(l, \psi \right) = \arg\max_{a \in \{0,1\}} \gamma^{0}\left(l, a, \psi \right) = I\left(\psi_0 + \psi_1 l > 0 \right)$
and the regret $E\left[Y_{d_{op}} - Y_a | L = l, \psi \right] = \left\{ I\left(\psi_0 + \psi_1 l > 0 \right) - a \right\} \left(\psi_0 + \psi_1 l \right)$.
Thus in our optimal drSNMM approach, we take our beliefs as to the
functional form of the dose response $E\left[Y | L = l, A = 1 \right] - E\left[Y | L = l, A = 0 \right]$
as primary. We encode these beliefs in a regression model $\gamma^{0}\left(l, a, \psi \right)$ for
$E\left[Y | L = l, A = a \right] - E\left[Y | L = l, A = 0 \right]$ and then derive the optimal regime
and the regret function from our regression model. I believe that most sci-
entists would use this same approach in working out their beliefs about the
likely functional form of the regret.

Murphy's approach is just the converse. She specifies a model $d_{op}(l, \beta_{regime}) = I(l > \beta_{regime})$ for the optimal regime and for the regret $E\left[Y_{d_{op}} - Y_a | L = l, \psi\right] = \beta_{scale}\left\{a - d_{op}(l, \beta_{regime})\right\}^2$. This of course induces an optimal dr SNMM
$$\gamma^0_{Murphy}(l, a, \beta) = u(l, 0, \beta) - u(l, 1, \beta)$$
$$= a\left\{\beta_{scale} I(l > \beta_{regime}) - \beta_{scale} I(l \leq \beta_{regime})\right\} = a\beta_{scale}\left[2I(l > \beta_{regime}) - 1\right]$$
for $E[Y | L = l, A = a] - E[Y | L = l, A = 0] = \gamma^0(l, a)$. Written in terms of the regression function $\gamma^0(l, a)$, one can immediately see how substantively unusual Murphy's regret model is with a jump discontinuity at β_{regime}, and why smooth optimization methods cannot be applied without approximation. In contrast, in section 4.1.1, we have seen how to obtain closed form g-estimates of the parameters of the semiparametric linear model $\gamma^0(l, a, \psi) = a(\psi_0 + \psi_1 l)$ when the treatment probabilities $p(a|l)$ are known or can be modelled.

We have seen it is easy to derive the optimal drSNMM model $\gamma^0_{Murphy}(l, a, \beta)$ implied by Murphy's regret model. We now show the converse is not true. That is the functional form of Murphy's regret model implied by the simple optimal drSNMM model $\gamma^0(l, a, \psi) = a(\psi_0 + \psi_1 l)$ for $\gamma^0(l, a) = E[Y | L = l, A = a] - E[Y | L = l, A = 0]$ is tedious to derive. Above we saw that the regret is
$$\{I(\psi_0 + \psi_1 l > 0) - a\}(\psi_0 + \psi_1 l).$$ But this is not in the Murphy form of a sum over j of functions $u_j(l, a, \beta) = \eta_j(l, \beta_{j,scale}) f_j\{a - d_{op,j}(l, \beta_{j,regime})\}$ with $\eta_j(l, \beta_{scale})$ nonnegative and $f_j(u)$ minimized at $u = 0$. To put it in the Murphy form we define $\beta_1 = |\psi_1|, \beta_2 = -\psi_0/\psi_1, \beta_3 = I(\psi_1 > 0)$. Then some tedious algebra shows that the regret $\{I(\psi_0 + \psi_1 l > 0) - a\}(\psi_0 + \psi_1 l)$
$$= \sum_{j=1}^4 \eta_j(l, \beta_{j,scale}) f_j\{a - d_{j,op}(l, \beta_{j,regime})\} \text{ where } f_j(u) = u^2 \text{ for all}$$
j,

$\eta_1(l, \beta_{1,scale}) = (1 - \beta_3) I(\beta_2 > 0) \beta_1 |1 - \beta_2 l|,$
$d_{op,1}(l, \beta_{1,regime}) = I\{l < \beta_2\}; \eta_2(l, \beta_{2,scale}) = \beta_3 I(\beta_2 > 0) \beta_1 |1 - \beta_2 l|,$
$d_{op,2}(l, \beta_{2,regime}) = I\{l \geq \beta_2\};$
$\eta_3(l, \beta_{3,scale}) = \beta_3 I(\beta_2 \leq 0) \beta_1 |1 - \beta_2 l|,$
$d_{op,3}(l, \beta_{3,regime}) = 1; \eta_4(l, \beta_{4,scale}) = (1 - \beta_3) I(\beta_2 \leq 0) \beta_1 |1 - \beta_2 l|,$
$d_{op,4}(l, \beta_{4,regime}) = 0$. Note in particular that $\beta_{1,scale}$ and $\beta_{1,regime}$ are not variation independent and that $\beta_{3,regime}$ and $\beta_{4,regime}$ do not exist. Given we choose $f_j(u) = u^2$, this is the unique expression for the regret in the Murphy parametrization. Further if we were given the model only in its Murphy parametrization with parameters buried within indicator functions, it would not be immediately obvious without some calculations that we could obtain closed form estimates of the parameter vector β by reexpressing the model in its alternative form $E[Y | L = l, A = a] - E[Y | L = l, A = 0] = a(\psi_0 + \psi_1 l)$ with ψ and β related as described above and then fitting using g-estimation. Indeed, we can obtain closed form dr-lse estimates as described in section 4.

To summarize we note that any optimal drSNMM model $\gamma^{\overline{0}}(\overline{l}_m, \overline{a}_m, \psi)$ for
$$E\left[Y_{\overline{a}_m, \underline{d}_{op,m+1}} - Y_{\overline{a}_{m-1}, 0_m, \underline{d}_{op,m+1}} | \overline{L}_{\overline{a}_{m-1}, m} = \overline{l}_m\right] \text{ induces a } \overline{d}_{op} - srSNNM$$

$$\varrho^{\overline{d}_{op}}\left(\overline{l}_m, \overline{a}_m, \psi\right)$$
$$= \gamma^{\overline{0}}\left(\overline{l}_m, \overline{a}_m, \psi\right) - \gamma^{\overline{0}}\left(\overline{l}_m, \overline{a}_{m-1}, d_{op,m}\left(\overline{l}_m, \overline{a}_{m-1}\right), \psi\right)$$

for $E\left[Y_{\overline{a}_m, \underline{d}_{op,m+1}} - Y_{\overline{a}_{m-1}, \underline{d}_{op,m}} | \overline{L}_{\overline{a}_{m-1}, m} = \overline{l}_m\right]$, which is the negative regret. Further the induced regret model $-\varrho^{\overline{d}_{op}}\left(\overline{L}_m, \overline{A}_m, \psi\right)$ can, after some tedious calculation, always be reparametrized $u_m\left(\overline{l}_m, \overline{a}_m, \beta\right)$ where $u_m\left(\overline{l}_m, \overline{a}_m, \beta\right)$ satisfies Murphy's parametrization $u_m\left(\overline{l}_m, \overline{a}_m, \beta\right)$
$= \eta_m\left(\overline{l}_m, \overline{a}_{m-1}, \beta_{scale}\right) f\left(a_m - d_{op,m}\left(\overline{l}_m, \overline{a}_{m-1}, \beta_{regime}\right)\right)$. Conversely any Murphy regret model $u_m\left(\overline{l}_m, \overline{a}_m, \beta\right)$ induces a optimal drSNMM model $\gamma^{\overline{0}}\left(\overline{l}_m, \overline{a}_m, \beta\right)$ via $\gamma^{\overline{0}}\left(\overline{l}_m, \overline{a}_m, \beta\right) = u_m\left(\overline{l}_m, \overline{a}_{m-1}, 0_m, \beta\right) - u_m\left(\overline{l}_m, \overline{a}_m, \beta\right)$. It follows that there is a clear sense in which optimal drSNMM models and Murphy regret models are mathematically equivalent. In my opinion, however, the advantages of optimal drSNMM models are that (i) it is easier to directly specify scientifically meaningful models for a) the mean effect $\gamma^{\overline{d}_{op}, \overline{0}}\left(\overline{l}_m, \overline{a}_m\right)$ of treatment level a_m (versus level "zero") at m before following $\overline{d}_{op}$ from $m+1$ onwards than for b1) the scale component $\eta_m\left(\overline{l}_m, \overline{a}_{m-1}\right)$ and b2) the optimal treatment regime $d_{op,m}\left(\overline{l}_m, \overline{a}_{m-1}\right)$ of the Murphy parametrized regret $u_m\left(\overline{l}_m, \overline{a}_m\right)$ for given a function $f\left(\cdot\right)$, (ii) it is straightforward to compute both the optimal regime $d_{op,m}\left(\overline{l}_m, \overline{a}_{m-1}\right) = argmax_{a_m}\gamma^{\overline{d}_{op}, \overline{0}}\left(\overline{l}_m, \overline{a}_m\right)$ and the regret $\gamma^{\overline{d}_{op}, \overline{0}}\left(\overline{l}_m, \overline{a}_{m-1}, d_{op,m}\left(\overline{l}_m, \overline{a}_{m-1}\right)\right) - \gamma^{\overline{d}_{op}, \overline{0}}\left(\overline{l}_m, \overline{a}_m\right)$ from $\gamma^{\overline{d}_{op}, \overline{0}}\left(\overline{l}_m, \overline{a}_m\right)$, (iii) the map from $\gamma^{\overline{d}_{op}, \overline{0}}\left(\overline{l}_m, \overline{a}_m\right)$ to Murphy's $u_m\left(\overline{l}_m, \overline{a}_m\right)$ is tedious to compute and of no additional utility, and (iv) for a dr SNMM it is usually immediately obvious when it is possible to obtain sequential closed form estimates of the model parameters by noting whether $\gamma^{\overline{0}}\left(\overline{l}_m, \overline{a}_m, \psi\right)$ can be embedded in a model $\gamma^{\overline{0}}\left(\overline{l}_m, \overline{a}_m, \psi_m^*, \underline{\psi}_{m+1}^*\right)$ linear in ψ_m^* with ψ a function of $\underline{\psi}_0^*$.

6.2 Comparison of Optimal drSNMMS with DP-regression SNMMs

Estimation of an Optimal Regime with DP-regression SNMMs

In this subsection we describe how to use a DP-like regression model applied to an estimated srSNMM or drSNMM to estimate the optimal treatment regime. In the following subsection we compare and contrast the optimal regime drSNMM methodology with this DP-regression SNMM methodology.

To avoid complex notation we will study the case where our SNMM is a srSNMM and the single regime is the regime that is always 0. It may be a standard or non-standard $\overline{0}$ regime. Generalization to other srSNMMs and drSNMMs is straightforward and is given explicitly in Section 7.3 . Recall the srSNMM $\gamma^{\overline{0}}\left(\overline{l}_m, \overline{a}_m, \psi\right)$ is a model for for $\gamma^{\overline{0}, \overline{0}}\left(\overline{l}_m, \overline{a}_m\right)$. If $\gamma^{\overline{0}}\left(\overline{l}_m, \overline{a}_m, \psi\right)$ is smooth in ψ we can obtain lse-dr estimators of $\psi^\dagger$ as described in Section

3. We now provide a DP-like algorithm for computing the optimal treatment regime from knowledge of $\gamma^0 \left(\bar{l}_m, \bar{a}_m, \psi\right)$. It is a special case of Theorem 7.6 below. It can also be seen as the consequence of part (iii) of Theorem 3.3.

Theorem 6.1: Under sequential randomization (2.5), the following recursive DP-like algorithm computes $\bar{d}_{op}$. Define

$$q\left(\bar{L}_K, \bar{A}_{K-1}, a_K\right) = \gamma^{0,0}\left(\bar{L}_K, \bar{A}_{K-1}, a_K\right)$$

For $m = K, ..., 0$ set

$$d_{op,m}\left(\bar{L}_m, \bar{A}_{m-1}\right) = \arg\max_{a_m} q\left(\bar{L}_m, \bar{A}_{m-1}, a_m\right),$$

$$j\left(\bar{L}_m, \bar{A}_{m-1}\right) = q\left(\bar{L}_m, \bar{A}_{m-1}, d_{op,m}\left(\bar{L}_m, \bar{A}_{m-1}\right)\right),$$

$$q\left(\bar{L}_{m-1}, \bar{A}_{m-2}, a_{m-1}\right) = E\left[j\left(\bar{L}_m, \bar{A}_{m-1}\right) | \bar{L}_{m-1}, \bar{A}_{m-2}, A_{m-1} = a_{m-1}\right] + \gamma^{0,0}\left(\bar{L}_{m-1}, \bar{A}_{m-2}, a_{m-1}\right)$$

Further $j\left(\bar{L}_m, \bar{A}_{m-1}\right) = E\left[Y_{\bar{A}_{m-1}, \underline{d}_{op,m}} - Y_{\bar{A}_{m-1}, \underline{0}_m} | \bar{L}_m, \bar{A}_{m-1}\right]$ and thus $E\left[Y_{\bar{d}_{op}}\right] = E\left[j\left(\bar{L}_0, \bar{A}_{-1}\right)\right] + E\left[Y_{\bar{0}}\right].$

Note $j\left(\bar{L}_m, \bar{A}_{m-1}\right)$ measures the difference in average utility of subjects with observed history $\left(\bar{L}_m, \bar{A}_{m-1}\right)$ were they were to follow the optimal regime from time t_m onward rather than the 0 regime. The above theorem motivates the following.

DP-regression srSNMM Fitting Algorithm: Let $\hat{\psi}$ be a dr-lse efficient estimator of the parameter $\psi^\dagger$ of a srSNMM calculated under the union model of Theorem 3.4. For $m = K, ..., 1$, we specify regression models

$$E\left[j\left(\bar{L}_m, \bar{A}_{m-1}\right) | \bar{L}_{m-1}, \bar{A}_{m-2}, A_{m-1} = a_{m-1}\right] = r\left(\bar{L}_{m-1}, \bar{A}_{m-2}, a_{m-1}; \beta_m\right)$$

and compute $Q_K\left(\hat{\psi}, a_K\right) = \gamma^0\left(\bar{L}_K, \bar{A}_{K-1}, a_K, \hat{\psi}\right)$. Then recursively, for $m = K, ..., 0$, (with β_{K+1} the null set),

$$d_{op,m}\left(\bar{L}_m, \bar{A}_{m-1}, \hat{\psi}, \underline{\hat{\beta}}_{m+1}\right) = \arg\max_{a_m} Q_m\left(\hat{\psi}, a_m, \underline{\hat{\beta}}_{m+1}\right),$$

$$J_m\left(\hat{\psi}, \underline{\hat{\beta}}_{m+1}\right) = Q_m\left(\hat{\psi}, d_{op,m}\left(\bar{L}_m, \bar{A}_{m-1}, \hat{\psi}, \underline{\hat{\beta}}_{m+1}\right), \underline{\hat{\beta}}_{m+1}\right),$$

$$Q_{m-1}\left(\hat{\psi}, a_{m-1}; \underline{\hat{\beta}}_m\right) = r\left(\bar{L}_{m-1}, \bar{A}_{m-2}, a_{m-1}; \hat{\beta}_m, \hat{\psi}, \underline{\hat{\beta}}_{m+1}\right) + \gamma^0\left(\bar{L}_{m-1}, \bar{A}_{m-2}, a_{m-1}, \hat{\psi}\right),$$

where $\hat{\beta}_m$ is the possibly non-linear least squares estimate of β_m from the regression of $J_m\left(\hat{\psi}, \underline{\hat{\beta}}_{m+1}\right)$ on $\bar{L}_{m-1}, \bar{A}_{m-2}, A_{m-1} = a_{m-1}$ based on the regression function $r\left(\bar{L}_{m-1}, \bar{A}_{m-2}, a_{m-1}; \beta_m\right)$.

Finally calculate

$$\widehat{E}_{\widehat{\psi},\widehat{\underline{\beta}}_0}\left[Y_{\overline{a}_{op,m}}\right] = P_n\left[J_0\left(\widehat{\psi},\widehat{\underline{\beta}}_1\right)\right] + P_n\left[H_0^{0,0}\left(\widehat{\psi}\right)\right]$$

Note that if the $H_m^{0,0}(\psi)$ are linear in ψ as for the model $\gamma^0\left(\bar{l}_m, \bar{a}_m, \psi\right) = a_m\left(1, l_m, a_{m-1}\right)\psi$, then $\widehat{\psi}$ will exist in closed form. If the $q\left(\overline{L}_{m-1}, \overline{A}_{m-2}, a_{m-1}; \beta_m\right)$ are linear in β_m and $\widehat{\beta}_m$ is the OLS estimator, then $d_{op,m}\left(\overline{L}_m, \overline{A}_{m-1}, \widehat{\psi}, \widehat{\underline{\beta}}_{m+1}\right)$ will exist in closed form (provided the argmax function can be evaluated in closed form). However the model will share the inferential difficulties we noted in our study of the closed-form inefficient estimator of an optimal drSNMM. Specifically although the parameter ψ of our srSNMM, in contrast to that of an optimal drSNMM, is a regular parameter, the parameters $\beta_m = \beta_m\left(\psi, \underline{\beta}_{m+1}\right)$ for $m < K$ are not, as $\beta_m\left(\psi, \underline{\beta}_{m+1}\right)$ is not an everywhere differentiable function of $\left(\psi, \underline{\beta}_{m+1}\right)$. Specifically, $J_m\left(\widehat{\psi}, \widehat{\underline{\beta}}_{m+1}\right) = Q_m\left(\widehat{\psi}, d_{op,m}\left(\overline{L}_m, \overline{A}_{m-1}, \widehat{\psi}, \widehat{\underline{\beta}}_{m+1}\right), \widehat{\underline{\beta}}_{m+1}\right)$ and, for dichotomous A_m, $d_{op,m}\left(\overline{L}_m, \overline{A}_{m-1}, \widehat{\psi}, \widehat{\underline{\beta}}_{m+1}\right)$ will jump from 1 to 0 or vice-versa as $\widehat{\psi}$ or $\underline{\beta}_{m+1}$ are continuously varied. However a large sample confidence interval for $\overline{d}_{op,m}$ can be obtained because (i) $d_{op,m}$ is a function of $\left(\psi, \underline{\beta}_{m+1}\right)$ and (ii) a joint large sample confidence interval for $(\psi, \beta) = \left(\psi, \underline{\beta}_1\right)$ can be obtained based on inverting a χ^2 statistic for the joint estimating functions for (ψ, β) (which for β are the least squares normal equations). Because the estimating functions for ψ do not depend on β, the confidence interval is guaranteed to be valid under the g-null hypothesis when the union model of theorem 3.4 is correct.

It follows that the misspecification of the regression model $E\left[j\left(\overline{L}_m, \overline{A}_{m-1}\right) | \overline{L}_{m-1}, \overline{A}_{m-2}, A_{m-1}\right] = r\left(\overline{L}_{m-1}, \overline{A}_{m-2}, A_{m-1}; \beta_m\right)$ does not lead to bias in estimating $d_{op,m}\left(\overline{L}_m, \overline{A}_{m-1}\right)$ or $E\left[Y_{\overline{d}_{op,m}}\right]$ under the g-null hypothesis that $\psi^\dagger$ is zero as $q\left(\overline{L}_m, \overline{A}_{m-1}, a_m\right)$ and $j\left(\overline{L}_m, \overline{A}_{m-1}\right)$ are identically zero. To obtain a consistent estimate of $\overline{d}_{op}$ under the alternative $\psi^\dagger \neq 0$, correct specification of this regression model will be necessary, which is not feasible due to the high dimension of the vector $\left(\overline{L}_{m-1}, \overline{A}_{m-1}\right)$. However, I do not consider this to be a major shortcoming of the DP-regression srSNMM methodology compared to the optimal drSNMM methodology for the following reason. To obtain a consistent estimate of $\overline{d}_{op}$ under an optimal drSNMM, the optimal drSNMM $\gamma^0\left(\bar{l}_m, \bar{a}_m, \psi\right)$ for $\gamma^{\overline{d}_{op},0}\left(\bar{l}_m, \bar{a}_m\right)$ must be correct, but this is also not feasible due to the high dimension of $\left(\overline{L}_m, \overline{A}_m\right)$. That is, because of the high dimensionality of the problem, no method can provide a consistent estimator for $\overline{d}_{op}$ under the alternative, even when the treatment probabilities are known. The question is then do we expect to obtain less biased estimates of $\overline{d}_{op}$ with the DP-regression srSNMM methodology that requires us to specify models for both $\gamma^{\bar{0},\bar{0}}\left(\bar{l}_m, \bar{a}_m\right)$ and $E\left[j\left(\bar{L}_m, \bar{A}_{m-1}\right)|\bar{L}_{m-1}, \bar{A}_{m-2}, A_{m-1} = a_{m-1}\right]$ or with the optimal drSNMM that requires a model for $\gamma^{\bar{d}_{op},\bar{0}}\left(\bar{l}_m, \bar{a}_m\right)$. In general that will depend on whether it is easier to use our substantive subject-matter knowledge to model $\gamma^{\bar{d}_{op},\bar{0}}\left(\bar{l}_m, \bar{a}_m\right)$ or to model both $\gamma^{\bar{0},\bar{0}}\left(\bar{l}_m, \bar{a}_m\right)$ and $E\left[j\left(\bar{L}_m, \bar{A}_{m-1}\right)|\bar{L}_{m-1}, \bar{A}_{m-2}, A_{m-1} = a_{m-1}\right]$. There is no general rule as to which is easier even when we use a standard (i.e. substantively mean-ingful) zero regime. To understand why it is only an issue about the ease of applying substantiative knowledge, I will now show there is a precise sense in which fitting optimal drSNMM models and DP- srSNMM models can be made algebraically equivalent. To do so I shall use the following Lemma.

Lemma 6.1: Under sequential randomization (2.5),

$$\gamma^{\bar{d}_{op},\bar{0}}\left(\bar{L}_m, \bar{A}_m\right) - \gamma^{\bar{d}_{op},\bar{0}}\left(\bar{L}_m, \bar{A}_{m-1}, d_{op,m}\left(\bar{L}_m, \bar{A}_{m-1}\right)\right)$$
$$= \gamma^{\bar{0},\bar{0}}\left(\bar{L}_m, \bar{A}_m\right) + j\left(\bar{L}_m, \bar{A}_{m-1}\right) - E\left[j\left(\bar{L}_{m+1}, \bar{A}_m\right)|\bar{L}_m, \bar{A}_m\right]$$
$$= j\left(\bar{L}_m, \bar{A}_{m-1}\right) + q\left(\bar{L}_m, \bar{A}_m\right).$$

Further

$$H_m^{\bar{d}_{op},\bar{0}} - E\left[H_m^{\bar{d}_{op},\bar{0}}|\bar{L}_m, \bar{A}_{m-1}\right] = H_m^{\bar{0},\bar{0}} - E\left[H_m^{\bar{0},\bar{0}}|\bar{L}_m, \bar{A}_{m-1}\right] + Z_m,$$

with

$$Z_m = \sum_{j=m+1}^{K} j\left(\bar{L}_j, \bar{A}_{j-1}\right) - E\left[j\left(\bar{L}_j, \bar{A}_{j-1}\right)|L_{j-1}, \bar{A}_{j-1}\right] -$$

$$E\left[\sum_{j=m+1}^{K} j\left(\bar{L}_j, \bar{A}_{j-1}\right) - E\left[j\left(\bar{L}_j, \bar{A}_{j-1}\right)|L_{j-1}, \bar{A}_{j-1}\right]|\bar{L}_m, \bar{A}_{m-1}\right]$$

Proof: By definition $\gamma^{\bar{d}_{op},\bar{0}}\left(\bar{L}_m, \bar{A}_m\right) - \gamma^{\bar{d}_{op},\bar{0}}\left(\bar{L}_m, \bar{A}_{m-1}, d_{op,m}\left(\bar{L}_m, \bar{A}_{m-1}\right)\right) - \gamma^{\bar{0},\bar{0}}\left(\bar{L}_m, \bar{A}_m\right)$

$$= -E\left[Y_{\bar{A}_{m-1},\underline{d}_{op,m}} - Y_{\bar{A}_m,\underline{d}_{op,m+1}} + Y_{\bar{A}_m,\underline{0}_{m+1}} - Y_{\bar{A}_{m-1},\underline{0}_m}|\bar{L}_m, \bar{A}_m\right]$$
$$= -E\left[Y_{\bar{A}_{m-1},\underline{d}_{op,m}} - Y_{\bar{A}_{m-1},\underline{0}_m}|\bar{L}_m, \bar{A}_m\right] + E\left[-Y_{\bar{A}_m,\underline{d}_{op,m+1}} + Y_{\bar{A}_m,\underline{0}_{m+1}}|\bar{L}_m, \bar{A}_m\right]$$
$$= -\left\{j\left(\bar{L}_m, \bar{A}_{m-1}\right) - E\left[j\left(\bar{L}_{m+1}, \bar{A}_m\right)|\bar{L}_m, \bar{A}_m\right]\right\}, \text{ where we have used}$$

sequential randomization in the final step. Thus by Lemma 6.1, a model $\gamma^{\bar{0},\bar{0}}\left(\bar{L}_m, \bar{A}_m, \psi\right)$ for $\gamma^{\bar{0},\bar{0}}\left(\bar{L}_m, \bar{A}_m\right)$ plus regression models

$$E\left[j\left(\bar{L}_m, \bar{A}_{m-1}\right)|\bar{L}_{m-1}, \bar{A}_{m-1}\right] = r\left(\bar{L}_{m-1}, \bar{A}_{m-1}; \beta_m\right),$$

$m = K, ..., 1$, induce a model $\gamma^{\bar{d}_{op},\bar{0}}\left(\bar{L}_m, \bar{A}_m, \psi, \underline{\beta}_m\right)$ for $\gamma^{\bar{d}_{op},\bar{0}}\left(\bar{L}_m, \bar{A}_m\right)$. Conversely a model $\gamma^{\bar{d}_{op},\bar{0}}\left(\bar{L}_m, \bar{A}_m, \psi\right)$ for $\gamma^{\bar{d}_{op},\bar{0}}\left(\bar{L}_m, \bar{A}_m\right)$ plus regres-sion models $E\left[j\left(\bar{L}_m, \bar{A}_{m-1}\right)|\bar{L}_{m-1}, \bar{A}_{m-1}\right] = r\left(\bar{L}_{m-1}, \bar{A}_{m-1}; \beta_m\right)$ induces a model $\gamma^{\bar{0},\bar{0}}\left(\bar{L}_m, \bar{A}_m, \psi, \underline{\beta}_m\right)$ for $\gamma^{\bar{0},\bar{0}}\left(\bar{L}_m, \bar{A}_m\right)$.

Given models $\gamma^{\bar{0},\bar{0}}\left(\bar{L}_m,\bar{A}_m,\psi\right)$ for $\gamma^{\bar{0},\bar{0}}\left(\bar{L}_m,\bar{A}_m\right)$ plus regression models $E\left[j\left(\bar{L}_m,\bar{A}_{m-1}\right)|\bar{L}_{m-1},\bar{A}_{m-1}\right]=r\left(\bar{L}_{m-1},\bar{A}_{m-1};\beta_m\right)$ an alternative way to estimate $\psi^\dagger$ would be to solve an estimating equation based on the induced optimal drSNMM model. For example we can solve $0=P_n\left[U^{\dagger\bar{d}_{op},\bar{0}}\left(\psi,\widehat{\underline{\beta}}_0\left(\psi\right),s,c^{s,\bar{d}_{op},\bar{0}},\widehat{\varsigma}\right)\right]$ where $\widehat{\underline{\beta}}_0\left(\psi\right)$ is obtained as in the DP srSNMM fitting algorithm. But from Lemma (6.1), this will equal

$$P_n\left[U^{\dagger\bar{0},\bar{0}}\left(\psi,s,c^{s,\bar{0},\bar{0}},\widehat{\varsigma}\right)\right]+$$

$$P_n\left[\sum_{m=0}^{K}Z_m\left(\psi,\widehat{\underline{\beta}}_{m+1}\left(\psi\right),\widehat{\varsigma}\right)\left\{S_m\left(A_m\right)-E\left[S_m\left(A_m\right)\mid\bar{A}_{m-1},\bar{L}_m\right]\right\}\right].$$

We can always choose our regression models $E\left[j\left(\bar{L}_m,\bar{A}_{m-1}\right)|\bar{L}_{m-1},\bar{A}_{m-1}\right]=r\left(\bar{L}_{m-1},\bar{A}_{m-1};\beta_m\right)$ such that $P_n\left[\sum_{m=0}^{K}Z_m\left(\psi,\widehat{\underline{\beta}}_{m+1}\left(\psi\right),\widehat{\varsigma}\right)\left\{S_m\left(A_m\right)-E\left[S_m\left(A_m\right)\mid\bar{A}_{m-1},\bar{L}_m\right]\right\}\right]$ is zero with probability one. Specifically we choose $r\left(\bar{L}_{m-1},\bar{A}_{m-1};\beta_m\right)=\beta_m^T W_m$ with W_m including each $\left\{S_j\left(A_j\right)-E\left[S_j\left(A_j\right)\mid\bar{A}_{j-1},\bar{L}_j\right]\right\}$ as a covariate for every $j<m$.

This will guarantee that we obtain the exact same estimates of ψ and $\bar{d}_{op}$ by directly solving the induced optimal drSNMM estimating equation $0=P_n\left[U^{\dagger\bar{d}_{op},\bar{0}}\left(\psi,\widehat{\underline{\beta}}_0\left(\psi\right),s,c^{s,\bar{d}_{op},\bar{0}},\widehat{\varsigma}\right)\right]$ as by first solving $P_n\left[U^{\dagger\bar{0},\bar{0}}\left(\psi,s,c^{s,\bar{0},\bar{0}},\widehat{\varsigma}\right)\right]=0$ and then implementing the DP srSNMM fitting algorithm. Thus the only issue is whether it is an easier substantive task to model $\gamma^{\bar{d}_{op},\bar{0}}\left(\bar{l}_m,\bar{a}_m\right)$ or to model both $\gamma^{\bar{0},\bar{0}}\left(\bar{l}_m,\bar{a}_m\right)$ and $E\left[j\left(\bar{L}_m,\bar{A}_{m-1}\right)|\bar{L}_{m-1},\bar{A}_{m-2},A_{m-1}=a_{m-1}\right]$, as either model can then be fit using the methods described in section 4 for fitting optimal drSNMM models. Thus the only issue is whether it is an easier substantive task to model $\gamma^{\bar{d}_{op},\bar{0}}\left(\bar{l}_m,\bar{a}_m\right)$

An example of a setting in which it might be easier to model $\gamma^{\bar{d}_{op},\bar{0}}\left(\bar{l}_m,\bar{a}_m\right)$ is one in which one believes that current medical practice fluctuates around the optimal regime, because the direct experience of clinicians will then be with subjects who followed treatment plans close to the optimal, providing a basis for developing a good intuition for the functional form of $\gamma^{\bar{d}_{op},\bar{0}}\left(\bar{l}_m,\bar{a}_m\right)$.

7 Sensitivity Analysis and Decisions with Information Loss:

In subsections 7.1 and 7.2 we no longer assume that sequential randomization holds and develops a sensitivity analysis methodology. In the next subsection, we develop two simple methods for estimating a $\left(\bar{d},\bar{d}^*\right)$ drSNMM model $\gamma^{\bar{d}^*}\left(\bar{l}_m,\bar{a}_m;\psi\right)$ and the corresponding regime -specific mean $E\left[Y^{\bar{d}}\right]$ in the absence of sequential randomization. The first method requires us to treat as known two different nonidentifiable functions unless $\bar{d} = \bar{d}^*$. These functions are then varied in a sensitivity analysis. The second, more parsimonious, method only requires us to treat as known a single nonidentifiable function. However we shall see in section 7.2 that two nonidentifiable functions will always be required to estimate $E\left[Y^{\bar{d}_{op}}\right]$ precisely because $\bar{d}_{op}$ is not known. In Section 7.2 and 7.3, we consider settings in which the decison maker can only use a subset of the past information to make a current decision.

7.1 Regime Specific SNMMs

Method 1:

We turn to our first method. Under the assumption of sequential randomization, the following function is identically zero for each m. Define

$$r^{\bar{d},\bar{d}^*}\left(\overline{L}_m, \overline{A}_{m-1}, a_m\right) = r^{\underline{d}_m, d_m^*}\left(\overline{L}_m, \overline{A}_{m-1}, a_m\right) =$$
$$E\left[Y_{\overline{A}_{m-1}, a_m, \underline{d}_{m+1}} - Y_{\overline{A}_{m-1}, d_m^*, \underline{d}_{m+1}} \middle| \overline{L}_m, \overline{A}_{m-1}, A_m = a_m\right] - \qquad (7.1)$$
$$E\left[Y_{\overline{A}_{m-1}, a_m, \underline{d}_{m+1}} - Y_{\overline{A}_{m-1}, d_m^*, \underline{d}_{m+1}} \middle| \overline{L}_m, \overline{A}_{m-1}, A_m \neq a_m\right]$$

We refer to $r^{\underline{d}_m, d_m^*}\left(\overline{L}_m, \overline{A}_{m-1}, a_m\right)$ as a regime $d - specific$ current treatment interaction function since, among subjects with history $\left(\overline{L}_m, \overline{A}_{m-1}\right)$, it compares the magnitude of the effect of a last blip of treatment of dose a_m compared to dose $d_m^*\left(\overline{L}_m, \overline{A}_{m-1}\right)$ before following regime d among those who received treatment a_m to the same effect among those who did not receive the treatment a_m. If, as in this section, we do not assume sequential randomization but do assume the support of $each$ counterfactual response may be the whole real line, then the function $r^{\underline{d}_m, d_m^*}\left(\overline{L}_m, \overline{A}_{m-1}, a_m\right)$ is completely nonidentified in the sense that the distribution of the observed data O places no restrictions on $r^{\underline{d}_m, d_m^*}\left(\overline{L}_m, \overline{A}_{m-1}, a_m\right)$ except for the definitional restriction that $r^{\underline{d}_m, d_m^*}\left(\overline{L}_m, \overline{A}_{m-1}, a_m\right) = 0$ if $a_m = d_m^*\left(\overline{L}_m, \overline{A}_{m-1}\right)$. This is immediately evident because there can be no data evidence restricting the mean of $Y_{\overline{A}_{m-1}, a_m, \underline{d}_{m+1}}$ among subjects with $A_m \neq a_m$. Thus we will regard the unidentified function $r^{\underline{d}_m, d_m^*}\left(\overline{L}_m, \overline{A}_{m-1}, a_m\right)$ as known and vary it in a sensitivity analysis. Note that under the non-identifiable assumption of additive local rank preservation $r^{\underline{d}_m, d_m^*}\left(\overline{L}_m, \overline{A}_{m-1}, a_m\right) \equiv 0$. Further $r^{\underline{d}_m, d_m^*}\left(\overline{L}_m, \overline{A}_{m-1}, a_m\right) \equiv 0$ under the sharp null hypothesis that $Y_{\bar{a}} = Y$ for all $\bar{a} \in \overline{\mathcal{A}}$ w.p.1 of no treatment effect. Thus if one wishes to test the sharp null hypothesis one must do so assuming $r^{\underline{d}_m, d_m^*}\left(\overline{L}_m, \overline{A}_{m-1}, a_m\right) \equiv 0$. Define the function $r^{\underline{d}_m, d_m^*}\left(\overline{L}_m, \overline{A}_{m-1}\right)$ of $\left(\overline{L}_m, \overline{A}_{m-1}\right)$ by

$$r^{\underline{d}_m, d_m^*}\left(\overline{L}_m, \overline{A}_{m-1}\right) \equiv r^{\underline{d}_m, d_m^*}\left(\overline{L}_m, \overline{A}_{m-1}, d_m\left(\overline{L}_m, \overline{A}_{m-1}\right)\right).$$

The following theorem states that knowledge of $r^{\underline{d}_m,d_m^*}\left(\overline{L}_m,\overline{A}_{m-1}\right)$ plus identification of $\gamma^{\overline{d},\overline{d}^*}\left(\overline{L}_m,\overline{A}_{m-1},a_m\right)$ suffices to identify $E\left[Y^{\overline{d}}\right]$ and more generally $E\left[Y_{\overline{A}_{m-1},\underline{d}_m}|\overline{L}_m,\overline{A}_{m-1}\right]$. Note by the definition of $\gamma^{\overline{d},\overline{d}^*}\left(\overline{L}_m,\overline{A}_{m-1},a_m\right)$,

$$r^{\underline{d}_m,d_m^*}\left(\overline{L}_m,\overline{A}_{m-1}\right) =$$
$$\gamma^{\overline{d},\overline{d}^*}\left(\overline{L}_m,\overline{A}_{m-1},d_m\left(\overline{L}_m,\overline{A}_{m-1}\right)\right) -$$
$$E\left[Y_{\overline{A}_{m-1},d_m,\underline{d}_{m+1}} - Y_{\overline{A}_{m-1},d_m^*,\underline{d}_{m+1}}|\overline{L}_m,\overline{A}_{m-1},A_m \neq d_m\left(\overline{L}_m,\overline{A}_{m-1}\right)\right]$$

We shall need the following definitions which reduce to our previous definitions (3.5) under sequential randomization. Let $\gamma^{\overline{d}*}*\left(\overline{L}_m,\overline{A}_m\right)$ satisfy (3.6) and define $a_m = d_m\left(\overline{L}_m,\overline{A}_{m-1}\right)$ for the remainder of this paragraph. Define
$$H_{K+1}\left(\gamma^{\overline{d}^**}\right) = Y,$$

$$H_K\left(\gamma^{\overline{d}^**}\right) = Y - \gamma^{\overline{d}^**}\left(\overline{L}_K,\overline{A}_K\right) +$$
$$\gamma^{\overline{d}^**}\left(\overline{L}_K,\overline{A}_{K-1},d_K\left(\overline{L}_K,\overline{A}_{K-1}\right)\right) - r^{\underline{d}_K,d_K^*}\left(\overline{L}_K,\overline{A}_{K-1}\right)\left\{1 - f\left(a_K|\overline{L}_K,\overline{A}_{K-1}\right)\right\}$$

$$H_m^{\underline{d}_m}\left(\gamma^{\overline{d}^**}\right) =$$
$$H_{m+1}^{\underline{d}_{m+1}}\left(\gamma^{\overline{d}^**}\right) + \gamma^{\overline{d}^**}\left(\overline{L}_m,\overline{A}_{m-1},d_m\left(\overline{L}_m,\overline{A}_{m-1}\right)\right) -$$
$$r^{\underline{d}_m,d_m^*}\left(\overline{L}_m,\overline{A}_{m-1}\right)\left\{1 - f\left(a_m|\overline{L}_m,\overline{A}_{m-1}\right)\right\} - \gamma^{\overline{d}^**}\left(\overline{L}_m,\overline{A}_m\right)$$
$$= Y - \sum_{j=m}^K \gamma^{\overline{d}^**}\left(\overline{L}_j,\overline{A}_j\right) +$$
$$\sum_{j=m}^K \gamma^{\overline{d}^**}\left(\overline{L}_j,\overline{A}_{j-1},d_j\left(\overline{L}_j,\overline{A}_{j-1}\right)\right) - r^{\underline{d}_j,d_j^*}\left(\overline{L}_j,\overline{A}_{j-1}\right)\left\{1 - f\left(a_j|\overline{L}_j,\overline{A}_{j-1}\right)\right\}$$

Note $H_m^{\underline{d}_m}\left(\gamma^{\overline{d},\overline{d}^*}\right)$ depends only on the data O and the functions $r^{\underline{d}_m,d_m^*}$ and $\gamma^{\overline{d},\overline{d}^*}$. In appendix 3 we prove the following.

Theorem 7.1: With $H_m^{\underline{d}_m}\left(\gamma^{\overline{d}^**}\right)$ as defined in the previous paragraph,
$$E\left[H_m^{\underline{d}_m}\left(\gamma^{\overline{d}^**}\right)|\overline{L}_m,\overline{A}_m\right] = E\left[Y_{\overline{A}_{m-1},\underline{d}_m}|\overline{L}_m,\overline{A}_m\right] \text{ for all } m \text{ if and only if}$$

$$\gamma^{\overline{d}^**}\left(\overline{L}_m,\overline{A}_m\right) = \gamma^{\overline{d},\overline{d}^*}\left(\overline{L}_m,\overline{A}_m\right) \text{ w.p.1 for all } m \qquad (7.2)$$

In particular $E\left[Y_{\overline{d}}\right] = E\left[H_0\left(\gamma^{\overline{d}}\right)\right]$.

To see why we require $r^{\underline{d}_K, d_K^*}\left(\overline{L}_K, \overline{A}_{K-1}\right)$ in addition to $\gamma^{\overline{d}, \overline{d}^*}\left(\overline{l}_m, \overline{a}_m\right)$ to identify $E\left[Y_{\overline{A}_{K-1}, d_K} | \overline{L}_K, \overline{A}_{K-1}\right]$ first note that knowledge of $\gamma^{\overline{d}, \overline{d}^*}\left(\overline{l}_K, \overline{a}_K\right)$ allows us to identify $E\left[Y_{\overline{A}_{K-1}, d_K^*} | \overline{L}_K, \overline{A}_{K-1}, A_K = a_K\right]$ for each a_K and thus to identify $E\left[Y_{\overline{A}_{K-1}, d_K^*} | \overline{L}_K, \overline{A}_{K-1}\right]$. Since we know

$$E\left[Y_{\overline{A}_{K-1}, d_K} - Y_{\overline{A}_{K-1}, d_K^*} | \overline{L}_K, \overline{A}_{K-1}, A_K = d_K\left(\overline{L}_K, \overline{A}_{K-1}\right)\right],$$ knowledge of $r^{\underline{d}_K, d_K^*}\left(\overline{L}_K, \overline{A}_{K-1}\right)$ allows us to calculate

$$E\left[Y_{\overline{A}_{K-1}, d_K} - Y_{\overline{A}_{K-1}, d_K^*} | \overline{L}_K, \overline{A}_{K-1}, A_K \neq d_K\left(\overline{L}_K, \overline{A}_{K-1}\right)\right]$$ and, using the law of O, $E\left[Y_{\overline{A}_{K-1}, d_K} - Y_{\overline{A}_{K-1}, d_K^*} | \overline{L}_K, \overline{A}_{K-1}\right]$ as well. Thus we can compute $E\left[Y_{\overline{A}_{K-1}, d_K} | \overline{L}_K, \overline{A}_{K-1}\right]$.

In the absence of sequential randomization, knowledge of $r^{\underline{d}_m, d_m^*}\left(\overline{L}_m, \overline{A}_{m-1}\right)$ is not sufficient to identify $\gamma^{\overline{d}, \overline{d}^*}\left(\overline{L}_m, \overline{A}_m\right)$ from the law of O. Now under sequential randomization the function

$$v^{\overline{d}, \overline{d}^*}\left(\overline{L}_m, \overline{A}_m\right) = E\left[Y_{\overline{A}_{m-1}, d_m^*, \underline{d}_{m+1}} | \overline{L}_m, \overline{A}_m\right] -$$
$$E\left[Y_{\overline{A}_{m-1}, d_m^*, \underline{d}_{m+1}} | \overline{L}_m, \overline{A}_{m-1}, A_m = d_m^*\left(\overline{L}_m, \overline{A}_{m-1}\right)\right]$$

takes the value zero. Hence $v^{\overline{d}, \overline{d}^*}\left(\overline{L}_m, \overline{A}_m\right)$ is a measure of the magnitude of confounding due to unmeasured factors among subjects with history $\left(\overline{L}_m, \overline{A}_{m-1}\right)$, as it compares the mean of the same counterfactual in those who received treatment A_m to that in those who received treatment $d_m^*\left(\overline{L}_m, \overline{A}_{m-1}\right)$ at t_m. Further knowledge of the law of O and of $r^{\underline{d}_m, d_m^*}\left(\overline{L}_m, \overline{A}_{m-1}\right)$ together place no restrictions on $v^{\overline{d}, \overline{d}^*}\left(\overline{L}_m, \overline{A}_m\right)$ beyond the definitional restriction that $v^{\overline{d}, \overline{d}^*}\left(\overline{L}_m, \overline{A}_m\right) = 0$ if $A_m = d_m^*\left(\overline{L}_m, \overline{A}_{m-1}\right)$. Thus we will regard the unidentified functions $r^{\underline{d}_m, d_m^*}\left(\overline{L}_m, \overline{A}_{m-1}\right)$ and $v^{\overline{d}, \overline{d}^*}\left(\overline{L}_m, \overline{A}_m\right)$ both as known and vary both in a sensitivity analysis. The following theorem, proved in Appendix 3, states that knowledge of $v^{\overline{d}, \overline{d}^*}\left(\overline{L}_m, \overline{A}_m\right)$ and $r^{\underline{d}_m, d_m^*}\left(\overline{L}_m, \overline{A}_{m-1}\right)$ identifies $\gamma^{\overline{d}, \overline{d}^*}\left(\overline{L}_m, \overline{A}_m\right)$ and thus by Theorem 7.1 $E\left[Y^{\overline{d}}\right]$ as well.

Theorem 7.2: Let $H_{m+1}^{\underline{d}_m}\left(\gamma^{\overline{d}^*}\right)$ be defined as in Theorem 7.1. Then

$$E\left[H_{m+1}^{\underline{d}_m}\left(\gamma^{\overline{d}^*}\right) - \gamma^{\overline{d}^*}\left(\overline{L}_m, \overline{A}_m\right) - v^{\overline{d}, \overline{d}^*}\left(\overline{L}_m, \overline{A}_m\right) | \overline{L}_m, \overline{A}_m\right]$$

is not a function of A_m for all m if and only if Eq (7.2) of Theorem 7.1 holds if and only if $E[H_m^{\underline{d}_m}\left(\gamma^{\overline{d}^*}\right) - v^{\overline{d}, \overline{d}^*}\left(\overline{L}_m, \overline{A}_m\right) | \overline{L}_m, \overline{A}_m]$ is not a function of A_m for all m.

Inference under Method 1:

The following two corollaries are special cases of Theorem 4.3 in Robins and Rotnizky (2003)

Corollary 7.2a: Consider again the semiparametric models (a.1) - (a.3) of Theorem 3.3, except now the assumption of sequential randomization is replaced by the assumption that the functions $v^{\bar{d},\bar{d}^*}\left(\bar{L}_m,\bar{A}_m\right)$ and $r^{\underline{d}_m,d^*_m}\left(\bar{L}_m,\bar{A}_{m-1}\right)$ are known (but may be non-zero). Then,

a) part *(i)* of Theorem 3.3 remains true if we replace $H^{\bar{d},\bar{d}^*}_m\left(\psi\right)$ in Eq. (3.9) with $H^{\bar{d},\bar{d}^*}_m\left(\psi\right) - v^{\bar{d},\bar{d}^*}\left(\bar{L}_m,\bar{A}_m\right)$ where (a) $H^{\bar{d},\bar{d}^*}_m\left(\psi\right)$ is now $H^{\underline{d}_m}_{m+1}\left(\gamma^{\bar{d}^*}*\right)$ as defined before Theorem 7.1 with $\gamma^{\bar{d}^**}\left(\bar{L}_m,\bar{A}_m\right) = \gamma^{\bar{d},\bar{d}^*}\left(\bar{L}_m,\bar{A}_m,\psi\right)$ being the dr SNMM model $\gamma^{\bar{d},\bar{d}^*}\left(\bar{L}_m,\bar{A}_m,\psi\right)$ for $\gamma^{\bar{d},\bar{d}^*}\left(\bar{L}_m,\bar{A}_m\right)$. However, part *(ii)* and (iii) must be modified as follows.

b) When $v^{\bar{d},\bar{d}^*}\left(\bar{L}_m,\bar{A}_m\right)$ and $r^{\underline{d}_m,d^*_m}\left(\bar{L}_m,\bar{A}_{m-1}\right)$ are identically zero, (ii) of Theorem 3.3 holds. However, if $v^{\bar{d},\bar{d}^*}\left(\bar{L}_m,\bar{A}_m\right)$ and $r^{\underline{d}_m,d^*_m}\left(\bar{L}_m,\bar{A}_{m-1}\right)$ are not identically zero, then $\widehat{\psi}\left(s,c^s\right) \equiv \widehat{\psi}\left(s,c^s,a^\dagger\right)$ has asymptotic variance less than or equal to that of $\widehat{\psi}\left(s,c^s,\widehat{\alpha}\right)$ which has an asymptotic variance less than or equal to that of $\widehat{\psi}\left(s,c^s,\widehat{\alpha}_{smooth}\right)$. Further

$$C^s_m - E\left[C^s_m|\bar{A}_{m-1},\bar{L}_m\right] \neq E\left[U_m\left(\psi^\dagger,s\right) \mid \bar{A}_m,\bar{L}_m\right] - E\left[U_m\left(\psi^\dagger,s\right)|\bar{A}_{m-1},\bar{L}_m\right]$$

and thus

$$C^s \neq \tilde{C}^s \equiv \sum_m \tilde{C}^s_m - E\left[\tilde{C}^s_m|\bar{A}_{m-1},\bar{L}_m\right] \text{ with } \tilde{C}^s_m = E\left[U_m\left(\psi^\dagger,s\right) \mid \bar{A}_m,\bar{L}_m\right]$$

Explicit expressions for the influence functions are as follows. $\widehat{\psi}\left(s,c\right)$ has influence function $I^{-1}U^\dagger\left(s,c\right)$ with variance $I^{-1}\left\{E\left[U^\dagger\left(s,c\right)^{\otimes 2}\right]\right\}I^{-1,T}$ where

$$E\left[U^\dagger\left(s,c\right)^{\otimes 2}\right] = E\left[U^\dagger\left(s,c^s\right)^{\otimes 2}\right] + E\left[\left(C_s - C\right)^{\otimes 2}\right], \widehat{\psi}\left(s,c,\widehat{\alpha}\right) \text{ has influence}$$

function $I^{-1}\left\{U^\dagger\left(s,c\right) + E[\partial U^\dagger\left(s,c,\alpha\right)/\partial\alpha]\left\{E\left(S^{\otimes 2}_{part}\right]\right\}^{-1}S_{part}\right\}$ with variance $I^{-1}\times$

$$\left\{E\left[U^\dagger\left(s,c^s\right)^{\otimes 2}\right] + E\left[\left\{C_s - C + E\left[\partial U^\dagger\left(s,c,\alpha\right)/\partial\alpha\right]\left[S^{\otimes 2}_{part}\right]^{-1}S_{part}\right\}^{\otimes 2}\right]\right\}I^{-1,T}$$

Finally, $\widehat{\psi}\left(s,c,\widehat{\alpha}_{smooth}\right)$ has has influence function $I^{-1}U^\dagger\left(s,\tilde{c}^s\right)$ with variance $I^{-1}\left\{E\left[U^\dagger\left(s,\tilde{c}^s\right)^{\otimes 2}\right]\right\}I^{-1,T}$.

c) When $v^{\bar{d},\bar{d}^*}\left(\bar{L}_m,\bar{A}_m\right)$ and $r^{\underline{d}_m,d^*_m}\left(\bar{L}_m,\bar{A}_{m-1}\right)$ are identically zero, (iii) of Theorem 3.3 holds. However, if $v^{\bar{d},\bar{d}^*}\left(\bar{L}_m,\bar{A}_m\right)$ and $r^{\underline{d}_m,d^*_m}\left(\bar{L}_m,\bar{A}_{m-1}\right)$ are not identically zero, the semiparametric variance bound is smallest in model (a.1) and greatest in model (a.3). The bound in model (a.3) is equal to the asymptotic variance of $\widehat{\psi}\left(s_{eff}, \widetilde{c}^{s_{eff}}\right)$. However a simple explicit expression for s_{eff} is no longer available since even when

$$var\left(H_m\left(\psi^\dagger\right) - v^{\overline{d},\overline{d}^*}\left(\overline{L}_m, \overline{A}_m\right) | \overline{L}_m, \overline{A}_m\right)$$
$$= var\left(H_m\left(\psi^\dagger\right) - v^{\overline{d},\overline{d}^*}\left(\overline{L}_m, \overline{A}_m\right) | \overline{L}_m, \overline{A}_{m-1}\right)$$

does not depend on A_m for all m, it is no longer the case that, when $v^{\overline{d},\overline{d}^*}\left(\overline{L}_m, \overline{A}_m\right)$ is non-zero, $E\left[U_m^\dagger\left(s, \widetilde{c}\right) U_j^\dagger\left(s, \widetilde{c}\right) | \overline{L}_m, \overline{A}_m\right] = 0$ for $m \neq j$ where $U_m^\dagger\left(s, \widetilde{c}\right) = U_m\left(s\right) - \left\{\widetilde{C}_m^s - E\left[\widetilde{C}_m^s | \overline{A}_{m-1}, \overline{L}_m\right]\right\}$.

Next consider a model $\varsigma^T W_m$ for $E\left[H_m\left(\psi^\dagger\right) - v^{\overline{d},\overline{d}^*}\left(\overline{L}_m, \overline{A}_m\right) | \overline{L}_m, \overline{A}_{m-1}\right]$ where $W_m = w_m\left(\overline{A}_{m-1}, \overline{L}_m\right)$ is a known vector function of $\left(\overline{A}_{m-1}, \overline{L}_m\right)$ and ς is an unknown parameter. Define $\widehat{\psi}\left(s, \widetilde{c}^s; \widehat{\alpha}, \widehat{\varsigma}\right)$ to be a solution to $P_n\left[U^\dagger\left(\psi^\dagger, s, \widetilde{c}^s; \widehat{\alpha}, \widehat{\varsigma}\right)\right] = 0$ where

$$U^\dagger\left(\psi^\dagger, s, \widetilde{c}^s; \widehat{\alpha}, \widehat{\varsigma}\right) = \sum_{m=0}^{K}\left\{H_m\left(\psi\right) - v^{\overline{d},\overline{d}^*}\left(\overline{L}_m, \overline{A}_m\right) - \widehat{\varsigma}^T\left(\psi\right) W_m\right\} \times$$
$$\left\{S_m\left(A_m\right) - E\left[S_m\left(A_m\right) | \overline{A}_{m-1}, \overline{L}_m\right]\right\}$$

and $\widehat{\varsigma}^T\left(\psi\right)$ solves the OLS estimating equation $P_n\left[\sum_{m=0}^{K}\left(\left\{H_m\left(\psi\right) - v^{\overline{d},\overline{d}^*}\left(\overline{L}_m, \overline{A}_m\right)\right\} - \varsigma^T W_m\right) W_m\right] = 0$. The following Corollary describes the so called "double-robustness" properties of $\widehat{\psi}\left(s, \widetilde{c}^s; \widehat{\alpha}, \widehat{\varsigma}\right)$ and $U^\dagger\left(\psi^\dagger, s, \widetilde{c}^s; \widehat{\alpha}, \widehat{\varsigma}\right)$.

Corollary 7.2b : Consider the $\overline{d}, \overline{d}^*$"union" model characterized by (a) $v^{\overline{d},\overline{d}^*}\left(\overline{L}_m, \overline{A}_m\right)$ and $r^{\underline{d}_m, \underline{d}_m^*}\left(\overline{L}_m, \overline{A}_{m-1}\right)$ known , (b) a correctly specified $\left(\overline{d}, \overline{d}^*\right)$-double-regime-specific SNMM $\gamma\left(\overline{l}_m, \overline{a}_m, \psi\right)$ and (c) that either (but not necessarily both) the parametric model $p_m\left[A_m | \overline{L}_m, \overline{A}_{m-1}; \alpha\right]$ for $p_m\left[A_m | \overline{L}_m, \overline{A}_{m-1}\right]$ is correct or the regression model $\varsigma^T W_m$ for $E\left[H_m\left(\psi^\dagger\right) - v^{\overline{d},\overline{d}^*}\left(\overline{L}_m, \overline{A}_m\right) | \overline{L}_m, \overline{A}_{m-1}\right]$ is correct. Then, under standard regularity conditions, the conclusions (i) and (ii) of Theorem 3.4 hold when we replace c by $\widetilde{c}$.

It follows that the algorithm following Theorem 3.4 can be used if we replace c by $\widetilde{c}$ and $H_m\left(\psi\right)$ by $H_m\left(\psi\right) - v^{\overline{d},\overline{d}^*}\left(\overline{L}_m, \overline{A}_m\right)$ as defined above. Of course the resulting estimator will only be locally efficient when $v^{\overline{d},\overline{d}^*}\left(\overline{L}_m, \overline{A}_m\right)$ is zero. Further we can also choose to replace $H_m\left(\psi\right)$ by $H_{\text{mod},m}\left(\psi\right)$.

Method 2:

In the special case that $\overline{d} = \overline{d}^*$ we, of course, do not need to vary $r^{\underline{d}_m, \underline{d}_m^*}\left(\overline{L}_m, \overline{A}_{m-1}\right)$ as it is 0 by definition. This raises the question if we might circumvent the need for $r^{d_m,d_m^*}\left(\overline{L}_m,\overline{A}_{m-1}\right)$ to identify $E\left[Y_{\overline{d}}\right]$ even when $\overline{d}\neq\overline{d}^*$. We shall now show this is possible if we define a modified version $\gamma_{\text{mod}}^{\overline{d},\overline{d}^*}\left(\overline{L}_m,\overline{A}_m\right)$ of $\gamma^{\overline{d},\overline{d}^*}\left(\overline{L}_m,\overline{A}_m\right)$, which equals $\gamma^{\overline{d},\overline{d}^*}\left(\overline{L}_m,\overline{A}_m\right)$ under sequential randomization or when $\overline{d}=\overline{d}^*$. In Section 7.2 we will see that, in the absence of sequential randomization, it is $\gamma_{\text{mod}}^{\overline{d}_{op},\overline{d}^*}\left(\overline{L}_m,\overline{A}_m\right)$, rather than $\gamma^{\overline{d}_{op}\overline{d}^*}\left(\overline{L}_m,\overline{A}_m\right)$, that is the essential function we shall need to estimate in order to find the optimal treatment regime d_{op}.

Define

$$\gamma_{\text{mod}}^{\overline{d},\overline{d}^*}\left(\overline{L}_m,\overline{A}_m\right) =$$

$$\gamma^{\overline{d},\overline{d}^*}\left(\overline{L}_m,\overline{A}_m\right) + E\left[Y_{\overline{A}_{m-1},d_m,\underline{d}_{m+1}} - Y_{\overline{A}_{m-1},d_m^*,\underline{d}_{m+1}}|\overline{L}_m,\overline{A}_{m-1},A_m\right] -$$

$$E\left[Y_{\overline{A}_{m-1},d_m,\underline{d}_{m+1}} - Y_{\overline{A}_{m-1},d_m^*,\underline{d}_{m+1}}|\overline{L}_m,\overline{A}_{m-1},A_m = d_m^*\left(\overline{L}_m,\overline{A}_{m-1}\right)\right]$$

$$= E\left[Y_{\overline{A}_m,\underline{d}_{m+1}}|\overline{L}_m,\overline{A}_m\right] -$$

$$E\left[Y_{\overline{A}_{m-1},d_m^*,\underline{d}_{m+1}}|\overline{L}_m,\overline{A}_{m-1},A_m = d_m^*\left(\overline{L}_m,\overline{A}_{m-1}\right)\right] -$$

$$m^{\overline{d},\overline{d}^*}\left(\overline{L}_m,\overline{A}_m\right),$$

where $m^{\overline{d},\overline{d}^*}\left(\overline{L}_m,\overline{A}_m\right) = E\left[Y_{\overline{A}_{m-1},\underline{d}_m}|\overline{L}_m,\overline{A}_m\right] -$

$$E\left[Y_{\overline{A}_{m-1},\underline{d}_m}|\overline{L}_m,\overline{A}_{m-1},A_m = d_m^*\left(\overline{L}_m,\overline{A}_{m-1}\right)\right].$$

Under sequential randomization the function $m^{\overline{d},\overline{d}^*}\left(\overline{L}_m,\overline{A}_m\right)$ takes the value zero. Hence $m^{\overline{d},\overline{d}^*}\left(\overline{L}_m,\overline{A}_m\right)$, like $v^{\overline{d},\overline{d}^*}\left(\overline{L}_m,\overline{A}_m\right)$, is a measure of the magnitude of confounding due to unmeasured factors among subjects with history $\left(\overline{L}_m,\overline{A}_{m-1}\right)$, as it compares the mean of the same counterfactual in those who received treatment A_m to that in those who received treatment $d_m^*\left(\overline{L}_m,\overline{A}_{m-1}\right)$ at t_m. In one case the counterfactual being compared is $Y_{\overline{A}_{m-1},d_m^*,\underline{d}_{m+1}}$ and in the other $Y_{\overline{A}_{m-1},\underline{d}_m}$. We have the following.

Theorem 7.3: Let $H_m^{\underline{d}_m}\left(\gamma^{\overline{d}^**}\right)$ again be defined as in equation (3.5). Then Theorem 7.1 and 7.2 hold when we replace $\gamma^{\overline{d},\overline{d}^*}\left(\overline{L}_m,\overline{A}_m\right)$ by $\gamma_{\text{mod}}^{\overline{d},\overline{d}^*}\left(\overline{L}_m,\overline{A}_m\right)$ and $v^{\overline{d},\overline{d}^*}\left(\overline{L}_m,\overline{A}_m\right)$ by $m^{\overline{d},\overline{d}^*}\left(\overline{L}_m,\overline{A}_m\right)$.

Proof: We only prove $\Leftarrow$ since the proof of $\Rightarrow$ mimics the proof of $\Rightarrow$ in Theorems 7.1 and 7.2 given in the Appendix.

¿From the definition of $\gamma_{\text{mod}}^{\overline{d},\overline{d}^*}\left(\overline{L}_m,\overline{A}_m\right)$, we have

$$\gamma_{\text{mod}}^{\overline{d},\overline{d}^*}\left(\overline{L}_m,\overline{A}_{m-1},d_m^*\left(\overline{L}_m,\overline{A}_{m-1}\right)\right) - \gamma_{\text{mod}}^{\overline{d},\overline{d}^*}\left(\overline{L}_m,\overline{A}_m\right)$$

$$= E\left[Y_{\overline{A}_{m-1},\underline{d}_m}|\overline{L}_m,\overline{A}_m\right] - E\left[Y_{\overline{A}_m,\underline{d}_{m+1}}|\overline{L}_m,\overline{A}_m\right].$$

We proceed by induction in reverse time order.

Case 1:
$$m = K : H_K\left(\gamma_{\text{mod}}^{\overline{d},\overline{d}^*}\right) = Y_{\overline{A}_K} - E\left[Y_{\overline{A}_K}|\overline{L}_K,\overline{A}_K\right] + E\left[Y_{\overline{A}_{K-1,\underline{d}_K}}|\overline{L}_K,\overline{A}_K\right],$$
so $E\left[H_K\left(\gamma_{\text{mod}}^{\overline{d},\overline{d}^*}\right)|\overline{L}_K,\overline{A}_K\right] = E\left[Y_{\overline{A}_{K-1,\underline{d}_K}}|\overline{L}_K,\overline{A}_K\right].$

Case 2: $m < K$: Assume $E\left[H_{m+1}\left(\gamma_{\text{mod}}^{\overline{d},\overline{d}^*}\right)|\overline{L}_{m+1},\overline{A}_{m+1}\right]$
$$= E\left[Y_{\overline{A}_{m,\underline{d}_{m+1}}}|\overline{L}_{m+1},\overline{A}_{m+1}\right]. \text{ By definition } H_m\left(\gamma_{\text{mod}}^{\overline{d},\overline{d}^*}\right) = H_{m+1}\left(\gamma_{\text{mod}}^{\overline{d},\overline{d}^*}\right) +$$
$$\gamma_{\text{mod}}^{\overline{d},\overline{d}^*}\left(\overline{L}_m,\overline{A}_{m-1},d_m^*\left(\overline{L}_m,\overline{A}_{m-1}\right)\right) - \gamma_{\text{mod}}^{\overline{d},\overline{d}^*}\left(\overline{L}_m,\overline{A}_m\right)$$
$$= \left\{H_{m+1}\left(\gamma_{\text{mod}}^{\overline{d},\overline{d}^*}\right) - E\left[Y_{\overline{A}_{m,\underline{d}_{m+1}}}|\overline{L}_m,\overline{A}_m\right]\right\} + E\left[Y_{\overline{A}_{m-1,\underline{d}_m}}|\overline{L}_m,\overline{A}_m\right].$$
So

$$E\left[H_m\left(\gamma_{\text{mod}}^{\overline{d},\overline{d}^*}\right)|\overline{L}_m,\overline{A}_m\right]$$
$$= E\left\{E\left[Y_{\overline{A}_{m,\underline{d}_{m+1}}}|\overline{L}_{m+1},\overline{A}_{m+1}\right]|\overline{L}_m,\overline{A}_m\right\} -$$
$$E\left[Y_{\overline{A}_{m,\underline{d}_{m+1}}}|\overline{L}_m,\overline{A}_m\right] + E\left[Y_{\overline{A}_{m-1,\underline{d}_m}}|\overline{L}_m,\overline{A}_m\right]$$
$$= E\left[Y_{\overline{A}_{m-1,\underline{d}_m}}|\overline{L}_m,\overline{A}_m\right],$$

proving the analogue of Theorem 7.1.
Thus

$$E\left[H_m\left(\gamma_{\text{mod}}^{\overline{d},\overline{d}^*}\right)|\overline{L}_m,\overline{A}_m\right] - m^{\overline{d},\overline{d}^*}\left(\overline{L}_m,\overline{A}_m\right)$$
$$= E\left[Y_{\overline{A}_{m-1,\underline{d}_m}}|\overline{L}_m,\overline{A}_m\right] - m^{\overline{d},\overline{d}^*}\left(\overline{L}_m,\overline{A}_m\right)$$
$$= E\left[Y_{\overline{A}_{m-1,\underline{d}_m}}|\overline{L}_m,\overline{A}_{m-1},A_m = d_m^*\left(\overline{L}_m,\overline{A}_{m-1}\right)\right]$$

which is not a function of A_m, proving the analogue of Theorem 7.2.
Corollary 7.3: Given $m^{\overline{d},\overline{d}^*}\left(\overline{L}_m,\overline{A}_m\right)$, both $\gamma_{\text{mod}}^{\overline{d},\overline{d}^*}\left(\overline{L}_m,\overline{A}_m\right)$ and $E\left[Y_{\overline{d}}\right]$ are identified.
Note knowledge of $r^{\underline{d}_m,d_m^*}\left(\overline{L}_m,\overline{A}_{m-1}\right)$ is no longer required for identification as, in contrast with Theorems 7.1 and 7.2, $H_m^{\underline{d}_m}\left(\gamma^{\overline{d}^*}*\right)$ in Theorem 7.3 is not a function of $r^{\underline{d}_m,d_m^*}\left(\overline{L}_m,\overline{A}_{m-1}\right)$.

Inference under Method 2:

Under method 2, we can use a drSNMM model $\gamma^{\overline{d}^*}\left(\overline{l}_m,\overline{a}_m;\psi\right)$ to model and estimate $\gamma_{\text{mod}}^{\overline{d},\overline{d}^*}\left(\overline{L}_m,\overline{A}_m\right)$ and $E\left[Y^{\overline{d}}\right]$ since $\gamma_{\text{mod}}^{\overline{d},\overline{d}^*}\left(\overline{L}_m,\overline{A}_m\right)$, like $\gamma^{\overline{d},\overline{d}^*}\left(\overline{L}_m,\overline{A}_m\right)$, is only restricted by the definitional constraint $\gamma_{\text{mod}}^{\overline{d},\overline{d}^*}\left(\overline{L}_m,\overline{A}_{m-1},d_m^*\left(\overline{L}_m,\overline{A}_{m-1}\right)\right)$ $= 0$. Specifically it follows from Theorem 4.3 in Robins and Rotnitzky (2003) that Corollary 7.2a and 7.2b continue to hold when we replace $v^{\overline{d},\overline{d}^*}\left(\overline{L}_m,\overline{A}_m\right)$ by $m^{\overline{d},\overline{d}^*}\left(\overline{L}_m,\overline{A}_m\right)$, references to $r^{\underline{d}_m,d_m^*}\left(\overline{L}_m,\overline{A}_{m-1}\right)$ are deleted, $H_m^{\underline{d}_m}\left(\gamma^{\overline{d}^*}*\right)$

is again defined as in equation (3.5), and $\gamma^{\bar{d}^*}\left(\bar{l}_m, \bar{a}_m; \psi\right)$ is interpreted as a model for $\gamma^{\bar{d}, \bar{d}^*}_{\text{mod}}\left(\bar{l}_m, \bar{a}_m\right)$.

Instrumental Variable Estimation under Method 2:

Suppose $A_m = (A_{pm}, A_{dm})$ where A_{pm} is the prescribed dose of a medicine and A_{dm} is the actual consumed dose. Since we often have good measures of why doctors prescribe a given dose but poor measures of why patients comply, it would often be reasonable to assume Eq (2.5) was false but the *partial sequential randomization* assumption

$$\{\bar{L}_{\bar{a}}; \bar{a} \in \bar{\mathcal{A}}\} \coprod A_{Pk} \mid \bar{L}_k, \bar{A}_{k-1} \text{ w.p.1, for } k = 0, 1, \ldots, K \qquad (7.3)$$

was true. Under this assumption we can estimate $\gamma^{\bar{d}, \bar{d}^*}_{\text{mod}}\left(\bar{l}_m, \bar{a}_m\right)$ and, by Theorem 7.3, $E\left[Y_{\bar{d}}\right]$ as well using Theorems 3.3 and 3.4 plus the algorithm following 3.4. Specifically given a correctly specified drSNMM model $\gamma^{\bar{d}^*}\left(\bar{l}_m, \bar{a}_m; \psi\right)$ for $\gamma^{\bar{d}, \bar{d}^*}_{\text{mod}}\left(\bar{l}_m, \bar{a}_m\right)$, it follows from Theorem 7.3 that $H_m\left(\gamma^{\bar{d}, \bar{d}^*}_{\text{mod}}\right) \equiv H^{\bar{d}, \bar{d}^*}_m\left(\psi^\dagger\right)$ satisfies $E\left[H^{\bar{d}, \bar{d}^*}_m\left(\psi^\dagger\right) | \bar{L}_m, \bar{A}_m\right] = E\left[Y_{\bar{A}_{m-1}, \underline{d}_m} | \bar{L}_m, \bar{A}_m\right]$. Hence $E\left[H^{\bar{d}, \bar{d}^*}_m\left(\psi^\dagger\right) | \bar{L}_m, \bar{A}_{m-1}, A_{Pm}\right]$ does not depend on A_{Pm} under partial sequential randomization. Thus, when $\psi^\dagger$ is identified, we can estimate the parameter $\psi^\dagger$ of our model for $\gamma^{\bar{d}, \bar{d}^*}_{\text{mod}}\left(\bar{l}_m, \bar{a}_m\right)$ using Theorems 3.3 and 3.4 plus the algorithm following 3.4, provided we use functions $S_m\left(A_{Pm}\right) \equiv s_m\left(A_{Pm}, \bar{A}_{m-1}, \bar{L}_m\right)$ that only depend on A_m only through A_{pm} and our models for treatment indexed by parameter α are models for $p_m\left(A_{Pm} | \bar{A}_{m-1}, \bar{L}_m\right)$ rather than for $p_m\left(A_m | \bar{A}_{m-1}, \bar{L}_m\right)$. If the exclusion restriction that $\gamma^{\bar{d}, \bar{d}^*}_{\text{mod}}\left(\bar{l}_m, \bar{a}_m\right)$ is a function of a_m only through actual dose a_{dm} holds, we say the A_{pm} are "instrumental variables" for the A_{dm}.

Remark: Even though under assumption (7.3) the function $\gamma^{\bar{d}, \bar{d}^*}_{\text{mod}}\left(\bar{l}_m, \bar{a}_m\right)$ is not non-parametrically identified from the law of the observed data, nonetheless the parameter $\psi^\dagger$ of most models for $\gamma^{\bar{d}, \bar{d}^*}_{\text{mod}}\left(\bar{l}_m, \bar{a}_m\right)$ will be identified provided the dimension of $\psi^\dagger$ is not too great. Robins(1994) gives precise conditions for identification.

7.2 Optimal Regime SNMM

Recall that, by definition,

$$d_{op,K} = d_{op,K}\left(\bar{L}_K, \bar{A}_{K-1}\right) = \arg \max_{a_K \in \mathcal{A}_K} E\left[Y_{\bar{A}_{K-1}, a_K} | \bar{L}_K, \bar{A}_{K-1}\right]$$

and for $m = K - 1, \ldots 0$, $d_{op,m} = d_{op,m}\left(\bar{L}_m, \bar{A}_{m-1}\right) =$ $\arg \max_{a_m \in \mathcal{A}_m} E\left[Y_{\bar{A}_{m-1}, a_m, \underline{d}_{op,m+1}} | \bar{L}_m, \bar{A}_{m-1}\right]$ where

$\underline{d}_{op,m+1} = (d_{op,m+1}, ..., d_{op,K})$. In Theorem 7.6 and 7.7, we will show that $\bar{d}_{op}$ is identified if, for a pair of regimes $\bar{d}$ and $\bar{d}^*$, the nonidentifiable functions $m^{\bar{d},\bar{d}^*}(\overline{L}_m, \overline{A}_m)$ and

$g^{\bar{d}_{op},\bar{d}^*}(\overline{L}_m, \overline{A}_{m-1}, a_m) = g^{\underline{d}_{op,m}\cdot \underline{d}_m^*}(\overline{L}_m, \overline{A}_{m-1}, a_m)$ are known where $g^{\bar{d},\bar{d}^*}(\overline{L}_m, \overline{A}_{m-1}, a_m)$ is a generalization of $r^{\bar{d},\bar{d}^*}(\overline{L}_m, \overline{A}_{m-1}, a_m)$ of Eq. 7.1 that is identically 0 under sequential randomization. Specifically, we define $g^{\bar{d},\bar{d}^*}(\overline{L}_m, \overline{A}_{m-1}, a_m) =$

$$E\left[Y_{\overline{A}_{m-1}, a_m, \underline{d}_{m+1}} - Y_{\overline{A}_{m-1}, \underline{d}_m^*} | \overline{L}_m, \overline{A}_{m-1}, A_m = a_m\right] -$$

$$E\left[Y_{\overline{A}_{m-1}, a_m, \underline{d}_{m+1}} - Y_{\overline{A}_{m-1}, \underline{d}_m^*} | \overline{L}_m, \overline{A}_{m-1}, A_m \neq a_m\right]$$

$$= r^{\bar{d},\bar{d}^*}(\overline{L}_m, \overline{A}_{m-1}, a_m) +$$

$$E\left[Y_{\overline{A}_{m-1}, \underline{d}_m^*, \underline{d}_{m+1}} - Y_{\overline{A}_{m-1}, \underline{d}_m^*} | \overline{L}_m, \overline{A}_{m-1}, A_m = a_m\right] -$$

$$E\left[Y_{\overline{A}_{m-1}, \underline{d}_m^*, \underline{d}_{m+1}} - Y_{\overline{A}_{m-1}, \underline{d}_m^*} | \overline{L}_m, \overline{A}_{m-1}, A_m \neq a_m\right]$$

so that $g^{\bar{d},\bar{d}^*}(\overline{L}_m, \overline{A}_m - 1, a_m) = r^{\bar{d},\bar{d}^*}(\overline{L}_m, \overline{A}_m - 1, a_m)$ if $\bar{d} = \bar{d}^*$. Note that $g^{\bar{d},\bar{d}^*}(\overline{L}_m, \overline{A}_m - 1, a_m)$ is identically zero under the sharp null hypothesis of no effect of treatment. In this sense $g^{\bar{d},\bar{d}^*}(\overline{L}_m, \overline{A}_m - 1, a_m)$, like $r^{\bar{d},\bar{d}^*}(\overline{L}_m, \overline{A}_m - 1, a_m)$, is a measure of treatment interaction.

However, as discussed in remark 4.1, in the absence of sequential randomization, $\bar{d}_{op}$ may not be the optimal regime in the sense that $\bar{d}_{op}$ may not be the maximizer of $E\left[Y^{\bar{d}}\right]$ over $\bar{d} \in \overline{\mathcal{D}}$ and thus methods based on backward induction may not be available. We now characterize those settings in which $\bar{d}_{op}$ is the maximizer of $E\left[Y^{\bar{d}}\right]$

Definition: We say the backward induction feasibility assumption holds if for all m, all a_m, and any $\underline{d}_{m+1} \in \mathcal{D}_{m+1}$,

$$E\left[Y_{\overline{A}_{m-1}, a_m, \underline{d}_{op,m+1}} - Y_{\overline{A}_{m-1}, a_m, \underline{d}_{m+1}} | \overline{L}_m, \overline{A}_{m-1}, A_m = a_m\right] \times \quad (7.4)$$

$$E\left[Y_{\overline{A}_{m-1}, a_m, \underline{d}_{op,m+1}} - Y_{\overline{A}_{m-1}, a_m, \underline{d}_{m+1}} | \overline{L}_m, \overline{A}_{m-1}\right] \geq 0$$

so that the two factors never have opposite signs.

This nonidentifiable assumption implies that if $\underline{d}_{op,m+1}$ is the optimal regime among subjects with observed history $(\overline{L}_m, \overline{A}_{m-1}, A_m = a_m)$ then it is the optimal regime from time t_{m+1} onwards for subjects with observed history $(\overline{L}_m, \overline{A}_{m-1})$ when they are forced to take treatment a_m at t_m. In Appendix 3, we prove the following.

Theorem 7.4: The regime $\underline{d}_{op,m}$ maximizes

$E\left[Y_{\overline{A}_{m-1}, \underline{d}_m} | \overline{L}_m, \overline{A}_{m-1}\right]$ over all regimes $\underline{d}_m \in \mathcal{D}_m$ for each m and $\bar{d}_{op} =$

$\underline{d}_{op,0}$ maximizes $E\left[Y_{\overline{d}}\right]$ over all $\overline{d} \in \overline{\mathcal{D}}$ if and only if the backward induction feasibility assumption holds.

Note that under sequential randomization the backward induction feasibility assumption holds and so $\overline{d}_{op}$ is the optimal regime. Further knowledge of $m^{\overline{d},\overline{d}^{*}}\left(\overline{L}_m, \overline{A}_m\right)$, $r^{\underline{d}_{op,m+1},d_m^*}\left(\overline{L}_m, \overline{A}_{m-1}, a_m\right)$ and the law of O do not determine whether the backward induction feasibility assumption holds. We will not consider the problem of estimating the true optimal regime when this assumption does not hold and thus $\overline{d}_{op}$ is not the optimal regime, because the computational problem of estimating the true optimal regime is then intractable without strong additional assumptions.

When sequential randomization does not hold, additional problematic issues arise even in the case of single stage decisions (i.e. the special case of $K = 0$). Specifically $E\left[Y_{d_{op}}|L_0\right]$ may be less than $E\left[Y|L_0\right]$ and thus $E\left[Y_{d_{op}}\right]$ may be less than $E\left[Y\right]$. This possibility reflects the fact that by definition any deterministic regime assigns the same treatment to all subjects with a given value of L_0. Thus it might be preferable to allow each subject to choose their own treatment than to impose the optimal treatment $d_{op}\left(L_0\right)$. For example, this will be the true when randomization does not hold because for a subgroup with a common L_0, the best treatment varies among individuals, and each individual is aware of some unmeasured factor that allows her to self-select the best treatment. Under the non-identifiable assumption of additive local rank preservation, the backward feasibility assumption always holds and $E\left[Y_{d_{op}}|L_0\right]$ can never be less than $E\left[Y|L_0\right]$.

Optimal w-compatible treatment regimes: We will actually prove identifiability of $\overline{d}_{op}$ given $m^{\overline{d},\overline{d}^{*}}\left(\overline{L}_m, \overline{A}_m\right)$ and $g^{\overline{d}_{op},\overline{d}}\left(\overline{L}_m, \overline{A}_{m-1}, a_m\right)$ in a broader setting. Specifically we no longer assume that decision rule at t_m can necessarily depend on the entire past history $\left(\overline{L}_m, \overline{A}_{m-1}\right)$. Rather we assume there exists a known vector-valued function $W_m = w_m\left(\overline{L}_m, \overline{A}_{m-1}\right)$ representing the data available at time t_m on which a decision is to be based. This would be the case if either (i) rules that can based on all of the data $\left(\overline{L}_m, \overline{A}_{m-1}\right)$ are viewed as too complex or (ii) because in the future, after the study is finished, the subject-specific data available to the decision makers (i.e. physicians) at t_m months from, say, onset of HIV infection will only be a subset $w_m\left(\overline{L}_m, \overline{A}_{m-1}\right)$ of the data $\left(\overline{L}_m, \overline{A}_{m-1}\right)$ available to the investigators who analyzed the study data. Let w_m denote a realization of W_m.

Let $\overline{d}_{op}^{w} = \left(\overline{d}_{op,1}^{w}, ..., \overline{d}_{op,K}^{w}\right)$ be the regime defined recursively as follows.

$$\overline{d}_{op,K}^{w}\left(W_K\right) = \arg\max_{a_K} E\left[Y_{\overline{A}_{K-1},a_K}|W_K\right],$$

$$\overline{d}_{op,m}^{w}\left(W_m\right) = \arg\max_{a_m} E\left[Y_{\overline{A}_{m-1},a_m,\underline{d}_{op,m+1}}|W_m\right]$$

We say a regime $\overline{d} = \overline{d}^{w} \in \overline{\mathcal{D}}$ is $w - compatible$ if $d_m\left(\overline{L}_m, \overline{A}_{m-1}\right) = d_m\left(W_m\right)$ for each m and we let $\overline{\mathcal{D}}^{w}$ denote the set of $w - compatible$ regimes. We say the regime $\overline{d}_{op}^{w}$ is $w - optimal$ if $\underline{d}_{op,m}^{w}$ maximizes

$E\left[Y_{\overline{A}_{m-1},\underline{d}_m}|W_m\right]$ over all regimes $\underline{d}^w{}_m \in \underline{\mathcal{D}}^w{}_m$ for each m and $\overline{d}^w_{op} = \underline{d}^w_{op,0}$ maximizes $E\left[Y_{\overline{d}^w}\right]$ over all $\overline{d}^w \in \overline{\mathcal{D}}^w$. We say w is increasing if (W_m, A_m) is a function of W_{m+1} with probability one, i.e., there is no 'forgetting'. We recover our previous set-up when W_m is equal to $(\overline{L}_m, \overline{A}_{m-1})$ so no information has been lost. We then have:

Theorem 7.5: The regime $\overline{d}^w_{op}$ is $w - optimal$ if w is increasing and for all m, all a_m, and any $\underline{d}^w_{m+1} \in \underline{\mathcal{D}}^w_{m+1}$,

$$E\left[Y_{\overline{A}_{m-1},a_m,\underline{d}^w_{op,m+1}} - Y_{\overline{A}_{m-1},a_m,\underline{d}^w_{m+1}}|W_m, A_m = a_m\right] \geq 0 \qquad (7.5)$$

$$\Rightarrow E\left[Y_{\overline{A}_{m-1},a_m,\underline{d}^w_{op,m+1}} - Y_{\overline{A}_{m-1},a_m,\underline{d}^w_{m+1}}|W_m\right] \geq 0.$$

The proof of theorem 7.5 is analogous to that of 7.4. It is well known that, even under sequential randomization, backward induction cannot be used to compute the true $w - optimal$ regime unless w is increasing.

Now let $\overline{d}, \overline{d}^*$ be two other regimes, either or both of which may themselves equal $\overline{d}^w_{op}$ or one another.

Theorem 7.6 : Given the non-identifiable functions $g^{\overline{d}^w_{op},\overline{d}}\left(\overline{L}_m, \overline{A}_{m-1}, a_m\right)$ and $\gamma^{\overline{d},\overline{d}^*}_{\text{mod}}\left(\overline{L}_m, \overline{A}_m\right)$, the quantities

$$\overline{d}^w_{op}, E\left[Y_{\overline{A}_{m-1},a_m,\underline{d}^w_{op,m+1}}|\overline{L}_m, \overline{A}_{m-1}\right], E\left[Y_{\overline{A}_{m-1},a_m,\underline{d}^w_{op,m+1}}|W_m\right], E\left[Y_{\overline{d}^w_{op}}\right]$$

are identified from the law of $O = (\overline{L}, \overline{A})$.

Proof: Define

$$q\left(\overline{L}_m, \overline{A}_{m-1}, a_m\right) = E\left[Y_{\overline{A}_{m-1},a_m,\underline{d}^w_{op,m+1}} - Y_{\overline{A}_{m-1},\underline{d}_m}|\overline{L}_m, \overline{A}_{m-1}\right]$$

$$= E\left[Y_{\overline{A}_{m-1},a_m,\underline{d}^w_{op,m+1}} - Y_{\overline{A}_{m-1},\underline{d}_m}|\overline{L}_m, \overline{A}_{m-1}, A_m = a_m\right] -$$

$$\left\{1 - f\left(a_m|\overline{L}_m, \overline{A}_{m-1}\right)\right\} g^{\overline{d}^w_{op},\overline{d}}\left(\overline{L}_m, \overline{A}_{m-1}, a_m\right),$$

$$\text{and } j\left(\overline{L}_m, \overline{A}_{m-1}\right) = q\left(\overline{L}_m, \overline{A}_{m-1}, d^w_{op,m}\left(\overline{L}_m, \overline{A}_{m-1}\right)\right) \qquad (7.6)$$

$$= E\left[Y_{\overline{A}_{m-1},\underline{d}^w_{op,m}} - Y_{\overline{A}_{m-1},\underline{d}_m}|\overline{L}_m, \overline{A}_{m-1}\right].$$

Note , from their definitions, $E\left[Y|\overline{L}_K, \overline{A}_K\right] = E\left[Y_{\overline{A}_{K-1},A_K}|\overline{L}_K, \overline{A}_K\right]$ equals

$$\gamma^{\overline{d},\overline{d}^*}_{\text{mod}}\left(\overline{L}_K, \overline{A}_K\right) - \gamma^{\overline{d},\overline{d}^*}_{\text{mod}}\left(\overline{L}_K, \overline{A}_{K-1}, d_K\left(\overline{L}_K, \overline{A}_{K-1}\right)\right) + E\left[Y_{\overline{A}_{K-1},d_K}|\overline{L}_K, \overline{A}_K\right].$$

Hence $E\left[Y_{\overline{A}_{K-1},d_K}|\overline{L}_K, \overline{A}_K\right]$ is identified. Further

$$d^w_{op,K}\left(W_K\right) = \arg\max_{a_K} E\left[Y_{\overline{A}_{K-1},a_K} - Y_{\overline{A}_{K-1},d_K}|W_K\right]$$

$$= \arg\max_{a_K} E\left[q\left(\overline{L}_K, \overline{A}_{K-1}, a_K\right)|W_K\right]$$

But $q\left(\overline{L}_K, \overline{A}_{K-1}, a_K\right)$ is identified by

$$q\left(\overline{L}_K, \overline{A}_{K-1}, a_K\right) \tag{7.7}$$
$$= \gamma_{\mathrm{mod}}^{\overline{d},\overline{d}^*}\left(\overline{L}_K, \overline{A}_{K-1}, a_K\right) - \gamma_{\mathrm{mod}}^{\overline{d},\overline{d}^*}\left(\overline{L}_K, \overline{A}_{K-1}, d_K\left(\overline{L}_K, \overline{A}_{K-1}\right)\right) -$$
$$\left\{1 - f\left(a_K | \overline{L}_K, \overline{A}_{K-1}\right)\right\} g^{\overline{d}_{op}^w, \overline{d}}\left(\overline{L}_K, \overline{A}_{K-1}, a_K\right).$$

Thus $d_{op,K}^w\left(W_K\right)$, $j\left(\overline{L}_K, \overline{A}_{K-1}\right)$, and
$E\left[Y_{\overline{A}_{K-1}, d_{op,K}^w} | \overline{L}_K, \overline{A}_{K-1}\right] = E\left[Y_{\overline{A}_{K-1}, d_K} | \overline{L}_K, \overline{A}_K\right] + j\left(\overline{L}_K, \overline{A}_{K-1}\right)$ are identified.

We now proceed by reverse induction. Specifically we show that if $j\left(\overline{L}_{m+1}, \overline{A}_m\right)$ is identified then $E\left[Y_{\overline{A}_{m-1}, a_m, \underline{d}_{op,m+1}^w} - Y_{\overline{A}_{m-1}, \underline{d}_m} | \overline{L}_m, \overline{A}_{m-1}, A_m = a_m\right]$ is identified and hence $q\left(\overline{L}_m, \overline{A}_{m-1}, a_m\right)$,

$$d_{op,m}^w\left(W_m\right) = \arg\max_{a_m} E\left[q\left(\overline{L}_m, \overline{A}_{m-1}, a_m\right) | W_m\right] \tag{7.8}$$

and $j\left(\overline{L}_m, \overline{A}_{m-1}\right) = q\left(\overline{L}_m, \overline{A}_{m-1}, d_{op,m}^w\left(\overline{L}_m, \overline{A}_{m-1}\right)\right)$ are identified. Write

$$E\left[Y_{\overline{A}_{m-1}, a_m, \underline{d}_{op,m+1}^w} - Y_{\overline{A}_{m-1}, \underline{d}_m} | \overline{L}_m, \overline{A}_{m-1}, A_m = a_m\right]$$
$$= E\left[Y_{\overline{A}_{m-1}, a_m, \underline{d}_{op,m+1}^w} - Y_{\overline{A}_{m-1}, a_m, \underline{d}_{m+1}} | \overline{L}_m, \overline{A}_{m-1}, A_m = a_m\right] +$$
$$E\left[Y_{\overline{A}_{m-1}, a_m, \underline{d}_{m+1}} - Y_{\overline{A}_{m-1}, \underline{d}_m} | \overline{L}_m, \overline{A}_{m-1}, A_m = a_m\right]$$
$$= E\left\{\frac{E\left[Y_{\overline{A}_{m-1}, a_m, \underline{d}_{op,m+1}^w} - Y_{\overline{A}_{m-1}, a_m, \underline{d}_{m+1}} | \overline{L}_{m+1}, \overline{A}_{m-1}, A_m = a_m\right] |}{\overline{L}_m, \overline{A}_{m-1}, A_m = a_m}\right\} +$$
$$\gamma_{\mathrm{mod}}^{\overline{d},\overline{d}^*}\left(\overline{L}_m, \overline{A}_{m-1}, a_m\right) - \gamma_{\mathrm{mod}}^{\overline{d},\overline{d}^*}\left(\overline{L}_m, \overline{A}_{m-1}, d_m\left(\overline{L}_m, \overline{A}_{m-1}\right)\right)$$
$$= E\left\{j\left(\overline{L}_{m+1}, \overline{A}_{m-1}, a_m\right) | \overline{L}_m, \overline{A}_{m-1}, A_m = a_m\right\} +$$
$$\gamma_{\mathrm{mod}}^{\overline{d},\overline{d}^*}\left(\overline{L}_m, \overline{A}_{m-1}, a_m\right) - \gamma_{\mathrm{mod}}^{\overline{d},\overline{d}^*}\left(\overline{L}_m, \overline{A}_{m-1}, d_m\left(\overline{L}_m, \overline{A}_{m-1}\right)\right)$$

Thus, in particular, by (7.6),

$$q\left(\overline{L}_m, \overline{A}_{m-1}, a_m\right) = E\left\{j\left(\overline{L}_{m+1}, \overline{A}_{m-1}, a_m\right) | \overline{L}_m, \overline{A}_{m-1}, A_m = a_m\right\} +$$
$$\gamma_{\mathrm{mod}}^{\overline{d},\overline{d}^*}\left(\overline{L}_m, \overline{A}_{m-1}, a_m\right) - \gamma_{\mathrm{mod}}^{\overline{d},\overline{d}^*}\left(\overline{L}_m, \overline{A}_{m-1}, d_m\left(\overline{L}_m, \overline{A}_{m-1}\right)\right) - \tag{7.9a}$$
$$\left\{1 - f\left(a_m | \overline{L}_m, \overline{A}_{m-1}\right)\right\} g^{\overline{d}_{op}^w, \overline{d}}\left(\overline{L}_m, \overline{A}_{m-1}, a_m\right) =$$
$$E\left[q\left(\overline{L}_{m+1}, \left(\overline{A}_{m-1}, a_m\right), d_{op,m+1}^w\left(\overline{L}_{m+1}, \left\{\overline{A}_{m-1}, a_m\right\}\right)\right) | \overline{L}_m, \overline{A}_{m-1}, A_m = a_m\right] +$$
$$\gamma_{\mathrm{mod}}^{\overline{d},\overline{d}^*}\left(\overline{L}_m, \overline{A}_{m-1}, a_m\right) - \gamma_{\mathrm{mod}}^{\overline{d},\overline{d}^*}\left(\overline{L}_m, \overline{A}_{m-1}, d_m\left(\overline{L}_m, \overline{A}_{m-1}\right)\right) - \tag{7.9b}$$
$$\left\{1 - f\left(a_m | \overline{L}_m, \overline{A}_{m-1}\right)\right\} g^{\overline{d}_{op}^w, \overline{d}}\left(\overline{L}_m, \overline{A}_{m-1}, a_m\right)$$

Finally since identification of $q\left(\overline{L}_m, \overline{A}_{m-1}, a_m\right)$ and $E\left[Y_{\overline{A}_{m-1}, \underline{d}_m} | \overline{L}_m, \overline{A}_{m-1}\right]$ implies identification of $E\left[Y_{\overline{A}_{m-1}, a_m, \underline{d}_{op,m+1}^w} | \overline{L}_m, \overline{A}_m\right]$, to complete the proof it suffices to prove that if $E\left[Y_{\overline{A}_m,\underline{d}_{m+1}}|\overline{L}_{m+1},\overline{A}_{m+1}\right]$ is identified, then $E\left[Y_{\overline{A}_{m-1},\underline{d}_m}|\overline{L}_m,\overline{A}_m\right]$ is identified. This implication follows from the fact that, by definition,

$$E\left[Y_{\overline{A}_{m-1},\underline{d}_m}|\overline{L}_m,\overline{A}_m\right]$$
$$= E\left[Y_{\overline{A}_m,\underline{d}_{m+1}}|\overline{L}_m,\overline{A}_m\right] - \gamma_{\text{mod}}^{\overline{d},\overline{d}^*}\left(\overline{L}_{m+1},\overline{A}_{m+1}\right) +$$
$$\gamma_{\text{mod}}^{\overline{d},\overline{d}^*}\left(\overline{L}_{m+1},\overline{A}_m, d_{m+1}\left(\overline{L}_{m+1},\overline{A}_m\right)\right).$$

The following corollary is an immediate consequence of corollary 7.3.

Corollary 7.6 : Given the non-identifiable functions $g^{\overline{d}_{op}^w,\overline{d}}\left(\overline{L}_m,\overline{A}_{m-1},a_m\right)$ and $m^{\overline{d},\overline{d}^*}\left(\overline{L}_m,\overline{A}_m\right)$, we have that $\gamma_{\text{mod}}^{\overline{d},\overline{d}^*}\left(\overline{L}_m,\overline{A}_m\right)$ is identified and thus the conclusions of Theorem 7.6 hold.

Using Theorem 7.6 and Corollary 7.6 to Estimate $\overline{d}_{op}^w$ in Various Settings:

Our basic approach will be to estimate the unknown quantities in Eq (7.7) and then for $m = K, ..., 0$, to alternate estimating the unknown quantities in Eqs (7.8) and Eq (7.9a) (or equivalently Eq (7.9b)). Here are some specific examples.

(1):To generalize estimation of optimal drSNMMs to the setting where we do not assume sequential randomization but $W_m = \left(\overline{L}_m,\overline{A}_{m-1}\right)$ so there is no information loss, we would typically choose (i) $\overline{d} = \overline{d}_{op}$ which implies that a) from its definition, $g^{\overline{d}_{op}^w,\overline{d}_{op}^w}\left(\overline{L}_m,\overline{A}_{m-1},a_m\right)$ equals $r^{\overline{d}_{op}^w,\overline{d}_{op}^w}\left(\overline{L}_m,\overline{A}_{m-1},a_m\right)$), b) by Eq. (7.6), for all m, $j\left(\overline{L}_{m+1},\overline{A}_{m-1},a_m\right) \equiv 0$, and c), by Eq. (7.9a),

$$q\left(\overline{L}_m,\overline{A}_{m-1},a_m\right) = \gamma_{\text{mod}}^{\overline{d},\overline{d}^*}\left(\overline{L}_m,\overline{A}_{m-1},a_m\right) - \gamma_{\text{mod}}^{\overline{d},\overline{d}^*}\left(\overline{L}_m,\overline{A}_{m-1},d_m\left(\overline{L}_m,\overline{A}_{m-1}\right)\right)$$
$$- \left\{1 - f\left(a_m|\overline{L}_m,\overline{A}_{m-1}\right)\right\} r^{\overline{d}_{op}^w,\overline{d}}\left(\overline{L}_m,\overline{A}_{m-1},a_m\right), \quad (7.10)$$

and (ii) choose $\overline{d}^*$ to be the regime that is identically zero. Thus to estimate the optimal treatment regime $\overline{d}_{op}^w$, we treat $g^{\overline{d}_{op}^w,\overline{d}}\left(\overline{L}_m,\overline{A}_{m-1},a_m\right)$ as known (but vary it in a sensitivity analysis), specify and fit a model for $f\left(a_m|\overline{L}_m,\overline{A}_{m-1}\right)$, and finally carry out doubly robust estimation, as described in the last subsection, of a drSNMM model $\gamma^{\overline{d}^*}\left(\overline{l}_m,\overline{a}_m;\psi\right)$ for $\gamma_{\text{mod}}^{\overline{d},\overline{d}^*}\left(\overline{L}_m,\overline{A}_m\right)$ either by assuming $m^{\overline{d},\overline{d}^*}\left(\overline{L}_m,\overline{A}_m\right)$ is a known function (to be varied in a sensitivity analysis) or, if $\overline{A}_m$ has two components $\left(\overline{A}_{pm},\overline{A}_{dm}\right)$, possibly, by assuming partial sequential randomization. Note that although based on Theorem 3.4 and its extensions discussed in the last subsection we can obtain doubly robust estimators of $\psi^\dagger$ and thus of $\gamma_{\text{mod}}^{\overline{d},\overline{d}^*}\left(\overline{L}_m,\overline{A}_m\right)$, we cannot obtain doubly robust estimators of $\overline{d}_{op}^w$ when $g^{\overline{d}_{op}^w,\overline{d}}\left(\overline{L}_m,\overline{A}_{m-1},a_m\right)$ is not assumed to be identically zero, since consistent estimation of $f\left(a_m | \overline{L}_m, \overline{A}_{m-1}\right)$ is then required.

Remark : Because $j\left(\overline{L}_{m+1}, \overline{A}_{m-1}, a_m\right) \equiv 0$ when $\overline{d} = \overline{d}_{op}$, we did not have to specify and fit $DP-like$ regression models for $E\left\{j\left(\overline{L}_{m+1}, \overline{A}_m\right) | \overline{L}_m, \overline{A}_m\right\}$ in Eq (7.9a).

(2): To generalize estimation of DP-regression srSNMMs with the single regime being the identically zero treatment regime to the setting where we do not assume sequential randomization but assume $W_m = \left(\overline{L}_m, \overline{A}_{m-1}\right)$, we would typically choose $\overline{d}^* = \overline{d}$ to be the zero regime $\overline{0}$ and proceed as in (1) just above except now we would have to fit $DP-$ regression models for $E\left\{j\left(\overline{L}_{m+1}, \overline{A}_m\right) | \overline{L}_m, \overline{A}_m\right\}$ in Eq (7.9a). Inference can proceed as described under the DP- srSNMM fitting algorithm of Section 6 except as modified below under (3).

Remark: The only simplifications due to choosing $\overline{d}^* = \overline{d}$ are that $\gamma_{\mathrm{mod}}^{\overline{d},\overline{d}^*}\left(\overline{L}_m, \overline{A}_{m-1}, d_m\left(\overline{L}_m, \overline{A}_{m-1}\right)\right) = 0$ in Eq (7.9a) and that $\gamma_{\mathrm{mod}}^{\overline{d},\overline{d}^*}\left(\overline{L}_m, \overline{A}_m\right) = \gamma^{\overline{d},\overline{d}^*}\left(\overline{L}_m, \overline{A}_m\right)$

(3):For estimation of DP-regression drSNMMs with $W_m = \left(\overline{L}_m, \overline{A}_{m-1}\right)$ we proceed as under (2), except now $\gamma_{\mathrm{mod}}^{\overline{d},\overline{d}^*}\left(\overline{L}_m, \overline{A}_{m-1}, d_m\left(\overline{L}_m, \overline{A}_{m-1}\right)\right) \neq 0$ and we make the appropriate substitutions of regimes $\overline{d}, \overline{d}^*$ for the regimes $\overline{0}, \overline{0}$ in the DP- srSNMM fitting algorithm of Section 6. Specifically now

$$Q_K\left(\widehat{\psi}, a_K\right) = \tag{7.11}$$

$$\gamma_{\mathrm{mod}}^{\overline{d},\overline{d}^*}\left(\overline{L}_K, \overline{A}_{K-1}, a_K, \widehat{\psi}\right) - \gamma_{\mathrm{mod}}^{\overline{d},\overline{d}^*}\left(\overline{L}_K, \overline{A}'_{K-1}, d_K\left(\overline{L}_K, \overline{A}_{K-1}\right), \widehat{\psi}\right) -$$
$$\left\{1 - f\left(a_K | \overline{L}_K, \overline{A}_{K-1}, \widehat{\alpha}\right)\right\} g^{\overline{d}_{op}^w, \overline{d}}\left(\overline{L}_K, \overline{A}_{K-1}, a_K\right),$$

$$Q_{m-1}\left(\widehat{\psi}, a_{m-1}, \widehat{\beta}_m\right) = \tag{7.12}$$

$$r\left\{\overline{L}_{m-1}, \overline{A}_{m-2}, a_{m-1}; \widehat{\beta}_m, \widehat{\psi}, \widehat{\beta}_{m+1}\right\} + \gamma_{\mathrm{mod}}^{\overline{d},\overline{d}^*}\left(\overline{L}_{m-1}, \overline{A}_{m-2}, a_{m-1}; \widehat{\psi}\right) -$$
$$\gamma_{\mathrm{mod}}^{\overline{d},\overline{d}^*}\left(\overline{L}_{m-1}, \overline{A}_{m-2}, d_m\left(\overline{L}_{m-1}, \overline{A}_{m-2}\right); \widehat{\psi}\right) -$$
$$\left\{1 - f\left(a_{m-1} | \overline{L}_{m-1}, \overline{A}_{m-2}\right)\right\} g^{\overline{d}_{op}^w, \overline{d}}\left(\overline{L}_{m-1}, \overline{A}_{m-2}, a_{m-1}\right)$$

(4): Consider again Murphy's regret model $u_m\left(\overline{l}_m, \overline{a}_m, \beta^\dagger\right)$

$$= E\left[Y_{\overline{a}_{m-1}, \underline{d}_{op,m}} - Y_{\overline{a}_m, \underline{d}_{op,m+1}} | \overline{L}_{\overline{a}_{m-1,m}} = \overline{l}_m\right] \text{ where}$$

$u_m\left(\overline{l}_m, \overline{a}_m, \beta\right) = \eta_m\left(\overline{l}_m, \overline{a}_{m-1}, \beta_{scale}\right) f\left(a_m - d_{op,m}\left(\overline{l}_m, \overline{a}_{m-1}, \beta_{regime}\right)\right)$, $\beta = \left(\beta_{scale}, \beta_{regime}\right)$ is a finite dimensional parameter vector, $f\left(\cdot\right)$ is a known non-negative function satisfying $f\left(0\right) = 0$, and $\eta_m\left(\overline{l}_m, \overline{a}_{m-1}, \beta_{scale}\right)$ is a known non-negative scale function. Suppose $W_m = \left(\overline{L}_m, \overline{A}_{m-1}\right)$ so there is no information loss. Murphy only considered her regret model in the case of sequential randomization. Since under sequential randomization

$$E\left[Y_{\overline{a}_{m-1},\underline{d}_{op,m}} - Y_{\overline{a}_m,\underline{d}_{op,m+1}}|\overline{L}_{\overline{a}_{m-1},m} = \overline{l}_m\right] \tag{7.13}$$

$$= E\left[Y_{\overline{a}_{m-1},\underline{d}_{op,m}} - Y_{\overline{a}_m,\underline{d}_{op,m+1}}|\overline{L}_m = \overline{l}_m, \overline{A}_{m-1} = \overline{a}_{m-1}\right]$$

$$= E\left[Y_{\overline{a}_{m-1},\underline{d}_{op,m}} - Y_{\overline{a}_m,\underline{d}_{op,m+1}}|\overline{L}_m = \overline{l}_m, \overline{A}_{m-1} = \overline{a}_{m-1}, A_m = a_m\right],$$

Murphy's regret model is also a model for

$$E\left[Y_{\overline{a}_{m-1},\underline{d}_{op,m}} - Y_{\overline{a}_m,\underline{d}_{op,m+1}}|\overline{L}_m = \overline{l}_m, \overline{A}_{m-1} = \overline{a}_{m-1}\right] \text{ and for}$$

$$E\left[Y_{\overline{a}_{m-1},\underline{d}_{op,m}} - Y_{\overline{a}_m,\underline{d}_{op,m+1}}|\overline{L}_m = \overline{l}_m, \overline{A}_{m-1} = \overline{a}_{m-1}, A_m = a_m\right]. \text{ In the ab-}$$
sence of sequential randomization, none of the equalities in Eq.(7.13) necessarily hold and we must choose which quantity $u_m\left(\overline{l}_m, \overline{a}_m, \beta\right)$ to model.

We now argue that the appropriate generalization of Murphy's regret model to the setting without sequential randomization is as a model $u_m\left(\overline{l}_m, \overline{a}_m, \beta\right)$ for $E\left[Y_{\overline{a}_{m-1},\underline{d}_{op,m}} - Y_{\overline{a}_m,\underline{d}_{op,m+1}}|\overline{L}_m = \overline{l}_m, \overline{A}_{m-1} = \overline{a}_{m-1}\right]$. The reason is that we would like to be able to determine the optimal treatment strategy beginning at t_m for a new subject who has data on $\overline{L}_m, \overline{A}_{m-1}$ available and who is exchangeable with the subjects in our study, but on whom we are unable to intervene with an optimal strategy prior to time t_m (say, because we did not have the ability to apply our optimal strategy prior to time t_m). It follows from Theorem 7.4 that given the the backward induction feasibility assumption holds, we can succeed in achieving this goal if we can successfully model the quantity $E\left[Y_{\overline{a}_{m-1},\underline{d}_{op,m}} - Y_{\overline{a}_m,\underline{d}_{op,m+1}}|\overline{L}_m = \overline{l}_m, \overline{A}_{m-1} = \overline{a}_{m-1}\right]$.

Consider then the model

$$u_m\left(\overline{l}_m, \overline{a}_m, \beta^\dagger\right) = E\left[Y_{\overline{a}_{m-1},\underline{d}_{op,m}} - Y_{\overline{a}_m,\underline{d}_{op,m+1}}|\overline{L}_m = \overline{l}_m, \overline{A}_{m-1} = \overline{a}_{m-1}\right].$$
$$\tag{7.14}$$
Recall $u_m\left(\overline{l}_m, \overline{a}_m, \beta\right)$ attains its minimum of 0 at $a_m = d_{op,m}\left(\overline{l}_m, \overline{a}_{m-1}, \beta_{regime}\right)$. Further, from our definitions, we have $\gamma_{mod}^{\overline{d}_{op}^w, \overline{d}_{op}^w}\left(\overline{L}_m, \overline{A}_m\right) = \gamma^{\overline{d}_{op}^w, \overline{d}_{op}^w}\left(\overline{L}_m, \overline{A}_m\right)$ is given by

$$\gamma^{\overline{d}_{op}^w, \overline{d}_{op}^w}\left(\overline{L}_m, \overline{A}_m\right)$$

$$= -u_m\left(\overline{L}_m, \overline{A}_m, \beta^\dagger\right) - r^{\overline{d},\overline{d}^*}\left(\overline{L}_m, \overline{A}_{m-1}, A_m\right)\left\{1 - f\left(A_m|\overline{L}_m, \overline{A}_{m-1}\right)\right\}.$$

Thus $\gamma^{\overline{d}_{op}^w, \overline{d}_{op}^w}\left(\overline{L}_m, \overline{A}_m\right)$ may not be either maximized or minimized at $A_m = d_{op,m}\left(\overline{L}_m, \overline{A}_{m-1}\right)$. To estimate the model $u_m\left(\overline{l}_m, \overline{a}_m, \beta\right)$, we put $\overline{d}^* = \overline{d} = \overline{d}_{op}^w$, and note our model $\gamma^{\overline{d}_{op}^w, \overline{d}_{op}^w}\left(\overline{L}_m, \overline{A}_m, \psi\right)$ is given by $-u_m\left(\overline{L}_m, \overline{A}_m, \beta\right) - r^{\overline{d}_{op}^w, \overline{d}_{op}^w}\left(\overline{L}_m, \overline{A}_{m-1}, A_m\right)\left\{1 - f\left(A_m|\overline{L}_m, \overline{A}_{m-1}; \alpha\right)\right\}$ for $\psi = (\beta, \alpha)$. We then regard $r^{\overline{d}_{op}^w, \overline{d}_{op}^w}\left(\overline{L}_m, \overline{A}_{m-1}, A_m\right)$ as known (but vary it in a sensitivity analysis), estimate α with the maximum partial likelihood estimator $\hat{\alpha}$, and finally estimate the remaining component β of ψ as in (1) above. The remarks found under both (1) and (2) apply in this setting. Furthermore the maximization in Eq (7.8) need not be explicitly carried out, as it will always return $d_{op,m}\left(\overline{L}_m, \overline{A}_{m-1}, \beta_{regime}\right)$ for the current value of β_{regime}.

(5) When $W_m \neq (\overline{L}_m, \overline{A}_{m-1})$ so there is information loss, we proceed as described in (1)-(4), except now, for each m, we estimate the unknown random function $B(a_m) = E[q(\overline{L}_m, \overline{A}_{m-1}, a_m) | W_m]$ of a_m in Eq.(7.8) by specifying a multivariate parametric regression model for the mean of the vector $\{B(a_m); a_m \in \mathcal{A}_m\}$ given W_m. We then regress the vector $\{B(a_m); a_m \in \mathcal{A}_m\}$ (or an estimate thereof) on W_m under this model. Note that a_m is fixed rather than random in the regression so a regression model for $B(a_m)$ given W_m would be a function of a_m, W_m, and a regression parameter.

7.3 Optimal Marginal drSNMMs vs. Optimal drSNMMs for Estimation of Optimal w-compatible treatment regimes:

Suppose the sequential randomization assumption (2.5) holds and we want to estimate $\overline{d}_{op}^w$ for an increasing w with $W_m \neq (\overline{L}_m, \overline{A}_{m-1})$, so there is information loss. In this section we will compare the approach described in the last subsection of specifying a optimal drSNMM model $\gamma^{\overline{d}_{op}^w, \overline{0}}(\overline{L}_m, \overline{A}_m, \psi)$ for $\gamma^{\overline{d}_{op}^w, \overline{0}}(\overline{L}_m, \overline{A}_m) = E\left[Y_{\overline{A}_{m-1}, A_m, \underline{d}_{op,m+1}^w} - Y_{\overline{A}_{m-1}, 0_m, \underline{d}_{op,m+1}^w} | \overline{L}_m, \overline{A}_{m-1}\right]$ versus modelling $\gamma^{\overline{d}_{op}^w, \overline{0}}(W_m) = E\left[Y_{\overline{A}_{m-1}, A_m, \underline{d}_{op,m+1}^w} - Y_{\overline{A}_{m-1}, 0_m, \underline{d}_{op,m+1}^w} | W_m\right]$ directly with a drSNMM model $\gamma^{\overline{d}_{op}^w, \overline{0}}(W_m, A_m, \omega)$ with parameter ω, say, and thus avoiding the need to specify a multivariate regression model for $B(a_m) = E[q(\overline{L}_m, \overline{A}_{m-1}, a_m) | W_m] = E[\gamma^{\overline{d}_{op}^w, \overline{0}}(\overline{L}_m, \overline{A}_{m-1}, a_m) | W_m] - \gamma^{\overline{d}_{op}^w, \overline{0}}(\overline{L}_m, \overline{A}_{m-1}, d_m(\overline{L}_m, \overline{A}_{m-1}))$ in order to evaluate $d_{op,m}^w(W_m) = \arg\max_{a_m} E[q(\overline{L}_m, \overline{A}_{m-1}, a_m) | W_m]$ in (7.8). Note, however, that if $\gamma^{\overline{d}_{op}^w, \overline{0}}(\overline{L}_m, \overline{A}_m, \psi)$ has the functional form $A_m r(\overline{L}_m, \overline{A}_{m-1}, \psi)$ for some given function $r(\overline{L}_m, \overline{A}_{m-1}, \psi)$, then $\gamma^{\overline{d}_{op}^w, \overline{0}}(\overline{L}_m, \overline{A}_m, \psi)$ is linear in A_m, and

$$d_{op,m}^w(W_m) = \max\{a_m \in \mathcal{A}_m\} I\left\{E[r(\overline{L}_m, \overline{A}_{m-1}, \psi^\dagger) | W_m] > 0\right\} + \min\{a_m \in \mathcal{A}_m\} I\left\{E[r(\overline{L}_m, \overline{A}_{m-1}, \psi^\dagger) | W_m] \leq 0\right\}.$$

It then follows that we only need to specify a univariate regression model for $E[r(\overline{L}_m, \overline{A}_{m-1}, \psi^\dagger) | W_m]$ in order to estimate $d_{op,m}^w(W_m)$ even though $\mathcal{A}_m$ might be an uncountable set.

Under (2.5), using ideas in van der Laan, Murphy, and Robins (2003) summarized in van der Laan and Robins (2002, Chapter 6), we could estimate the model $\gamma^{\overline{d}_{op}^w, \overline{0}}(W_m, A_m, \omega)$ (which, by an extension of their nomenclature should be referred to a optimal marginal drSNMM) directly by (i) creating a pseudo-data set with WT_i copies of each subject i, where

$$WT = \prod_{m=0}^{K} 1/f(A_m | \overline{L}_m, \overline{A}_{m-1}) \text{ if } f(A_m | \overline{L}_m, \overline{A}_{m-1}) \text{ is known or with } \widehat{WT}_i$$

copies where $\widehat{WT} = \prod_{m=0}^{K} 1/f\left(A_m|\overline{L}_m,\overline{A}_{m-1};\widehat{\alpha}\right)$ if $f\left(A_m|\overline{L}_m,\overline{A}_{m-1}\right)$ is unknown and must be modelled, (ii) retaining in the pseudo -data set only the data $(W_K, A_K, Y) = \left(\overline{V}_K, \overline{A}_K, Y\right)$ where $V_m = W_m \backslash (\overline{A}_{m-1} \cup W_{m-1})$ are the non-treatment components of W_m that were not in W_{m-1} (since by w increasing, $\overline{A}_{m-1}$ is a function of W_m and (W_m, A_m) can be written as $\left(\overline{V}_m, \overline{A}_m\right)$), and (iii) fitting the optimal marginal drSNMM model $\gamma^{\overline{d}_{op}^w,\overline{0}}(W_m, A_m, \omega) = \gamma^{\overline{d}_{op}^w,\overline{0}}\left(\overline{V}_m, \overline{A}_m, \omega\right)$ to the retained part of the pseudo -data set as in Section 4 except with $\overline{V}_m$ replacing $\overline{L}_m$ and ω replacing ψ. This approach succeeds because (2.5) holding in the actual population implies that, in the pseudo-poulation based on weighting by WT_i, (2.5) holds with L replaced by V and $V_{K+1} \equiv Y$.

However when $f\left(A_m|\overline{L}_m,\overline{A}_{m-1}\right)$ is unknown and must be modelled, the approach based on modelling $\gamma^{\overline{d}_{op}^w,\overline{0}}\left(\overline{L}_m, \overline{A}_m\right)$ may be preferred to that based on modelling $\gamma^{\overline{d}_{op}^w,\overline{0}}(W_m)$ directly, because the former approach has robustness properties under the g-null mean hypothesis not shared by the latter. To see this sharply, imagine the L_m are discrete with only a moderate number of levels and the A_m are continuous. Then, even with $f\left(A_m|\overline{L}_m,\overline{A}_{m-1}\right)$ totally unrestricted , an asymptotically distribution-free test of $\psi^{\dagger} = 0$ (and thus of g-null mean hypothesis) exists based on the model $\gamma^{\overline{d}_{op}^w,\overline{0}}\left(\overline{L}_m, \overline{A}_m, \psi\right)$, but, because of the curse of dimensionality, not based on the model $\gamma^{\overline{d}_{op}^w,\overline{0}}\left(\overline{V}_m, \overline{A}_m, \omega\right)$. Specifically, suppose in the interest of robustness to misspecification, we use model (a.3) that regards $f\left(A_m|\overline{L}_m,\overline{A}_{m-1}\right)$ as completely unknown and also use the empirical conditional distribution of $f\left(A_m|\overline{L}_m,\overline{A}_{m-1}\right)$ as its estimator. Then our test of the hypothesis $\psi^{\dagger} = 0$ reduces to a nonparametric test of independence of Y and A_0 within strata (where each $l_0 \in \mathcal{L}_0$ defines a separate stratum), because at times other than t_0 no two subjects have the same history $\overline{L}_m, \overline{A}_{m-1}$ so $S\left(A_m\right) - \widehat{E}\left[S\left(A_m\right)|\overline{L}_m,\overline{A}_{m-1}\right]$ will be zero for $m > 0$. This test will have some, although limited, power to detect alternatives with $\psi^{\dagger} \neq 0$. In contrast, as discussed in Robins (1999), a test of $\omega^{\dagger} = 0$ will have the correct $\alpha - level$ even asymptotically only if WT can be uniformly consistently estimated which requires we can uniformly consistently estimate $f\left(A_m|\overline{L}_m,\overline{A}_{m-1}\right)$ for all m which is not possible under model (a.3). Quite generally when estimating $\psi^{\dagger}$ we can trade off efficiency in return for protection against bias caused by possible model misspecification in a way that is not available when we are estimating $\omega^{\dagger}$.

On the other hand, the approach based on modelling $\gamma^{\overline{d}_{op}^w,\overline{0}}(W_m)$ may be preferred to that based on modelling $\gamma^{\overline{d}_{op}^w,\overline{0}}\left(\overline{L}_m, \overline{A}_m\right)$ if it is important that we succeed in specifying a correct or nearly correct blip model because the dimension of $\left(\overline{L}_m, \overline{A}_m\right)$ vastly exceeds that of W_m. For example if based on prior beliefs we are essentially certain $\gamma^{\overline{d}_{op}^w,\overline{0}}(W_m)$ only depends on on $W_m = w_m\left(\overline{L}_m, \overline{A}_{m-1}\right)$ through the few components of W_m that are functions of the data (L_j, A_{j-1}) obtained at times for $j = m, m-1, m-2$ and W_m is discrete, it is possible we could fit a model saturated in those few components of W_m, thus avoiding major worries about model misspecification. See the Remark on Marginal drSNMMs in Section 9.1 below.

7.4 Bayesian Decision Making in the Prescence of Unmeasured Confounding:

In this section we go beyond sensitivity analysis and consider optimal Bayes decision making in the presence of unmeasured confounding, although we only consider the single occasion setting.

The Single Decision Problem:

Consider again the setting in which we have a single time-independent treatment $(K = 0)$. Thus assume the data are $L = L_0, A = A_0, Y = L_1$ with A dichotomous, L multivariate with continuous components and Y continuous. Suppose we have a known correct linear model $\gamma(l, a, \psi) = ar(l, \psi) = a\psi^T w(L) = a\psi^T W$ with true value $\psi^\dagger$ for $\gamma(l, a) = E[Y_a - Y_0 | L = l, A = a]$ and for simplicity assume that it is known that $E[Y_a - Y_0 | L = l, A = a] = E[Y_a - Y_0 | L = l, A \neq a]$ so $r^{\bar{d}, \bar{0}}(l, a)$ of (7.1) is identically 0. Then $d_{op}(l) = \arg\max_a \gamma(l, a, \psi) = I\{r(l, \psi) > 0\}$. Further suppppose that there may be unmeasured confounding with $v^{\bar{d}, \bar{0}}(l, a) = E[Y_0 | L = l, A = a] - E[Y_0 | L = l, A = 0] = a\delta^{\dagger, T} W$ with $\delta^\dagger$ unknown. Then if we define $\theta = \psi + \delta$, $H(\theta) = Y - A\theta^T W$, we have that

$$E\left[H\left(\theta^\dagger\right) | L, A\right] = E\left[H\left(\theta^\dagger\right) | L\right], \quad \theta^\dagger = \psi^\dagger + \delta^\dagger \qquad (7.15)$$

It follows from (7.15) if we define $\widehat{Z}_t^\circ\left(\theta, \widehat{s}_{eff}, c^{\widehat{s}eff}, \widehat{\alpha}, \widehat{\varsigma}, \widehat{\varkappa}, \widehat{\zeta}\right)$ exactly as we did $\widehat{Z}_t\left(\psi, \widehat{s}_{eff}, c^{\widehat{s}eff}, \widehat{\alpha}, \widehat{\varsigma}, \widehat{\varkappa}, \widehat{\zeta}\right)$ except with θ everywhere replacing ψ, we obtain an asymptotic approximation $\pi_{post}\left(\theta^\dagger\right)$ to the posterior for $\theta^\dagger$ given the stochastic process $\widehat{Z}_t^\circ\left(\cdot, \widehat{s}_{eff}, c^{\widehat{s}eff}, \widehat{\alpha}, \widehat{\varsigma}, \widehat{\varkappa}, \widehat{\zeta}\right)$ indexed by θ given by

$$\pi_{post}\left(\theta^\dagger\right) \qquad (7.16)$$
$$= \frac{I\left\{\theta^\dagger; \left\|\widehat{Z}_t^\circ\left(\theta^\dagger\right)\right\| < t \dim\left(\theta^\dagger\right)^{1/2}\right\} \exp\left(-\widehat{Z}_t^\circ\left(\theta^\dagger\right)^T \widehat{Z}_t^\circ\left(\theta^\dagger\right)/2\right)\pi\left(\theta^\dagger\right)}{\int_{\left\{\theta^\dagger; \|\widehat{Z}_t^\circ(\theta^\dagger)\| < t \dim(\theta^\dagger)^{1/2}\right\}} \exp\left(-\widehat{Z}_t^\circ\left(\theta^\dagger\right)^T \widehat{Z}_t^\circ\left(\theta^\dagger\right)/2\right)\pi\left(\theta^\dagger\right)d\theta^\dagger}.$$

Thus since $\psi^\dagger$ is independent of $\widehat{Z}_t^\circ\left(\cdot, \widehat{s}_{eff}, c^{\widehat{s}eff}, \widehat{\alpha}, \widehat{\varsigma}, \widehat{\varkappa}, \widehat{\zeta}\right)$ given $\theta^\dagger$, we have that

$$\pi_{post}\left(\psi^\dagger\right) = \int \pi_{post}\left(\theta^\dagger\right)\pi\left(\psi^\dagger | \theta^\dagger\right)d\theta^\dagger$$

where $\pi\left(\psi^\dagger|\theta^\dagger\right)$ is the conditonal prior of $\psi^\dagger$ given $\theta^\dagger = \psi^\dagger + \delta^\dagger$. The optimal Bayes decison rule is, of course,

$$d_{bayes}\left(l\right) = \arg \max_{a \in \mathcal{A} = \{0,1\}} \int ar\left(l,\psi^\dagger\right) \pi_{post}\left(\psi^\dagger\right) d\psi^\dagger$$

Assume a correct model for either $E\left[H\left(\theta^\dagger\right)|L\right]$ or $f(A|L)$, so that $\theta^\dagger$ is estimated at rate $n^{1/2}$. Then $\pi_{post}\left(\theta^\dagger\right)$ charges a volume with radius $O\left(n^{-1/2}\right)$. It follows that if $\pi\left(\psi^\dagger|\theta^\dagger\right)$ charges a volume of radius $O\left(1\right)$ [as would be the case if $\psi^\dagger$ and $\delta^\dagger$ were apriori independent with priors charging a volume of radius $O\left(1\right)$] $\pi_{post}\left(\psi^\dagger\right)/\pi\left(\psi^\dagger|\theta^\dagger\right)$ is approximately 1 . If $\psi^\dagger$ and $\delta^\dagger$ were apriori independent with $\pi\left(\psi^\dagger\right)$ charging a volume of radius $O\left(n^{-1/2}\right)$ and $\pi\left(\delta^\dagger\right)$ charging a volume of radius $O\left(1\right)$, then $\pi_{post}\left(\psi^\dagger\right)/\pi\left(\psi^\dagger\right)$ is approximately 1. A limitation of the above analysis is that we assumed $v^{\bar{d},\bar{0}}\left(l,a\right) = a\delta^{\dagger,T}W$ and $\gamma\left(l,a,\psi\right) = a\psi^{\dagger,T}W$ had the same functional form so that the approximate distribution of $\widehat{Z}_t^\circ\left(\cdot,\widehat{s}_{eff},c^{\widehat{s}_{eff}},\widehat{\alpha},\widehat{\varsigma},\widehat{\varkappa},\widehat{\zeta}\right)$ depended on $\left(\delta^\dagger,\psi^\dagger\right)$ only through their sum $\theta^\dagger$. This limitation is more apparent than real as it can be modified by appropriate specification of the joint prior $\pi\left(\delta^\dagger,\psi^\dagger\right)$. For example suppose suppose that W was 20 dimensional and one believed that $\gamma\left(l,a\right)$ only depended on the first 2 components of W but $v^{\bar{d},\bar{0}}\left(l,a\right)$ depended on all 20. Then one could take $\pi\left(\psi^\dagger\right)$ to place all its mass on the last 18 components of $\psi^\dagger$ being 0. Note that in such a case, since $\theta^\dagger$ is estimated at rate $n^{1/2}$, we obtain $n^{1/2} - consistent$ estimates of the last 18 components of $\delta^\dagger$.

8 Continuous Time Optimal drSNMMs

Continuous Time drSNMMs: To extend some of our results to continuous time, let $A\left(u\right)$ and $L\left(u\right)$ be recorded treatment and covariates at time u, where in this section we use parentheses rather than subscripts to denote the time of an event. We shall assume that a subject's observed data $O = \left(\overline{L}\left(K\right),\overline{A}\left(K\right)\right)$ with $\overline{L}\left(t\right) = \{L\left(u\right);0 \leq u \leq t\}$ and $\overline{A}\left(t\right) = \{A\left(u\right);0 \leq u \leq t\}$ are generated by a marked point process such that (i) $L\left(t\right)$ and $A\left(t\right)$ have sample paths that are CADLAG step functions, i.e. they are right-continuous with left-hand limits and we write $\left(\overline{A}\left(t^-\right),\overline{L}\left(t^-\right)\right)$ for a subject's history up to but not including t ; (ii) the $L\left(t\right)$ and $A\left(t\right)$ process do not jump simultaneously or both in an interval of time $o\left(1\right)$; and (iii) both processes have continuous time bounded intensities so the total number of jumps K^* of the joint $\left(\overline{A}\left(t\right),\overline{L}\left(t\right)\right)$ process in $[0,K]$ is random and finite, occurring at random times $T_1,\ldots,T_{K^*}$. That is we assume $\lambda_A\left(t\mid\overline{A}\left(t^-\right),\overline{L}\left(t^-\right)\right) = \lim_{\delta t \to 0} pr[A\left(t+\delta t\right) \neq A\left(t^-\right)\mid$ $\overline{A}\left(t^-\right),\overline{L}\left(t^-\right)]/\delta t$ and $\lambda_L\left(t\mid\overline{A}\left(t^-\right),\overline{L}\left(t^-\right)\right) = \lim_{\delta t \to 0} pr[L\left(t+\delta t\right) \neq L\left(t^-\right)\mid$ $\overline{A}\left(t^-\right),\overline{L}\left(t^-\right)]/\delta t$ are bounded and measurable on $[0,K]$ where, for example, $A\left(t^-\right) = \lim_{u \uparrow t} A\left(u\right)$ is well defined because the sample path have left hand limits. We choose this restricted class of sample paths because their statistical properties are well understood.

We only consider the case of sequential randomization. Generalizations similar to those in Section 7 are straightforward. The assumption (2.5) of sequential randomization becomes

$$\lambda_A\left[t\mid \overline{L}\left(t^-\right),\overline{A}\left(t^-\right),\{\overline{L_{\overline{a}}};\overline{a}\in\overline{\mathcal{A}}\}\right]=\lambda_A\left[t\mid \overline{L}\left(t^-\right),\overline{A}\left(t^-\right)\right] \qquad (8.1)$$

and

$$f[A\left(t\right)\mid \overline{L}\left(t^-\right),\overline{A}\left(t^-\right),A\left(t\right)\neq A\left(t^-\right),\{\overline{L_{\overline{a}}};\overline{a}\in\overline{\mathcal{A}}\}]= \qquad (8.2)$$
$$f\left[A\left(t\right)\mid \overline{L}\left(t^-\right),\overline{A}\left(t^-\right),A\left(t\right)\neq A\left(t^-\right)\right].$$

Eq. (8.1) says that given past treatment and confounder history, the probability that the A process jumps at t does not depend on the joint counterfactual histories $\overline{L}_{\overline{a}}=\{L_{\overline{a}}\left(u\right);0\leq u\leq K\}$ corresponding to the non-dynamic treatment histories $\overline{a}=\{a\left(u\right);0\leq u\leq K\}\in\overline{\mathcal{A}}$. Eq. (8.2) says that given that the treatment process did jump at t, the probability it jumped to a particular value of $A\left(t\right)$ does not depend on the counterfactual histories.

A regime $\overline{d}=\left\{d\left(t,\overline{l}\left(t^-\right),\overline{a}\left(t^-\right)\right);t\in[0,K]\right\}$ is a collection of functions $d\left(t,\overline{l}\left(t^-\right),\overline{a}\left(t^-\right)\right)$ indexed by t mapping $\left(\overline{l}\left(t^-\right),\overline{a}\left(t^-\right)\right)\in\overline{L}\left(t^-\right)\times\overline{A}\left(t^-\right)$ into the support $A\left(t\right)$ of $A\left(t\right)$ such that the law $f_{res}\left(o\right)f_{tr,\overline{d}}\left(o\right)$ that replaces the observed treatment process $f_{tr,\overline{p}_{obs}}$ with the deterministic process $f_{tr,\overline{d}}\left(o\right)$ has sample paths satisfying (i)-(iii) above with probability one. This is a limitation on the collection of functions that can constitute a valid regime $\overline{d}$. Let $\overline{\mathcal{D}}$ denote the collection of all such regimes. We assume all regimes are feasible in the sense that $f\left[a\left(t\right)\mid \overline{L}\left(t^-\right),\overline{A}\left(t^-\right),A\left(t\right)\neq A\left(t^-\right)\right]$ is non-zero w.p.1 for all $a\left(t\right)\in A\left(t\right)\setminus\{A\left(t^-\right)\}$.

Example 8.1: Suppose $A(t)$ is Bernoulli and consider $d\left(t,\overline{L}\left(t^-\right),\overline{A}\left(t^-\right)\right)=I\left[A\left(t-\delta\right)<1/2\right]=1-A\left(t-\delta\right)$ for a given known $\delta>0$ where $A\left(t\right)=0$ w.p.1 for $t<0$. Then a subject starts treatment at time 0 and is to take treatment until time δ, to take no treatment from δ to 2δ, to again take treatment from 2δ to 3δ and continue alternating thereafter. Suppose we tried to replace $A\left(t-\delta\right)$ by $A\left(t-\right)=\lim_{\delta\uparrow t}A\left(\delta\right)$ but kept the same parameter values. We will call such a replacement the case $\delta=0$. Then we have a contradiction as the regime for a subject starting from time zero is not defined, because treatment cannot alternate infinitely quickly at all t. So the regime $\delta=0$ is not in $\overline{\mathcal{D}}$.

Given a treatment regime $\overline{d}$, let $\underline{d}(u)=\left\{d\left(t,\overline{l}\left(t^-\right),\overline{a}\left(t^-\right)\right);t\in[u,K]\right\}$. Then, given $h\geq 0$, $\overline{d}$ and $\overline{a}\left(t^-\right)$, and a define $\left(\overline{a}\left(t^-\right),a,\underline{d}(t+h)\right)$ to be the regime in which the nondynamic regime $\overline{a}\left(t^-\right)$ is followed on $[0,t)$, the constant dose a is given on $[t,t+h)$ and $\overline{d}$ is followed from $t+h$.

Let $Y=y\left(\overline{L}\left(K\right),\overline{A}\left(K\right)\right)$ be a utility and $Y_{\overline{d}}$ be its counterfactual version under a regime $\overline{d}$. Let $V^{\overline{d},\overline{0}}\left(t,h,a\right)$
$$=E\left[Y_{\left(\overline{A}(t^-),a,\underline{d}(t+h)\right)}-Y_{\left(\overline{A}(t^-),0,\underline{d}(t+h)\right)}\mid \overline{L}\left(t\right),\overline{A}\left(t^-\right)\right]$$ be the mean causal

effect on subjects with observed history $\left(\overline{L}\left(t\right),\overline{A}\left(t^{-}\right)\right)$ of a final blip of constant treatment a in the interval $[t,t+h)$ compared to no treatment before changing to the regime $\overline{d}$ at $t+h$. Note $V^{\overline{d},\overline{0}}\left(t,h,0\right)=0$. We restrict attention to treatments for which an instantaneously brief bit of treatment has a negligible effect on Y. We formalize this as follows.

Assumption Of Negligible Instantaneous Effects: We assume that, for all $\overline{d}\in\overline{\mathcal{D}}$, (i) $V^{\overline{d},\overline{0}}\left(t,h,a\right)$ is continuous in h and $M^{\overline{d},\overline{0}}\left(t,a\right)\equiv\lim_{h\downarrow0}V^{\overline{d},\overline{0}}\left(t,h,a\right)/h$ exists for all $t\in[0,K)$ and (ii) with probability one, $M^{\overline{d},\overline{0}}\left(t,a\right)=\partial V^{\overline{d},\overline{0}}\left(t,0,a\right)/\partial h$ is continuous in t (uniformly over $\overline{d}\in\overline{\mathcal{D}},a\in\mathcal{A}\left(t\right)$ and $t\in[0,K)$) for all $t\in[T_m,T_{m+1}),m=0,\ldots,K^*+1$ where $T_0\equiv0,T_{K^*+1}\equiv K$.

$V^{\overline{d},\overline{0}}\left(t,h,a\right)$ and $M^{\overline{d},\overline{0}}\left(t,a\right)$ may be discontinuous in t at the jump times T_m because of the abrupt change in the conditioning event defining $V^{\overline{d},\overline{0}}\left(t,h,a\right)$ at $t=T_m$. Note $M^{\overline{d},\overline{0}}\left(t,a\right)dt$ is the effect on the mean of Y of a last blip of treatment a compared to no treatment both sustained for "instantaneous" time dt before resorting to regime $\overline{d}$. Hence, $M^{\overline{d},\overline{0}}\left(t,A(t)\right)\equiv m^{\overline{d},\overline{0}}\left(t,\overline{L}\left(t\right),\overline{A}\left(t\right)\right)$ is the instantaneous version of the function $\gamma^{\overline{d},\overline{0}}\left(\overline{L}_m,\overline{A}_m\right)$ of Sec. 3.

Define $H^{\overline{d},\overline{0}}\left(u\right)=Y+\int_u^K\left[M^{\overline{d},\overline{0}}\left\{t,d\left(t,\overline{L}\left(t^{-}\right),\overline{A}\left(t^{-}\right)\right)\right\}-M^{\overline{d},\overline{0}}\left\{t,A(t)\right\}\right]dt$ and define $H^{\overline{d},\overline{0}}$ to be $H^{\overline{d},\overline{0}}\left(0\right)$. Then our main result is the following which is proved exactly like it analogue in the appendix of Robins (1998).

Theorem 8.1: Under sequential randomization (8.1)-(8.2) and the Assumption of negligible instantaneous effects, if $\overline{d}\in\overline{\mathcal{D}}$, then

$$E\left[H^{\overline{d},\overline{0}}\left(t\right)\mid\overline{L}\left(t\right),\overline{A}\left(t\right)\right]=E\left[Y_{\left(\overline{A}(t^{-}),\underline{d}(t)\right)}\mid\overline{L}\left(t\right),\overline{A}\left(t\right)\right]\text{ and}$$

$E\left[Y_{\left(\overline{A}(t^{-}),\underline{d}(t)\right)}\mid\overline{L}\left(t\right),\overline{A}\left(t\right)\right]$ is not a function of $A\left(t\right)$. In particular,

$$E\left(H^{\overline{d},\overline{0}}\left(0\right)\right)=E\left[Y_{\overline{d}}\right].$$

We say the data follows a continuous-time drSNMM $M^{\overline{d},\overline{0}}\left(t,a,\psi\right)$ if $M^{\overline{d},\overline{0}}\left(t,a\right)\equiv m^{\overline{d},\overline{0}}\left(t,\overline{L}\left(t\right),\overline{A}\left(t^{-}\right),a\right)$ equals $M^{\overline{d},\overline{0}}\left(t,a,\psi^{\dagger}\right)\equiv m^{\overline{d},\overline{0}}\left(t,\overline{L}\left(t\right),\overline{A}\left(t^{-}\right),a,\psi^{\dagger}\right)$ where $\psi^{\dagger}$ is an unknown parameter to be estimated and $M^{\overline{d},\overline{0}}\left(t,a,\psi\right)$ is a known random function continuous in t on $[T_m,T_{m+1})$ satisfying $M^{\overline{d},\overline{0}}\left(t,a,\psi\right)=0$ if $\psi=0$ or $a=0$.

First suppose that $A\left(t\right)$ is Bernoulli and let $H^{\overline{d},\overline{0}}\left(t,\psi\right)$ be $H^{\overline{d},\overline{0}}\left(t\right)$ with $M^{\overline{d},\overline{0}}\left(t,a,\psi\right)$ replacing $M^{\overline{d},\overline{0}}\left(t,a\right)$. Given a Cox model for jumps in the treatment process

$$\lambda_A\left(t\mid\overline{L}\left(t^{-}\right),\overline{A}\left(t^{-}\right)\right)=\lambda_0\left(t\right)\exp\left[\alpha'W\left(t\right)\right]\qquad(8.3)$$

where $W\left(t\right)$ is a vector function of $\left\{\overline{L}\left(t^{-}\right),\overline{A}\left(t^{-}\right)\right\}$, α is an unknown vector parameter, and $\lambda_0\left(t\right)$ is an unrestricted baseline hazard function, we obtain a G-estimate of the parameter ψ of the continuous-time drSNMM $M^{\overline{d},\overline{0}}\left(t,a,\psi\right)$ by adding the term $\theta'H^{\overline{d},\overline{0}}\left(t,\psi\right)b\left(t,\overline{L}\left(t^{-}\right),\overline{A}\left(t^{-}\right)\right)$ to model (8.3) where

$b\left(t,\bar{l}\left(t^{-}\right),\bar{a}\left(t^{-}\right)\right)$ is a known vector function of the dimension of ψ chosen by the investigator. Specifically, the G-estimate $\widehat{\psi}_{ge}$ is the value of ψ for which the Cox partial likelihood estimator $\widehat{\theta}=\widehat{\theta}\left(\psi\right)$ of θ in the expanded model

$$\lambda_{A}\left(t\mid\bar{L}\left(t^{-}\right),\bar{A}\left(t^{-}\right)\right) \tag{8.4}$$
$$=\lambda_{0}\left(t\right)\left\{\exp\left[\alpha'W\left(t\right)\right]+\theta'H^{\bar{d},\bar{0}}\left(t,\psi\right)b\left(t,\bar{L}\left(t^{-}\right),\bar{A}\left(t^{-}\right)\right)\right\}$$

is zero. Then, under sequential randomization, Theorem 8.1 can be used to show that $\widehat{\psi}_{ge}$ and $n^{-1}\sum_{i}H_{i}\left(0,\widehat{\psi}_{ge}\right)$ will be $n^{\frac{1}{2}}$-consistent for $\psi^{\dagger}$ and $E\left[Y_{\bar{d}}\right]$ provided the drSNMM $M^{\bar{d},\bar{0}}\left(t,a,\psi\right)$ and the Cox model (8.3) are correctly specified. It is also possible to construct doubly robust estimators of $\psi^{\dagger}$. In addition, confidence intervals for $\psi^{\dagger}$ and $E\left[Y_{\bar{d}}\right]$ can also be obtained. Futhermore, if $A\left(t\right)$ is not a dichotomous random variable, then we can obtain more efficient estimators of $\psi^{\dagger}$ and $E\left[Y_{\bar{d}}\right]$ by exploiting (8.2). Technical details will be presented elsewhere.

Example 8.1 (cont): Suppose again $d\left(t,\bar{L}\left(t^{-}\right),\bar{A}\left(t^{-}\right)\right)=1-A\left(t-\delta\right)$. Further $M^{\bar{d},\bar{0}}\left(t,a,\psi\right)=ar\left(t,\bar{L}\left(t\right),\bar{A}\left(t^{-}\right),\psi\right)$ with

$$r\left(t,\bar{L}\left(t\right),\bar{A}\left(t^{-}\right),\psi\right)=\left(1,A\left(t-\delta\right)\right)\psi=\psi_{1}+\psi_{3}A\left(t-\delta\right)$$

where δ is the same known non-negative number. Then $H^{\bar{d},\bar{0}}\left(t,\psi\right)=Y+\psi_{1}cum_{1,\delta}\left(\underline{A}\left(t\right)\right)-\left(\psi_{1}+\psi_{3}\right)cum_{2,\delta}\left(\underline{A}\left(t-\delta\right)\right)$ where $cum_{1,\delta}\left(\underline{A}\left(t\right)\right)$ is the measure of the set $\{u;u\in\left[t,K\right]$ and $A\left(u\right)=A\left(u-\delta\right)=0\}$ and $cum_{2,\delta}\left(\underline{A}\left(t-\delta\right)\right)$ is the measure of the set $\{u;u\in\left[t,K\right]$ and $A\left(u\right)=A\left(u-\delta\right)=1\}$.

Extension to Continuous Time Optimal drSNMMs: The proof of the existence of an optimal regime under our assumptions is subtle and will be given elsewhere. Here we will simply suppose there exists an optimal regime $\bar{d}_{op}$ i.e. a regime $\bar{d}_{op}\in\mathcal{D}$ satisfying $E\left[Y_{\bar{A}\left(t^{-}\right),\underline{d}_{op}\left(t\right)}\mid\bar{L}\left(t^{-}\right),\bar{A}\left(t^{-}\right)\right]\geq E\left[Y_{\bar{A}\left(t^{-}\right),\underline{d}\left(t\right)}\mid\bar{L}\left(t^{-}\right),\bar{A}\left(t^{-}\right)\right]$ for all $\bar{d}\in\mathcal{D}$.

Remark: To see why it is not completely trivial to prove the existence of an optimal regime, given a regime $\bar{d}$, define $z_{op}\left(t,\bar{L}\left(t\right),\bar{A}\left(t^{-}\right),\bar{d}^{*}\right)=\arg\max_{a}m^{\bar{d}^{*},\bar{0}}\left(t,\bar{L}\left(t\right),\bar{A}\left(t^{-}\right),a\right)$. Define

$$d_{op}\left(t,\bar{L}\left(t^{-}\right),\bar{A}\left(t^{-}\right),\bar{d}^{*}\right)$$
$$=\arg\max_{a}E\left[m^{\bar{d}^{*},\bar{0}}\left(t,a,\bar{L}\left(t\right),\bar{A}\left(t^{-}\right)\right)\mid\bar{L}\left(t^{-}\right),\bar{A}\left(t^{-}\right)\right]$$
$$=z_{op}\left(t,\bar{L}\left(t^{-}\right),L\left(t\right)=L\left(t^{-}\right),\bar{d}^{*}\right)$$

where the last equality follows from the fact that the event $L\left(t\right)=L\left(t^{-}\right)$ has probability one (because the probability the covariate process jumps at any given t is zero). Informally $d_{op}\left(t,\overline{L}\left(t^{-}\right),\overline{A}\left(t^{-}\right),\overline{d}^{*}\right)$ is the optimal treatment decision at t given the information in $\overline{L}\left(t^{-}\right),\overline{A}\left(t^{-}\right)$ if one is to follow $\overline{d}^{*}$ from $t+h$ onwards for h sufficiently small. But since the number of times t are now uncountable we cannot use simple backward induction to define $d_{op}\left(t,\overline{L}\left(t^{-}\right),\overline{A}\left(t^{-}\right)\right)$ in terms of the $d_{op}\left(t,\overline{L}\left(t^{-}\right),\overline{A}\left(t^{-}\right),\overline{d}^{*}\right)$. The smoothness assumptions embedded in the Assumption of negligible instantaneous effects will be needed.

We now consider an optimal drSNMM model $M^{\overline{d}_{op},\overline{0}}\left(t,a,\psi\right)=m^{\overline{d}_{op},\overline{0}}\left(t,\overline{L}\left(t\right),\overline{A}\left(t^{-}\right),a,\psi\right)$ for $M^{\overline{d}_{op},\overline{0}}\left(t,a\right)$. Then, we define

$$H^{\overline{d}_{op},\overline{0}}\left(u,\psi\right)=Y+\int_{u}^{K}\left[M^{\overline{d}_{op},\overline{0}}\left\{t,d_{op}\left(t,\overline{L}\left(t^{-}\right),\overline{A}\left(t^{-}\right),\psi\right)\right\}-M^{\overline{d}_{op},\overline{0}}\left\{t,A(t),\psi\right\}\right]$$

where

$$d_{op}\left(t,\overline{L}\left(t^{-}\right),\overline{A}\left(t^{-}\right),\psi\right)=\arg\max_{a}E\left[m^{\overline{d}_{op},\overline{0}}\left(t,\overline{L}\left(t\right),\overline{A}\left(t^{-}\right),a,\psi\right)|\overline{L}\left(t^{-}\right),\overline{A}\left(t^{-}\right)\right]$$
$$=z_{op}(t,\overline{L}\left(t^{-}\right),L\left(t\right)=L\left(t^{-}\right),\psi)$$

and $z_{op}(t,\overline{L}\left(t^{-}\right),L\left(t\right),\psi)=\arg\max_{a}m^{\overline{d}_{op},\overline{0}}\left(t,a,\overline{L}\left(t\right),\overline{A}\left(t^{-}\right),\psi\right)$. We estimate $\psi^{\dagger}$ and $E\left[Y_{\overline{d}_{op}}\right]$ by g-estimation as in the paragraph above.

Example 8.1 (cont): Consider the model $M^{\overline{d}_{op},\overline{0}}\left(t,a,\psi\right)=ar\left(t,\overline{L}\left(t\right),\overline{A}\left(t^{-}\right),\psi\right)$ with $r\left(t,\overline{L}\left(t\right),\overline{A}\left(t^{-}\right),\psi\right)=\left(1,L\left(t\right),A\left(t-\delta\right)\right)\psi$ where δ is the same non-negative number. Then

$$d_{op}\left(t,\overline{L}\left(t^{-}\right),\overline{A}\left(t^{-}\right),\psi\right)=I\left(r\left(t,\overline{L}\left(t^{-}\right),L\left(t\right)=L\left(t^{-}\right),\overline{A}\left(t^{-}\right),\psi\right)>0\right)$$
$$=I\left(\left(1,L\left(t^{-}\right),A\left(t-\delta\right)\right)\psi>0\right).$$

Thus $d_{op}\left(t,\overline{L}\left(t^{-}\right),\overline{A}\left(t^{-}\right),\psi\right)=I\left[A\left(t-\delta\right)<\left\{\psi_{1}+\psi_{2}L\left(t\right)\right\}/\psi_{3}\right]$ if $\psi_{3}<0$. Suppose that $\psi_{3}^{\dagger}=2\,\psi_{1}^{\dagger}<0$ and $\psi_{2}^{\dagger}=0$ so $d_{op}\left(t,\overline{L}\left(t^{-}\right),\overline{A}\left(t^{-}\right),\psi^{\dagger}\right)=I\left[A\left(t-\delta\right)<1/2\right]$. Then the optimal regime for a subject starting at time 0 is to take treatment until time δ, to take no treatment from δ to 2δ, to again take treatment from 2δ to 3δ and continue alternating thereafter as we saw before. Suppose we tried to replace $A\left(t-\delta\right)$ by $A\left(t-\right)=\lim_{\delta\uparrow t}A\left(\delta\right)$ but kept the same parameter values. Then as above, we have a contradiction as the optimal regime for a subject starting from time zero is not defined, because treatment cannot alternate infinitely quickly.

9 Some Important Alternative Approaches:

Results in Sections 1-8 rely on two assumptions that will never be strictly correct: the first that our optimal drSNMM is correct and the second that either (but not necessarily both) a low dimensional model for the conditional law of treatment or a low dimensional model for the mean of the counterfactual utility given the past is correct. In this section, we relax both assumptions, although not simultaneously. To accomplish this, we use recent results of van der Laan and Dudoit (2003) on model selection via cross-validation and of Robins and van der Vaart (2003,2004) on adaptive non-parametric confidence intervals and inference based on higher order influence functions. Robins and van der Vaart (2004) consider simultaneously relaxing both assumptions.

Selection of a Candidate Optimal Treatment Regime by Cross-Validation

In this section we study a frequentist approach to selecting a single best candidate for the optimal treatment regime using cross-validation regime. The motivation for the method relies heavily on recent work by Wegkamp (2003) and, more particularly and crucially, van der Laan and Dudoit (2003) on model selection by cross-validation. For the remainder of this subsection we assume sequential randomization (i.e. no unmeasured confounders). A major limitation of the methods we proposed in sections 1-5 is the assumption that we have a correctly specified parametric dr SNMM model $\gamma^{\overline{d}^*}\left(\overline{l}_m, \overline{a}_m; \psi\right)$ with true parameter $\psi^\dagger$ for the very high dimensional function $\gamma^{\overline{d}, \overline{d}^*}\left(\overline{l}_m, \overline{a}_m\right)$ determining the optimal regime. Here rather than assuming a single correct model we will assume a large list of candidate models $\gamma^j\left(\overline{l}_m, \overline{a}_m; \psi^j\right)$, $j = 1, ..., J$ for the optimal regime where we have dropped the $\overline{d}^*$ from the notation and ψ^j denotes the parameter vector corresponding to the jth model. Further, we will no longer assume that any of the J models are true. Rather our approach will be as follows. We will randomly split the n study subjects into two subsamples - the estimation subsample and the validation subsample. We will obtain estimates $\widehat{\psi}^j$ by fitting each of the J models to the estimation subsample. We will use the validation subsample to select among the candidates.

The Single Decision Problem:

We begin with the single occassion problem. Thus suppose we have n iid copies of data $O = (A, L, Y)$. Then $d_{op}(l) = \arg\max_{a \in \mathcal{A}} \gamma(l, a)$ where $\gamma(l, a) = E\left(Y_a | L = l\right) - E\left(Y_{a=0} | L = l\right)$. We assume sequential randomization but now leave $\gamma(l, a)$ unspecified. In terms of the distribution F_O of the observables randomization implies that

$$E\left(Y | A = a, L = l\right) - E\left(Y | A = 0, L = l\right) = \gamma(l, a) \tag{9.1}$$

and thus that $E\left[Y - \gamma(L, A) | A, L\right] = E\left\{Y - \gamma(L, A) | L\right\} = E\left(Y | A = 0, L = l\right) = E\left(Y_{a=0} | L = l\right)$, i.e., $E\left[H | A, L\right] = E\left[H | L\right] =$ with $H = Y - \gamma(L, A)$.

A First Risk Function:

The key to the first approach employed in this section is the following characterization theorem for $\gamma(l, a)$ of (9.1). Let $E\left[\cdot\right]$ denote expectation with respect to the distribution F_O generating the data and let $E^*[\cdot]$ denote an expectation with respect to an arbitary distribution F^*. Then we have the following.

Theorem 9.1:(i): If $E^*[Y - \gamma(L, A)|L] = E[Y - \gamma(L, A)|L]$, then, for any $g(l)$ such that $g(L) \neq 0$ w.p.1, $\gamma(l, a)$ of (9.1) is the unique function $c(L, A)$ minimizing

$$E\left[g^2(L)\{Y - c(L, A) - E^*[Y - c(L, A)|L]\}^2\right] \qquad (9.2)$$

subject to $c(L, 0) = 0$;

(ii): For all functions $b(l)$ and $g(l)$ such that $g(L) \neq 0$ w.p.1, $\gamma(l, a)$ of (9.1) is the unique function $c(L, A)$ minimizing

$$E\left[g^2(L)\{Y - c(L, A) + E[c(L, A)|L] - b(L)\}^2\right] \qquad (9.3)$$

subject to $c(L, 0) = 0$

Proof: To prove (ii), write $\{Y - c(L, A)\}g(L) - g(L)b(L) + E[g(L)c(L, A)|L]$ as $R + S(c)$, where $R = \{Y - \gamma(L, A)\}g(L) - g(L)b(L) + E[g(L)\gamma(L, A)|L]$ and $S(c) = \{\gamma(L, A) - c(L, A)\}g(L) - E[g(L)\gamma(L, A)|L] + E[g(L)c(L, A)|L]$. Then (9.3) is $E[R^2] + 2E[RS(c)] + E[S^2(c)]$. Thus $c(L, A)$ minimizing (9.3) is the minimizer of $2E[RS(c)] + E[S^2(c)]$. But $E[RS(c)] = 0$ because $E[S(c)|L] = 0$ so $E[RS(c)] = E[\{Y - \gamma(L, A)\}g(L)S(c)] = E[E\{Y - \gamma(L, A)|L, A\}g(L)S(c)]$
$= E[E(Y|A = 0, L)g(L)E[S(c)|L]] = 0$. Finally $E[S^2(c)]$ takes it minimum at 0 when $\gamma(L, A) = c(L, A)$.

To prove (i), write $\{Y - c(L, A)\}g(L) - g(L)E^*[Y - c(L, A)|L]$ as $R^* + S^*(c)$ where $R^* = \{Y - \gamma(L, A)\}g(L) - g(L)E^*[Y - \gamma(L, A)|L]$ and $S^*(c) = \{\gamma(L, A) - c(L, A)\}g(L) - g(L)E^*[\gamma(L, A) - c(L, A)|L]$. Note $R^* = \{Y - \gamma(L, A)\}g(L) - g(L)E[Y - \gamma(L, A)|L]$ under the supposition of the theorem. Thus $c(L, A)$ minimizing (9.2) is the minimizer of $2E[R^*S^*(c)] + E[S^{*2}(c)]$. But $E[R^*S^*(c)] = 0$ because $E[R^*|A, L] = 0$. Finally $E[S^{*2}(c)]$ takes it minimum at 0 when $\gamma(L, A) = c(L, A)$.

Corollary 9.1: Doubly Robust Minimizer of Risk:
If $E^*[Y - \gamma(L, A)|L] = E[Y - \gamma(L, A)|L]$ or $E^*[c(L, A)|L] = E[c(L, A)|L]$ for all $c(L, A)$, then for all functions $g(l)$ such that $g(L) \neq 0$ w.p.1, $\gamma(l, a)$ of (9.1) is the unique function $c(L, A)$ minimizing $risk(c, F^*, g) = E[Loss(c, F^*, g)]$ with $Loss(c, F^*, g) = loss(O, c, F^*, g) =$

$$g^2(L)\{[Y - c(L, A)] - E^*[Y - c(L, A)|L]\}^2 \qquad (9.4)$$

subject to $c(L, 0) = 0$.

Proof: If $E^*[Y - \gamma(L, A)|L] = E[Y - \gamma(L, A)|L]$ this follows immediately from Theorem 9.1(i). If $E^*[c(L, A)|L] = E[c(L, A)|L]$, the corollary follows from Theorem 9.1(ii) upon writing $risk(c, F^*, g)$ as

$$E\left[\{[Y - c(L, A)]g(L) + g(L)E^*[c(L, A)|L] - g(L)b(L)\}^2\right] \text{ with } b(L) = E^*[Y|L].$$

Corollary 9.1 provides a characterization of $\gamma(L, A)$ as the minimizer over functions $c(L, A)$ of the particular risk function $risk(c, F^*, g)$. Suppose we have data from a randomized trial with known randomization probabilities $p(a|l)$, say $p(a|l) = 1/2$, and choose F^* such that $F^*_{A|L}$ is $F_{A|L}$ generating the data and $E^*(Y|L)$ is set to a fixed function $b(L)$. We use $F_{A|L}, b$ as shorthand for this F^* and so write $risk(c, F^*, g)$ as $risk(c, F_{A|L}, b, g)$.

Suppose one is given J candidates models $\gamma^j(L, A, \psi^j), j = 1, ..., J$, for $\gamma(L, A)$ where the dimension of ψ^j and the function $\gamma^j(.,.,.)$ can vary with j, and, based only on the estimation (i.e training) sample data, locally efficient estimators $\widehat{\psi}^j$ of ψ^j and thus $\widehat{\gamma}^j(L, A) = \gamma^j\left(L, A, \widehat{\psi}^j\right)$ of $\gamma^j(L, A, \psi^j)$ are obtained as in Sections 3 and 4. Then given user-supplied functions $b(l)$ and $g(l)$ we select the index $\widehat{j}$ minimizing $\widehat{risk}\left(\widehat{\gamma}^j, F_{A|L}, b, g\right) = P^{val}_{n^{val}}\left[Loss\left(\widehat{\gamma}^j, F_{A|L}, b, g\right)\right] =$

$P^{val}_{n^{val}}\left[g^2(L)\left\{Y - \widehat{\gamma}^j(L, A) - b(L) + E\left[\widehat{\gamma}^j(L, A)|L\right]\right\}^2\right]$ over the J candidates functions $\widehat{\gamma}^j$ where $P^{val}_{n^{val}}[\cdot]$ is the sample average over the validation sample. Let j_{oracle} be the j minimizing $risk\left(\widehat{\gamma}^j, F_{A|L}, b, g\right)$

$= E\left[g^2(L)\left\{Y - \widehat{\gamma}^j(L, A) - b(L) + E\left[\widehat{\gamma}^j(L, A)|L\right]\right\}^2\right]$. If our goal were to minimize $risk\left(\widehat{\gamma}^j, F_{A|L}, b, g\right)$ over our J candidates, $\widehat{\gamma}^{j_{oracle}}(L, A)$ is the optimal but unobtainable solution. However van der Laan and Dudoit (1993) show that, with high probability, provided the number of models J is not too large compared to n, $risk\left(\widehat{\gamma}^{\widehat{j}}, F_{A|L}, b, g\right)$ is very close to $risk\left(\widehat{\gamma}^{j_{oracle}}, F_{A|L}, b, g\right)$ even though $\widehat{j}$ only minimized $\widehat{risk}\left(\widehat{\gamma}^j, F_{A|L}, b, g\right)$. Indeed, the number of candidates J can increase as $e^{(n^\alpha)}$ with $\alpha < 1$ and yet, under regularity conditions, $risk\left(\widehat{\gamma}^{\widehat{j}}, F_{A|L}, b, g\right)/risk\left(\widehat{\gamma}^{j_{oracle}}, F_{A|L}, b, g\right)$ will still approach 1 as $n \to \infty$.

One might reasonably wonder why, if we are nearly certain that model j is misspecified, we use the locally efficient estimator $\widehat{\psi}^j$ to estimate the parameter ψ^j, since the desirable properties of $\widehat{\psi}^j$ described above only hold if model j is correctly specified. Our justification is (i) $\widehat{\psi}^j$ should perform well if model j is correct or nearly correct and (ii) if model j is far wrong our cross validation procedure will appropriately eliminate model j from consideration.

Remark on Marginal drSNMMs: The usefulness of having $\widehat{\psi}^j$ correct or nearly correct suggests one might use as candidates at least some optimal marginal drSNMMs with discrete W_m for the reasons described in the final paragraph of Section 7.3.

Minus Expected Utility As A Better Risk Function:

Given these encouraging results for our cross-validated selected model, the question becomes: Is minimizing $risk\left(\widehat{\gamma}^j, F_{A|L}, b, g\right)$ over our J candidates really the optimization criteria we wish to use when the true optimal function of interest $\gamma = \gamma(A, L)$ is unknown. Now, of course, our goal is not to minimize $risk\left(\widehat{\gamma}^{j}, F_{A|L}, b, g\right)$ over our J available candidates but rather to maximize expected utility $E\left[Y_{\widehat{d}_{op}^{j}}\right]$ (i.e to minimize the risk $E\left[-Y_{\widehat{d}_{op}^{j}}\right]$ of the loss $-Y_{\widehat{d}_{op}^{j}}$) over the J candidates $\widehat{\gamma}^{j}$ where, we write $\widehat{d}_{op}^{j}$ (or sometimes even d_{op}^{j}) as short-hand for $d_{op}^{\widehat{\gamma}^{j}}$ and, as usual, $d_{op}^{\widehat{\gamma}^{j}} = d_{op}^{\widehat{\gamma}^{j}}(l) = \arg\max_{a}\widehat{\gamma}^{j}(a, l)$. To be explict about the distinction, suppose that we have a dichotomous treatment only taking the values 1 or 0 so $\gamma(A, L)$ can be written $A\gamma(L)$ for some function $\gamma(L)$. Then any candidate function $c(a, l) = ac(l)$ for $\gamma(a, l)$ is associated with a candidate optimal regime $d_{op}^{c}(l) = \arg\max_{a} c(a, l) = I\{c(l) > 0\}$ while the true optimal regime $d_{op}(l) = d_{op}^{\gamma}(l)$ is $I\{\gamma(l) > 0\}$. Now the expected utility of c is $E\left[Y_{d_{op}^{c}}\right] = E[I\{c(L) > 0\}Y_{a=1}] + E[I\{c(L) \le 0\}Y_{a=0}] = E[I\{c(L) > 0\}\gamma(L)] + E[Y_{a=0}]$ while $E\left[Y_{d_{op}}\right] = E[I\{\gamma(L) > 0\}\gamma(L)] + E[Y_{a=0}]$. Thus it is clear that $\sup_{c}E\left[Y_{d_{op}^{c}}\right] = E\left[Y_{d_{op}}\right]$ and that the supremum is attained not only at γ but at any c^{*} for which the sets $\{l; c^{*}(l) > 0\} = \{l; \gamma(l) > 0\}$ on which c^{*} and γ are positive are equal. Thus one also can characterize the optimal regime(s) as the maximizer over c of $E[I\{c(L) > 0\}c^{*}(L)] + E[Y_{a=0}]$ as well as the oracle maximizer $\widehat{\gamma}^{j_{util-orac}}$ of the expected utility $E[I\{c(L) > 0\}\gamma(L)] + E[Y_{a=0}]$. However this last result does not imply that, if one has only J candidates $\widehat{\gamma}^{j}(a, l)$ available (none of which typically includes any optimal regime), the oracle $\widehat{\gamma}^{j^{*}}$ that maximizes $E[I\{\widehat{\gamma}^{j}(L) > 0\}c^{*}(L)]$ will have expected utility $E\left[Y_{\widehat{d}_{op}^{j^{*}}}\right]$ close to the expected utility $E\left[Y_{\widehat{d}_{op}^{j_{util-orac}}}\right]$ of the oracle maximizer $\widehat{\gamma}^{j_{util-orac}}$ of expected utility $E[I\{\widehat{\gamma}^{j}(L) > 0\}\gamma(L)] + E[Y_{a=0}]$ over $j = 1, ..., J$.

Likewise, the maximizer $\widehat{\gamma}^{j_{oracle}}$ of $risk\left(\widehat{\gamma}^{j}, F_{A|L}, b, g\right)$ over the J candidates may have expected utility $E\left[Y_{\widehat{d}_{op}^{j_{oracle}}}\right]$ much less than $E\left[Y_{\widehat{d}_{op}^{j_{util-orac}}}\right]$, even though $risk\left(c, F_{A|L}, b, g\right)$, $E[I\{c(L) > 0\}c^{*}(L)]$ and $E[I\{c(L) > 0\}\gamma(L)]$ are all maximized over all c by γ. The result in the preceding clause is only useful in an asymptopia which, with realistic sized samples and L high dimesional, we can never reach.

Remark A: The point being made here is different from the equally valid point that even if we are fortunate and one of the J models $\gamma^{j}\left(L, A, \psi^{j}\right)$ happens to be correctly specifed, i.e., $\gamma^{j_{correct}}\left(\cdot, \cdot, \psi^{\dagger j_{correct}}\right) = \gamma(\cdot, \cdot)$ for some $j_{correct}$ and some parameter value $\psi^{\dagger j_{correct}}$, if $\psi^{\dagger j_{correct}}$ is sufficiently high dimensional, the huge variability of $\widehat{\psi}^{j_{correct}}$ compared to the smaller variablity of the $\widehat{\psi}^{j}$ of incorrectly specified lower dimensional models may mean that, with high probability, $\widehat{\gamma}^{j_{correct}}$ does much worse with respect to $risk\left(c, F_{A|L}, b, g\right)$, $E[I\{c(L) > 0\}c^{*}(L)]$ and $E[I\{c(L) > 0\}\gamma(L)]$ than the corresponding aforementioned oracles.

If we had an unbiased estimator of expected utility $E\left[Y_{d_{op}^{c}}\right] = E[I\{c(L) > 0\}\gamma(L)] + E[Y_{a=0}]$ or $E[I\{c(L) > 0\}\gamma(L)]$ we could use cross validation, as we did with $risk\left(c, F_{A|L}, b, g\right)$, to obtain an estimator whose expected utility was close to that of the oracle maximizer $\widehat{\gamma}^{j_{util-orac}}$ and all would seem well.

Now for any $d = d(l)$ an unbiased estimator of $E[Y_d]$ under sequential randomization with $p(a|l)$ known and A discrete is the Horvitz-Thompson-like estimator $P_n[YI\{A = d(L)\}/p(A|L)]$. Thus for any candidate $c(a,l)$ for $\gamma(a,l)$ with associated candidate optimal regime

$d_{op}^c(l) = \arg\max_a c(a,l)$, $P_n[YI\{A = d_{op}^c(L)\}/p(A|L)]$ is an unbiased estimator of $E\left[Y_{d_{op}^c}\right]$. Thus, under van der Laan and Dudoit's regularity conditions, the $\widehat{\gamma}^{j_{util}}$ maximizing $P_{n_{val}}^{val}\left[YI\{A = d_{op}^{\widehat{\gamma}^j}(L)\}/p(A|L)\right]$ has expected utility $E\left[Y_{d_{op}^{\widehat{\gamma}^{j_{util}}}}\right]$ close to expected utility $E\left[Y_{d_{op}^{\widehat{\gamma}^{j_{util-orac}}}}\right]$ of the utility oracle, provided J is not too large. Thus it appears, at least in the one occasion problem, we have developed a quite reasonable approach that selects $d_{op}^{\widehat{\jmath}_{util}}(l) = \arg\max_a \gamma^{\widehat{\jmath}_{util}}\left(a,l,\widehat{\psi}^{\widehat{\jmath}_{util}}\right)$ as the estimated optimal regime with which to treat new patients.

Remaining philosophical and practical difficulties:

But there are remaining philosophical and practical difficulties. For example consider using the data from a study of a population with distribution F to determine the optimal regime for a new and different population in which Y_a has the same conditional distribution given L as the study population but $f_{new}(l) \neq f(l)$. The expected utility of a candidate optimal regime $c(l,a)$ in the new population is then $E\left[\{YI\{A = d_{op}^c(L)\}/p(A|L)\}w(L)\right]$ with weight function $w(L) = f_{new}(L)/f(L)$ which is still maximized over all c at $c = \gamma$ but is no longer necessarily maximixed over the J candidates $\widehat{\gamma}^j$ at $\widehat{\gamma}^{j_{util-orac}}$ because of the weight function $w(L) = f_{new}(L)/f(L)$. Thus, all would agree that cross validation of the $\widehat{\gamma}^j$ should be done by maximizing $P_{n_{val}}^{val}\left[\{YI\{A = d_{op}^{\widehat{\gamma}^j}(L)\}/p(A|L)\}w(L)\right]$ if reasonable smooth and reliable estimates of the densities $f_{new}(L)$ and $f(L)$ can be obtained.

The Single Patient Problem : But now consider a single new patient with $L_{new} = l$ for whom a physician needs to select a treatment. The patient certainly constitutes a population with a point mass at $L = l$. Now even if there were a validation sample member with $L = l$, the above maximization would be based on just that one validation sample member, and thus is too variable to be useful. But why should the physician be interested in the loss $-E\left[Y_{d_{op}^{\widehat{\gamma}^j}}\right]$ for a candidate regime $\widehat{\gamma}^j$ rather than, for example, $-E\left[Y_{d_{op}^{\widehat{\gamma}^j}}|L \in rel\right]$ where rel is a subset of covariate values that includes his patient's l, excludes values of l the physician believes irrelevant for determining treatment for his patient, and that contains a sufficiently large fraction of the validation sample so that the expected utility of the $\widehat{\gamma}^j$ selected by cross-validation restricted to validations member with $L \in rel$ will be close to the oracle maximizer over the $\widehat{\gamma}^j$ of $E\left[Y_{d_{op}^{\widehat{\gamma}^j}}|L \in rel\right]$. For example in an AIDS study suppose the CD4 count of the patient was 100. Then the physician might include in rel only the 60%, say, of validation subjects with CD4 counts less than 250. The use of rel is a special case of a more general strategy wherein the physician would use $d_{op}^{\widehat{j}_w}$ with $\widehat{j}_w$ the j that maximizes $P_{n^{val}}^{val}\left[\left\{YI\left\{A=d_{op}^{\widehat{\gamma}^j}(L)\right\}/p(A|L)\right\}w(L)\right]$ for a weight function $w(l)$ supplied by the physician that attains its maximum height at his patient's l, and has relatively less height at those l's the physician believes less relevant to his patient. Determining how quickly $w(l)$ plummets from its maximum is a classic variance bias trade off since the more peaked is $w(l)$ (i) the greater is the probability (owing to sampling variability) that the w-risk $E\left[\left\{YI\left\{A=d_{op}^{\widehat{j}_w}(L)\right\}/p(A|L)\right\}w(L)\right]$ of the selected model $\widehat{\gamma}^{\widehat{j}_w}$ differs greatly from the $w-risk$ $E\left[\left\{YI\left\{A=d_{op}^{j_w,util-orac}(L)\right\}/p(A|L)\right\}w(L)\right]$ of the $w-$oracle regime $\widehat{\gamma}^{j_w,util-orac}$ that maximizes $E\left[\left\{YI\left\{A=d_{op}^{\widehat{\gamma}^j}(L)\right\}/p(A|L)\right\}w(L)\right]$, but (ii) the less the (doctor's subjective) probability of large bias where we measure bias as the absolute difference between the oracle $w-$risk and the oracle $patient$-risk $\max_j E\left[\left\{YI\left\{A=d_{op}^{\widehat{\gamma}^j}(L)\right\}/p(A|L)\right\}w_{patient}(L)\right]$ and the patient-risk $E\left[\left\{YI\left\{A=d_{op}^{j_w,util-orac}(L)\right\}/p(A|L)\right\}w_{patient}(L)\right]$ of the $w-$oracle regime $\widehat{\gamma}^{j_w,util-orac}$, where $w_{patient}(l)=0$ for all l other than the patient's. To help understand the doctor's subjective probability of bias suppose, after defining the subset rel based on his own knowledge base, the doctor was persuaded by others that the (i) some of the proposers of the optimal regime SNNMs $\gamma^j\left(a,l,\psi^j\right)$ had an understanding of the relevant biology superior to his and, therefore, (ii) to the extent their models $\gamma^j\left(a,l,\psi\right)$ borrow information from subjects with $l \notin rel$ to estimate the effect of treatment at his patient's $l \in rel$ (say, by assuming $\gamma^j\left(a,l,\psi^j\right)=a\gamma^j\left(l,\psi^j\right)$ had a quadratic dependence $\psi_1^j CD4 + \psi_2^j CD4^2$ over the entire CD4 range), this decison to borrow is based on sound biological knowledge. In that case the physician might assume that the oracle $w-$risk even for $w(l)$ constant would not differ greatly from the oracle $patient$-risk so to decrease variability the doctor would choose treatment simply by maximizing $P_{n^{val}}^{val}\left[\left\{YI\left\{A=d_{op}^{\widehat{\gamma}^j}(L)\right\}/p(A|L)\right\}\right]$. But if the doctor could not be so persuaded he would use a non-constant weight function. Software to allow the doctor to input a his preferred weight function and to select among the J offered treatment by cross-validation could be implemented. Clearly it would be important to derive the distribution of and confidence intervals for the difference between the w-risk $E\left[\left\{YI\left\{A=d_{op}^{\widehat{j}_w}(L)\right\}/p(A|L)\right\}w(L)\right]$ of the randomly selected model $\widehat{\gamma}^{\widehat{j}_w}$ and the oracle $w-risk$

$E\left[\left\{YI\left\{A=d_{op}^{j_w,util-orac}\left(L\right)\right\}/p\left(A|L\right)\right\}w\left(L\right)\right]$, as a function of $J, n, w\left(\cdot\right)$, and various other parameters. This is an open statistical problem.

Adding Regimes by Voting : When one is given a collection of J candidate regimes $d_{op}^{\hat{\gamma}^j}\left(l\right)$ it is natural to add one or more regimes to the collection before choosing among them using the above methods. Specifically we add the "vote regime" $d_{op}^{vote}\left(l\right)$ that selects $\arg\max_a\left(\sum_j I\left(d_{op}^{\hat{\gamma}^j}\left(l\right)=a\right)\right)$ that selects the most recommended regime. If several values of a tie at a given l then add both regimes, unless the combinatorics from ties at different values of l would add a prohibitively large numer of *vote* regimes; in that case, one can select randomly among ties.

Continuous Treatment: Suppose now that the treatment A is continuous with conditional density given L absolutely continuous wrt Lebesgue measure rather than binary. For example A may represent the number of milligrams of a drug that one takes and all take some, but differing amounts of the drug. In that case even when $p\left(A|L\right)$ is known, there exists no unbiased estimator of $E\left[Y_d\right]=E\left[E\{Y|A=d\left(L\right),L\}\right]$. For example $P_{n^{val}}^{val}\left[YI\left\{A=d\left(L\right)\right\}/p\left(A|L\right)\right]$ is undefined since the event $I\left\{A=d\left(L\right)\right\}$ is 0 with probability one. Nonetheless $P_{n^{val}}^{val}\left[Loss\left(c,F_{A|L},b,g\right)\right]$ remains an unbiased estimate of $risk\left(c,F_{A|L},b,g\right)=E\left[Loss\left(c,F_{A|L},b,g\right)\right]$ so we can continue to estimate the less desirable risk function $risk\left(c,F_{A|L},b,g\right)$. An alternative, perhaps preferred, approach based on ideas in Murphy, van der Laan, and Robins (1998) and Gill and Robins (2001) is given a candidate $c\left(a,l\right)$ to convert d_{op}^c to a random regime p^c in which when $L=l$ we treat with A drawn from $p^c\left(a|l\right)$, where, say, $p^c\left(a|l\right)$ could be a uniform distribution with support on $\left(d_{op}^c\left(l\right)-\sigma,d_{op}^c\left(l\right)+\sigma\right)$ or more precisely on $\left(min\left\{d_{op}^c\left(l\right)-\sigma,a_{\min}\right\},min\left\{d_{op}^c\left(l\right)+\sigma,a_{\max}\right\}\right)$ where $a_{\min}$ and $a_{\max}$ are the extremes of ethically allowed doses and σ is a positive constant. Letting Y_{p^c} represent the counterfactual response under the random regime, the expected utility $E\left[Y_{p^c}\right]$ under $p^c\left(a|l\right)$ is $\int E\{Y|A=a,L\}p^c\left(a|L\right)dadF\left(l\right)=E\left[p^c\left(A|L\right)Y/p\left(A|L\right)\right]$ which admits the unbiased estimator $P_{n^{val}}^{val}\left[p^c\left(A|L\right)Y/p\left(A|L\right)\right]$ since $p^c\left(a|l\right)$ is absoutely continuous with respect to $p\left(a|l\right)$. Now we would wish to choose σ very small so that the $E\left[Y_{p^{\hat{\gamma}^j}}\right]$ approximate the $E\left[Y_{d^{\hat{\gamma}^j}}\right]$, our utilities of interest. However this is not generally possible since σ must be chosen large enough for the expected utility of the random regime $p^{\hat{\gamma}^j}$ maximizing $P_{n^{val}}^{val}\left[Yp^{\hat{\gamma}^j}\left(A|L\right)/p\left(A|L\right)\right]$ over J to be close to oracle utility $max_j E\left[Yp^{\hat{\gamma}^j}\left(A|L\right)/p\left(A|L\right)\right]$. Having selected $\hat{\gamma}^j$ the question then remains whether to treat randomly with $p^{\hat{\gamma}^j}$ or deterministically with $d_{op}^{\hat{\gamma}^j}$ I would opt for the latter but with no strong justification.

Attempts to Acheive Double Robustness : Assume again A is binary and $w\left(L\right)=1$, but now suppose that, as in an observational study, $p\left(A|L\right)$ is unknown. Then, following van der Laan and Dudoit, we might try to construct doubly robust estimators of the risk $E\left[Y_{d_{op}^c}\right]$ of a candidate regime $c(a,l) =$ $ac(l)$ based on the following double robust identity (9.5).

Theorem (9.2): Let F^* be an arbitrary distribution. Then, under the assumption of no unmeasured confounders, if $p^*(A|L) = p(A|L)$ or $E^*[Y|A = d_{op}^c(L),L] = E[Y|A = d_{op}^c(L),L]$ then $E\left[Y_{d_{op}^c}\right]$ is given by

$$E\left[Y_{d_{op}^c}\right] \tag{9.5a}$$

$$= E\left[\frac{YI\left(A = d_{op}^c(L)\right)}{p^*(A|L)} - E^*[Y|A = d_{op}^c(L),L]\left(\frac{I\left(A = d_{op}^c(L)\right)}{p^*(A|L)} - 1\right)\right]$$

$$= E\left[\frac{I\left(A = d_{op}^c(L)\right)\left\{Y - E^*[Y|A = d_{op}^c(L),L]\right\}}{p^*(A|L)} + E^*[Y|A = d_{op}^c(L),L]\right]$$

$$\tag{9.5b}$$

It follows that the cross validated estimate of expected utility

$$P_{n^{val}}^{val}$$

$$\left[\frac{YI\{A = d_{op}^c(L)\}}{p(A|L;\widehat{\alpha})} - E[Y|A = d_{op}^c(L),L;;\widehat{\eta}]\left(\frac{I\left(A = d_{op}^c(L)\right)}{p(A|L;\widehat{\alpha})} - 1\right)\right]$$

will be a $n^{1/2}$ CAN estimator of $E\left[Y_{d_{op}^c}\right]$ if we have estimated from estimation sample or validation sample data parametric models $E[Y|A,L;\eta]$ and $p(A|L;\alpha)$ for $E[Y|A,L]$ and $p(A|L)$ and either (but not necessarily both) are correct. But note that $E[Y|A,L] = \{\gamma(A,L) + E[Y|A = 0,L]\}$. Now given a correct model $\gamma(A,L;\psi)$ for $\gamma(A,L)$, we are familiar from Sections 3 and 4 of having to model $p(A|L)$ or $E[Y|A = 0,L]$ correctly to obtain CAN estimates of the parameter ψ and thus of $\gamma(A,L)$ and $d_{op}(l)$. But now we find, that if our model for $E[Y|A = 0,L]$ is correct and our model for $p(A|L)$ is mispecified, we must still model $\gamma(A,L)$ correctly to obtain CAN estimates of the expected utilities $E\left[Y_{d_{op}^c}\right]$ of candidate regimes $d_{op}^c(l) = \arg\max_a c(a,l)$. One might suppose this is of no help for if we could specify a correct model $\gamma^{j_{correct}}(A,L,\psi^{j_{correct}})$ for $\gamma(A,L)$ and a correct model for $E[Y|A = 0,L]$, we could immediately obtain a CAN estimate $d_{op}(L)$, namely $\arg\max_a \gamma\left(A,L;\widehat{\psi}\right)$, where $\widehat{\psi}$ is the DR estimator of sections 3 and 4 without needing to resort to cross-validation. However, as discussed in Remark A just above, since our goal is to minimize expected utility based on a sample of size n if $\psi^{j_{correct}}$ is high dimesional so that $\widehat{\psi}^{j_{correct}}$ is highly variable, the model $j_{util-orac}$ that maximizes expected utility might not be the model $j_{correct}$ and thus our cross validation procedure would correctly and usefully fail to select model $j_{correct}$. Thus there is a meaningful, sense in which we can obtain useful cross-validated DR estimators of $E\left[Y_{d_{op}^c}\right]$ that are robust to misspecification of the model for $p(A|L)$.

The situation appears to be different if we decide to use $risk(c, F^*, g) = E[Loss(c, F^*, g)]$ as a criterion, where we recall that

$Loss(c, F^*, g) = loss(O, c, F^*, g) = g^2(L)\{[Y - c(L, A)] - E^*[Y - c(L, A)|L]\}^2$

and that, by Corollary (9.1), $\gamma(L, A)$ is the minimizer of $risk(c, F^*, g)$ over all c if (i) either $E^*[Y - \gamma(L, A)|L] = E[Y - \gamma(L, A)|L]$ or (ii) $E^*[c(L, A)|L] = E[c(L, A)|L]$ for all $c(L, A)$. Thus if we have estimated, from the estimation sample or validation sample data, a correct parametric model $p(A|L; \alpha)$ for $p(A|L)$, then

$\widehat{risk}\left(c, \widehat{F}_{A|L}, b, g\right) = P_{n^{val}}^{val}\left[g^2(L)\{Y - c(L, A) - b(L) + E[c(L, A)|L; \widehat{\alpha}]\}^2\right]$

is a CAN estimator of $risk(c, F^*, g)$ where $F^* = (F_{A|L}, b)$ satisifies (ii). If, separately for each candidate $c(L, A)$, we obtain, from estimation sample data or validation sample data, an estimate $\widehat{\varsigma}(c)$ of the fit of a correct parametric model $b(L; \varsigma)$ for $E[Y|A = 0, L]$ based on regressing $Y - c(L, A)$ on L wiith regression function $b(L; \varsigma)$, then $\widehat{risk}\left(c, \widehat{F}_{Y|A=0, L}, g\right) = P_{n^{val}}^{val}\left[g^2(L)\{Y - c(L, A) - b(L; \widehat{\varsigma}(c))\}^2\right]$

is a CAN estimator of $risk(c, F^*(c), g)$ where $F^*(c) = \left(F_{Y|A=0, L}^*(c)\right)$ satisifies (i) (since $F_{Y|A=0, L}^*(\gamma) = F_{Y|A=0, L}$). Thus, we see that, unlike when we used expected utility as a criterion, we can obtain a CAN estimator of a risk function $risk(c, F^*(c), g)$ that is minimized over c at $\gamma(L, A)$ if we have a correct model for $E[Y|A = 0, L]$. However in contrast to the spirit of the doubly robust estimators of $\gamma(L, A)$ studied in Sections 3 and 4, we cannot obtain a CAN estimator of a risk function $risk(c, F^*(c), g)$ that is minimized over c at $\gamma(L, A)$ when either (but not necessarily both) of the parametric models $b(L; \varsigma)$ and $p(A|L; \alpha)$ for $E[Y|A = 0, L]$ and $p(A|L)$ are correct. Thus a true double robustness property is lacking.

Beyond Double Robustness:

Heretofore we have assumed that we have been able to correctly specify either (but not necessarily both) models for the law of treatment A_m given the past or a model for the mean of $H_m(\psi^\dagger)$. With high dimensional data such an assumption will never be exactly true and so the question arises as to whether we can obtain additional robustness to misspecification beyond double robustness and if so what will be the cost in terms of variance. We investigate that question in this section using a new theory of higher dimensional influence functions based on $U-$ statistics due to Robins and van der Vaart (2004). We consider the simplest example in order to make the ideas clear. For more general examples see Robins and van der Vaart (2004). We do not consider the estimation of nonparametric $\gamma(A, L)$ as above but rather assume $\gamma(A, L) = \psi A$ and focus on estimating ψ.

Consider the analysis of the normal semiparametric regression model based on n iid observations $O_i = (Y_i, A_i, X_i)$

$$Y = \psi^\dagger A + b\left(X; \eta^\dagger\right) + e \tag{9.6}$$

where $e \sim N(0, 1)$, $b\left(X; \eta^\dagger\right)$ is an unknown function, and A is dichotomous. For simplicity we will assume the law of e is known. The law $F\left(a|X; \alpha^\dagger\right)$ of $A|X$ is unknown as is the law $F\left(x; \omega^\dagger\right)$ of X. We consider first the case with X discrete with either finite or countable support. All quantities will be allowed to depend on the sample size n, including the support of X and the true parameters generating the data. We suppress the dependence on n in the notation except for emphasis.

The likelihood with respect to a dominating measure for one observation is

$$f\left(O; \theta = (\psi, \eta, \alpha, \omega)\right) \tag{9.7}$$
$$= \phi\{Y - \psi A - b\left(X; \eta\right)\} f\left(A|X; \alpha\right) f\left(X; \omega\right); \theta \in \Theta = \Psi \times \mathcal{N} \times \mathring{A} \times \Omega$$

The following argument suggests that there should exist estimators that are superior to our doubly robust estimators. Our doubly robust estimators of $\psi^\dagger$ are (i) $n^{1/2}-$ consistent estimators if we succeed in specifying a correct lower dimensional model for either $b\left(X; \eta^\dagger\right)$ or $f\left(A|X; \alpha^\dagger\right)$ but (ii) our estimators are inconsistent if both models are incorrect. It seems logical to suppose that by specifying larger models for $b\left(X; \eta^\dagger\right)$ and/or $f\left(A|X; \alpha^\dagger\right)$ we should be able to obtain doubly robust confidence intervals and point estimators whose length and standard deviation are $n^{-\alpha}$ for $\alpha < 1/2$, thus allowing us to give up efficiency for further protection against bias. We shall see that this is indeed possible. Indeed this approach can result in triply robust or even infinitely robust (i.e. exactly unbiased) estimating functions in certain settings.

We will analyze this model using a new theory of higher order influence functions due to Robins and van der Vaart (2004) that extends the first order semiparametric efficiency theory of Bickel et al. (1993) and van der Vaart (1991) by incorporating the theory of higher order scores and Bhattacharrya bases due to McLeish and Small (1994) and Lindsay and Waterman (1996). The following follows the development in McLeish and Small (1994) in many aspects.

A Theory of Higher Order Influence Functions :

Suppose we observe n iid observations $O_i, i = 1, ..., n$, from a model $M(\Theta) = \{F(o; \theta), \theta \in \Theta\}$ and we wish to make inference on a particular functional $\widetilde{\psi}(F) \in R^{p^*}$ or equivalently $\psi(\theta) = \widetilde{\psi}(F(\theta))$. In general the functional $\widetilde{\psi}(F)$ can infinite dimensional but here for simplicity we only consider consider the finite dimensional case.

Given a possibly vector valued function $b(\varsigma)$, $\varsigma = \{\varsigma_1, ..., \varsigma_p\}^T$, define for $m = 0, 1, 2$, $b_{\backslash i_1 ... i_m}(\varsigma) = \partial^m b(\varsigma) / \partial \varsigma_{i_1} ... \partial \varsigma_{i_m}$ with $i_s \in \{1, ..., p\}$, for $s = 1, 2, ..., m$ where the $\backslash$ symbol denotes differentiation by the variables occurring to its right. Given a sufficiently smooth $p-$ dimensional parametric submodel $\widetilde{\theta}(\varsigma)$ mapping $\varsigma \in R^p$ injectively into Θ, define $\psi_{\backslash i_1 ... i_m}(\theta)$ to be

$$\left(\psi \circ \widetilde{\theta}\right)_{\backslash i_1 \ldots i_m}(\varsigma)\big|_{\varsigma = \widetilde{\theta}^{-1}\{\theta\}} \text{ and } f_{\backslash i_1 \ldots i_m}(\mathbf{O};\theta) \text{ to be } \left(f \circ \widetilde{\theta}\right)_{\backslash i_1 \ldots i_m}(\varsigma)\big|_{\varsigma = \widetilde{\theta}^{-1}\{\theta\}}$$

where $f(\mathbf{O};\theta) \triangleq \prod_{i=1}^{n} f(O_i;\theta)$ and each $i_s \in \{1,...,p\}$.

Definition of a kth order estimation influence function: A vector U-statistic $U_k(\theta) = u_k(\mathbf{O};\theta)$ of order k, dimension of p^* of $\psi(\theta)$ and finite variance is said to be an kth order estimation influence function for $\psi(\theta)$ if (i) $E_\theta[U_k(\theta)] = 0$, $\theta \in \Theta$ and (ii) for $m = 1, 2, \ldots, k$, and every suitably smooth p dimensional parametric submodel $\widetilde{\theta}(\varsigma)$, $p = 1, 2, \ldots$,

$$\psi_{\backslash i_1 \ldots i_m}(\theta) = E_\theta\left[U_k(\theta) S_{i_1 \ldots i_m}(\theta)\right]$$

where $S_{i_1 \ldots i_m}(\theta) \triangleq f_{\backslash i_1 \ldots i_m}(\mathbf{O};\theta)/f(\mathbf{O};\theta)$. We refer to $S_{i_1 \ldots i_m}(\theta)$ as an mth order score associated with the model $\widetilde{\theta}(\varsigma)$. If $\psi_{\backslash i_1 \ldots i_m}(\theta) = 0$, we refer to $S_{i_1 \ldots i_m}(\theta)$ as an estimation nuisance score.

Remark: The scores $S_{i_1 \ldots i_m}(\theta)$ are U statistics of order m. For later use it will be useful here to collect formula for the an arbitrary score $S_{i_1 \ldots i_s}(\theta)$ of order s in terms of the subject specific scores $S_{i_1 \ldots i_m, j}(\theta) = f_{/i_1 \ldots i_m, j}(O_j;\theta)/f_j(O_j;\theta), j = 1, \ldots, n$ for $s = 1, 2, 3$. Resullts in Waterman and Lindsay (1996) imply

$$S_{i_1} = \sum_j S_{i_1, j} \tag{9.8a}$$

$$S_{i_1 i_2} = \sum_j S_{i_1 i_2, j} + \sum_{l \neq j} S_{i_1, j} S_{i_2, l} \tag{9.8b}$$

$$S_{i_1 i_2 i_3} = \sum_j S_{i_1 i_2 i_3, j} + \sum_{l \neq j} S_{i_1 i_2, j} S_{i_3, l} + S_{i_3 i_2, j} S_{i_1, l} + S_{i_1 i_3, j} S_{i_2, l} + \sum_{l \neq j \neq t} S_{i_1, j} S_{i_2, l} S_{i_3, t} \tag{9.8c}$$

Note these formulae are examples of the following canonical representation of an arbitrary s^{th} order U statistic.

$$U_m = \sum_{m=1}^{m=s} D_m \tag{9.9}$$

$$D_m(\theta) = \sum_{\{i_1 \neq i_2 \neq \ldots \neq i_m; i_l \in \{1,2,\ldots,n\}, l \in =1,\ldots,m\}} d_m(O_{i_1}, O_{i_2}, \ldots, O_{i_m}),$$

For all m and $l, 1 \leq l \leq m$, with $O_{-i_l} = \left(O_{i_1}, \ldots O_{i_{l-2}}, O_{i_{l-1}}, O_{i_{l+1}}, O_{i_{l+2}} \ldots, O_{i_m}\right)$

$$E\left[d_m(O_{i_1}, O_{i_2}, \ldots, O_{i_m})|O_{-i_l}\right] = 0,$$

$d_m(O_{i_1}, O_{i_2}, \ldots, O_{i_m})$ need not be symmetric in $O_{i_1}, O_{i_2}, \ldots, O_{i_m}$

We also consider a U statistic of order $m < s$ to also be a U statistic of order s with $d_j\left(O_{i_1}, O_{i_2}, \ldots, O_{i_j}\right) = 0$ for $s \geq j > m$.

Estimation influence functions will be useful for deriving point estimators of ψ with small bias and for deriving interval estimators centered on an estimate of ψ. We also define testing influence functions both to test hypotheses about ψ and to form confidence intervals for ψ whose expected length may be less than that of intervals based on an estimation influence function.

Definition of a kth order testing influence function: A U-statistic $U_k(\theta) = u_k(\mathbf{O};\theta)$ of order k, dimension p^*, and finite variance is said to be an kth order testing influence function for testing $\psi(\theta) = \psi^\dagger$ if in the restricted model $M(\Theta(\psi^\dagger)) = M(\Theta) \cap \{F; \widetilde{\psi}(F) = \psi^\dagger\}$ (i.e the submodel with parameter space $\Theta(\psi^\dagger) = \Theta \cap \{\theta; \psi(\theta) = \psi^\dagger\}$) (i) $E_\theta[U_k(\theta)] = 0$, $\theta \in \Theta(\psi^\dagger)$ and (ii) for $m = 1, 2, ..., k$, and every suitably smooth p dimensional parametric submodel $\widetilde{\theta}(\varsigma)$ with range $\Theta(\psi^\dagger)$, $p = 1, 2, ..., \psi_{\backslash i_1...i_m}(\theta) = E_\theta[U_k(\theta) S_{i_1...i_m}(\theta)]$ where $S_{i_1...i_m}(\theta) \triangleq f_{\backslash i_1...i_m}(\mathbf{O};\theta)/f(\mathbf{O};\theta)$. Since in model $M(\Theta(\psi^\dagger))$, $\psi_{\backslash i_1...i_m}(\theta) = 0$ for all $S_{i_1...i_m}(\theta)$, all scores are nuisance scores.

Remark: Suppose that $\psi(\theta) = \psi^\dagger$ and $U_k(\theta)$ is a kth order estimation influence function, then it is a kth order testing influence function, since every smooth submodel through θ in model $M(\Theta(\psi^\dagger))$ is a smooth submodel through θ in model $M(\Theta)$. Further the set of estimation nuisance scores includes the set of testing scores. The converses need not be true.

Remark: Henceforth, in any statement in which we do not mention whether the parameter space under consideration is $M(\Theta(\psi^\dagger))$ or $M(\Theta)$, our results hold for for both. When we wish to distinguish the 2 cases we use 'est' and 'test' to discriminate.

Definition of the Bias Function of a kth order influence function: We call $B_k[\theta^\dagger, \theta] = E_{\theta^\dagger}[U_k(\theta)]$ the bias function of $U_k(\theta)$.

Given a parametric submodel $\widetilde{\theta}(\varsigma)$, define $B_{k,i_1^*...i_m^* i_{m+1}...i_s}[\theta, \theta]$

$= \partial^s B_k\left[\widetilde{\theta}(\varsigma^*), \widetilde{\theta}(\varsigma)\right]/\partial\varsigma_{i_1}^* ... \partial\varsigma_{i_m}^* \partial\varsigma_{i_{m+1}} ... \partial\varsigma_{i_s}\big|_{\varsigma^*=\widetilde{\theta}^{-1}\{\theta\}, \varsigma=\widetilde{\theta}^{-1}\{\theta\}}$ where we reserve $*$ for differentiation with respect to the first argument of $B_k[\cdot, \cdot]$. Thus, under regularity conditions, by the definition of a kth order influence function $U_k(\theta)$, $B_{k,i_1^*...i_s^*}[\theta, \theta] = \psi_{\backslash i_1...i_s}(\theta)$.

The following Theorem is closely analagous to related results in McLeish and Small (1994).

Extended Information Equality Theorem: Given a kth order influence function $U_k(\theta)$, for all smooth submodels $\widetilde{\theta}(\varsigma)$ and all $i_1^*...i_m^* i_{m+1}...i_s$, $s \leq k$, (i) $B_{k,i_1^*...i_m^* i_{m+1}...i_s}[\theta, \theta] = 0$ if $s > m > 0$, but (ii) $B_{k,i_1^*...i_m^* i_{m+1}...i_s}[\theta, \theta] \equiv B_{k,i_1...i_s}[\theta, \theta] = -\psi_{\backslash i_1...i_s}(\theta)$ if $m = 0$

Proof: See Robins and van der Vaart (2004).

Let $V_m(\theta) = S_{i_1...i_m}(\theta)$ denote a generic m^{th} order score at θ in model Let $\{V_m(\theta)\}$ be the set of mth order scores at θ as we vary over both the parametric submodels $\widetilde{\theta}(\varsigma)$ of our model and the indices $i_1...i_m$. Let $\cup_{l=1}^{l=m}\{V_l(\theta)\}$ be the collection of scores of order m or less and $\overline{B}_m(\theta)$ be the closed linear span of $\cup_{l=1}^{l=m}\{V_l(\theta)\}$ in the Hilbert space $\mathcal{U}_m$ composed of all $U - statistics$ of order m with mean zero and finite variance and dimension of p^* of ψ with inner product defined by covariances with respect to the product measure $F^n(\cdot;\theta)..$ We refer to $\overline{B}_m(\theta)$ as the mth order tangent space for the model. $\overline{B}_m(\theta)$ is parametrization invariant and thus a "geometric quantity."

Repeating the above for the estimation nuisance scores $V_m^{est,nuis}(\theta)$ in the 'estimation' model with parameter space $M(\Theta)$, we refer to the closed linear span $\overline{\Lambda}_m(\theta)$ of $\cup_{l=1}^{l=m}\{V_m^{est,nuis}(\theta)\}$ to be the mth order estimation nuisance tangent space. We write $\overline{B}_m^{est}(\theta)$ and $\overline{\Lambda}_m^{est}(\theta)$ for the tangent space and nuisance tangent space in model $M(\Theta)$..We write $\overline{B}_m^{test}(\theta)$ for the tangent space in model $M(\Theta(\psi^\dagger))$. Note $\overline{B}_m^{test}(\theta) \subseteq \overline{\Lambda}_m^{est}(\theta) \subseteq \overline{B}_m^{est}(\theta)$.

Given any kth order estimation influence function $U_k^{est}(\theta)$, define $IF_k^{est}(\theta) = \Pi_\theta\left[U_k(\theta)|\overline{B}_k^{est}(\theta)\right]$ where the projection operator $\Pi_\theta[\cdot|\cdot]$ is the projection operator in the Hilbert space $\mathcal{U}_k(\theta)$. .

Efficient Influence Function Theorem : (i)$IF_k^{est}(\theta)$ is unique in the sense that for any two kth order influence functions $\Pi_\theta\left[U_k^{est(1)}(\theta)|\overline{B}_k^{est}(\theta)\right]$ and $\Pi_\theta\left[U_k^{est(2)}(\theta)|\overline{B}_k^{est}(\theta)\right]$ are equal almost surely.

(ii) $IF_k^{est}(\theta)$ is a kth order estimation influence function and has variance less than or equal to any other kth order estimation influence function.

(iii)$U_k(\theta)$ is a kth order estimation influence function if and only if $U_k(\theta) \in \left\{IF_k^{est}(\theta) + \overline{B}_k^{est,\perp}(\theta) ; \overline{B}_k^{est,\perp}(\theta) \in \overline{B}_k^{est,\perp}(\theta)\right\}$ where $\overline{B}_k^{est,\perp}(\theta)$ is the ortho-complement of $\overline{B}_k^{est}(\theta)$

(iv) For $m < k, \Pi\left[IF_k^{est}(\theta)|\overline{B}_m^{est}(\theta)\right] = IF_m^{est}(\theta)$

Proof: See Robins and van der Vaart (2004):

Definition of the kth order efficient influence function and variance: $IF_k^{est}(\theta)$ is referred to as the the kth order efficient estimation influence function and its variance as the kth order efficient estimation variance.

Consider again model $M(\Theta)$ with parameter space Θ. When the parameter space $\Theta = \prod_{r=1}^{r=R}\Theta_r$ is a cartesian product of sets Θ_r, so $\theta = (\theta_1,...\theta_R), \theta_r \in \Theta_r$,we say a parametric submodel $\tilde{\theta}(\varsigma), \varsigma \in \mathcal{Z}$, is variation independent wrt the Θ_r if $\varsigma = (\varsigma_1,...,\varsigma_R), \varsigma_r \in \mathcal{Z}_r, \mathcal{Z} = \prod_{r=1}^{r=R}\mathcal{Z}_r$, and $\tilde{\theta}(\varsigma) = \left(\tilde{\theta}_1(\varsigma),...,\tilde{\theta}_R(\varsigma)\right) = \left(\tilde{\theta}_1(\varsigma_1),...,\tilde{\theta}_R(\varsigma_R)\right)$ with $\tilde{\theta}_r(\varsigma_r) \in \Theta_r$. An m dimensional score $S_{i_1...i_m}(\theta)$ of a variation independent submodel is a member of a particular set of scores B_{mt_m} with generic member $V_{\theta_1^{t_{m1}},...,\theta_R^{t_{mR}}}$ where the t_{mr} are components of an R-vector $t_m = (t_{m1},...,t_{mR})$ satisfying $\sum_{r=1}^{R}t_{mr} = m$ with t_{mr} determined by $S_{i_1...i_m}(\theta)$ via $t_{mr} = \sum_{j=1}^{m}I(\varsigma_{i_j} \in \mathcal{Z}_r)$. The components t_{mr} tell how many of the m derivatives in $S_{i_1...i_m}(\theta)$ were with respect to components of ς that lay in $\mathcal{Z}_r$. We let $B_{mt_m} = \left\{V_{\theta_1^{t_{m1}},...,\theta_R^{t_{mR}}}\right\}$ denote the set of all order m scores of variation independent parametric submodels with a given value of t_m. Then in general $\overline{B}_k$ is the closed linear span of the union $\cup_{m=1}^{k}\cup_{\{t_m\}}B_{mt_m}$ of variation independent scores where $\cup_{\{t_m\}}refers$

to the *union* over all vectors of length R with nonnegative integer components whose components sum to m.

Example: If $m = 2$ and $R = 4$, the number of sets B_{2t_2} is 10 as there are 10 vectors of length 4 with nonnegative integer components whose components sum to 2.

Suppose the model can be parametrized as $\theta = (\psi, \gamma)$, $\psi \in \Psi, \gamma \in \Gamma, \Theta = \Psi \times \Gamma$ (at least locally). That is, in the above notation, with $\Theta = \prod_{r=1}^{r=2} \Theta_r$, we can then take $\Theta_1 = \Psi$ and $\Theta_2 = \Gamma$. We refer to the 1st order $(m = 1)$ scores $V_\gamma = V_{\gamma^1}$ as (pure) nuisance scores and $V_\psi = V_{\psi^1}$ as the score for ψ. For $m > 1$, we refer to generic scores (i) V_{γ^m} as mth order pure nuisance scores ; (ii) V_{ψ^m} as mth order scores for ψ and (iii) $V_{\psi^c \gamma^{m-c}}, m > c > 0$ as mth order mixed scores. The closed linear span of $\cup_{m=1}^k \{V_{\gamma^m}\}$ of all pure nuisance scores of order k or less is $\overline{B}_k^{test}$. The closed linear span $\left[\cup_{m=1}^k \{V_{\gamma^m}\}\right] \cup \left[\cup_{m=2}^k V_{\psi^m}\right] \cup \left[\cup_{m=1}^k \cup_{c=1}^{c=m-1} \{V_{\psi^c \gamma^{m-c}}\}\right]$ of all scores excepting the 1st order $(m = 1)$ score V_ψ for ψ is the estimation nuisance tangent space $\overline{\Lambda}_k^{est}(\theta)$. Finally the estimation tangent space $\overline{B}_k^{est}(\theta)$ is the closed linear span of all the scores of order k or less. Note if $\Theta = \prod_{r=1}^{r=R} \Theta_r$ and the likelihood for one observation factors as $f(O; \theta) = \prod_{r=1}^{r=R} L_r(\theta_r)$ and $S_{i_1 \dots i_R, j}(\theta)$ is a mixed score $V_{\theta_1 \theta_2 \dots \theta_R}$, then $S_{i_1 \dots i_R, j} = \prod_{r=1}^{r=R} S_{i_r, j}$.

Definition of the kth order efficient testing and estimation scores and information: Suppose $\theta = (\psi, \gamma)$, $\psi \in \Psi, \gamma \in \Gamma, \Theta = \Psi \times \Gamma$ (at least locally). We define the kth order efficient testing score $ES_k^{test}(\theta) = \Pi_\theta \left[V_\psi(\theta) | \overline{B}_k^{test, \perp}\right]$ to be the projection of the first order score $V_\psi(\theta)$ on the orthogonal complement in $\mathcal{U}_k(\theta)$ of the kth order testing tangent space. We define the kth order efficient estimation score $ES_k^{est}(\theta) = \Pi_\theta \left[V_\psi(\theta) | \overline{\Lambda}_k^{est \perp}(\theta)\right]$ to be the projection of the first order score $V_\psi(\theta)$ on the orthogonal complement in $\mathcal{U}_k(\theta)$ of the kth order estimation nuisance tangent space. We call the variances $E_\theta \left[ES_k^{test}(\theta) ES_k^{test}(\theta)^T\right]$ and $E_\theta \left[ES_k^{est}(\theta) ES_k^{est}(\theta)^T\right]$ of the kth order efficient scores the kth order testing and estimation efficient informations.

Remark: Note that $E_\theta \left[ES_k^{test}(\theta) ES_k^{test}(\theta)^T\right] \geq E_\theta \left[ES_k^{est}(\theta) ES_k^{est}(\theta)^T\right]$ since $\overline{\Lambda}_k^{est \perp} \subseteq \overline{B}_k^{test, \perp}$ so the efficient testing information is greater than or equal to the efficient estimation information. For $k = 1$, $\overline{\Lambda}_k^{est \perp} = \overline{B}_k^{test, \perp}$, so $ES_1^{test}(\theta) = ES_1^{est}(\theta)$

Efficient Score Lemma: Suppose the model can be parametrized as $\theta = (\psi, \gamma)$, $\psi \in \Psi, \gamma \in \Gamma, \Theta = \Psi \times \Gamma$ (at least locally), then $IF_k(\theta) = \left\{E_\theta \left[ES_k^{est}(\theta) ES_k^{est}(\theta)^T\right]\right\}^{-1} ES_k^{est}(\theta)$, so the kth order estimation efficient variance is the inverse $\left\{E_\theta \left[ES_k^{est}(\theta) ES_k^{est}(\theta)^T\right]\right\}^{-1}$ of the kth order estimation information.

Proof: see Robins and van der Vaart (2004).

The main ideas: Here are the main ideas behind using higher order influence functions in models in which they exist. [In models which are so large that higher order influence functions do not exist, we will consider a lower dimensional working model that admits higher order influence functions and allow the dimension of the working model (the sieve) to increase with sample size. A worked example is given later.] Consider the estimator $\widehat{\psi}_k = \psi\left(\widehat{\theta}\right) + U_k\left(\widehat{\theta}\right)$ based on a sample size n where $\widehat{\theta}$ is an initial estimator of θ from a separate sample (based on random sample splitting) that perhaps obtains the optimal rate of convergence for θ and $U_k(\theta)$ is a kth order estimation influence function. It would be optimal to choose $U_k(\theta)$ equal to $IF_k^{est}(\theta)$. Expanding and evaluating conditonally on $\widehat{\theta}$, we have

$$\widehat{\psi}_k - \psi(\theta) = \left\{\psi\left(\widehat{\theta}\right) - \psi(\theta) + U_k\left(\widehat{\theta}\right) - U_k(\theta)\right\} + U_k(\theta)$$

$$= U_k(\theta) + \left\{U_k\left(\widehat{\theta}\right) - U_k(\theta) - E_\theta\left[U_k\left(\widehat{\theta}\right) - U_k(\theta)|\widehat{\theta}\right]\right\} +$$

$$\left\{\psi\left(\widehat{\theta}\right) - \psi(\theta) + E_\theta\left[U_k\left(\widehat{\theta}\right)|\widehat{\theta}\right]\right\}$$

Now under weak conditions $var\left\{U_k\left(\widehat{\theta}\right) - U_k(\theta)|\widehat{\theta}\right\} / var\left[U_k(\theta)\right] = o_p(1)$ unconditonally since we assume, with unconditional probability approaching one, $\left\|\widehat{\theta} - \theta\right\| \to 0$ as $n \to \infty$ for a norm on Θ for which $var\left\{U_k\left(\widehat{\theta}\right) - U_k(\theta)|\widehat{\theta}\right\} / var\left[U_k(\theta)\right]$ is continuous in $\widehat{\theta}$ at θ. Thus given $\widehat{\theta}$, the distance $d\left(\widehat{\psi}_k - \psi(\theta), U_k(\theta) + \left\{\psi\left(\widehat{\theta}\right) - \psi(\theta) + E_\theta\left[U_k\left(\widehat{\theta}\right)\right]\right\}\right)$ is converging to 0 where $d(\cdot, \cdot)$ is a distance that metrizes weak convergence. If $\psi\left(\widehat{\theta}\right) - \psi(\theta) + E_\theta\left[U_k\left(\widehat{\theta}\right)\right]$ has $k+1$ Frechet derivatives in $\widehat{\theta}$ in a neighborhood of $\widehat{\theta} = \theta$, then by part (ii) of the extended information equality theorem, we expect that the multilinear operator of m arguments corresponding to the mth Frechet derivative at $\widehat{\theta} = \theta$ would be zero for $m = 1, ..., k$. Hence $\psi\left(\widehat{\theta}\right) - \psi(\theta) + E_\theta\left[U_k\left(\widehat{\theta}\right)\right]$ [and thus the bias of $\widehat{\psi}_k - \psi(\theta)$] will be $O_p\left(\left\|\widehat{\theta} - \theta\right\|^{k+1}\right)$, which decreases with k for fixed n. On the other hand, in view of part (iv) of the efficient influence function theorem, we know the variance $var[U_k(\theta)]$ increases with k. Thus the rate of convergence of $\widehat{\psi}_k$ to $\psi(\theta)$ is minimized at $k(n)$ equal to $k_{balance} = k_{balance}(n)$ at which the squared bias and the variance are of the same order. Further the shortest conservative uniform asymptotic confidence intervals will be based on $\widehat{\psi}_{k_{conf}} \pm var\left[U_{k_{conf}}\left(\widehat{\theta}\right)|\widehat{\theta}\right]^{1/2} z_\alpha c_{est}$ where $k_{conf} = k_{conf}(n)$ is the smallest value of k such that $var[U_k(\theta)]$ is of higher order than the squared bias and $c_{est}, c_{est} \geq 1$, is an appropriate constant chosen to guarantee coverage $1 - \alpha$, as $U_k\left(\widehat{\theta}\right)$ may not be normal and we might use a tail bound based on, say, Markov's inequality.

In this same setting if the model can be parametrized as $\theta = (\psi, \gamma)$, then, for an appropriate choice of k, conservative uniform asymptotic confidence intervals can be constructed as

$$\left\{\psi; \left|ES_k^{test}\left(\psi, \widehat{\gamma}\left(\psi\right)\right) / \sqrt{\widehat{var}}\left[ES_k^{test}\left(\psi, \widehat{\gamma}\left(\psi\right)\right) \middle| \widehat{\gamma}\left(\psi\right)\right]^{1/2}\right| < z_\alpha c_{test}\right\}$$

where $\widehat{var}\left[ES_k^{test}\left(\psi, \widehat{\gamma}\left(\psi\right)\right) \middle| \widehat{\gamma}\left(\psi\right)\right]$ is an appropriate variance estimator and c_{test} is similiar to c_{est}. Because $ES_k^{test}\left(\psi, \gamma\right)$ is not orthogonal to the higher order scores for ψ and the mixed $\psi - \gamma$ scores, in an expansion of $ES_k^{test}\left(\psi^*, \widehat{\gamma}\left(\psi^*\right)\right)$ around $\psi^\dagger$, the ψ-derivative $ES_{k,\psi}^{test}\left(\dagger, \widehat{\gamma}\left(\psi^\dagger\right)\right)$ will typically be of the same order as the mixed derivatives $ES_{k,\psi^c\gamma^{m-c}}^{test}\left(\psi^\dagger, \widehat{\gamma}\left(\psi^\dagger\right)\right)$ and the higher order ψ-derivatives $ES_{k,\psi^m}^{test}\left(\psi^\dagger, \widehat{\gamma}\left(\psi^\dagger\right)\right)$. Nonetheless, because in the expansion $ES_{k,\psi^c\gamma^{m-c}}^{test}\left(\psi^\dagger, \widehat{\gamma}\left(\psi^\dagger\right)\right)$ is multiplied by $\left(\psi^* - \psi^\dagger\right)^c \left(\widehat{\gamma}\left(\psi^*\right) - \widehat{\gamma}\left(\psi^\dagger\right)\right)^{m-c}$ and $ES_{k,\psi^m}^{test}\left(\psi^\dagger, \widehat{\gamma}\left(\psi^\dagger\right)\right)$ is multiplied by $\left(\psi^* - \psi^\dagger\right)^m, m > 1$, but $ES_{k,\psi}^{test}\left(\psi^\dagger, \widehat{\gamma}\left(\psi^\dagger\right)\right)$ is only multiplied by $\left(\psi^* - \psi^\dagger\right)$, the asymptotic distribution of the solution $\widehat{\psi}_{eff,k}^{test}$ to $ES_k^{test}\left(\psi, \gamma\right) = 0$ will often be unaffected by the fact that $ES_k^{test}\left(\psi, \gamma\right)$ is not orthogonal to the higher order scores for ψ and the mixed $\psi - \gamma$ scores. Thus $\widehat{\psi}_{eff,k_{conf}}^{test}$ may have smaller limiting variance than the solution $\widehat{\psi}_{eff,k_{conf}}^{est}$ to $ES_k^{est}\left(\psi, \widehat{\gamma}\left(\psi\right)\right) = 0$ without incurring greater bias. Under further regularity conditions, for an appropriate choice of k, $\widehat{\psi}_{eff,k}^{test}$ will typically have 'limiting' variance $\left\{var_{(\psi,\gamma)}\left[ES_k^{test}\left(\psi, \gamma\right)\right]\right\}^{-1}$. Note, for $m \leq k$,

$$\left\{var_{(\psi,\gamma)}\left[ES_k^{test}\left(\psi, \gamma\right)\right]\right\}^{-1} = \tau_{km}^{-1}var_{(\psi,\gamma)}\left[ES_k^{test}\left(\psi, \gamma\right)\right]\tau_{km}^{-1,T}$$

$$\tau_{km} = E_{(\psi,\gamma)}\left[ES_k^{test}\left(\psi, \gamma\right)ES_m^{test}\left(\psi, \gamma\right)^T\right]$$

The lesson here is that for a given functional $\psi\left(\theta\right)$ the optimal procedure is not necessarily based on $IF_k^{est}\left(\theta\right)$ for any k as one only needs to consider those components of θ that can make the bias exceed the variance. As an example we have just seen that when $\theta = (\psi, \gamma)$ it is often not important to be orthogonal to the nuisance scores corresponding to the higher order scores for ψ and the mixed $\psi - \gamma$ scores, even though it may be important to be orthogonal to higher order scores for some or all components of γ (depending on the rate at which particular components are estimable).

We now apply this methodology to our semiparametric regression model. In Robins and van der Vaart (2003, 2004) we used this methodology (i) to obtain an alternative derivation of some results due to Ritov and Bickel (1988), Laurent and Massart (2000), and Laurent (1996) concerning the estimation of $\int f^2\left(x\right) dx$, (ii) to construct conditonal interval estimates for the functionals

$\int \left[\hat{f}(x) - f(x) \right]^2 dx$ and $\int \left[\hat{E}\left[Y|X = x\right] - E\left[Y|X = x\right] \right]^2 dx$, obtaining as a by-product improved adaptive confidence intervals for $f(x)$ and $E[Y|X = x]$ compared to those of Lepski and Hoffmann (2002), and (iii) to construct point and interval estimators for finite dimensional parameters in complex missing and censored data models that improve on the doubly robust estimators of Robins, Rotnitzky and van der Laan (2000) and van der Laan and Robins (2002).

Application To Semiparametric Regression: We are now ready to return to the semiparametric regression example. $\Theta = \prod_{r=1}^{r=4} \Theta_r = \Psi \times \mathcal{N} \times \mathring{A} \times \Omega$. Let $\Delta(\alpha) = A - E_\alpha(A|X)$, $e(\psi, \eta) = Y - \psi A - b(X; \eta)$. Then the generic subject -specific first order scores for $\Psi, \mathcal{N}, \mathring{A}$, and Ω are $V_{\psi i}(\psi, \eta) = Ae_i(\psi, \eta)$, $V_{\eta i}(\psi, \eta, g_\eta) = g_\eta(X_i) e_i(\psi, \eta)$, $V_{\alpha i}(\alpha, g_\alpha) = g_\alpha(X_i) \Delta_i(\alpha)$, $V_{\omega i}(\omega, g_\omega) = g_\omega(X_i)$, where $E_\omega[g_\omega(X_i)] = 0$. Thus the set of composite first order scores evaluated at the truth $\theta^\dagger$ are

$$\left\{ \sum_i V_{\psi i} \right\} = \left\{ \sum_i Ae_i \right\} \tag{9.10a}$$

$$\left\{ \sum_i V_{\eta i}(g_\eta) \right\} = \left\{ \sum_i g_\eta(X_i) e_i; g(.) \ unrestricted \right\} \tag{9.10b}$$

$$\left\{ \sum_i V_{\alpha i}(g_\alpha) \right\} = \left\{ \sum_i g_\alpha(X_i) \Delta_i; \Delta = A - E_{\alpha^\dagger}(A|X), g_\alpha(.) unrestricted \right\} \tag{9.10c}$$

$$\left\{ \sum_i V_{\omega i}(g_\omega) \right\} = \left\{ g_\omega(X_i); E_{\omega^\dagger}[g_\omega(X_i)] = 0 \right\} \tag{9.10d}$$

The first order estimation and testing tangent space $\overline{\mathcal{B}}_1^{est}$ is the closed linear span (cls) of the union of the sets (9.10a)-(9.10d). The first order estimation nuisance tangent space $\overline{\mathcal{B}}_1^{test}$ and the first order testing nuisance tangent space $\overline{\Lambda}_1^{est}$ equal the cls of (9.10b)-(9.10d) The second order estimation tangent $\overline{\mathcal{B}}_2^{est}$ space is the cls of the union of $\overline{\mathcal{B}}_1^{est}$ and the 10 sets of second order scores.

$$\{V_{\psi\psi}\} = \left\{ \sum_i V_{\psi i} V_{\psi i} - A_i^2 + \sum\sum_{i \neq j} V_{\psi i} V_{\psi j} \right\}$$

$$\{V_{\psi\eta}(g_\eta)\} = \left\{ \sum_i V_{\psi i} V_{\eta i}(g_\eta) - g_\eta(X_i) A_i + \sum\sum_{i \neq j} V_{\psi i} V_{\eta j}(g_\eta) \right\}$$

$$\{V_{\psi\omega}(g_\omega)\} = \left\{ \sum_i V_{\psi i} V_{\omega i}(g_\omega) + \sum\sum_{i \neq j} V_{\psi i} V_{\omega j}(g_\omega) \right\}$$

$$\{V_{\alpha\psi}(g_\alpha)\} = \left\{ \sum_i V_{\alpha i}(g_\alpha) V_{\psi i} + \sum\sum_{i \neq j} V_{\alpha i}(g_\alpha) V_{\psi j} \right\}$$

$$= \left\{ \sum_i g_\alpha(X_i) \Delta_i e_i A_i + \sum\sum_{i \neq j} g_\alpha(X_i) \Delta_i e_j A_j \right\}$$

$$\{V_{\eta\omega}(g_\eta, g_\omega)\} = \left\{ \sum_i V_{\eta i}(g_\eta) V_{\omega i}(g_\omega) + \sum\sum_{i \neq j} V_{\eta i}(g_\eta) V_{\omega j}(g_\omega) \right\}$$

$$\{V_{\alpha\omega}(g_\alpha, g_\omega)\} = \left\{\sum_i V_{\alpha i}(g_\alpha) V_{\omega i}(g_\omega) + \sum\sum_{i\neq j} V_{\alpha i}(g_\alpha) V_{\omega j}(g_\omega)\right\}$$

$$\{V_{\alpha\eta}((g_\eta, g_\alpha))\} = \left\{\sum_i V_{\alpha i}(g_\alpha) V_{\eta i}(g_\eta) + \sum\sum_{i\neq j} V_{\alpha i}(g_\alpha) V_{\eta j}(g_\eta)\right\}$$

$$\{V_{\eta\eta}(g_\eta, g_\eta^*, g_\eta^{**})\}$$

$$= \left\{\sum_i [e_i^2 - 1]g_\eta(X_i) g_\eta^*(X_i) + e_i g_\eta^{**}(X_i)] + \sum\sum_{i\neq j} g_\eta(X_i) e_i e_j g_\eta^*(X_j)\right\}$$

$$\{V_{\alpha\alpha}(g_\alpha, g_\alpha^*, g_\alpha^{**})\} = \left\{\sum_i \Delta_i g_\alpha^{**}(X_i) + \sum\sum_{i\neq j} g_\alpha(X_i) g_\alpha^*(X_i) \Delta_i \Delta_j\right\}$$

$$\{V_{\omega\omega}(g_\omega, g_\omega^*, g_\omega^{**})\} = \left\{\sum_i g_\omega^{**}(X_i) + \sum\sum_{i\neq j} g_\omega(X_i) g_\omega^*(X_i)\right\},$$

with $g_\omega^{**}(X_i), g_\omega(X_i)$, and $g_\omega^*(X_i)$ having mean zero. The second estimation nuisance tangent $\overline{\Lambda}_2^{est}$ space is the cls of the union of $\overline{\Lambda}_1^{est}$ and the 10 sets of second order scores. The second order testing tangent space is the cls of the union of $\overline{\mathcal{B}}_1^{test}$ and the 6 sets of second order scores that do not involve ψ.

The first order efficient (testing and estimation) score ES_1 for ψ is easily seen to be $\Pi\left[V_\psi|\Lambda_1^\perp\right] = \sum_i \Delta_i e_i$. The following Lemma proved in Robins and van der Vaart (2004) gives ES_2^{test}. Recall X is discrete.

Lemma: Let $c^*(X_i) = \{1 + (n-1)f(X_i)\}^{-1}, v(X_i) = var(A_i|X_i)$

$$ES_2^{test} = ES_1 - \Pi\left[ES_1|\overline{\{V_{\alpha\eta}\}}\right] \tag{9.11}$$

$$= \sum_i \Delta_i e_i\{(n-1)f(X_i)\}c^*(X_i) - \sum\sum_{i\neq j}\Delta_i e_j I(X_i = X_j)c^*(X_i)$$

Remark: ES_2^{test} differs from ES_1 because ES_1 is not orthogonal to the scores $\{V_{\alpha\eta}\}$. Robins and van der Vaart also show that ES_2^{test} differs from ES_2^{est} because ES_2^{test} is not orthogonal to the mixed scores $\{V_{\alpha\psi}\}$ and the use of ES_2^{est} may result in a loss of efficiency. ES_1 and ES_2^{test} are the same whether the marginal distribution X is known, known to lie in a low dimensional model, or completely unknown. Recall $ES_1(\psi, \alpha, \eta)$ is doubly robust in the sense $E_{(\psi^\dagger, \alpha^\dagger, \eta^\dagger, \omega^\dagger)}\left[ES_1(\psi^\dagger, \alpha^\dagger, \eta)\right] = E_{(\psi^\dagger, \alpha^\dagger, \eta^\dagger, \omega^\dagger)}\left[ES_1(\psi^\dagger, \alpha, \eta^\dagger)\right].$ Strikingly ES_2^{test} is triply robust in that it has mean 0 if one of the three nuisance parameters $(\alpha^\dagger, \eta^\dagger, \omega^\dagger)$ are correct. That is,

$$E_{(\psi^\dagger, \alpha^\dagger, \eta^\dagger, \omega^\dagger)}\left[ES_2^{test}(\psi^\dagger, \alpha^\dagger, \eta, \omega)\right] = E_{(\psi^\dagger, \alpha^\dagger, \eta^\dagger, \omega^\dagger)}\left[ES_2^{test}(\psi^\dagger, \alpha, \eta^\dagger, \omega)\right] \tag{9.12}$$

$$= E_{(\psi^\dagger, \alpha^\dagger, \eta^\dagger, \omega^\dagger)}\left[ES_2^{test}(\psi^\dagger, \alpha, \eta, \omega^\dagger)\right] = 0$$

ES_2^{test} has variance

$$E\left[v(X)f^2(X)\left\{b^\cdot(X_i)\right\}^2(n-1)^2 n + f(X_i)v(X)\left\{b^\cdot(X_i)\right\}^2(n-1)n\right]$$

$$= E\left[\frac{(n-1)f(X_i)}{\{1 + (n-1)f(X_i)\}}n[v(X)]\right]$$

while ES_1 has the greater variance $E[v(X)n]$. It is interesting to consider the case where X_i has n^ρ levels and $f(X_i) = n^{-\rho}$. Then $\{var[ES_1]\}^{-1}$ is always $O(n^{-1})$ while $var[ES_2^{test}]$ is $O(\min\{n, n^2/n^\rho\})$ and $\{var[ES_2^{test}]\}^{-1}$ is

$O\left(\max\left\{n^{-1}, n^{\rho}/n^2\right\}\right)$. On the other hand the conditional bias of $ES_1\left(\psi, \widehat{\eta}, \widehat{\alpha}\right)$ (i.e., $E\left[ES_1\left(\psi, \widehat{\eta}, \widehat{\alpha}\right) | \widehat{\eta}, \widehat{\alpha}\right]$), where $(\widehat{\eta}, \widehat{\alpha})$ is obtained from an independent sample, is $n\sum_l\left\{p\left(l, \alpha_l^{\dagger}\right) - p\left(l, \widehat{\alpha}_l\right)\right\}\left\{b\left(l, \eta_l^{\dagger}\right) - b\left(l, \widehat{\eta}_l\right)\right\}$. If $\rho < 1$ and $b\left(l, \widehat{\eta}_l\right)$ is the empirical mean of $Y - \psi A$ in statum l and $p\left(l, \widehat{\alpha}_l\right)$ is the empirical mean of A in stratum l, the conditional bias is approximated by

$$n\left\{E\left[var\left\{p\left(L, \widehat{\alpha}_L\right) | L\right\}^{1/2} var\left\{b\left(L, \widehat{\eta}_L\right) | L\right\}^{1/2}\right]\right\} = nO\left(\left[\left\{n^{-(1-\rho)}\right\}^{1/2}\right]^2\right) =$$

$O\left(n^{\rho}\right)$. Now to be able to set conditional confidence intervals given $(\widehat{\alpha}, \widehat{\eta})$ based on $ES_1\left(\psi, \widehat{\eta}, \widehat{\alpha}\right)$ we need the bias squared of $O\left(n^{2\rho}\right)$ to be less than the variance of $O\left(n\right)$, thus requiring $\rho < 1/2$. In contrast the bias of $ES_2^{test}\left(\psi, \widehat{\eta}, \widehat{\alpha}, \omega^{\dagger}\right)$ is always zero when $\omega^{\dagger}$ is known and has variance $O\left(\min\left\{n, n^2/n^{\rho}\right\}\right)$. In fact $ES_2^{test}\left(\psi, \widehat{\eta}, \widehat{\alpha}, \omega^{\dagger}\right)$ has variance converging to the first order efficient information $E\left[v\left(X\right)n\right]$ for $\rho < 1$. Let $\widehat{\psi}_1\left(\widehat{\eta}, \widehat{\alpha}\right)$ be the solution to $ES_1\left(\psi, \widehat{\eta}, \widehat{\alpha}\right) = 0$. Conditional on $(\widehat{\eta}, \widehat{\alpha})$, the estimator $\widehat{\psi}_2^{test}\left(\widehat{\eta}, \widehat{\alpha}\right)$ solving $ES_2^{test}\left(\psi, \widehat{\eta}, \widehat{\alpha}, \omega^{\dagger}\right) = 0$, with $\omega^{\dagger}$ assumed known, is semiparametric efficent for $\rho < 1$, $n^{1/2} - consistent$ for $\rho = 1$, converges at rate $n^{1-\rho/2}$ for $2 > \rho \geq 1$, and is inconsistent for $2 > \rho$.

In summary, conditional on $(\widehat{\eta}, \widehat{\alpha})$, our 2nd order $U - statistic$ is necessary to obtain first order semiparametric efficiency for $1/2 \leq \rho < 1$, because the bias of our usual doubly robust estimator $\widehat{\psi}_1\left(\widehat{\eta}, \widehat{\alpha}\right)$ is too large. Our second order estimator corrects the bias without adding to the limiting variability of $\widehat{\psi}_1\left(\widehat{\eta}, \widehat{\alpha}\right)$ for $1/2 \leq \rho < 1$. Results exactly analogous to ours have been obtained for other quadratic functions by a number of other investigators such as Bickel and Ritov (1988) and Laurent and Massart (2000).

The reason that it is not possible to obtain a consistent estimator if $\rho > 2$ is that to control bias, it was necessary that in the "degenerate" part of the U-statistic, the pair i and j only contribute if they have the same value of X. When we toss n subjects randomly onto a grid with $n^{\rho}, \rho > 1$, compartments, one can show that the number of compartments containing more than one subject goes as $n^{(2-\rho)}$ and thus we will obtain an infinite amount of information as $n \to \infty$ only if $\rho \leq 2$.

Suppose now we do not know the law of X apriori. When $f\left(X\right)$ (i.e., $\psi^{\dagger}$) is known ES_2^{test} is uncorrelated with $\overline{B}_k^{test}$ for $k \geq 2$, since $E_{(\psi^{\dagger}, \alpha^{\dagger}, \eta^{\dagger}, \omega^{\dagger})}\left[ES_2^{test}\left(\psi^{\dagger}, \alpha, \eta, \omega^{\dagger}\right)\right] = 0$ for all (α, η). However when $\omega^{\dagger}$ is unknown, the third order scores

$$V_{\alpha\eta\omega}\left(g_\omega, g_\alpha, g_\eta\right)$$

$$= \sum_i g_\omega\left(X_i\right) g_\alpha\left(X_i\right) g_\eta\left(X_i\right) \Delta_i e_i + \sum\sum_{i\neq j} g_\omega\left(X_i\right) g_\alpha\left(X_i\right) g_\eta\left(X_j\right) \Delta_i e_j +$$

$$\sum\sum_{i\neq j} g_\omega\left(X_i\right) g_\alpha\left(X_j\right) g_\eta\left(X_j\right) \Delta_j e_j + g_\omega\left(X_j\right) g_\alpha\left(X_i\right) g_\eta\left(X_j\right) \Delta_i e_j +$$

$$\sum\sum\sum_{i\neq j\neq s} g_\omega\left(X_s\right) g_\alpha\left(X_i\right) \Delta_i e_j g_\eta\left(X_j\right)$$

are correlated with ES_2^{test}, i.e., $E\left[ES_2^{test} V_{\alpha\eta\omega}\left(g_\omega, g_\alpha, g_\eta\right)\right] \neq 0$, implying third order bias. We could elimate the third order bias by calculating $ES_3^{test} = \Pi\left[ES_2^{test}|\overline{B}_3^{test,\perp}\right]$. However rather than take this approach define $ES_2^{test}\left(c\right) = \sum_i \Delta_i e_i \left\{(n-1) f\left(X_i\right)\right\} c\left(X_i\right) - \sum\sum_{i\neq j} \Delta_i e_j I\left(X_i = X_j\right) c\left(X_i\right)$ for any $c\left(X_i\right)$. Note $f\left(X_i\right)$ appears only at one place in $ES_2^{test}\left(c\right)$. Let $ES_2^{test}\left(\psi, \widehat{\eta}, \widehat{\alpha}, \widehat{\omega}_-; c\right)$ be $ES_2^{test}\left(\psi, \widehat{\eta}, \widehat{\alpha}, \omega^\dagger\right)$ with c replacing c^* and with $f\left(X_i\right)$ replaced by

$$\widehat{f}_{-i}\left(X_i\right) = \sum_{\{j; j\neq i\}} I\left(X_j = X_i\right) / (n-1).$$

Define $H\left(\psi\right) = Y - \psi A$, $e_i\left(\psi, \widehat{\eta}\right) = H\left(\psi\right) - b\left(X, \widehat{\eta}\right)$, and $\Delta_i\left(\widehat{\alpha}\right) = A_i - E_{\widehat{\alpha}}\left[A|X_i\right]$. Then

$$ES_2^{test}\left(\psi, \widehat{\eta}, \widehat{\alpha}, \widehat{\omega}_-; c\right)$$

$$= \sum_i \Delta_i\left(\widehat{\alpha}\right) e_i\left(\psi, \widehat{\eta}\right) \widehat{f}_{-i}\left(X_i\right) c\left(X_i\right) (n-1) -$$

$$\sum\sum_{i\neq j} c\left(X_i\right) I\left(X_i = X_j\right) \Delta_i\left(\widehat{\alpha}\right) e_j\left(\psi, \widehat{\eta}\right) \tag{9.13a}$$

$$= ES_2^{test}\left(\psi, \widehat{\eta}, \widehat{\alpha}, \omega^\dagger; c\right) + \sum\sum_{i\neq j} \left\{I\left(X_i = X_j\right) - f\left(X_i\right)\right\} c\left(X_i\right) \Delta_i\left(\widehat{\alpha}\right) e_i\left(\psi, \widehat{\eta}\right)$$

$$\tag{9.13b}$$

$$= \sum\sum_{i\neq j} I\left(X_i = X_j\right) c\left(X_i\right) H_i\left(\psi\right) \left(A_i - A_j\right) \tag{9.13c}$$

where $|\mathcal{X}|$ is the cardinality of the support $\mathcal{X}$ of X. Note that (9.13b) shows that $ES_2^{test}\left(\psi, \widehat{\eta}, \widehat{\alpha}, \widehat{\omega}_-; c\right)$ has mean zero and (9.13c) shows that $ES_2^{test}\left(\psi, \widehat{\eta}, \widehat{\alpha}, \widehat{\omega}_-; c\right) = ES_2^{test}\left(\psi, \widehat{\omega}_-; c\right)$ does not depend on the nuisance parameters (η, ω, α) and thus is orthogonal to $\overline{B}_k^{test}$ regardless of the order k. That is, $ES_2^{test}\left(\psi, \widehat{\omega}_-; c\right)$ is exactly unbiased for 0. [This would not be the case had we estimated $f\left(X_i\right)$ by $\widehat{f}\left(X_i\right) = \sum_{j=1}^{n} I\left(X_j = X_i\right) / n$]. However even though $ES_2^{test}\left(\psi, \widehat{\omega}_-; c\right)$ is orthogonal to the 3rd order testing nuisance tangent space $\overline{B}_3^{test}$, nonetheless $ES_2^{test}\left(\psi, \widehat{\omega}_-; c\right)$ with $c\left(X_i\right) = c^*\left(X_i\right)$ is not the residual from the projection of ES_2^{test} on $\overline{B}_3^{test}$, so it is not fully third order efficient.

Remark: Define $\overline{Z}_x = \sum_i Z_i I\left(X_i = x\right) / \sum_i I\left(X_i = x\right)$ for any Z_i and $\overline{Z}_{x,-j} = \sum_{\{i;i\neq j\}} Z_i I\left(X_i = x\right) / \sum_{\{i;i\neq j\}} I\left(X_i = x\right)$. Let $\widetilde{\eta}\left(x\right) = \overline{H}_x\left(\psi\right), \widetilde{\alpha}\left(x\right) = \overline{A}_x$. Note that the statistic
$ES_2^{test}\left(\psi, \widehat{\omega}_-; c\right) = \sum_{x=1}^{|\mathcal{X}|} \sum_i I\left(X_i = x\right) c\left(x\right) H_i\left(\psi\right)\left(n-1\right)\left(A_i - \overline{A}_{x,-i}\right)$. Hence, it is closely related to the statisitic $ES_1\left(\psi, \widetilde{\eta}, \widetilde{\alpha}\right) =$

$$\sum_{x=1}^{|\mathcal{X}|} \sum_i I\left(X_i = x\right)\left(H_i\left(\psi\right) - \overline{H}_x\left(\psi\right)\right)\left(A_i - \overline{A}_x\right)$$

$$= \left\{\frac{n-1}{n}\right\}^2 \sum_{x=1}^{|\mathcal{X}|}\sum_i I\left(X_i = x\right)\left(H_i\left(\psi\right) - \overline{H}_{x,-i}\left(\psi\right)\right)\left(A_i - \overline{A}_{x,-i}\right)$$

$$= \left\{\frac{n-1}{n^2}\right\} ES_2^{test}\left(\psi, \widehat{\omega}_-; c\right) - \left\{\frac{n-1}{n}\right\}^2 \sum_{x=1}^{|\mathcal{X}|}\sum_i I\left(X_i = x\right)\overline{H}_{x,-i}\left(\psi\right)\left(A_i - \overline{A}_{x,-i}\right)$$

that uses the same sample rather than a different sample to estimate (η, α). $ES_1\left(\psi, \widetilde{\eta}, \widetilde{\alpha}\right)$ is thus also orthogonal to all $\overline{B}_k^{test}$ and is unbiased for 0 (Donald and Newey, 1994). $ES_2^{test}\left(\psi, \widehat{\omega}_-; c\right)$ and $ES_2^{test}\left(\psi, \widehat{\omega}_-; c\right)$ are asymptotically normal under weak conditions. To see this let
$R\left(x\right) = \sum_i I\left(X_i = x\right)\left(H_i - \overline{H}_x\right)\left(A_i - \overline{A}_x\right)$ and $N\left(x\right) = \sum_i I\left(X_i = x\right)$.
Then, given
$\mathbf{X} = \{X_1, ..., X_n\}$, $ES_1\left(\psi, \widetilde{\eta}, \widetilde{\alpha}\right) = \sum_{x=1}^{|\mathcal{X}|} R\left(x\right) = \sum_{x=1}^{|\mathcal{X}|} I\left\{N\left(x\right) \geq 2\right\} R\left(x\right)$ is a sum of $IS = \sum_{x=1}^{|\mathcal{X}|} I\left\{N\left(x\right) \geq 2\right\}$ independent mean zero random variables $I\left\{N\left(x\right) \geq 2\right\} R\left(x\right)$ with $IS \to \infty$ as $n \to \infty$ provided $|\mathcal{X}| = O\left(n^\rho\right), 0 < \rho < 2$. The ability to substitute an 'own' sample estimate of η and α into $ES_1\left(\psi, \eta, \alpha\right)$ without incurring bias results from our assuming that $H\left(\psi^\dagger\right)$ and A are (mean) independent given X and will not happen in most models. For example, suppose we had defined $\psi^\dagger = E\left\{Var\left[A|X\right]\right\}^{-1} E\left\{Cov\left[Y, A|X\right]\right\}$ to be the unique solution to

$$E\left[\left\{Y - A\psi - E\left[Y - A\psi|X\right]\right\}\left\{A - E\left[A|X\right]\right\}\right] = 0$$

in the nonparametric model that does not assume $E\left[Y - A\psi^\dagger|A, X\right] = E\left[Y - A\psi^\dagger|X\right]$. In this nonparametric model, $ES_1\left(\psi, \eta, \alpha\right)$ is still the first order efficient score for ψ and $ES_2^{test}\left(\psi, \widehat{\omega}_-; c\right)$ is still an unbiased estimating function. But, if $E\left[Y - A\psi^\dagger|A, X\right] = E\left[Y - A\psi^\dagger|X\right]$ is false, then, owing to the terms $I\left(X_i = x\right)\overline{H}_{x,-i}\left(\psi\right)\left(A_i - \overline{A}_{x,-i}\right)$, $ES_1\left(\psi, \widetilde{\eta}, \widetilde{\alpha}\right)$ will not be unbiased for 0 and will have second order bias if the number of levels of X exceed $n^{1/2}$. An analogous remark applies to the continuous covariate case discussed below.

The ability to obtain an unbiased estimator in our semiparametric regression model by estimating the nuisance parameters in ES_1 using "own" sample estimates is not only unusual but obscures the fundamental connection of the inference problem to the need for orthogonality with higher order nuisance scores. By using "independent" sample estimates of nuisance parameters and considering inference conditional on these, the underlying general structure of the inference problem is revealed.

Continuous Covariates: Consider the analysis of the semiparametric regression model

$$Y = \psi^\dagger A + b^\dagger (X) + e$$

with $e \tilde{} N(0,1)$ having a known distribution, X absolutely continuous wrt Lesbegue measure on $[0,1]$, and A dichotomous based on n iid observations $O_i = (Y_i, A_i, L_i)$. Let $F_X(X; \omega^\dagger)$ be the marginal of X

Consider the model with likelihood with respect to a dominating measure

$$f(O; \theta = (\psi, \eta, \alpha, \omega))$$
$$= \phi_{std-n} \{e(\psi, \eta, \omega)\} p(X; \alpha, \omega)^A \{1 - p(X; \alpha, \omega)\}^{1-A} f(X; \omega)$$
$$= \theta \in \Theta = \Psi \times N \times \mathring{A} \times \Omega$$

with $e(\psi, \eta, \omega) = Y - \psi A - b(X, \eta, \omega)$,
$p(X; \alpha, \omega) = E[A|X; \alpha, \omega]$

where we use the model

$$b(x, \eta, \omega) = b^*(x, \eta) / f(x; \omega), b^*(x, \eta) \in \left\{ \sum_{r=1}^{k_\eta} \eta_r \varphi_r(x) \right\}, \quad (9.14a)$$

$$p(x; \alpha, \omega) = p^*(x; \alpha) / f(x; \omega), p^*(x; \alpha) \in \left\{ \sum_{r=1}^{k_\alpha} \alpha_r \varphi_r(x) \right\}, \quad (9.14b)$$

$$\int \varphi_r(x) \varphi_j(x) dx = I(r = j), \quad \{\varphi_r(x), \text{ a complete orthonormal basis for } L_2(\mu)\}$$

We assume k_η and k_α are known functions of n that may be infinite for all n. When k_η and k_α are infinite we consider 2 kinds of models

$$mod\,el\ (i): \sum_{r=1}^{\infty} \eta_r^2 < C_\eta, \sum_{r=1}^{\infty} \alpha_r^2 < C_\alpha \qquad (9.14c)$$

$$mod\,el\ (ii): \ p = 1, \sum_{r=1}^{\infty} \eta_r^2 r^{2\beta_\eta} < C_\eta, \sum_{r=1}^{\infty} \alpha_r^2 r^{2\beta_\alpha} < C_\alpha \qquad (9.14d)$$

If we let $k_\eta = k_\alpha = \infty$, and chose model (i) so the only restriction is that $h^*(x; \eta^\dagger)$ and $p^*(x; \alpha)$ are in L_2 balls, $\psi^\dagger$ is not a kth order pathwise differentiable parameter except for the case $k = 1$ and this case is misleading in the sense that the first order asymptotic bound (the Cramer Rao bound) is not attainable. In fact no uniformly consistent estimators of $\psi^\dagger$ exist (Ritov and Bickel,1990). Thus we use model (ii) for some apriori choice of (β_η, C_η) and (β_α, C_α). In model (ii), $\psi^\dagger$ still does not have a kth order influence function with finite variance for $k > 1$. But we can make progress by considering a sequence of (misspecified) working models (sieves) changing with n with finite $k_\eta(n)$ and $k_\alpha(n)$ in such a way that the bias due to setting coefficients past $k_\eta(n)$ and $k_\alpha(n)$ to 0 is properly controlled. Thus we first study models with a finite $k_\eta(n)$ and $k_\alpha(n)$. These models have kth order influence functions with finite variance for $k > 1$.

Here we only give detailed results for the case where the marginal of X (i.e., $\omega^\dagger$ is known). leaving the general case to Robins and van der Vaart (2004). Robins and van der Vaart show that $U_1^{test}(\theta) = \sum_i e_i \Delta_i$ is a 1st order testing influence function and that it equals ES_1^{test} when $k_\alpha \leq k_\eta$. Further with $k^* = \min(k_\alpha, k_\eta)$,

$$U_2^{test}(\psi, \eta, \alpha, \omega) = \sum_i \Delta_i(\alpha, \omega) e_i(\psi, \eta, \omega) f(X_i; \omega)(n-1) -$$

$$\sum_{l=1}^{k^*} \sum \sum_{i \neq j} e_i(\psi, \eta, \omega) \varphi_l(X_i) \Delta_j(\alpha, \omega) \varphi_l(X_j)$$

is a 2nd order testing influence function under law $(\psi, \eta, \alpha, \omega)$ with ω known. Further $U_2^{test}(\psi, \eta, \alpha, \omega)$ is strongly doubly robust in the sense that

$$E_{(\psi^\dagger, \alpha^\dagger, \eta^\dagger, \omega^\dagger)}\left[U_2^{test}(\psi^\dagger, \alpha, \eta, \omega^\dagger)\right] = 0, \tag{9.15}$$

but only for $p^*(x; \alpha)$ and $h^*(x; \eta)$ in model $(9.14a - 9.14b)$. That is, $U_2^{test}(\psi^\dagger, \alpha, \eta, \omega^\dagger)$ has mean zero even if both α and η are incorrect.

Sketch of proof: Note that, with $\omega^\dagger$ known, double robustness in the sense of (9.15) implies U_2^{test} is a 2nd order testing influence function as it implies orthogonality to $\{V_{\alpha\eta}\}, \{V_\alpha\}$, and $\{V_\eta\}$. Now suppressing dependence on the true parameter values and setting $H = Y - \psi^\dagger A$, $E\left[U_2^{test}(\psi^\dagger, \alpha, \eta, \omega^\dagger)\right] =$

$$nE\left[(n-1)\left\{H - b(X, \eta, \omega^\dagger)\right\} f(X; \omega^\dagger)\left\{A - p(X, \alpha, \omega^\dagger)\right\}\right] -$$

$$n(n-1)\sum_{l=1}^{k^*} E\left[\left\{H - b(X, \eta, \omega^\dagger)\right\}\varphi_l(X)\right] E\left[\left\{A - p(X, \alpha, \omega^\dagger)\right\}\varphi_l(X)\right]$$

Now

$$E\left[\{H - b\left(X, \eta, \omega^\dagger\right)\} f\left(X; \omega^\dagger\right) \{A - p\left(X, \alpha, \omega^\dagger\right)\}\right]$$

$$= E\left[\{b\left(X, \eta^\dagger, \omega^\dagger\right) - b\left(X, \eta, \omega^\dagger\right)\} f\left(X; \omega^\dagger\right) \{p\left(X, \alpha^\dagger, \omega^\dagger\right) - p\left(X, \alpha, \omega^\dagger\right)\}\right]$$

$$= E\left[\begin{array}{l} \{\sum_{r=1}^\infty \left(\eta_r^\dagger - \eta_r I\left(r < k_\eta\right)\right) \varphi_r\left(X\right)/f\left(X; \omega^\dagger\right)\} f\left(X; \omega^\dagger\right) \times \\ \{\sum_{r=1}^\infty I\left(r < k_\alpha\right) \left(\alpha_r^\dagger - \alpha_r I\left(r < k_\alpha\right)\right) \varphi_r\left(X\right)/f\left(X; \omega^\dagger\right)\} \end{array} \right]$$

$$= \sum_{r=1}^\infty \left(\eta_r^\dagger - \eta_r I\left(r < k_\eta\right)\right) \left(\alpha_r^\dagger - \alpha_r I\left(r < k_\alpha\right)\right) =$$

$$\sum_{r=1}^{\min(k_\eta, k_\alpha)} \left(\eta_r^\dagger - \eta_r\right) \left(\alpha_r^\dagger - \alpha_r\right) + \sum_{\min(k_\eta, k_\alpha)+1}^\infty \eta_r^\dagger \alpha_r^\dagger - \tag{9.16}$$

$$\sum_{\min(k_\eta, k_\alpha)+1}^{k_\alpha} \eta_r^\dagger \alpha_r - \sum_{\min(k_\eta, k_\alpha)+1}^{k_\eta} \eta_r \alpha_r^\dagger$$

When $\eta_r^\dagger = \eta_r = 0$ for $r > k_\eta$ and $\alpha_r^\dagger = \alpha_r = 0$ for $r > k_\alpha$, (9.16) equals $\sum_{r=1}^{\min(k_\eta, k_\alpha)} \left(\eta_r^\dagger - \eta_r\right) \left(\alpha_r^\dagger - \alpha_r\right)$. The following calculation completes the proof.

$$\sum_{l=1}^{k^*} E\left[\{H - b\left(X, \eta, \omega^\dagger\right)\} \varphi_l\left(X\right)\right] E\left[\{A - p\left(X, \alpha, \omega^\dagger\right)\} \varphi_l\left(X\right)\right]$$

$$= \sum_{l=1}^{k^*} E\left[\{\sum_{r=1}^\infty \left(\eta_r^\dagger - \eta_r I\left(r < k_\eta\right)\right) \varphi_r\left(X\right)/f\left(X; \omega^\dagger\right)\} \varphi_l\left(X\right)\right] \times$$

$$E\left[\{\sum_{r=1}^\infty \left(\alpha_r^\dagger - \alpha_r I\left(r < k_\alpha\right)\right) \varphi_r\left(X\right)/f\left(X; \omega^\dagger\right)\} \varphi_l\left(X\right)\right]$$

$$= \sum_{l=1}^{k^*} \left(\eta_l^\dagger - \eta_l I\left(l < k_\eta\right)\right) \left(\alpha_l^\dagger - \alpha_l I\left(l < k_\alpha\right)\right) \tag{9.17}$$

When $\eta_r^\dagger = \eta_r = 0$ for $r > k_\eta$ and $\alpha_r^\dagger = \alpha_r = 0$ for $r > k_\alpha$, (9.17) equals $\sum_{r=1}^{\min(k_\eta, k_\alpha)} \left(\eta_r^\dagger - \eta_r\right) \left(\alpha_r^\dagger - \alpha_r\right)$ for $k^* = \min\left(k_\alpha, k_\eta\right)$.

Thus since the variance of the estimator solving $0 = U_2^{test}\left(\psi^\dagger, \alpha, \eta, \omega^\dagger\right)$ is $O\left(n^{-1} + k^*/n^2\right)$ it has rate of convergence $n^{1/2}$ if $\min\left(k_\alpha, k_\eta\right)$ is $O\left(n\right)$ and convergence rate $n^{1-\rho/2}$ if $\min\left(k_\alpha, k_\eta\right) = n^\rho, 1 < \rho < 2$.

We now turn our attention to model (9.14d) which allows $\eta_r^\dagger$ and $\alpha_r^\dagger$ to exceed 0 for all r. Suppose $\beta_\eta \leq \beta_\alpha$. We shall still choose a "working" model of the form $(9.14a - 9.14b)$ in which $\eta_r = 0$ and $\alpha_r = 0$ for $r > k^* = k_\eta = k_\alpha$. Then (9.17) equals $\sum_{r=1}^{k^*} \left(\eta_r^\dagger - \eta_r\right) \left(\alpha_r^\dagger - \alpha_r\right)$ and (9.16) equals $\sum_{r=1}^\infty \left(\eta_r^\dagger - \eta_r I\left(r < k_\eta\right)\right) \left(\alpha_r^\dagger - \alpha_r I\left(r < k_\alpha\right)\right)$ so the squared bias is $\left(\sum_{k^*+1}^\infty \eta_r^\dagger \alpha_r^\dagger\right)^2$ which is less than or equal to $\sum_{k^*+1}^\infty \left(\eta_r^\dagger\right)^2 \sum_{k^*+1}^\infty \left(\alpha_r^\dagger\right)^2 < \left(k^*\right)^{-2(\beta_\eta+\beta_\alpha)}$. Thus the maximum squared bias of $U_2^{test}\left(\psi^\dagger, \alpha, \eta, \omega^\dagger\right)$ is $\{n\left(n-1\right)\}^2 \left(k^*\right)^{-2(\beta_\eta+\beta_\alpha)}$. Since the variance of $U_2^{test}\left(\psi^\dagger, \alpha, \eta, \omega^\dagger\right)$ is $O\left(n + k^*\right)$,

the maximum bias squared and variance are balanced for $k^*_{balance} = O\left[n^{1/(\frac{1}{2}+\beta_\eta+\beta_\alpha)}\right]$.
To construct confidence intervals we would choose k^* slightly larger. The order of the length of those confidence intervals would just exceed

$$O\left[\{\kappa^{-2} var\left(U_2^{test}\left(\psi^\dagger,\alpha,\eta,\omega^\dagger\right)\right)\}^{1/2}\right] = O\left[\min\left(n^{-1/2},\{k^*_{balance}/n^2\}^{1/2}\right)\right] =$$
$$O\left[\min\left(n^{-1/2},n^{-2(\beta_\eta+\beta_\alpha)/1+2(\beta_\eta+\beta_\alpha)}\right)\right] \text{ where } \kappa =$$

$$E\left[\partial U_2^{test}\left(\psi^\dagger,\alpha,\eta,\omega^\dagger\right)/\partial\psi\right]$$
$$= E\left[U_2^{test}\left(\psi^\dagger,\alpha,\eta,\omega^\dagger\right)ES_1\right]$$
$$= E\left[U_2^{test}\left(\psi^\dagger,\alpha,\eta,\omega^\dagger\right)ES_2^{test}\right]$$

Remark: If we do not wish to assume β_η and β_α are known apriori we can use the data itself to choose these parameters and thereby obtain adaptive estimators of $\psi^\dagger$. See Robins and van der Vaart (2004). However, although one can obtain adaptive point estimators, it is not possible to obtain adaptive confidence intervals for $\psi^\dagger$.

The theory of higher order influence functions and their associated U-statistics can, in certain cases, be used to improve upon the cross-validation results of van der Laan and Dudoit (2003) by replacing their loss functions, which are first order U-statistics, by loss functions that are higher order U-statistics, thereby decreasing sensitivity to the bias in estimators of the unknown parameters in the loss function. This will be true even when van der Laan and Dudoit's loss functions are doubly robust. Indeed van der Laan and Dudoit's results for first order U-statistic loss functions can be fairly straightforwardly generalized to higher order U-statistics by replacing the maximal inequalities used in their proofs by maximal inequalities for higher order U-statistics.

In addition our theory of inference based on higher order U statistics can be applied to data generated under exceptional laws at which the parameter $\psi(\theta)$ is not differentiable by using a higher order generalization of Theorem 5.1.

Unknown marginal for X : When the marginal of X is unknown, Robins and van der Vaart (2004) show that when $\beta_\eta + \beta_\alpha > 1/2$, root-n estimation of $\psi^\dagger$ is possible with no assumptions on the rate at which rate the density $f(x)$ is estimable (a result previously obtained by Donald and Newey (1994)). However if $\beta_\eta + \beta_\alpha < 1/2$, the optimal rate of estimation of $\psi^\dagger$ depends not only on $\beta_\eta + \beta_\alpha$, but also on the rate at which the density $f(x)$ can be estimated. Thus for valid confidence interval construction, we require that, in addition to β_η and β_α, we be given β_ω specifying the maximum apriori complexity of $f(x)$.

Confidence Intervals After Selection:

Intervals based on Negative Utility as A Loss Function and $\hat{d}^j_{op^{util}}(l)$ as Input : Suppose again that A is binary, sequential randomization holds, and $p(a|l)$ is known. Recall that of the J candidate regimes $\widehat{\gamma}^j$, $\widehat{\gamma}^j_{util}$ maximizes $P^{val}_{nval}\left[YI\left\{A = d^{\widehat{\gamma}^j}_{op}(L)\right\}/p(A|L)\right]$ and will have expected utility $E\left[Y_{d^j_{op^{util}}}\right]$ close to expected utility $E\left[Y_{d^{j_{util-orac}}_{op}}\right]$ of the utility oracle, provided J is not too large. Suppose rather than using $d^{j}_{op^{util}}(l)$ to determine our treatment choice, we wish to use $d^{\widehat{j}}_{op^{util}}(l)$ to 'center' in some sense a $(1 - \alpha)$ confidence set for the unknown $d_{op} = d^{\gamma}_{op} = \arg\max_a \gamma(l, a)$, under the theory that (i) one should report confidence intervals to show the regimes compatible with the data and (ii) one's 'best' estimate should be used to center a confidence interval.

We shall see go in this direction and shall fail. But the failure will point us in a better direction. We assume that we have available a third group of subjects the confidence group, for which we assume no unmeasured confounders. We will construct confidence intervals for this group's optimal regime $d^{\gamma}_{op}(l)$ which will be a confidence interval for the estimation and validation sample's $d^{\gamma}_{op}(l)$ as well if $\gamma(l, a)$ for the confidence group equals the common $\gamma(l, a)$ in the other groups. [Most often the confidence group will have arisen by a random division of the original study into the three groups - estimation, validation, and confidence.]

To begin we shall be satisfied with constructing a confidence interval for $d^{\gamma}_{op}(l)$ only at the n_{conf} values of l in the set $OLC = \{l_i; i \in \text{confidence group}\}$ corresponding to the observed values of l in the confidence group, where we have assumed no ties. [Thus, for the present, we view L as having support OLC and a regime $d(l)$ is a n_{conf} vector of $0's$ and $1's$ corresponding to whether on not to treat at each $l \in OLC$.] To do so we will use a new construction due to Robins and van der Vaart (2003) to form conservative uniform $(1 - \alpha)$ large sample confidence region for $d^{\gamma}_{op}(l)$ for $l \in OLC$. In the following expectations and probabilities are wrt the distribtion of the confidence population. First note that since $E\left[YI\left\{A = d^{\widehat{j}}_{op^{util}}(L)\right\}/p(A|L)|L\right] = \gamma(L)d^{\widehat{j}}_{op^{util}}(L) + E[Y|L, A = 0]$ where $\gamma(L) = \gamma(L, 1)$, we have that

$$n^{1/2}_{conf}P^{conf}_{n_{conf}}\left[Y\frac{\left[I\{A = 0\} - I\left\{A = d^{\widehat{j}}_{op^{util}}(L)\right\}\right]}{p(A|L)} + \gamma(L)d^{\widehat{j}}_{op^{util}}(L)\}\right]$$

$$= n^{1/2}_{conf}P^{conf}_{n_{conf}}\left[Y\frac{\{1 - 2A\}d^{\widehat{j}}_{op^{util}}(L)}{p(A|L)} + \gamma(L)d^{\widehat{j}}_{op^{util}}(L)\right]$$

is conditionally asymptotically normal with mean 0 conditional on the estimation, and validation sample and the the set OLC of confidence sample $L's$ (so the support of L is OLC.) The conditional variance

$$\tau^2 = P^{conf}_{n_{conf}}\left\{Var\left[Y\frac{\{1-2A\}d^{j}_{op^{util}}(L)}{p(A|L)}|L\right]\right\} \text{ is } O_p(1). \text{ Thus}$$

$$C_\gamma (1 - \alpha) = \left\{ \begin{array}{l} \gamma^* (L) ; P_{n_{conf}}^{conf} \left[-\gamma^* (L) \, \widehat{d_{op}^{\tilde{j}}}^{util} (L) \right] \\ < n^{-1/2} \tau z_\alpha + P_{n_{conf}}^{conf} \left[Y \frac{\{1-2A\} \widehat{d_{op}^{\tilde{j}}}^{util}(L)}{p(A|L)} \right] \end{array} \right\}$$

is a uniform $1 - \alpha$ asymptotic confidence for the true $\gamma(L)$, where z_α is the upper α quantile of a standard normal so $z_{.05} = 1.64$. Thus

$$C_{d_{op}} (1 - \alpha) = \{ d^* (L) = I \{ \gamma^* (L) > 0 \} ; \gamma^* (L) \in C_\gamma (1 - \alpha) \}$$

is a uniform $1 - \alpha$ asymptotic confidence for the true $d_{op} (L) = I \{ \gamma (L) > 0 \}$.

We shall see this confidence set has terrible power properties, failing to exclude $d^* (L)$ that are far from d_{op}. To understand what the confidence set $C_{d_{op}} (1 - \alpha)$ looks like note that it follows from above that

$$P_{n_{conf}}^{conf} \left[Y \frac{\{1-2A\} \widehat{d_{op}^{\tilde{j}}}^{util}(L)}{p^*(A|L)} \right] = P_{n_{conf}}^{conf} \left[-\gamma(L) \, \widehat{d^{\tilde{\gamma j}}}^{util} (L) \right] + \tau n^{-1/2} Z + o_p \left(n^{-1/2} \right)$$

where Z is independent standard normal.

Thus

$$C_\gamma (1 - \alpha)$$
$$= \left\{ \gamma^* (L) ; P_{n_{conf}}^{conf} \left[(\gamma(L) - \gamma^*(L)) \, \widehat{d_{op}^{\tilde{j}}}^{util} (L) \} \right] < n^{-1/2} \tau (z_\alpha + Z) + o_p \left(n^{-1/2} \right) \right\}$$

Now consider the extreme "perfect" case in which $\widehat{d_{op}^{\tilde{j}}}^{util} (L) = d_{op} (L)$. Suppose the subset $POS = \{ l_1, ..., l_{100} \}$ of OLC on which $\gamma(L) > 0$ contains 100 points and at each such point $\gamma(L) = 100$. Consider now $\gamma^* (L)$ such that $\gamma^* (l_1) = 10^5$ and $\gamma^* (l_k) = -101$ for the remaining 99 l_k in POS. Then $P_{n_{conf}}^{conf} \left[(\gamma(L) - \gamma^*(L)) \, \widehat{d_{op}^{\tilde{j}}}^{util} (L) \} \right]$ will be less than -7×10^4 so $\gamma^* (L)$ will be in $C_\gamma (1 - \alpha)$ and thus $d^* (L) = I (\gamma^* (L) > 0)$ in $C_{d_{op}} (1 - \alpha)$ even though $d^* (L)$ incorrectly withholds treatment at all but one l_k in POS. Part of the problem is the input $\widehat{d_{op}^{\tilde{j}}}^{util} (L)$, even when optimal, does not contain enough information to sufficiently constrain the possible $\gamma^* (L)$ that could have generated the data. That is although $d_{op} (L) = I (\gamma(L) > 0)$ solves (i) $\text{argmax}_{c(L)} E \left[I (c(L) > 0) \gamma(L) \right]$, $\gamma(L)$ does not solve (ii) $\text{argmax}_{c(L)} E \left[I (\gamma(L) > 0) c(L) \right]$, and indeed a $c(L)$ that, with high probability, differs in sign from $\gamma(L)$ can have $E \left[I (\gamma(L) > 0) c(L) \right] \gg E \left[I (\gamma(L) > 0) \gamma(L) \right]$. The good properties of $\widehat{\gamma^j}_{util}$ derives from the fact that it approximately solves (i). The bad properties of the above confidence interval derives from the fact that it is based on 'approximately solving' (ii).

Intervals based on $Loss \left(c, F_{A|L}, b, g \right)$ **as A Loss Function and an Estimate of** γ **as Input :**

The Fixed L Case: One lesson of the last subsection is that if we wish our confidence regions to be sufficiently small that they have the power to exclude implausible candidates $d^* (l)$ for $d_{op} (l)$, we at least need a confidence procedure that uses as input the full information contained in a cross-validated selected approximation, such as $\widehat{\gamma^j}_{util}(l)$, to $\gamma(l)$ rather than the lesser information contained in, say, $\widehat{d_{op}^{util}}(l) = I\left[\widehat{\gamma^j}_{util}(l) > 0\right]$. To do so we consider intervals based based on

$$Loss\left(\widehat{\gamma}, F_{A|L}, b, g\right) = \left[g^2(L)\left\{Y - \widehat{\gamma}(L, A) - b(L) + E\left[\widehat{\gamma}(L, A)|L\right]\right\}^2\right]$$

where $\widehat{\gamma}$ is some cross-validated selected estimate such as $\widehat{\gamma^j}_{util}(l)$ or $\widehat{\gamma^j}$ that we hope might be a good approximation to the true γ. We will use the construction due to Robins and van der Vaart (2003) to form conservative uniform $(1-\alpha)$ large sample confidence region for γ and thus $d_{op}^{\gamma}(l)$ for $l \in OLC$. We will see that the size is adaptive in the sense that the set of regimes contained in the confidence set for d_{op}^{γ} will be few if $\widehat{\gamma}$ is a good estimate of γ but will be many if the estimate $\widehat{\gamma}$ is poor. Recall that

$$R = g(L)\left[\{Y - \gamma(L, A)\} - b(L) + E[\gamma(L, A)|L]\right]$$
$$= g(L)\left[\{Y - \gamma(L, A)\} - E[\{Y - \gamma(L, A)\}|L]\right] + g(L)\left\{E[Y|L] - b(L)\right\}$$

and

$$S(c) = g(L)\left[\{\gamma(L, A) - c(L, A)\} - E[\gamma(L, A) - c(L, A)|L]\right]$$
$$= g(L)\left[\{\gamma(L) - c(L)\}\{A - E[A|L]\}\right].$$

Therefore $E\left[S^2(c)|L\right] = g^2(L)\{\gamma(L) - c(L)\}^2 var[A|L]$ and

$$E\left[R^2|L\right] = g^2(L)\left[\{var[Y - \gamma(L, A)|L]\} + \{E[Y|L] - b(L)\}^2\right].$$

We know from our prior results that

$$n_{conf}^{1/2} P_{n_{conf}}^{conf}\left[Loss\left(\widehat{\gamma}, F_{A|L}, b, g\right) - \{E[R^2|L] + E[S^2(\widehat{\gamma})|L]\}\right]$$

is conditionally asymptotically normal with mean 0 conditional on the estimation, and validation sample and the the set OLC of confidence sample $L's$ (so the support of L is OLC) because $Loss\left(\widehat{\gamma}, F_{A|L}, b, g\right)$ has conditional mean $E[R^2|L] + E[S^2(c)|L]$. The conditional variance $\tau^2 = \tau^2(\gamma^*) = P_{n_{conf}}^{conf}\left\{Var\left[Loss\left(\widehat{\gamma}, F_{A|L}, b, g\right)|L\right]\right\}$ is $O_p(1)$. Thus

$$C_\gamma(1-\alpha) = \begin{array}{l}\left\{\gamma^*(L); P_{n_{conf}}^{conf}\left[g^2(L)\left[\{\widehat{\gamma}(L) - \gamma^*(L)\}^2 var[A|L]\right]\right]\right.\\ \left. < n^{-1/2}\tau z_\alpha + P_{n_{conf}}^{conf}\left[Loss\left(\widehat{\gamma}, F_{A|L}, b, g\right) - E[R^2|L]\right]\right\}\end{array}$$

$$(9.18)$$

is a uniform $1 - \alpha$ asymptotic confidence for the true $\gamma(L)$, where z_α is the upper α quantile of a standard normal so $z_{.05} = 1.64$. Thus

$$C_{d_{op}}(1-\alpha) = \{d^*(L) = I\{\gamma^*(L) > 0\}; \gamma^*(L) \in C_\gamma(1-\alpha)\}$$

is a uniform $1 - \alpha$ asymptotic confidence for the true $d_{op}(L) = I\{\gamma(L) > 0\}$.

To understand what the confidence set $C_\gamma(1 - \alpha)$ looks like note that it follows from the above normal distributional result that

$$P_{n_{conf}}^{conf}\left[Loss\left(\widehat{\gamma}, F_{A|L}, b, g\right) - E\left[R^2|L\right]\right]$$
$$= P_{n_{conf}}^{conf}\left[g^2(L)\left[\{\widehat{\gamma}(L) - \gamma(L)\}^2 var[A|L]\right]\right] + \tau n^{-1/2}Z + o_p\left(n^{-1/2}\right)$$

where Z is independent standard normal.

Thus our interval (9.18) has the asymptotic expansion

$$C_\gamma(1 - \alpha) \tag{9.19a}$$
$$= \left\{\begin{array}{c} \gamma^*(L); P_{n_{conf}}^{conf}\left\{g^2(L)\left[\{\widehat{\gamma}(L) - \gamma^*(L)\}^2 var[A|L]\right]\right\} < n^{-1/2}\tau(z_\alpha + Z) \\ + P_{n_{conf}}^{conf}\left\{g^2(L)\left[\{\widehat{\gamma}(L) - \gamma(L)\}^2 var[A|L]\right]\right\} \end{array}\right\}$$
$$= \left\{\begin{array}{c} \gamma^*(L); P_{n_{conf}}^{conf}\left[var[A|L]g^2(L)\{\gamma^*(L) - \gamma(L)\}^2 + 2\{\gamma(L) - \widehat{\gamma}(L)\}\right] \\ < n^{-1/2}\tau(z_\alpha + Z) + o_p\left(n^{-1/2}\right) \end{array}\right\}$$
$$\tag{9.19b}$$

¿From (9.19a) we see that if we choose $g^2(L) = \{var[A|L]\}^{-1}$, then

$$C_\gamma(1 - \alpha) = \left\{\begin{array}{c} \gamma^*(L); P_{n_{conf}}^{conf}\left[\{\widehat{\gamma}(L) - \gamma^*(L)\}^2\right] < n^{-1/2}\tau(z_\alpha + Z) + \\ P_{n_{conf}}^{conf}\left[\{\widehat{\gamma}(L) - \gamma(L)\}^2\right] \end{array}\right\}.$$

If $P_{n_{conf}}^{conf}\left[\{\widehat{\gamma}(L) - \gamma(L)\}^2\right] = O_p\left(n^{-1/2}\right)$ then our confidence region $C_\gamma(1 - \alpha)$ is contained in a ball centered on $\widehat{\gamma}(L)$ of radius $n^{-1/4}$ and we cannot obtain a smaller radius even if $P_{n_{conf}}^{conf}\left[\{\widehat{\gamma}(L) - \gamma(L)\}^2\right]$ is smaller than $O_p\left(n^{-1/2}\right)$. [The proof that our confidence region is contained in a ball of radius $n^{-1/4}$ uses the fact that the dependence of τ on γ^* is negligible.] Li (1988) shows that no uniform $1 - \alpha$ asymptotic confidence ball for the $\gamma(L)$ can have radius less than $n^{-1/4}$. An $n^{-1/4}$ rate rather than the usual $n^{-1/2}$ rate is the price we pay for admitting that we cannot be certain that we have specified a correct finite dimensional parametric model for $\gamma(A, L) = A\gamma(L)$. The radius of our interval depends on how good an estimator $\widehat{\gamma}(L)$ is of the true $\gamma(L)$. If $O_p\left(n^{-1/2}\right) < P_{n_{conf}}^{conf}\left[\{\widehat{\gamma}(L) - \gamma(L)\}^2\right] = O_p\left(n^{-\beta}\right)$ for $0 < \beta < 1/2$, our intervals have radius $n^{-\beta/2}$, while if $o_p(1) < P_{n_{conf}}^{conf}\left[\{\widehat{\gamma}(L) - \gamma(L)\}^2\right] = O_p(1)$ so that $\widehat{\gamma}(L)$ was so poor an estimate that it was inconsistent, our intervals have radius $O(1)$.

A better choice of the user suppied function $g(L)$ can be made. Recall that we can chose $g(L)$ after knowing our candidate $\widehat{\gamma}(L)$ since $\widehat{\gamma}(L)$ is regarded as fixed in the analysis. Now to obtain a precise interval for $d_{op}(L) = I(\gamma(L) > 0)$, we only need to provide a very narrow interval for $\gamma(L)$ at values of L where it is near zero. Thus we can choose $g(L)$ large at those L

where our candidate $\widehat{\gamma}(L)$ is near zero, although we cannot go too far in this direction without inflating τ, which, by inflating the overall interval length will counteract the benefits of sharpening $g(L)$.

The above approach however is not altogether satisfactory. Not only does the serious problem of extrapolating our confidence interval for $d_{op}(L)$ to values of l not realized in the confidence group remain, but, in addition, we have swept one important difficulty under the rug. To compute the interval (9.18) requires that we know $\sigma^2(L) = var[Y - \gamma(L, A)|L]$ to be able to calculate the term $E(R^2 \mid L)$ Otherwise, we require an $n^{1/2} - consistent$ of estimator of $\sigma^2(L)$, say computed from the validation sample, for our interval to have the above stated properties (Baraud, 2000). This requirement is a prohibitive limitation since $\sigma^2(L)$ cannot be estimated without an estimate of the residual $Y - \gamma(L, A)$; but $\gamma(L, A)$ is unknown and is in fact the quantity we are constructing an interval for. In the next subsection we show how one can attack both these problems at once.

The Random L Case: We once again take L to be random with full support. Again we follow Robins and van der Vaart (2003). We assume $p(a|l)$ and $f(l)$ are known. The case where these are unknown is considered in Robins and van der Vaart (2004). We first assume we can specify a linear model $\theta^{*,T}W^* = \sum_{s=1}^{S^*} \theta_s^* W_s^*$ for $\xi(L) = \xi(L, \gamma) = g(L)\gamma(L)var[A|L]^{1/2}$ with $g(L)$ a user chosen function and with user chosen regressors $W_s^* = w_s^*(L)$ where S^* is sufficiently large that the approximation bias

$inf_{\theta^* = (\theta_s^*; s=1, \ldots S^*)} E\left[\left\{\xi(L) - \sum_{s=1}^{S^*} \theta_s^* w_s^*(L)\right\}^2\right]$ will be small compared to

the width of any confidence region for $\xi(L)$ and thus for $\gamma(L)$. By the population version of Gram-Schmidt orthogonalization we can replace $\gamma^*(L; \theta^*) \equiv \theta^{*,T}W^*$ by $\gamma(L; \theta) \equiv \theta^T W = \sum_{s=1}^{S} \theta_s W_s$ for $S \leq S^*$ such that $E[W_s W_p] = 0$ for $p \neq s$, $E[W_s W_s] = 1$ for $p = s$ and for each θ^* there exists a θ such that $\gamma(L; \theta) = \gamma^*(L; \theta^*)$ for all L. With $\widehat{\gamma}(L)$ again our cross-validated selected estimator of $\gamma(L)$ and $\widehat{\xi}(L) = g(L)\widehat{\gamma}(L)\{var(A|L)\}^{1/2}$, let

$$\xi\left(L; \widehat{\theta}\right) = \widehat{\theta}^T W = \sum_{s=1}^{S} \widehat{\theta}_s W_s = E\left[\widehat{\xi}(L)W\right] E\left[WW^T\right]^{-1} W \text{ and } \xi\left(L; \theta^\dagger\right) =$$

$\theta^{\dagger T}W = \sum_{s=1}^{S} \theta_s^\dagger W_s = E[\xi(L)W] E[WW^T]^{-1} W$ be the population least squares projections onto our model. Note $\theta_s^\dagger = E[\xi(L)W_s]$, $E[WW^T]^{-1}$ is the identity, and

$\xi(L; \theta^\dagger) = \theta^{*,\dagger T}W^*$, where

$$\theta^{*,\dagger} = \arg\min_{\theta^* = (\theta_s^*; s=1, \ldots S^*)} E\left[\left\{\xi(L) - \sum_{s=1}^{S^*} \theta_s^* w_s^*(L)\right\}^2\right]. \text{ We only con-}$$

sider the functions

$\gamma(L; \theta) = \xi(L; \theta) / \left[g(L)\{var(A|L)\}^{1/2}\right]$ as candidates for $\gamma(L)$ based on

our assumption, that S^* was chosen large enough to control approximation bias. Our approach to constructing a $(1 - \alpha)$ confidence interval for $\theta^\dagger$ and thus for $\gamma(L; \theta^\dagger)$ is as follows.

We will find a conservative uniform asymptotic $(1 - \alpha)$ confidence interval of the form $C_{\theta^\dagger}(1 - \alpha) = \left\{ \theta; \sum_{s=1}^{S} \left(\widehat{\theta}_s - \theta_s \right)^2 < Q^2 \right\}$ for $\theta^\dagger$ where the random variable Q^2 is chosen as described below. By orthonormality of the W_s,

$$\sum_{s=1}^{S} \left(\widehat{\theta}_s - \theta_s \right)^2 = E\left[\left\{ \xi\left(L; \theta\right) - \xi\left(L; \widehat{\theta}\right) \right\}^2 \right] =$$

$E[g^2(L)\left[\gamma\left(L; \theta\right) - \gamma\left(L; \widehat{\theta}\right)\right]^2 \{var\,(A|L)\}]$ so our confidence interval can also be written as the set

$$C_{\gamma(\cdot;\theta^\dagger)}(1 - \alpha) = \left\{ \gamma\left(\cdot; \theta\right); E[g^2(L)\left[\gamma\left(L; \theta\right) - \gamma\left(L; \widehat{\theta}\right)\right]^2 \{var\,(A|L)\}] < Q^2 \right\}.$$

Finally we obtain the interval

$$C_{d_{op}}(1 - \alpha) = \left\{ d^*(L) = I\left\{ \gamma\left(L; \theta\right) > 0 \right\}; \gamma\left(\cdot; \theta\right) \in C_{\gamma(\cdot;\theta^\dagger)}(1 - \alpha) \right\}$$

We next describe how we obtain Q.

Let $M = M\left(g, F_{A|L} \right) = g\left(L\right) \{Y \{A - E[A|L]\}\} \{var\,(A|L)\}^{-1/2}$. Note the estimator $\widetilde{\theta}_s = P_{n_{conf}}^{conf}[MW_s]$ has mean $E\left[g\left(L\right) \gamma\left(L\right) \{var\,(A|L)\}^{1/2} W_s \right] = \theta_s^\dagger$.

Further the estimator

$\mathcal{R}_s\left(\widehat{\theta} \right) = \sum \sum_{\{i \neq j, i,j = 1, \ldots, n_{conf}\}} \sum_{s=1}^{S} \left(M_i W_{s,i} - \widehat{\theta}_s \right) \left(M_j W_{s,j} - \widehat{\theta}_s \right)$ has mean $\sum_{s=1}^{S} \left(\widehat{\theta}_s - \theta_s^\dagger \right)^2$ conditional on the estimation and validation sample data (Laurent, 1996). Robins and van der Vaart show that we can take $Q^2 = \mathcal{R}_s\left(\widehat{\theta} \right) - c\left(S/(1 - \alpha)\, n_{conf}^2 \right)^{1/2}$ for $\alpha < 1/2$ where the constant c is explicit and given in Robins and van der Vaart.

Remark: Conditional on $\widehat{\theta}$, $\mathcal{R}_s\left(\widehat{\theta} \right) - \sum_{s=1}^{S} \left(\widehat{\theta}_s - \theta_s^\dagger \right)^2$ is the second order estimation influence function IF_2^{est} for the functional $\sum_{s=1}^{S} \left(\widehat{\theta}_s - \theta_s^\dagger \right)^2$ in the model satisfying the sole restrictions that $f\,(l)$ and $f\,(a \mid l)$ are known (Robins and van der Vaart, 2004).

Sequential Decisions:

We now generalize some of the above results on using cross validation to select the optimal treatment regime to the sequential decision problem. We only cover areas where the natural generalization from single to sequential decisions is either non apparent or somewhat suprising.

Voting Rule Additions: A natural additional candidate, the "vote regime", exists in the sequential problem as in the single decision problem if we have available the candidate functions $\widehat{\gamma}^j\left(\overline{L}_m, \overline{A}_m \right)$ for the optimal function $\gamma\left(\overline{L}_m, \overline{A}_m \right) = \gamma^{\overline{d}_{op},\overline{d}^*}\left(\overline{L}_m, \overline{A}_m \right)$ rather than simply the associated candidate regimes $d_{op}^{\widehat{\gamma}^j}$. Specifically given J candidates $\widehat{\gamma}^j\left(\bar{L}_m, \bar{A}_m\right)$ the "vote regime" d_{op}^{vote} is defined recursively as follows :

$$d_{op,0}^{vote}\left(l_0\right) = \arg\max_{a_0^*}\left(\sum_j I\left(\arg\max_{a_0}\widehat{\gamma}^j\left(\bar{l}_0, \bar{a}_0\right) = a_0^*\right)\right),$$

$$d_{op,m}^{vote}\left(\bar{l}_m, \bar{a}_{m-1} = d_{op,m-1}^{vote}\left(\bar{l}_{m-1}\right)\right)$$

$$= \arg\max_{a_m^*}\left(\sum_j I\left(\arg\max_{a_m}\widehat{\gamma}^j\left(\bar{l}_m, \bar{a}_{m-1} = d_{op,m-1}^{vote}\left(\bar{l}_{m-1}\right), a_m\right) = a_m^*\right)\right)$$

that selects the most recommended treatment given your value of $\bar{l}_m$ and that you have followed the vote regime through $\bar{l}_{m-1}$. Here, for simplicity, we have discounted the possibility of ties.

Unbiased Estimation of Expected Utility in Sequential Decision Problems:

Suppose that each A_m is binary but the number of time periods K is large, say 400, as would not be untypical in many epidemiologic settings. Now, under sequential randomization, for any candidate optimal regime $\bar{d}_{op}^c$ based on a candidate optimal blip function $c\left(\bar{l}_m, \bar{a}_m\right)$, $m = 0, ..., K$, an unbiased estimator of $E\left[Y_{\bar{d}_{op}^c}\right]$ with the $p\left(a_m | \bar{l}_m, \bar{a}_{m-1}\right)$ known is

$$P_{nval}^{val}\left[YI\left\{\bar{A}_K = \bar{d}_{op}^c\left(L_{K-1}\right)\right\} / \prod_{m=0}^K p\left(A_m | \bar{L}_m, \bar{A}_{m-1}\right)\right] \text{ with }$$

$I\left\{\bar{A}_K = \bar{d}_{op}^c\left(\bar{L}_{K-1}\right)\right\}$ the indicator that a subject followed the regime $\bar{d}_{op}^c$ through the end of the study. But for almost all regimes $\bar{d}_{op}^c$, there will be at most a few subjects and often none who followed the regime through K and thus the variance of the estimator is so large as to be useless. Again we might consider replacing the deterministic regime $\bar{d}_{op}^c$ with a random regime $\bar{p}^c$ in which given $\bar{L}_m = \bar{l}_m\ \bar{A}_{m-1} = \bar{a}_{m-1}$, we treat with a_m drawn from a conditional density p_m^c with $p_m^c\left(a_m | \bar{l}_m, \bar{a}_{m-1}\right)$ equal to $1-\sigma$ if $a_m = \bar{d}_{op}^c\left(\bar{l}_m, \bar{a}_{m-1}\right)$ and to σ otherwise for σ small and then estimate $E\left[Y_{\bar{p}^c}\right]$ with the unbiased estimator $\widehat{E}\left[Y_{\bar{p}^c}\right] = P_{nval}^{val}\left[Y\prod_{m=0}^K p_m^c\left(A_m | \bar{L}_m, \bar{A}_{m-1}\right) / \prod_{m=0}^K p\left(A_m | \bar{L}_m, \bar{A}_{m-1}\right)\right]$.

We must not choose σ too small in order to prevent $\widehat{E}\left[Y_{\bar{p}^c}\right]$ from being a highly variable estimate of $E\left[Y_{\bar{p}^c}\right]$. Now consider the case where $c\left(\bar{l}_m, \bar{a}_m\right)$ is $\widehat{\gamma}^j\left(\bar{l}_m, \bar{a}_m\right) = \gamma^j\left(\bar{l}_m, \bar{a}_m, \widehat{\psi}^j\right)$ based on a fit of the model $\gamma^j\left(\bar{l}_m, \bar{a}_m, \psi^j\right)$ to the estimation sample data so $d_{op}^{\widehat{\gamma}^j}\left(\bar{l}_m, \bar{a}_{m-1}\right) = \arg\max_{a_m}\gamma^j\left(\bar{l}_m, \bar{a}_m, \widehat{\psi}^j\right)$.

It seems wise to choose $\sigma = \sigma^j\left(\bar{l}_m, \bar{a}_{m-1}\right)$ as a function of $\left(\bar{l}_m, \bar{a}_{m-1}\right)$ and j. Specifically if the lower confidence limit for the absolute value $\left|\widehat{\gamma}^j\left(\bar{l}_m, \bar{a}_{m-1}, a_m = 1\right)\right|$ is far from 0 we could choose $\sigma^j\left(\bar{l}_m, \bar{a}_{m-1}\right)$ to be 0 (or very nearly 0) and (ii) if it includes 0 we choose $\sigma^j\left(\bar{l}_m, \bar{a}_{m-1}\right)$ to be large (but less than $1/2$). We then treat a new subject beginning at time of HIV infection t_0 with the regime $\bar{p}^{\widehat{\gamma}^{j_0}}$ that maximizes $\widehat{E}\left[Y_{\bar{p}^{\widehat{\gamma}^j}}\right]$ over the J candidates.

However for a subject who receives care in the community until the time t_k from infection with HIV and who presents to our optimal treatment clinic at that time with history $\left(\bar{L}_k, \bar{A}_{k-1}\right)$, we would treat with the regime $\underline{p}_k^{\widehat{\gamma}^{j_k}}$

that maximizes the unbiased estimator
$$P_{n^{val}}^{val} \left[Y \prod_{m=k}^{K} p_m^c \left(A_m | \overline{L}_m, \overline{A}_{m-1} \right) / \prod_{m=k}^{K} p \left(A_m | \overline{L}_m, \overline{A}_{m-1} \right) \right] \text{ of}$$

$$E\left[Y_{\overline{A}_{k-1}, \underline{p}_k^{\hat{\gamma}^j}} \right] = E\left\{ E\left[Y_{\overline{A}_{k-1}, \underline{p}_k^{\hat{\gamma}^j}} | \overline{L}_k, \overline{A}_{k-1} \right] \right\}.$$ The reason that the regime

$\underline{p}_k^{\hat{\gamma}^{jk}}$ can differ from the regime $\underline{p}_k^{\hat{\gamma}^{j0}}$ is that (i) the observed (i.e. community) data distribution of $\left(\overline{L}_k, \overline{A}_{k-1} \right)$ differs from the distribution of the counterfactual variables $\left(\overline{L}_{\overline{p}^{\hat{\gamma}^{j0}}, k}, \overline{A}_{\overline{p}^{\hat{\gamma}^{j0}}, k-1} \right)$ that would obtain upon following the regime $\overline{p}^{\hat{\gamma}^{j0}}$ from time t_0 and (ii) because none of the candidate regimes $\overline{p}^{\hat{\gamma}^j}$ are considered optimal for each value of $\left(\overline{L}_k, \overline{A}_{k-1} \right)$, the best choice among them from time k onwards will appropriately depend on the distribution of $\left(\overline{L}_k, \overline{A}_{k-1} \right)$ that will exist at time k. However there is a philosophical conundrum associated with this argument. Consider a subject i who receives care in the community until the time t_k and then presents to our optimal treatment clinic with history $\left(\overline{l}_{k,i}, \overline{a}_{k-1,i} \right)$ that is strongly compatible with following regime $\overline{p}^{\hat{\gamma}^{j0}}$ in the sense $a_{m,i} = \overline{d}_{op,m}^{\hat{\gamma}^{j0}} \left(\overline{l}_{m,i}, \overline{a}_{m-1,i} \right)$ for $m = 0, ..., k-1$. That is the patient would have the same data $\left(\overline{l}_{k,i}, \overline{a}_{k-1,i} \right)$ had he been treated deterministically with $\overline{d}_{op}^{\hat{\gamma}^{j0}}$ beginning at time t_0. In that case why should the subject be viewed as a random member of a population that has the observed data distribution of $\left(\overline{L}_k, \overline{A}_{k-1} \right)$ rather than as a random member of a population that has $\left(\overline{L}_k, \overline{A}_{k-1} \right)$ distributed as $\left(\overline{L}_{\overline{p}^{\hat{\gamma}^{j0}}, k}, \overline{A}_{\overline{p}^{\hat{\gamma}^{j0}}, k-1} \right)$. This conundrum is very analogous to the conundrum of the individual patient treatment decison discussed above and is a well recognized difficulty that arises in many guises in any frequentist theory of inference.

A Problem in the Generalization of Corollary 9.1: We first provide a partial generalization of Corollary (9.1) to the setting of optimal regime estimation in a sequential decision problem under the assumption of no unmeasured confounders. We then discuss problems with the partial generalization.

We first define the quantity $H_{\text{mod},m}^{d_{op,m}, \underline{d}_m^*} (c_m)$ in analogy to Eq. (3.19) except we substitute $c_m \left(\overline{L}_m, \overline{A}_m \right)$ for $\gamma^{d_{op}, \overline{d}^*} \left(\overline{L}_m, \overline{A}_m, \psi \right)$ and do not specify a model for $\gamma^{\overline{d}_{op}, \overline{d}^*} \left(\overline{L}_j, \overline{A}_j \right)$:

$$H_{\text{mod},m}^{d_{op,m}, \underline{d}_m^*} (c_m) = Y - c_m \left(\overline{L}_m, \overline{A}_m \right) - \qquad (9.20)$$

$$\sum_{j=m+1}^{K} \left\{ \gamma^{\overline{d}_{op}, \overline{d}^*} \left(\overline{L}_j, \overline{A}_{j-1}, d_{op,j} \left(\overline{L}_j, \overline{A}_{j-1} \right) \right) - \gamma^{\overline{d}_{op}, \overline{d}^*} \left(\overline{L}_j, \overline{A}_j \right) \right\},$$

where $d_{op,m} \left(\overline{L}_m, \overline{A}_{m-1} \right) = \arg\max_{a_m \in \mathcal{A}_m} \gamma^{\overline{d}_{op}, \overline{d}^*} \left(\overline{L}_m, \overline{A}_{m-1}, a_m \right).$

Let $H_{\text{mod},m}^{d_{op,m}, \underline{d}_m^*} \left(\gamma_m^{\overline{d}_{op}, \overline{d}^*} \right)$ be $H_{\text{mod},m}^{d_{op,m}, \underline{d}_m^*} (c_m)$ with $\gamma^{\overline{d}_{op}, \overline{d}^*} \left(\overline{L}_m, \overline{A}_m \right)$ replacing $c_m \left(\overline{L}_m, \overline{A}_m \right)$

Corollary 9.2: Assume (2.5) holds. Then recursively for $m = K, K -$
$1, ..., 0$, we have the following: if $E^* \left[H_{\text{mod},m}^{\bar{d}_{op,m},\underline{d}_m^*} \left(\gamma_m^{\bar{d}_{op},\bar{d}^*} \right) | \bar{L}_m, \bar{A}_{m-1} \right]$
$= E \left[H_{\text{mod},m}^{\bar{d}_{op,m},\underline{d}_m^*} \left(\gamma_m^{\bar{d}_{op},\bar{d}^*} \right) | \bar{L}_m, \bar{A}_{m-1} \right]$ or
$E^* \left[c \left(\bar{L}_m, \bar{A}_m \right) | \bar{L}_m, \bar{A}_{m-1} \right] = E \left[c \left(\bar{L}_m, \bar{A}_m \right) | \bar{L}_m, \bar{A}_{m-1} \right]$ for all $c \left(\bar{L}_m, \bar{A}_m \right)$,
then given any function $g \left(\bar{L}_m, \bar{A}_{m-1} \right)$ that is non-zero w.p1, $\gamma^{\bar{d}_{op},\bar{d}^*} \left(\bar{L}_m, \bar{A}_m \right)$
is the unique function $c \left(\bar{L}_m, \bar{A}_m \right)$ minimizing

$$E \left[g^2 \left(\bar{L}_m, \bar{A}_{m-1} \right) \left\{ H_{\text{mod},m}^{\bar{d}_{op,m},\underline{d}_m^*} \left(c_m \right) - E^* \left[H_{\text{mod},m}^{\bar{d}_{op,m},\underline{d}_m^*} \left(c_m \right) | \bar{L}_m, \bar{A}_{m-1} \right] \right\}^2 \right]$$
$$(9.21)$$

subject to $c \left(\bar{L}_m, \bar{A}_m \right) = 0$ if $A_m = 0$.

The proof is completely analogous to that of Corollary 9.1 and thus is
omitted. Further it holds if we replace d_{op} by any other regime d. Now in
practice one can see that to use this result to find $\gamma^{\bar{d}_{op},\bar{d}^*} \left(\bar{L}_m, \bar{A}_m \right)$ one must
precede recursively and have already found $\gamma^{\bar{d}_{op},\bar{d}^*} \left(\bar{L}_{m+1}, \bar{A}_{m+1} \right)$. One might
wonder whether a simultaneous minimization might work. For example, define
$H^{\bar{d},\bar{d}^*} \left(\bar{c} \right)$ to be the vector with components

$$H_m^{\bar{d},\bar{d}^*} \left(\bar{c}_m \right) = Y - c_m \left(\bar{L}_m, \bar{A}_m \right) -$$
$$\sum_{j=m+1}^{K} \left\{ c_j \left(\bar{L}_j, \bar{A}_{j-1}, d_{op,j}^{c_j} \left(\bar{L}_j, \bar{A}_{j-1} \right) \right) - c_j \left(\bar{L}_j, \bar{A}_j \right) \right\}$$

and $V \left(\bar{c} \right)$ to be the vector with components

$$V_m \left(\bar{c}_m \right) = g \left(\bar{L}_m, \bar{A}_{m-1} \right) \left\{ H_m^{\bar{d},\bar{d}^*} \left(\bar{c}_m \right) - E \left[H_m^{\bar{d},\bar{d}^*} \left(\bar{c}_m \right) | \bar{L}_m, \bar{A}_{m-1} \right] \right\}$$

Note one might have hoped that it would be the case that $V \left(\bar{c} \right)^T B V \left(\bar{c} \right)$ is
minimzed at $c_m \left(\bar{L}_m, \bar{A}_m \right) = \gamma^{\bar{d}_{op},\bar{d}^*} \left(\bar{L}_m, \bar{A}_m \right)$ for $m = 0, 1, .., K$ for some
positive definite matrix B. However a straightforward calculation shows this
is not the case.

The inability to do simultaneous minimization has some very unpleasant
implications when we acknowledge that none of our models $\gamma^j \left(\bar{l}_m, \bar{a}_m; \psi_m^j \right)$, $j =$
$1, ..., J$, $m = K, ..., 0$ for the optimal regimen are correct, where we assume the
ψ_m^j are variation independent as m varies to facilitate sequential fitting.). At
each time m we will consider the J candidates $\hat{\gamma}_m^j \left(\bar{l}_m, \bar{a}_m \right) = \gamma^j \left(\bar{l}_m, \bar{a}_m; \hat{\psi}_m^j \right)$
for $\gamma^j \left(\bar{l}_m, \bar{a}_m \right)$. Suppose, for subjects who receive care in the community until
the time t_K from infection and who presents to our optimal treatment clinic
with history $\left(\bar{L}_K, \bar{A}_{K-1} \right)$, we chose $\hat{\gamma}^{j_K} \left(\bar{l}_K, \bar{a}_K \right)$ minimizing, at $m = K$,

$$P_{n^{val}}^{val} \left[g^2 \left(\bar{L}_m, \bar{A}_{m-1} \right) \left\{ H_{\text{mod},m}^{\bar{d}_{op,m},\underline{d}_m^*} \left(\hat{\gamma}_m^j \right) - E^* \left[H_{\text{mod},m}^{\bar{d}_{op,m},\underline{d}_m^*} \left(\hat{\gamma}_m^j \right) | \bar{L}_m, \bar{A}_{m-1} \right] \right\}^2 \right]$$

for an agreed upon function $g\left(\overline{L}_K, \overline{A}_{K-1}\right)$. Then for subjects who begin following our final estimate $\widehat{d}_{op}$ of the optimal regime beginning at t_0 we would often wish to chose $\widehat{\gamma}^{j_0}\left(\overline{l}_K, \overline{a}_K\right)$ minimizing, at $m = K$, $P^{val}_{nval}[g^2\left(\overline{L}_m, \overline{A}_{m-1}\right) \times$

$$\left\{H^{d_{op},m,d_m^*}_{\text{mod},m}\left(\widehat{\gamma}^j_m\right) - E^*\left[H^{d_{op},m,d_m^*}_{\text{mod},m}\left(\widehat{\gamma}^j_m\right)|\overline{L}_m, \overline{A}_{m-1}\right]\right\}^2 w\left(\overline{L}_m, \overline{A}_{m-1}\right)]$$

with $w\left(\overline{l}_K, \overline{a}_{K-1}\right) = f_{\overline{L}_{\widehat{d}_{op},K}, \overline{A}_{\widehat{d}_{op},K-1}}\left(\overline{l}_K, \overline{a}_{K-1}\right) / f_{\overline{L}_K, \overline{A}_{K-1}}\left(\overline{l}_K, \overline{a}_{K-1}\right)$. But our final estimate $\widehat{d}_{op}$, much less an estimate of $f_{\overline{L}_{\widehat{d}_{op},K}, \overline{A}_{\widehat{d}_{op},K-1}}\left(\overline{l}_K, \overline{a}_{K-1}\right)$, is unknown to us at the time we are estimating $\widehat{\gamma}^{j_0}\left(\overline{l}_K, \overline{a}_K\right)$ since we estimate $\widehat{d}_{op}$ beginning with occassion K. Thus it is not at all straightforward to estimate an optimal regime using Corollary 9.2, suggesting that, in practice, we should use the cross-validation methods described in the previous subsection.

10 Appendix 1:

A1.1: Exceptional Laws:

In this Appendix we prove that under certain exceptional laws F_O (i) no regular estimators of the parameter $\psi^{\dagger}$ of an drSNMM $\gamma^{\overline{0}}\left(\overline{l}_m, \overline{a}_m, \psi^{\dagger}\right)$ for $\gamma^{\overline{d}_{op}}\left(\overline{l}_m, \overline{a}_m\right)$ exists and (ii) although $n^{1/2}$-consistent non-regular estimators exist, they will generally be asymptotically biased. As a consequence our estimators of $E\left[Y_{\overline{d}_{op}}\right]$ may also be non-regular and asymptotically biased.

In the interest of concreteness and with essentially no loss of generality, we will consider example 1 in the main text with $K = 1$, and $L_0 = 0$ wp1 (so we can disregard L_0), A_0, A_1, L_1 all Bernoulli, and $Y = L_2$ continuous. Thus we observe $O = (A_0, A_1, L_1, Y)$. Hence, dropping the $\overline{0}$ superscript from $\gamma^{\overline{0}}$, we have the model $\gamma\left(\overline{l}_1, \overline{a}_1, \psi\right) = a_1\left(1, l_1, a_0\right)\psi_1 = a_1\left(\psi_{11} + \psi_{21}l_1 + \psi_{31}a_0\right), \gamma\left(\overline{l}_0, \overline{a}_0, \psi\right) = \psi_0 a_0$, where we note $\overline{l}_1 = l_1$. We assume sequential randomization and that $f\left(a_m|\overline{l}_m, \overline{a}_{m-1}\right)$ is known. Let $\mathcal{F}$ denote all laws F_O with compact support and consistent with these assumptions. Then, by Eq. 3.8, we have that

$$\psi^{\dagger}_0 = \tag{A1.1}$$

$$[var\left\{A_0\right\}]^{-1} E\left[\left\{A_0 - E[A_0]\right\}\left\{Y + \left(I\left[(1, L_1, A_0)\psi^{\dagger}_1 > 0\right] - A_1\right)(1, L_1, A_0)\psi^{\dagger}_1\right\}\right]$$

We will prove that their is no regular estimator of $\psi^{\dagger}_0$ when $pr\left[(1, L_1, A_0)\psi^{\dagger}_1 = 0\right] \neq 0$, where before doing so it will be pedagogically useful to study the simplest example of the phenomenon.

A simple normal theory example: Consider estimation of the parameter $\psi^{\dagger} = \psi\left(\mu^{\dagger}\right) = \mu^{\dagger}I\left(\mu^{\dagger} > 0\right)$ from n i.i.d. observations X_i from a $N\left(\mu^{\dagger}, 1\right)$

distribution. By definition, a necessary condition for the existence of a regular estimator of $\psi\left(\mu^\dagger\right)$ at $\mu^\dagger$ is that $\psi\left(\mu\right)$ be differentiable at $\mu^\dagger$. As $\psi\left(\mu\right)$ is not differentiable at $\mu=0$, no regular estimator of $\psi^\dagger$ exists at $\mu^\dagger=0$ and we say that $\psi^\dagger$ is a non-regular parameter.

The MLE $I\left(X_{av}>0\right)X_{av}$ with $X_{av}=P_n\left(X\right)$ is an efficient RAL estimator of $\psi^\dagger$ at any non-zero $\mu^\dagger$. To see explicitly that $I\left(X_{av}>0\right)X_{av}$ is non-regular at $\mu^\dagger=0$, we compute its limiting distribution under the local data generating process (LDGP) $\mu=kn^{-1/2}$. Now regularity would mean that the limiting distribution of $V\left(k\right)$ does not depend on k where

$V\left(k\right)=n^{1/2}\left\{I\left(X_{av}>0\right)X_{av}-\psi\left(kn^{-1/2}\right)\right\}$
$=n^{1/2}\left\{I\left(X_{av}>0\right)X_{av}-I\left[kn^{-1/2}>0\right]kn^{-1/2}\right\}$
$=I\left(n^{1/2}\left(X_{av}-kn^{-1/2}\right)>-k\right)n^{1/2}\left(X_{av}-kn^{-1/2}\right)+$
$I\left(n^{1/2}\left(X_{av}-kn^{-1/2}\right)>-k\right)k-I\left[k>0\right]k$
$=I\left(Z>-k\right)Z+I\left(Z>-k\right)k-I\left[k>0\right]k$ where Z is a standard normal deviate. Thus $V\left(k\right)$ converges to the $N\left(0,1\right)$ distribution as $k\to\infty$, to a degenerate random variable with mass 1 at 0 as $k\to-\infty$, and to the law of $I\left(Z>0\right)Z$ for $k=0$. The asymptotic bias $asybias\left(k\right)$ of $I\left(X_{av}>0\right)X_{av}$ as an estimator of $\psi\left(kn^{-1/2}\right)$ is

$$asybias\left(k\right)=\left\{E\left[Z|Z>-k\right]+k\right\}pr\left[Z>-k\right]-I\left[k>0\right]k$$

so

$$asybias\left(0\right)=E\left[Z|Z>0\right]pr\left[Z>0\right]=1/\sqrt{2\pi}=.707\left(\sqrt{\pi}\right)^{-1}.$$

Note the asymptotic bias is bounded for all k. Standard attempts at bias correction such as bootstrapping do not result in an asymptotically unbiased estimator. The exact bias of the MLE $I\left(X_{av}>0\right)X_{av}$ is also $\int_{-n^{1/2}\mu}^{\infty}\left(z+n^{1/2}\mu\right)\phi\left(z\right)dz-\mu I\left(\mu>0\right)$. The parametric bootstrap estimate (i.e. MLE) of bias is thus $\int_{-n^{1/2}X_{av}}^{\infty}\left(z+n^{1/2}X_{av}\right)\phi\left(z\right)dz-X_{av}I\left(X_{av}>0\right)$ so the bootstrap biased corrected estimator of $\mu I\left(\mu>0\right)$ is $2X_{av}I\left(X_{av}>0\right)-\int_{-n^{1/2}X_{av}}^{\infty}\left(z+n^{1/2}X_{av}\right)\phi\left(z\right)dz$ which itself has bias $2\int_{-n^{1/2}\mu}^{\infty}\left(z+n^{1/2}\mu\right)\phi\left(z\right)dz-\mu I\left(\mu>0\right)-E\left[\int_{-n^{1/2}X_{av}}^{\infty}\left(z+n^{1/2}X_{av}\right)\phi\left(z\right)dz\right]$. Thus the asymptotic and exact bias of the bias corrected estimator at $\mu=0$ is

$$2\int_0^\infty z\phi\left(z\right)dz-\int_{-\infty}^\infty\int_{-x}^\infty\left\{z+x\right\}\phi\left(z\right)\phi\left(x\right)dzdx$$
$$=\left(\sqrt{\pi}\right)^{-1}\left(\sqrt{2}-1\right)=.41\left(\sqrt{\pi}\right)^{-1}$$

which is positive although less than the MLE's exact and asymptotic bias of $.707\left(\sqrt{\pi}\right)^{-1}$.

Consider next the submodel of our previous normal model in which we know that $\mu^\dagger>0$. Then for every value of $\mu^\dagger$ in the parameter space $\left(0,\infty\right)$, both the MLE $I\left(X_{av}>0\right)X_{av}$ and the estimator X_{av} of the now regular parameter $\psi^{\dagger} = \psi(\mu^{\dagger}) = \mu^{\dagger} I(\mu^{\dagger} > 0) = \mu^{\dagger}$ are RAL estimators with asymptotic variance 1 i.e. both $n^{1/2}\{I(X_{av} > 0) X_{av} - \psi(\mu^{\dagger} + kn^{-1/2})\}$ and $n^{1/2}\{X_{av} - \psi(\mu^{\dagger} + kn^{-1/2})\}$ converge in distribution to $N(0,1)$ random variable under the LDGP $\mu = \mu^{\dagger} + kn^{-1/2}$. However the MLE Wald interval $I(X_{av} > 0) X_{av} \pm z_{\alpha/2} n^{-1/2}$, in contrast to the interval $X_{av} \pm z_{\alpha/2} n^{-1/2}$, is neither an exact nor a uniform asymptotic $(1 - \alpha)$ conservative confidence interval for $\mu^{\dagger}$, although it is a non-uniform asymptotic $(1 - \alpha)$ confidence interval where we have used the following definitions.

Some Definitions: Suppose we observe n i.i.d copies of a random variable O whose distribution F_O lies in a set $\mathcal{F} = \{F(\psi, \rho) ; (\psi, \rho) \in \Psi \times \mathcal{R}\}$ of distributions indexed by a finite dimesional parameter of interest ψ and, a possibly infinite-dimesional, variation-independent nuisance parameter ρ. We shall need the following from Robins and Ritov (1997). Below, we abbreviate $\sup\limits_{(\psi,\rho) \in \Psi \times \mathcal{R}}$ by $\sup\limits_{(\psi,\rho)}$.

Definition: An estimator $\widehat{\psi}_n$ (with n indexing sample size) is uniformly regular Gaussian (URG) with uniform asymptotic variance $\sigma^2(\psi, \rho)$ if

$$\sup_{(\psi,\rho)} | \Pr_{(\psi,\rho)} \left[n^{\frac{1}{2}} \left(\widehat{\psi}_n - \psi \right) < t \right] - \Phi\left(t; \sigma^2(\psi,\rho)\right) | \to 0 \text{ as } n \to \infty \quad \text{(A1.2)}$$

where $\Phi(t; \sigma^2)$ is the cumulative distribution function of a normal random variable with mean zero and variance σ^2. If $\widehat{\psi}_n$ is a uniformly asymptotic linear estimator of ψ (i.e. the $o_p(1)$ term in the definition of an asymptotically linear estimator is uniformly $o_p(1)$ over all laws in $\Psi \times \mathcal{R}$), then $\widehat{\psi}_n$ is URG. However, $\widehat{\psi}_n$, a regular asymptotic linear (RAL) estimator, does not imply $\widehat{\psi}_n$ is URG.

Definition: The estimator $\widehat{\psi}_n$ is uniformly asymptotically normal and unbiased (UANU) for ψ if there exists a sequence $\sigma_n^2(\psi, \rho)$ such that the z-statistic $n^{\frac{1}{2}} \left(\widehat{\psi}_n - \psi \right) / \sigma_n(\psi, \rho)$ converges uniformly to a $N(0,1)$ random variable, i.e.

$$\sup_{(\psi,\rho)} | \Pr_{(\psi,\rho)} \left[n^{\frac{1}{2}} \left(\widehat{\psi}_n - \psi \right) / \sigma_n(\psi, \rho) < t \right] - \Phi(t; 1) | \to 0 \text{ as } n \to \infty .$$

$$\text{(A1.3)}$$

$\widehat{\psi}_n$ URG implies $\widehat{\psi}_n$ UANU but the converse is false. However, if $\widehat{\psi}_n$ is UANU and $\sigma_n(\psi, \rho)$ converges uniformly to $\sigma(\psi, \rho)$ i.e.

$$\sup_{(\psi,\rho)} | \sigma(\psi, \rho) / \sigma_n(\psi, \rho) - 1 | \to 0 \text{ as } n \to \infty \quad \text{(A1.4)}$$

the $\widehat{\psi}_n$ is URG. Furthermore, if $\widehat{\psi}_n$ is UANU and there exists an estimator $\widehat{\sigma}_n$ of $\sigma_n(\psi, \rho)$ such that $\sigma_n(\psi, \rho) / \widehat{\sigma}_n$ converges to one uniformly in probability, i.e. for all $\varepsilon > 0$

$$\sup_{(\psi,\rho)} \Pr_{(\psi,\rho)} [| 1 - \sigma_n(\psi, \rho) / \widehat{\sigma}_n | > \varepsilon] \to 0 \text{ as } n \to \infty \quad \text{(A1.5)}$$

then, by the uniform version of Slutzky's Theorem, the t-statistic $n^{\frac{1}{2}} \left(\widehat{\psi}_n - \psi \right) /$ $\widehat{\sigma}_n$ converges uniformly to a $N(0,1)$ random variable, and thus the "Wald" interval $C_n \equiv \widehat{\psi}_n \pm z_{\alpha/2} \widehat{\sigma}_n / \sqrt{n}$ is a uniform asymptotic $1 - \alpha$ confidence interval for ψ where $z_{\alpha/2}$ is the $\alpha/2$ quantile of a standard normal distribution, and we have the following definition.

Definition: C_n is a uniform asymptotic $1 - \alpha$ confidence interval for ψ if $\sup_{(\psi,\rho)} |\Pr_{(\psi,\rho)} [\psi \in C_n] - (1 - \alpha)| \to 0$ as $n \to \infty$.

Definiton: C_n is a conservative uniform asymptotic $1 - \alpha$ confidence interval for ψ if

$$\liminf_n \inf_{(\psi,\rho)} \left\{ \Pr_{(\psi,\rho)} [\psi \in C_n] - (1 - \alpha) \right\} \geq 0 \text{ as } n \to \infty$$

Note a uniform asymptotic $1 - \alpha$ confidence interval is a conservative uniform asymptotic $1 - \alpha$ confidence interval. We required uniformity in our definition of an asymptotic confidence interval to be consistent with the usual definition of a non-asymptotic confidence interval. Specifically, by definition, for each sample size n, a conservative $1 - \alpha$ (non-asymptotic) confidence interval C_n satisfies that for all $(\psi, \rho) \in \Psi \times \mathcal{R}$,

$$\Pr_{(\psi,\rho)} [\psi \in C_n] \geq 1 - \alpha.$$

Our definition of a uniform asymptotic confidence interval satisfies the following consistency condition: if there is no conservative (non-asymptotic) $1 - \alpha$ confidence interval for ψ whose length converges to 0 in probability as $n \to \infty$, then no conservative uniform asymptotic $1 - \alpha$ confidence interval for ψ exists whose length converges to 0 in probability as $n \to \infty$; in contrast, there may still exist a conservative asymptotic $1 - \alpha$ confidence interval for ψ whose length converges to 0 in probability as $n \to \infty$, where we have the following.

Definition: C_n is a conservative asymptotic $1 - \alpha$ confidence interval for ψ if for all $(\psi, \rho) \in \Psi \times \mathcal{R}$, $\liminf_n \left\{ \Pr_{(\psi,\rho)} [\psi \in C_n] - (1 - \alpha) \right\} \geq 0$ as $n \to \infty$

If $\widehat{\psi}$ is UANU and $\sigma_n(\psi, \rho) / \widehat{\sigma}_n$ converges uniformly to one, then the $\widehat{\psi}_n \pm z_{\alpha/2} \widehat{\sigma}_n / \sqrt{n}$ will be a uniform asymptotic $(1 - \alpha)$ confidence interval for ψ, even if $\widehat{\psi}_n$ is not URG. If $\widehat{\psi}_n$ is UANU but not URG, then even if $\sigma_n(\psi, \rho) \to \sigma(\psi, \rho)$ as $n \to \infty$ for all (ψ, ρ), this convergence cannot be uniform. Further, under mild regularity conditions, when $\widehat{\psi}_n$ is UANU, the non-parametric bootstrap estimator $\widehat{\sigma}_n$ of the standard error of $n^{\frac{1}{2}} \left(\widehat{\psi}_n - \psi \right)$ will satisfy (A1.5). Hence, if $\widehat{\psi}_n$ is UANU, then a Wald interval centered on $\widehat{\psi}_n$ and using a bootstrap estimate of the standard error will be an asymptotic uniform $(1 - \alpha)$ Wald confidence interval for ψ

The simple normal example continued: Returning to the simple normal example with $\mu^\dagger \in (0, \infty)$, the Wald interval $I(X_{av} > 0) X_{av} \pm z_{\alpha/2} n^{-1/2}$ is not a uniform asymptotic $(1 - \alpha)$ conservative confidence interval for $\mu^\dagger$ because $I(X_{av} > 0) X_{av}$, in contrast to X_{av}, is not URG. Indeed

$I(X_{av} > 0) X_{av}$ is not even UANU and thus cannot center a uniform asymptotic $(1 - \alpha)$ confidence interval even were its standard error estimated with the bootstrap. The reason that $I(X_{av} > 0) X_{av}$ is not UANU is that, at each sample size n, there exists a $\mu^\dagger \in (0, \infty)$ depending on n that is sufficiently close to 0 that $I(X_{av} > 0) X_{av}$ is significantly biased upwards as an estimator of $\psi^\dagger = \mu^\dagger$. However, if we took the parameter space for $\mu^\dagger$ to be (σ, ∞) for a fixed $\sigma > 0$, then $I(X_{av} > 0) X_{av}$ is UANU and can center a uniform asymptotic $(1 - \alpha)$ confidence interval. Returning to the case where the parameter space for $\mu^\dagger$ is the entire real line so no UANU estimator of $\psi^\dagger$ exists, we can nonetheless construct a conservative non-asymptotic $(1 - \alpha)$ confidence interval for $\psi^\dagger$ that is also a conservative uniform asymptotic $(1 - \alpha)$ confidence interval by intersecting the usual interval $X_{av} \pm z_{\alpha/2} n^{-1/2}$ for $\mu^\dagger$ with the non-negative real line to obtain $\{X_{av} \pm z_{\alpha/2} n^{-1/2}\} \cap [0, \infty)$.

Return to our optimal-regime SNMM example. In this example, the data distribution can be parametrized as follows: $f(Y, \overline{L}_1, \overline{A}_1; \psi_1, \theta) = f(\delta(\psi_1, \theta_1)|\overline{L}_1, \overline{A}_1; \theta_2) f(A_1|\overline{L}_1, A_0) f(L_1|A_0; \theta_3) f(A_0)$, where $\theta = (\theta_1, \theta_2, \theta_3)$, $\delta(\psi_1, \theta_1) = Y - A_1 (1, L_1, A_0) \psi_1 - \{q(L_1, A_0; \theta_1) - \int q(L_1, A_0; \theta_1) dF(L_1|A_0; \theta_3)\}$ and θ_1 indexes all functions $q(L_1, A_0; \theta_1)$ of (L_1, A_0) that satisfy $q(0, A_0; \theta_1) = 0$, θ_2 indexes all conditional densities $f(u|\overline{L}_1, \overline{A}_1; \theta_2)$ satisfying the conditional mean zero restriction $\int u f(u|\overline{L}_1, \overline{A}_1; \theta_2) = 0$, and θ_3 indexes all conditional densities $f(L_1|A_0; \theta_3)$. In this parametrization we view $\psi_0^\dagger$ as a function of $(\psi_1^\dagger, \theta^\dagger)$ determined by equation (A1.1). In the following discussion $\psi_0^\dagger$ and $\psi_1^\dagger$ are analogous to $\psi^\dagger$ and $\mu^\dagger$ respectively in our normal example. Consider a regular parametric submodel with θ fixed at its true value $\theta^\dagger$ and ψ_1 a free parameter with true value $\psi_1^\dagger$. Then $\psi_0(\psi_1) = [var\{A_0\}]^{-1} \times E_{\psi_1, \theta^\dagger} [\{A_0 - E[A_0]\} \{Y_{K+1} + (I[(1, L_1, A_0) \psi_1 > 0] - A_1)(1, L_1, A_0) \psi_1\}]$ and $\psi_0(\psi_1)$ is a differentiable function of ψ_1 at the truth $(\psi_1^\dagger, \theta^\dagger)$ w.p.1. if and only if the event $(1, L_1, A_0) \psi_1^\dagger = 0$ has probability 0 under $f(Y, \overline{L}_1, \overline{A}_1; \psi_1^\dagger, \theta^\dagger)$. It follows that if $pr_{\psi_1^\dagger, \theta^\dagger} [(1, L_1, A_0) \psi_1^\dagger = 0] \neq 0$, then ψ_0 is not a pathwise differentiable parameter and thus no regular estimator of ψ_0 exists under the data generating process $(\psi_1^\dagger, \theta^\dagger)$. If $pr_{\psi_1^\dagger, \theta^\dagger} [(1, L_1, A_0) \psi_1^\dagger = 0] = 0$ the closed form estimator estimator $\widetilde{\psi}_0$ of Sec. 4.2 is regular at $(\psi_1^\dagger, \theta^\dagger)$.

This raises the question as to the asymptotic distribution and asymptotic mean of $\widetilde{\psi}_0$ when $pr_{\psi_1^\dagger, \theta^\dagger} [(1, L_1, A_0) \psi_1^\dagger = 0] \neq 0$, i.e. under an exceptional law. [Analogous results apply to the non-closed form estimators of $\psi_0^\dagger$ discussed earlier; the advantage of considering the simpler $\widetilde{\psi}_0$ is that its behavior is relatively transparent.] Abbreviate $U_{mod, m}^{\overline{d}_{op}, \overline{0}}$ of Section 4.2 to U_m.

Recall

$$\tilde{\psi}_0 = \tilde{I}_0^{-1}$$

$$P_n \left[\{s_0(A_0) - E[s_0(A_0)]\} \left\{ Y + \left(I\left[(1, L_1, A_0)\,\tilde{\psi}_1 > 0\right] - A_1 \right)(1, L_1, A_0)\,\tilde{\psi}_1 \right\} \right]$$

with $\tilde{I}_0 = P_n \left[\{s_0(A_0) - E[s_0(A_0)]\} A_0\right]$. Recall $\tilde{\psi}_0$ solves

$$0 = n^{1/2} P_n \left[U_0 \left(\psi_0, s_0, \tilde{\psi}_1 \right) \right]$$

where

$$U_0 \left(\psi_0, s_0, \tilde{\psi}_1 \right) \qquad\qquad (A1.6)$$
$$= \{s_0(A_0) - E[s_0(A_0)]\} \times$$
$$\left\{ Y - \psi_0 A_0 + \left(I\left[(1, L_1, A_0)\,\tilde{\psi}_1 > 0\right] - A_1 \right)(1, L_1, A_0)\,\tilde{\psi}_1 \right\}.$$

Now

$$n^{1/2} P_n \left[U_0 \left(\psi_0, s_0, \tilde{\psi}_1 \right) \right]$$
$$= n^{1/2} P_n \left[U_0 \left(\psi_0, s_0, \psi_1^\dagger \right) \right] + n^{1/2} P_n \left[\Delta_0 \left(s_0, \tilde{\psi}_1, \psi_1^\dagger \right) \right],$$

where
$$\Delta_0 \left(s_0, \tilde{\psi}_1, \psi_1^\dagger \right) = I\left[(1, L_1, A_0)\,\psi_1^\dagger = 0\right] \{s_0(A_0) - E[s_0(A_0)]\} \times$$
$$\left(I\left[(1, L_1, A_0)\left(\tilde{\psi}_1 - \psi_1^\dagger\right) > 0\right] - A_1 \right)(1, L_1, A_0)\left(\tilde{\psi}_1 - \psi_1^\dagger\right) +$$
$$I\left[(1, L_1, A_0)\,\psi_1^\dagger \neq 0\right] \{s_0(A_0) - E[s_0(A_0)]\} \times$$
$$\left[\begin{array}{c} \left(I\left[(1, L_1, A_0)\,\tilde{\psi}_1 > 0\right] - A_1 \right)(1, L_1, A_0)\,\tilde{\psi}_1 - \\ \left(I\left[(1, L_1, A_0)\,\psi_1^\dagger > 0\right] - A_1 \right)(1, L_1, A_0)\,\psi_1^\dagger \end{array} \right].$$

To be concrete suppose that $\sum_{j=1}^3 \psi_{j1}^\dagger = 0$, but none of the $\psi_{j1}^\dagger$ are zero so $(1, L_1, A_0)\,\psi_1^\dagger = 0 \iff L_1 = A_0 = 1$ which we assume happens with positive probability so the law is exceptional. Then, we have $n^{1/2} P_n \left[\Delta_0 \left(s_0, \tilde{\psi}_1, \psi_1^\dagger \right) \right] =$

$$n^{1/2} P_n \left[\begin{array}{c} I\left[(1, L_1, A_0)\,\psi_1^\dagger = 0\right] \{s_0(A_0) - E[s_0(A_0)]\} \times \\ \left(I\left[\sum_{j=1}^3 \left(\tilde{\psi}_{j1} - \psi_{j1}^\dagger\right) > 0\right] - A_1 \right) \sum_{j=1}^3 \left(\tilde{\psi}_{j1} - \psi_{j1}^\dagger\right) \end{array} \right] +$$

$$n^{1/2} P_n \left[\begin{array}{c} I\left[(1, L_1, A_0)\,\psi_1^\dagger \neq 0\right] \{s_0(A_0) - E[s_0(A_0)]\} \times \\ \left(I\left[(1, L_1, A_0)\,\psi_1^\dagger > 0\right] - A_1 \right)(1, L_1, A_0)\left(\tilde{\psi}_1 - \psi_1^\dagger\right) \end{array} \right] + o_p(1).$$

To obtain this result we used the fact that, conditional on $\{(A_{0i}, L_{1i}); i = 1, ..., n\}$, when $(1, l_1, a_0) \psi_1^\dagger \neq 0$, $I\left[(1, l_1, a_0) \tilde{\psi}_1 > 0\right] = I\left[(1, l_1, a_0) \psi_1^\dagger > 0\right] + o_p(1)$ under any $F_O \in \mathcal{F}$. To prove this fact we reasoned as follows. Because, as argued below, with probability going to one, $\tilde{\psi}_1$ is $n^{1/2} - consistent$ for $\psi_1^\dagger$ conditional on $\{(A_{0i}, L_{1i}); i = 1, ..., n\}$, it follows that whenever $(1, l_1, a_0) \psi_1^\dagger \neq 0$, $(1, l_1, a_0) \tilde{\psi}_1$ and $(1, l_1, a_0) \psi_1^\dagger$ will have the same sign except on a set $C(l_1, a_0)$ with conditional probability given $\{(A_{0i}, L_{1i}); i = 1, ..., n\}$ converging to 0. That is

$$\text{for all } \left\{F_O; F_O \in \mathcal{F}, \ (1, l_1, a_0) \psi_1^\dagger (F_O) \neq 0\right\}, \qquad (A1.7)$$

$\cdot pr_{F_O} \left[\{O_i, i = 1, ..., n\} \in C(l_1, a_0) \mid \{(A_{0i}, L_{1i}); i = 1, ..., n\}\right] \to 0 \text{ as } n \to \infty.$

However it is important to note for later reference that this convergence is not uniform, i.e.,

$$\sup_{F_O \in \tilde{Q}} pr\left[\{O_i, i = 1, ..., n\} \in C(l_1, a_0) \mid \{(A_{0i}, L_{1i}); i = 1, ..., n\}\right] \qquad (A1.8)$$

$$\nrightarrow 0 \text{ as } n \to \infty,$$

$\tilde{Q} = \left\{F_O; F_O \in \mathcal{F}, \ (1, l_1, a_0) \psi_1^\dagger (F_O) \neq 0\right\}$, because for each sample size n and each (l_1, a_0), there exists a $F_O \in \mathcal{F}$ with $(1, l_1, a_0) \psi_1^\dagger \neq 0$ but $(1, l_1, a_0) \psi_1^\dagger$ within $O\left(n^{-1/2}\right)$ of 0. It follows that due to the $O\left(n^{-1/2}\right)$ fluctuations in $\tilde{\psi}_1$, $(1, l_1, a_0) \tilde{\psi}_1$ and $(1, l_1, a_0) \psi_1^\dagger$ will have different signs with probability substantially greater than 0.

To proceed in our analysis of $\tilde{\psi}_0$, we need to analyze $\tilde{\psi}_1$. By a Taylor expansion $\tilde{\psi}_1$ is a RAL estimator so that

$$n^{1/2} \left(\tilde{\psi}_1 - \psi_1^\dagger\right) = n^{1/2} P_n [IF_1] + o_p(1),$$

where

$$IF_1 = (IF_{11}, IF_{21}, IF_{31})^T$$

$$= I_1^{-1}(s_1) U_1\left(\psi_1^\dagger, s_1\right),$$

$$I_1(s_1) = -\partial E\left[U_1\left(\psi_1^\dagger, s_1\right)\right] / \partial \psi_1$$

Thus, by another Taylor expansion of around $\tilde{\psi}_1$ around $\psi_1^\dagger$,

$$n^{1/2} P_n\left[\Delta_0\left(s_0, \tilde{\psi}_1, \psi_1^\dagger\right)\right] = E\left[A_0 L_1 \{s_0(A_0) - E[s_0(A_0)]\} \times\right.$$

$$I\left[n^{1/2} P_n\left[\sum_{j=1}^3 IF_{j1}\right] > 0\right] n^{1/2} P_n\left[\sum_{j=1}^3 IF_{j1}\right] -$$

$$E\left[A_1 A_0 L_1 \{s_0(A_0) - E[s_0(A_0)]\}\right] n^{1/2} P_n\left[\sum_{j=1}^3 IF_{j1}\right] +$$

$$E\left[I\left[(1, L_1, A_0) \psi_1^\dagger \neq 0\right] \{s_0(A_0) - E[s_0(A_0)]\} \times\right.$$

$$\left(I\left[(1,L_1,A_0)\,\psi_1^\dagger > 0\right] - A_1\right)(1,L_1,A_0)\right]n^{1/2}P_n\left[IF_1\right] + o_p\,(1)\,.$$ Note in terms of the estimation of $\psi_1^\dagger$, $\{(A_{0i},L_{1i})\,;i=1,...,n\}$ is ancillary, so $\widetilde{\psi}_1$ is $n^{1/2} -$ *consistent* for $\psi_1^\dagger$ conditional on $\{(A_{0i},L_{1i})\,;i=1,...,n\}$.

Let $Z = \left(Z_0, Z_1^T\right)^T = (Z_0, Z_{11}, Z_{21}, Z_{31})^T$ be MVN with mean 0 and variance equal to that of $\left(U_0, IF_1^T\right)^T = (U_0, IF_{11}, IF_{21}, IF_{31})^T$ with $U_0 = U_0\left(\psi_0^\dagger, s_0, \psi_1^\dagger\right)$. Let $Z_{1+} = Z_{11} + Z_{21} + Z_{31}$. Then it follows from the expansion above that, under our assumption that for the F_O generating the data $A_0L_1 = 1 \Leftrightarrow I\left[(1,L_1,A_0)\,\psi_1^\dagger = 0\right]$, $n^{1/2}\left(\widetilde{\psi}_0 - \psi_0^\dagger\right)$ converges in law to the distribution of $I_0^{-1}\,(s_0)\times$

$$Z_0 + E\left[A_0L_1\left\{s_0\,(A_0) - E[s_0\,(A_0)]\right\}\right]I\left[Z_{1+} > 0\right]Z_{1+} -$$
$$\left\{E\left[A_1A_0L_1\left\{s_0\,(A_0) - E[s_0\,(A_0)]\right\}\right]Z_{1+}\right\} +$$
$$E\left[\left\{1 - A_0L_1\right\}\left\{s_0\,(A_0) - E[s_0\,(A_0)]\right\}\left(I\left[(1,L_1,A_0)\,\psi_1^\dagger > 0\right] - A_1\right)(1,L_1,A_0)\right]Z_1$$

where

$$I_0\,(s_0) = -\partial E\left[U_0\left(\psi_0, s_0, \psi_1^\dagger\right)\right]/\partial\psi_0 = E\left[\left\{s_0\,(A_0) - E[s_0\,(A_0)]\right\}A_0\right]\,.$$

Because of the term $E\left[A_0L_1\left\{s_0\,(A_0) - E[s_0\,(A_0)]\right\}\right]I\left[Z_{1+} > 0\right]Z_{1+}$, $\widetilde{\psi}_0$, although $n^{1/2}$-consistent, is neither asymptotically normal nor asymptotically unbiased. The asymptotic bias $asybias\,(0)$ is $I_0^{-1}\,(s_0)\left\{E\left[A_0L_1\left\{s_0\,(A_0) - E[s_0\,(A_0)]\right\}\right]\right\}E\left[Z_{1+}|Z_{1+} > 0\right]pr\left[Z_{1+} > 0\right]$. Thus

$$asybias\,(0) = I_0^{-1}\,(s_0)\,E\left[A_0L_1\left\{s_0\,(A_0) - E[s_0\,(A_0)]\right\}\right]\left\{var\left[Z_{1+}\right]\right\}^{1/2}/\sqrt{2\pi}\,.$$

To see that the estimator $\widetilde{\psi}_0$ is non-regular when $\psi_{11}^\dagger + \psi_{21}^\dagger + \psi_{31}^\dagger = 0$, (implied by our assumption $I\left[(1,L_1,A_0)\,\psi_1^\dagger = 0\right] \Longleftrightarrow L_1 = A_0 = 1$), consider the local data generating process $(\psi_1^T, \theta^\dagger) = \left(\psi_{11}, \psi_{21}^\dagger, \psi_{31}^\dagger, \theta^\dagger\right)$ with $\psi_{11} = \psi_{11}^\dagger + kn^{-1/2}$. Then
$$n^{1/2}P_n\left[U_0\left(\psi_0, s_0, \widetilde{\psi}_1\right)\right] = n^{1/2}P_n\left[U_0\left(\psi_0, s_0, \psi_1\right)\right] + n^{1/2}P_n\left[\Delta_0\left(s_0, \widetilde{\psi}_1, \psi_1\right)\right],$$
$$\Delta_0\left(s_0, \widetilde{\psi}_1, \psi_1\right) = I\left[(1,L_1,A_0)\,\psi_1^\dagger = 0\right]\left\{s_0\,(A_0) - E[s_0\,(A_0)]\right\}\times$$
$$\left(I\left[(1,L_1,A_0)\left(\widetilde{\psi}_1 - \psi_1^\dagger\right) > 0\right] - A_1\right)(1,L_1,A_0)\left(\widetilde{\psi}_1 - \psi_1^\dagger\right)\widetilde{\psi}_1$$
$$-I\left[(1,L_1,A_0)\,\psi_1^\dagger = 0\right]\left\{s_0\,(A_0) - E[s_0\,(A_0)]\right\}\left(I\left[kn^{-1/2} > 0\right] - A_1\right)kn^{-1/2} +$$
$$I\left[(1,L_1,A_0)\,\psi_1^\dagger \neq 0\right]\left\{s_0\,(A_0) - E[s_0\,(A_0)]\right\}\left[\left(I\left[(1,L_1,A_0)\,\widetilde{\psi}_1 > 0\right] - A_1\right)\times\right.$$
$$(1,L_1,A_0)\,\widetilde{\psi}_1 - (I\left[(1,L_1,A_0)\,\psi_1 > 0\right] - A_1)(1,L_1,A_0)\,\psi_1\right].$$

Thus $n^{1/2}P_n\left[\Delta_0\left(s_0, \widetilde{\psi}_1, \psi_1\right)\right] =$
$$n^{1/2}P_n\left[\begin{array}{c}A_0L_1\left\{s_0\,(A_0) - E[s_0\,(A_0)]\right\}\times \\ \left(I\left[\sum_{j=1}^3\left(\widetilde{\psi}_{1j} - \psi_{1j}^\dagger\right) > 0\right] - A_1\right)\sum_{j=1}^3\left(\widetilde{\psi}_{1j} - \psi_{1j}^\dagger\right)\end{array}\right]$$

$$-n^{1/2}P_n\left[I\left[(1,L_1,A_0)\,\psi_1^\dagger=0\right]\{s_0\,(A_0)-E[s_0\,(A_0)]\}\,(I\,[k>0]-A_1)\,kn^{-1/2}\right]+$$

$$n^{1/2}P_n\begin{bmatrix}I\left[(1,L_1,A_0)\,\psi_1^\dagger\neq0\right]\{s_0\,(A_0)-E[s_0\,(A_0)]\}\times\\\left(I\left[(1,L_1,A_0)\,\psi_1^\dagger>0\right]-A_1\right)(1,L_1,A_0)\left(\widetilde\psi_1-\psi_1\right)\end{bmatrix}$$

$$+o_p\,(1).$$

Now $\widetilde\psi_1$ is a RAL estimator so that $n^{1/2}\left(\widetilde\psi_1-\psi_1\right)$ has the same limiting distribution under $\left(\psi_1,\theta_1^\dagger\right)$ as $n^{1/2}\left(\widetilde\psi_1-\psi_1^\dagger\right)$ under $\left(\psi_1^\dagger,\theta_1^\dagger\right)$. Therefore noting

$$\left(I\left[\textstyle\sum_{j=1}^3\left(\widetilde\psi_{1j}-\psi_{1j}^\dagger\right)>0\right]-A_1\right)\sum_{j=1}^3\left(\widetilde\psi_{1j}-\psi_{1j}^\dagger\right)=$$
$$\left(I\left[\textstyle\sum_{j=1}^3\left(\widetilde\psi_{1j}-\psi_{1j}\right)>-kn^{-1/2}\right]-A_1\right)\left[\sum_{j=1}^3\left(\widetilde\psi_{1j}-\psi_{1j}\right)+kn^{-1/2}\right],\text{ let}$$

$Z=\left(Z_0,Z_1^T\right)^T=(Z_0,Z_{11},Z_{12},Z_{13})^T$ have the same distribution as above.

Then $n^{1/2}\left(\widetilde\psi_0-\psi_0\left(\psi_1^T,\theta^\dagger\right)\right)$ converges in law to the distribution of $I_0^{-1}\,(s_0)\times$

$$\begin{bmatrix}Z_0+E\left[A_0L_1\{s_0\,(A_0)-E[s_0\,(A_0)]\}\right]I\,[Z_{1+}>-k]\,[Z_{1+}+k]\\-E\left[A_1A_0L_1\{s_0\,(A_0)-E[s_0\,(A_0)]\}\right][Z_{1+}+k]\\+E\left[I\left[(1,L_1,A_0)\,\psi_1^\dagger=0\right]\{s_0\,(A_0)-E[s_0\,(A_0)]\}\,(I\,[k>0]-A_1)\right]k+Z_1\times\\E\left[I\left[(1,L_1,A_0)\,\psi_1^\dagger\neq0\right]\{s_0\,(A_0)-E[s_0\,(A_0)]\}\times\\\left(I\left[(1,L_1,A_0)\,\psi_1^\dagger>0\right]-A_1\right)(1,L_1,A_0)\right]\end{bmatrix}$$

which can be written $I_0^{-1}\,(s_0)\times$

$$\begin{bmatrix}Z_0+E\left[A_0L_1\{s_0\,(A_0)-E[s_0\,(A_0)]\}\right]I\,[Z_{1+}>-k]\,[Z_{1+}+k]\\-E\left[A_1A_0L_1\{s_0\,(A_0)-E[s_0\,(A_0)]\}\right]Z_{1+}\\+E\left[A_0L_1\{s_0\,(A_0)-E[s_0\,(A_0)]\}\right]k\,(I\,[k>0])+Z_1\times\\E\left[\{1-A_0L_1\}\{s_0\,(A_0)-E[s_0\,(A_0)]\}\left(I\left[(1,L_1,A_0)\,\psi_1^\dagger>0\right]-A_1\right)(1,L_1,A_0)\right]\end{bmatrix}.$$

Thus, the mean of the limiting distribution [i.e the asymptotic bias, $asybias\,(k)$, of $\widetilde\psi_0$] is

$$I_0^{-1}\,(s_0)\left\{\begin{matrix}E\left[A_0L_1\{s_0\,(A_0)-E[s_0\,(A_0)]\}\right]E\,[Z_{1+}+k|Z_{1+}>-k]\,pr\,[Z_{1+}>-k]\\+E\left[A_0L_1\{s_0\,(A_0)-E[s_0\,(A_0)]\}\right]k\,(I\,[k>0])\end{matrix}\right\}$$

Since the limiting distribution depends on k, $\widetilde\psi_0$ is not regular at exceptional laws. It follows that the nominal $(1-\alpha)$ Wald interval centered on $\widetilde\psi_0$ is not a conservative $(1-\alpha)$ uniform asymptotic confidence interval. Appropriate alternative methods for construction of uniform asymptotic confidence intervals for the entire vector $\psi^\dagger$ are discussed in Section 4.3 and for subvectors such as $\psi_0^\dagger$ in section 5.1.

Now suppose one objected to the above example by arguing that it is apriori unlikely that $\sum_{j=1}^3\psi_{j1}^\dagger=0$, when none of the $\psi_{j1}^\dagger$ are zero as such a fortuitous cancellation of parameter values would be apriori unlikely. If we apriori excluded such unlikely laws from our model then the only remaining exceptional laws would be those corresponding to the null hypothesis $\psi_{j1}^\dagger=0$ for $j=1,2,3$ that says treatment at time 1 has no effect. Suppose, however, that it was known from other considerations that this null hypothesis was false. Then we are led to consider the submodel of our original model in which we impose the additional apriori assumption that $(1, l_1, a_0)\,\psi_1^\dagger \neq 0$ for any (l_1, a_0). This model has no exceptional laws. In this setting, $\psi_0^\dagger$ is a regular parameter and $\tilde{\psi}_0$ is a RAL estimator at all laws in the model. However we now argue that $\tilde{\psi}_0$ is not UANU. Thus a nominal $(1 - \alpha)$ Wald interval centered on $\tilde{\psi}_0$ is not a conservative $(1 - \alpha)$ uniform asymptotic confidence interval, although it is a $(1 - \alpha)$ non-uniform asymptotic interval.

To see why we revisit our derivation of the large sample distribution of $\tilde{\psi}_0$ except now $I\left[(1, L_1, A_0)\,\psi_1^\dagger = 0\right]$ takes the value zero with probability one. Recall that in our derivation we proved that, asymptotically,

$$n^{1/2} P_n\left[\Delta_0\left(s_0, \tilde{\psi}_1, \psi_1^\dagger\right)\right] = n^{1/2} P_n\left[\{s_0\left(A_0\right) - E[s_0\left(A_0\right)]\} \times\right.$$
$$\left\{\left(I\left[(1, L_1, A_0)\,\tilde{\psi}_1 > 0\right] - A_1\right)(1, L_1, A_0)\,\tilde{\psi}_1 -\right.$$
$$\left.\left.\left(I\left[(1, L_1, A_0)\,\psi_1^\dagger > 0\right] - A_1\right)(1, L_1, A_0)\,\psi_1^\dagger\right\}\right]$$

did not have the random $\tilde{\psi}_1$ within an indicator function by using the fact that $I\left[(1, l_1, a_0)\,\tilde{\psi}_1 > 0\right] = I\left[(1, l_1, a_0)\,\psi_1^\dagger > 0\right] + o_p(1)$ under any $F_O \in \mathcal{F}$ leading to $n^{1/2} P_n\left[\Delta_0\left(s_0, \tilde{\psi}_1, \psi_1^\dagger\right)\right] =$

$$n^{1/2} P_n\left[\{s_0\left(A_0\right) - E[s_0\left(A_0\right)]\}\left(I\left[(1, L_1, A_0)\,\psi_1^\dagger > 0\right] - A_1\right)(1, L_1, A_0)\left(\tilde{\psi}_1 - \psi_1^\dagger\right)\right]$$

$+ o_p(1)$. But in (A1.8), we showed that these $o_p(1)$ terms were not uniform because for each n there exist $F_O \in \mathcal{F}$ with $(1, l_1, a_0)\,\psi_1^\dagger \neq 0$ but $(1, l_1, a_0)\,\psi_1^\dagger$ within $O\left(n^{-1/2}\right)$ of 0. As a consequence $n^{1/2} P_n\left[\Delta_0\left(s_0, \tilde{\psi}_1, \psi_1^\dagger\right)\right]$ and thus $n^{1/2}\left(\tilde{\psi}_0 - \psi_0^\dagger\right)$, although asymptotically normal, are not UANU because we cannot uniformly remove $\tilde{\psi}_1$ from within an indicator function. However, if we further reduced our model by assuming $\left|(1, l_1, a_0)\,\psi_1^\dagger\right| > \sigma > 0$ for some fixed σ and all (l_1, a_0), then $n^{1/2}\left(\tilde{\psi}_0 - \psi_0^\dagger\right)$ would be UANU and a nominal $(1 - \alpha)$ Wald interval centered on $\tilde{\psi}_0$ would be $(1 - \alpha)$ uniform asymptotic confidence interval.

What does all this asymptotics imply for practical finite sample inference in non toy examples? I believe the take home message is roughly as follows. (The task of backing up the statements in this paragraph through further theoretical work and simulation experiments remains to be done.) Consider the uniform asymptotic confidence interval $C_{op}(1 - \alpha)$ for the entire vector $\psi^\dagger$ discussed in Section 4.3. Let $H_{m,i} = card\left\{d_{op,m}\left(\overline{L}_{m,i}, \overline{A}_{m-1,i}, \psi\right); \psi \in C_{op}(1 - \alpha)\right\}$ be the number of potential optimal treatment strategies at time m for subject i based on his observed data $(\overline{L}_{m,i}, \overline{A}_{m-1,i})$ that are consistent with his observed data. If the fraction p_{op} of the $H_{m,i}$ in the set $\{H_{m,i}; i = 1, ..., n, \ m = 1, ..., K\}$ that exceed 1 is moderate to large (say, $p_{op} > .05$) then inferences based on ordinary Wald point and interval estimates are unreliable for frequentist inference and the methods of sections 4.3 and 5.1 should be used instead. In terms of our toy model, the fraction of the $H_{m,i}$ exceeding 1 is an informal upper bound on how often $I\left[(1, l_1, a_0)\, \widetilde{\psi}_1 > 0\right]$ might differ from $I\left[(1, l_1, a_0)\, \psi_1^\dagger > 0\right]$ over the set of $\psi_1^\dagger$ consistent with the observed data (as determined via the confidence interval $C_{op}(1 - \alpha)$). If p_{op} is small our finite sample inferences should agree with those based on an asymptotics that assumes $\left|(1, l_1, a_0)\, \psi_1^\dagger\right| > \sigma > 0$ and thus inference based on Wald intervals and asymptotic normality should be trustworthy. The governing idea is that we not worry about values of $\psi^\dagger$ that are incompatible with the data.

Indeed I believe a successful strategy with a potential for enormous savings in computing time is as follows. Compute the closed form estimate $\widetilde{\psi}$ and then the locally efficient one step update $\widetilde{\psi}^{(1)}$ of Section 4.2 and use $\widetilde{\psi}^{(1)}$ to center a Wald intervsal $C_{Wald-onestep}(1 - \alpha)$. Compute the fraction $p_{Wald-onestep}$ of the $H_{m,i}$ that exceed 1 but now using the easy to compute $C_{Wald-onestep}(1 - \alpha)$ in place of the hard to compute $C_{op}(1 - \alpha)$. Then base inferences on usual Wald statistics under the assumption of joint multivariate normality if $p_{Wald-onestep}$ is small. If $p_{Wald-onestep}$ is not small use the methods in Secs 4.3 and 5.1. Since $C_{Wald-onestep}(1 - \alpha)$ differs from $C_{op}(1 - \alpha)$ by at most $O\left(n^{-1/2}\right)$ the hope is that the qualitative sizes of $p_{Wald-onestep}$ and p_{op} will be the same even when p_{op} is large and thus quantitative inferences based on $C_{Wald-onestep}(1 - \alpha)$ are inappropriate. Here is an example where I believe this strategy would save lots of effort.

Suppose we modify our toy model such that L_1 is continuous and real-valued with distribution that is absolutely continuous wrt Lesbegue measure and approximately uniform on $(-5, 5)$. Suppose the true but unknown values of $\psi_{21}^\dagger$ and $\psi_{11}^\dagger$ are 1 and $\psi_{31}^\dagger = 0$ is known to be 0. Then the unknown parameters of our drSNMM model are $\left(\psi_{11}^\dagger, \psi_{21}^\dagger, \psi_0^\dagger\right)$. Thus $(1, L_1, A_0)\, \psi_1^\dagger = 0$ if and only if $\psi_{11}^\dagger + \psi_{21}^\dagger L_1 = 0$. Now the event $L_1 = -\psi_{11}^\dagger/\psi_{21}^\dagger = -1$ has probability zero. Further the event that $\left|\psi_{11}^\dagger + \psi_{21}^\dagger L_1\right| < O\left(n^{-1/2}\right)$ has probability $O\left(n^{-1/2}\right)$. Since $\left(\widetilde{\psi}_1 - \psi_1^\dagger\right) = O\left(n^{-1/2}\right)$, $I\left[(1, l_1, a_0)\, \widetilde{\psi}_1 > 0\right]$ will differ from $I\left[(1, l_1, a_0)\, \psi_1^\dagger > 0\right]$ with probability $O\left(n^{-1/2}\right)$ and as $O\left(n^{-1/2}\right)$ is also the radius of $C_{Wald-onestep}(1 - \alpha)$, we will find that $p_{Wald-onestep}$ is also $O\left(n^{-1/2}\right)$. Thus, with sample size n sufficiently large that the preceding calculations (which depended only on rates and not on constants) are valid approximations, Wald inferences centered on the one step estimator are valid and our diagnostic $p_{Wald-onestep}$ will have revealed this, preventing the need for a more difficult analysis.

A1.2: Locally Degenerate Distribution of a Stochastic Process in Our Toy Example :

Our goal is to show that for $(\psi - \psi^\dagger)$ of $O\left(n^{-1/2}\right)$, $n^{1/2} P_n \left[U_0 \left(\psi_0, s_0, \psi_1 \right) \right] = n^{1/2} P_n \left[U_0 \left(\psi_0^\dagger, s_0, \psi_1^\dagger \right) \right] + \kappa \left(\psi, \psi^\dagger, F_O \right) + o_p(1)$ where the $o_p(1)$ is uniform in F_O. and $\kappa \left(\psi, \psi^\dagger, F_O \right)$ is non-random. First note that if $(1, L_1, A_0) \psi_1$ and $(1, L_1, A_0) \psi_1^\dagger$ are not both positive or both negative, then, by continuity, the function $(1, L_1, A_0) \psi_1$ of ψ_1 has a zero at some point, say $\psi_1^* \left(L_1, A_0, \psi_1, \psi_1^\dagger \right)$, on the line connecting ψ_1 and $\psi_1^\dagger$. Further by $(\psi - \psi^\dagger) = O\left(n^{-1/2}\right)$, $\psi - \psi_1^* \left(L_1, A_0, \psi_1, \psi_1^\dagger \right)$ and $\psi_1^* \left(L_1, A_0, \psi_1, \psi_1^\dagger \right) - \psi^\dagger$ are $O_p\left(n^{-1/2}\right)$ Now from A1.6 we have

$$n^{1/2} P_n \left[U_0 \left(\psi_0, s_0, \psi_1 \right) \right] - n^{1/2} P_n \left[U_0 \left(\psi_0^\dagger, s_0, \psi_1^\dagger \right) \right]$$
$$= n^{1/2} \left(\psi_0 - \psi_0^\dagger \right) P_n \left[A_0 \left\{ s_0 \left(A_0 \right) - E[s_0 \left(A_0 \right)] \right\} \right] + n^{1/2} P_n \left[\Delta_0 \left(s_0, \psi_1, \psi_1^\dagger \right) \right]$$

But

$$n^{1/2} P_n \left[\Delta_0 \left(s_0, \psi_1, \psi_1^\dagger \right) \right]$$
$$= -n^{1/2} P_n \left[\left\{ s_0 \left(A_0 \right) - E[s_0 \left(A_0 \right)] \right\} A_1 \left(1, L_1, A_0 \right) \right] \left(\psi_1 - \psi_1^\dagger \right)$$
$$+ n^{1/2} P_n \left[\Delta_0^* \left(s_0, \psi_1, \psi_1^\dagger \right) \right]$$

where $n^{1/2} \Delta_0^* \left(s_0, \psi_1, \psi_1^\dagger \right) =$
$n^{1/2} \left[\left(I \left[(1, L_1, A_0) \psi_1 > 0 \right] \right) (1, L_1, A_0) \psi_1 - \left(I \left[(1, L_1, A_0) \psi_1^\dagger > 0 \right] \right) (1, L_1, A_0) \psi_1^\dagger \right\} =$
$I \left[(1, L_1, A_0) \psi_1 > 0 \right] I \left[(1, L_1, A_0) \psi_1^\dagger > 0 \right] (1, L_1, A_0) n^{1/2} \left\{ \psi_1 - \psi_1^\dagger \right\} +$
$I \left[(1, L_1, A_0) \psi_1 > 0 \right] I \left[(1, L_1, A_0) \psi_1^\dagger \le 0 \right] (1, L_1, A_0) n^{1/2} \left\{ \psi_1 - \psi_1^* \left(L_1, A_0, \psi_1, \psi_1^\dagger \right) \right\} +$
$I \left[(1, L_1, A_0) \psi_1 \le 0 \right] I \left[(1, L_1, A_0) \psi_1^\dagger > 0 \right] (1, L_1, A_0) n^{1/2} \left\{ \psi_1^* \left(L_1, A_0, \psi_1, \psi_1^\dagger \right) - \psi_1^\dagger \right\}$
is $O_p(1)$.

Thus $P_n \left[n^{1/2} \Delta_0^* \left(s_0, \psi_1, \psi_1^\dagger \right) \right] = E \left[n^{1/2} \Delta_0^* \left(s_0, \psi_1, \psi_1^\dagger \right) \right] + o_p(1)$ by the uniform law of large numbers.

Thus we have proved the claimed result with $\kappa \left(\psi, \psi^\dagger, F_O \right) = E \left[n^{1/2} \Delta_0^* \left(s_0, \psi_1, \psi_1^\dagger \right) \right]$
$+ E \left[A_0 \left\{ s_0 \left(A_0 \right) - E[s_0 \left(A_0 \right)] \right\} \right] n^{1/2} \left(\psi_0 - \psi_0^\dagger \right) -$
$E \left[\left\{ s_0 \left(A_0 \right) - E[s_0 \left(A_0 \right)] \right\} A_1 \left(1, L_1, A_0 \right) \right] n^{1/2} \left(\psi_1 - \psi_1^\dagger \right)$

Consider the special case where F_O is an exceptional law so $(1, L_1, A_0) \psi_1^\dagger = 0$. Assume as above, $(1, L_1, A_0) \psi_1^\dagger = 0 \Leftrightarrow L_1 = A_0 = 1$. Then $E\left[n^{1/2}\Delta_0^* \left(s_0, \psi_1, \psi_1^\dagger\right)\right]$

$$E\left\{ \begin{array}{l} I\left[\sum_j \psi_{j1} > 0\right] E\left[L_1 A_0 \left(1, L_1, A_0\right)\right] + \\ E\left[\{1 - L_1 A_0\} I\left[\left(1, L_1, A_0\right)\psi_1^\dagger > 0\right]\left(1, L_1, A_0\right)\right] \end{array} \right\} n^{1/2}\left\{\psi_1 - \psi_1^\dagger\right\}.$$

Thus $\partial E\left[U_0\left(\psi_0, s_0, \psi_1\right)\right]/\partial\psi_1^T = DER_{01}\left(\psi\right) =$

$$E\left\{ \begin{array}{l} I\left[\sum_j \psi_{j1} > 0\right] E\left[L_1 A_0 \left(1, L_1, A_0\right)\right] + \\ E\left[\{1 - L_1 A_0\} I\left[\left(1, L_1, A_0\right)\psi_1^\dagger > 0\right]\left(1, L_1, A_0\right)\right] \end{array} \right\}$$

$$-E\left[\{s_0\left(A_0\right) - E[s_0\left(A_0\right)]\} A_1\left(1, L_1, A_0\right)\right]$$

which converges to different limits depending on whether $\sum_j \psi_{j1}$ decreases from above or increases from below to $\sum_j \psi_{j1}^\dagger = 0$ so $DER_{01}\left(\psi^\dagger\right)$ is undefined. Note $\partial E\left[U_0\left(\psi_0, s_0, \widetilde{\psi}_1\right)\right]/\partial\psi_1^T$ will have variance $O\left(1\right)$ since $\sum_j \widetilde{\psi}_{j1}$ takes on both positive and negative values with positive probability as $n \to \infty$.

Even when the data are not generated under an exceptional law so $DER_{01}\left(\psi^\dagger\right)$ exists, the convergence of $DER_{01}\left(\psi\right)$ to $DER_{01}\left(\psi^\dagger\right)$ is non-uniform since, given any sequence $kn^{-1/2}$, there exists at each sample size n, ψ and $\psi^\dagger$ with $\sum_j \psi_{j1}^\dagger$ sufficiently close to 0 and $||\psi - \psi^\dagger|| = kn^{-1/2}$, such that $DER_{01}\left(\psi\right) - DER_{01}\left(\psi^\dagger\right) = O\left(1\right)$ because $\sum_j \psi_{j1}$ and $\sum_j \psi_{j1}^\dagger$ have different signs. However the Lebesgue measure of the set of $\psi^\dagger$ that has this property will decrease as n increases so that posterior associated with a smooth prior (that does not change with sample size) will be quadratic for n large.

11 Appendix 2:

Proof of Lemma 5.1: For some $\psi_2^* \in \left[\psi_2, \widehat{\psi}_2\right]$

$$n^{1/2}P_n\left[U_a\left(\psi_1, \widehat{\psi}_2\right)\right]$$
$$= n^{1/2}P_n\left[U_a\left(\psi_1, \psi_2\right)\right] + n^{1/2}P_n\left[\partial U_a\left(\psi_1, \psi_2\right)/\partial\psi_2\right]\left(\widehat{\psi}_2 - \psi_2\right) +$$
$$n^{1/2}P_n\left[\partial^2 U_a\left(\psi_1, \psi_2^*\right)/\partial^2\psi_2\right]\left(\widehat{\psi}_2 - \psi_2\right)^2$$
$$= n^{1/2}P_n\left[U_a\left(\psi_1, \psi_2\right)\right] + n^{1/2}P_n\left[\partial U_a\left(\psi_1, \psi_2\right)/\partial\psi_2\right]\left(\widehat{\psi}_2 - \psi_2\right) + o_p\left(1\right)$$

Similiarly

$$n^{1/2}P_n\left[U_b\left(\psi_1, \widehat{\psi}_2\right)\right] = n^{1/2}P_n\left[U_b\left(\psi_1, \psi_2\right)\right] +$$
$$n^{1/2}P_n\left[\partial U_b\left(\psi_1, \psi_2\right)/\partial\psi_2\right]\left(\widehat{\psi}_2 - \psi_2\right) + o_p\left(1\right)$$

Also

$$P_n \left[\partial U_a \left(\psi_1, \widehat{\psi}_2\right) / \partial \psi_2\right] \left\{P_n \left[\partial U_b \left(\psi_1, \widehat{\psi}_2\right) / \partial \psi_2\right]\right\}^{-1} n^{1/2} P_n \left[U_b \left(\psi_1, \psi_2\right)\right]$$

$$= P_n \left[\partial U_a \left(\psi_1, \psi_2\right) / \partial \psi_2\right] \left\{P_n \left[\partial U_b \left(\psi_1, \psi_2\right) / \partial \psi_2\right]\right\}^{-1} n^{1/2} P_n \left[U_b \left(\psi_1, \psi_2\right)\right] + o_p(1)$$

Hence,

$$n^{1/2} P_n \left[U_1 \left(\psi_1, \widehat{\psi}_2\right)\right] - n^{1/2} P_n \left[U_1 \left(\psi_1, \psi_2\right)\right]$$

$$= n^{1/2} P_n \left[\partial U_a \left(\psi_1, \psi_2\right) / \partial \psi_2\right] \left(\widehat{\psi}_2 - \psi_2\right) -$$

$$P_n \left[\partial U_a \left(\psi_1, \widehat{\psi}_2\right) / \partial \psi_2\right] \left\{P_n \left[\partial U_b \left(\psi_1, \widehat{\psi}_2\right) / \partial \psi_2\right]\right\}^{-1} n^{1/2} \times$$

$$P_n \left[\partial U_b \left(\psi_1, \psi_2\right) / \partial \psi_2\right] \left(\widehat{\psi}_2 - \psi_2\right) + o_p(1)$$

$$= n^{1/2} P_n \left[\partial U_a \left(\psi_1, \psi_2\right) / \partial \psi_2\right] \left(\widehat{\psi}_2 - \psi_2\right)$$

$$- P_n \left[\partial U_a \left(\psi_1, \psi_2\right) / \partial \psi_2\right] \left\{P_n \left[\partial U_b \left(\psi_1, \psi_2\right) / \partial \psi_2\right]\right\}^{-1} n^{1/2} \times$$

$$P_n \left[\partial U_b \left(\psi_1, \psi_2\right) / \partial \psi_2\right] \left(\widehat{\psi}_2 - \psi_2\right) + o_p(1)$$

$$= o_p(1)$$

12 Appendix 3:

Proof of Theorem 7.1: $\Leftarrow$ By induction in reverse time order.

Case 1: $m = K$. Let $a_K = d_K \left(\overline{L}_K, \overline{A}_{K-1}\right)$. Then $E \left[Y_{\overline{A}_{K-1}, a_K} | \overline{L}_K, \overline{A}_{K-1}\right] =$

$E \left[Y_{\overline{A}_{K-1}, a_K} | \overline{L}_K, \overline{A}_{K-1}, A_K = a_K\right] f \left(a_K | \overline{L}_K, \overline{A}_{K-1}\right) +$

$\left\{1 - f \left(a_K | \overline{L}_K, \overline{A}_{K-1}\right)\right\} E \left[Y_{\overline{A}_{K-1}, a_K} | \overline{L}_K, \overline{A}_{K-1}, A_k \neq a_K\right]$

$= \left\{E \left[Y_{\overline{A}_{K-1}, d_K^*} | \overline{L}_K, \overline{A}_{K-1}, A_K = a_K\right] + \gamma^{\overline{d}, \overline{d}^*} \left(\overline{L}_K, \overline{A}_{K-1}, a_K\right)\right\} \times$

$f \left(a_K | \overline{L}_K, \overline{A}_{K-1}\right) + \left\{1 - f \left(a_K | \overline{L}_K, \overline{A}_{K-1}\right)\right\} \times$

$\left\{E \left[Y_{\overline{A}_{K-1}, d_K^*} | \overline{L}_K, \overline{A}_{K-1}, A_K \neq a_K\right] + \gamma^{\overline{d}, \overline{d}^*} \left(\overline{L}_K, \overline{A}_{K-1}, a_K\right) - r^{\underline{d}_K, d_K^*} \left(\overline{L}_K, \overline{A}_{K-1}\right)\right\}$

$= E \left[Y_{\overline{A}_{K-1}, d_K^*} | \overline{L}_K, \overline{A}_{K-1}\right] + \gamma^{\overline{d}, \overline{d}^*} \left(\overline{L}_K, \overline{A}_{K-1}, a_K\right) -$

$\left\{1 - f \left(a_K | \overline{L}_K, \overline{A}_{K-1}\right)\right\} r^{\underline{d}_K, d_K^*} \left(\overline{L}_K, \overline{A}_{K-1}\right)$

$= E \left\{E \left[Y_{\overline{A}_{K-1}, A_K} - \gamma^{\overline{d}, \overline{d}^*} \left(\overline{L}_K, \overline{A}_K\right) | \overline{L}_K, \overline{A}_{K-1}, A_K\right] | \overline{L}_K, \overline{A}_{K-1}\right\} -$

$\left\{1 - f \left(a_K | \overline{L}_K, \overline{A}_{K-1}\right)\right\} r^{\underline{d}_K, d_K^*} \left(\overline{L}_K, \overline{A}_{K-1}\right) = E \left[H_K \left(\gamma^{\overline{d}, \overline{d}^*}\right) | \overline{L}_K, \overline{A}_{K-1}\right]$

where the first equality is by the law of total probability, the second by the definition of $\gamma^{\overline{d}, \overline{d}^*} \left(\overline{L}_K, \overline{A}_{K-1}, a_K\right)$ and $r^{\underline{d}_m, d_m^*} \left(\overline{L}_K, \overline{A}_{K-1}\right)$, the third by the law of total probability, the fourth by the definition of $\gamma^{\bar{d},\bar{d}^*}\left(\overline{L}_K,\overline{A}_K\right)$, and the 5th by the definition of $H_K\left(\gamma^{\bar{d},\bar{d}^*}\right)$.

Case 2: $m < K$. Let $a_m = d_m\left(\overline{L}_m,\overline{A}_{m-1}\right)$.

Then $E\left[Y_{\overline{A}_{m-1},a_m,\underline{d}_{m+1}}|\overline{L}_m,\overline{A}_{m-1}\right]$

$= E\left[Y_{\overline{A}_{m-1},a_m,\underline{d}_{m+1}}|\overline{L}_m,\overline{A}_{m-1},A_m = a_m\right]f\left(a_m|\overline{L}_m,\overline{A}_{m-1}\right)$

$+ \left\{1 - f\left(a_m|\overline{L}_m,\overline{A}_{m-1}\right)\right\}E\left[Y_{\overline{A}_{m-1},a_m,\underline{d}_{m+1}}|\overline{L}_m,\overline{A}_{m-1},A_m \neq a_m\right]$

$= \left\{E\left[Y_{\overline{A}_{m-1},d_m^*,\underline{d}_{m+1}}|\overline{L}_m,\overline{A}_{m-1},A_m = a_m\right] + \gamma^{\bar{d},\bar{d}^*}\left(\overline{L}_m,\overline{A}_{m-1},a_m\right)\right\} \times$

$f\left(a_m|\overline{L}_m,\overline{A}_{m-1}\right) + \left\{1 - f\left(a_m|\overline{L}_m,\overline{A}_{m-1}\right)\right\} \times$

$\left\{E\left[Y_{\overline{A}_{m-1},d_m^*,\underline{d}_{m+1}}|\overline{L}_m,\overline{A}_{m-1},A_m \neq a_m\right] + \gamma^{\bar{d},\bar{d}^*}\left(\overline{L}_m,\overline{A}_{m-1},a_m\right)\right.$

$\left. - r^{\underline{d}_m,d_m^*}\left(\overline{L}_m,\overline{A}_{m-1}\right)\right\}$

$= E\left[Y_{\overline{A}_{m-1},d_m^*,\underline{d}_{m+1}}|\overline{L}_m,\overline{A}_{m-1}\right] + \gamma^{\bar{d},\bar{d}^*}\left(\overline{L}_m,\overline{A}_{m-1},a_m\right) -$

$\left\{1 - f\left(a_m|\overline{L}_m,\overline{A}_{m-1}\right)\right\}r^{\underline{d}_m,d_m^*}\left(\overline{L}_m,\overline{A}_{m-1}\right) =$

$$E\left\{E\left[Y_{\overline{A}_{m-1},A_m,\underline{d}_{m+1}} - \gamma^{\bar{d},\bar{d}^*}\left(\overline{L}_m,\overline{A}_m\right)|\overline{L}_m,\overline{A}_{m-1},A_m\right]|\overline{L}_m,\overline{A}_{m-1}\right\}$$

(A3.1)

$- \left\{1 - f\left(a_m|\overline{L}_m,\overline{A}_{m-1}\right)\right\}r^{\underline{d}_m,d_m^*}\left(\overline{L}_m,\overline{A}_{m-1}\right)$

where the first equality is by the law of total probability, the second by the definition of $\gamma^{\bar{d},\bar{d}^*}\left(\overline{L}_m,\overline{A}_{m-1},a_m\right)$ and $r^{\underline{d}_m,d_m^*}\left(\overline{L}_m,\overline{A}_{m-1}\right)$, and the third by the law of total probability, the fourth by the definition of $\gamma^{\bar{d},\bar{d}^*}\left(\overline{L}_m,\overline{A}_m\right)$.

But $E\left[Y_{\overline{A}_{m-1},A_m,\underline{d}_{m+1}} - \gamma^{\bar{d},\bar{d}^*}\left(\overline{L}_m,\overline{A}_m\right)|\overline{L}_m,\overline{A}_{m-1},A_m\right]$

$= \int E\left[Y_{\overline{A}_{m-1},A_m,\underline{d}_{m+1}}|\overline{L}_{m+1},\overline{A}_{m-1},A_m\right]dF\left(L_{m+1}|\overline{L}_m,\overline{A}_m\right) - \gamma^{\bar{d},\bar{d}^*}\left(\overline{L}_m,\overline{A}_m\right)$

$= \int E\left[H_{m+1}^{\underline{d}_{m+1}}\left(\gamma^{\bar{d},\bar{d}^*}\right)|\overline{L}_{m+1},\overline{A}_m\right]dF\left(L_{m+1}|\overline{L}_m,\overline{A}_m,\right) - \gamma^{\bar{d},\bar{d}^*}\left(\overline{L}_m,\overline{A}_m\right)$

$= E\left[H_{m+1}^{\underline{d}_{m+1}}\left(\gamma^{\bar{d},\bar{d}^*}\right)|\overline{L}_m,\overline{A}_m\right] - \gamma^{\bar{d},\bar{d}^*}\left(\overline{L}_m,\overline{A}_m\right)$ where the first equality is by the law of total probability, the second by the induction hypothesis, and the last by the definition of $H_{m+1}^{\underline{d}_{m+1}}\left(\gamma^{\bar{d},\bar{d}^*}\right)$. We complete the proof by plugging this last expression back into (A3.1)

$\Rightarrow$ By contradiction. Let m^* be the largest value of m such that $\Delta\left(\overline{L}_m,\overline{A}_m\right) \equiv \gamma^{\bar{d}^**}\left(\overline{L}_m,\overline{A}_m\right) - \gamma^{\bar{d},\bar{d}^*}\left(\overline{L}_m,\overline{A}_m\right)$ is a function of A_m with positive probability. By the assumption that $\gamma^{\bar{d}^**}\left(\overline{L}_m,\overline{A}_m\right) = 0$ if $A_m = 0$, we are guaranteed that $m^* \geq 0$. It follows that $0 = E\left[H_{m^*}^{\underline{d}_{m^*}}\left(\gamma^{\bar{d},\bar{d}^*}\right)|\overline{L}_{m^*},\overline{A}_{m^*}\right]$ but $E\left[H_{m^*}^{\underline{d}_{m^*}}\left(\gamma^{\bar{d}^*}\right)|\overline{L}_{m^*},\overline{A}_{m^*}\right] = \gamma^{\bar{d}^**}\left(\overline{L}_{m^*},\overline{A}_{m^*}\right) - \gamma^{\bar{d},\bar{d}^*}\left(\overline{L}_{m^*},\overline{A}_{m^*}\right) \neq 0$ w.p1.

Corollary A3.1: $E\left[H_m^{\underline{d}_m}\left(\gamma^{\bar{d},\bar{d}^*}\right) - \gamma^{\bar{d},\bar{d}^*}\left(\overline{L}_{m-1},\overline{A}_{m-1}\right)|\overline{L}_{m-1},\overline{A}_{m-1}\right] =$

$E\left[Y_{\overline{A}_{m-2},d_m^*,\underline{d}_m}|\overline{L}_{m-1},\overline{A}_{m-1}\right].$

Proof: $E\left[H_m^{\underline{d}_m}\left(\gamma^{\overline{d},\overline{d}^*}\right) - \gamma^{\overline{d},\overline{d}^*}\left(\overline{L}_{m-1},\overline{A}_{m-1}\right)|\overline{L}_{m-1},\overline{A}_{m-1}\right]$

$= E\left[E\left[Y_{\overline{A}_{m-1},\underline{d}_m}|\overline{L}_m,\overline{A}_{m-1}\right] - \gamma^{\overline{d},\overline{d}^*}\left(\overline{L}_{m-1},\overline{A}_{m-1}\right)|\overline{L}_{m-1},\overline{A}_{m-1}\right]$

$= E\left[Y_{\overline{A}_{m-1},\underline{d}_m} - \gamma^{\overline{d},\overline{d}^*}\left(\overline{L}_{m-1},\overline{A}_{m-1}\right)|\overline{L}_{m-1},\overline{A}_{m-1}\right]$

$= E\left[Y_{\overline{A}_{m-2},d_m^*,\underline{d}_m}|\overline{L}_{m-1},\overline{A}_{m-1}\right]$

where the 1st equality is by theorem 7.1, the second by the law of total probability, and the third by the definition of $\gamma^{\overline{d},\overline{d}^*}\left(\overline{L}_{m-1},\overline{A}_{m-1}\right)$.

Proof of Theorem 7.2:

$\Leftarrow E\left[H_m^{\underline{d}_m}\left(\gamma^{\overline{d},\overline{d}^*}\right) - \gamma^{\overline{d},\overline{d}^*}\left(\overline{L}_{m-1},\overline{A}_{m-1}\right) - q^{\overline{d},\overline{d}^*}\left(\overline{L}_{m-1},\overline{A}_{m-1}\right)|\overline{L}_{m-1},\overline{A}_{m-1}\right]$

$= E\left[Y_{\overline{A}_{m-2},d_m^*,\underline{d}_m} - q^{\overline{d},\overline{d}^*}\left(\overline{L}_{m-1},\overline{A}_{m-1}\right)|\overline{L}_{m-1},\overline{A}_{m-1}\right] =$

$E\left[Y_{\overline{A}_{m-2},d_m^*,\underline{d}_m}|\overline{L}_{m-1},\overline{A}_{m-2},A_{m-1}=0\right]$ where the 1st equality is by Corollary A.1 and the second by the definition of $q^{\overline{d},\overline{d}^*}\left(\overline{L}_{m-1},\overline{A}_{m-1}\right)$.

$\Rightarrow$trivial

Proof of Theorem 7.4:$\Leftarrow$By induction

Case 1: $m = K$: Trivial since $Y_{\overline{A}_{m-1},a_m,\underline{d}_{m+1}}$ does not depend on $\underline{d}_{m+1}$.

Case 2: Assume it is true for $m + 1$ and we shall prove it for m. By the induction hypothesis for $\underline{d}_{m+1} \in \mathcal{D}_{m+1}$

$$E\left[Y_{\overline{A}_{m-1},a_m,\underline{d}_{op,m+1}} - Y_{\overline{A}_{m-1},a_m,\underline{d}_{m+1}}|\overline{L}_{m+1},\overline{A}_{m-1},A_m=a_m\right] \geq 0$$

Thus $E\left[Y_{\overline{A}_{m-1},a_m,\underline{d}_{op,m+1}} - Y_{\overline{A}_{m-1},a_m,\underline{d}_{m+1}}|\overline{L}_m,\overline{A}_{m-1},A_m=a_m\right] \geq 0$ after integrating over L_{m+1}. By the backward induction feasibility assumption this implies $E\left[Y_{\overline{A}_{m-1},a_m,\underline{d}_{op,m+1}} - Y_{\overline{A}_{m-1},a_m,\underline{d}_{m+1}}|\overline{L}_m,\overline{A}_{m-1}\right] \geq 0$. Hence since $d_{op,m}\left(\overline{L}_m,\overline{A}_{m-1}\right) = \arg\max_{a_m\in A_m} E\left[Y_{\overline{A}_{m-1},a_m,\underline{d}_{op,m+1}}|\overline{L}_m,\overline{A}_{m-1}\right]$, we conclude that $\underline{d}_{op,m}$ maximizes $E\left[Y_{\overline{A}_{m-1},\underline{d}_m}|\overline{L}_m,\overline{A}_{m-1}\right]$ over all regimes $\underline{d}_m \in \mathcal{D}_m$. The proof in the other direction is trivial.

Bibliography:

Baraud, Y. (2002). Confidence balls in Gaussian regression, (to appear).

Bertsekas, D.P. and Tsitsiklis, J.N. (1996). *Neuro-dynamic programming*. Belmont MA: Athena Scientific.

Bickel, P.J. and Ritov, Y. (1988). Estimating integrated squared density derivatives: sharp best order of convergence estimates. *Sankya Ser.*A 50: 381-393.

Bickel, P.J., Klaassen, C., Ritov, Y., and Wellner, J. (1993). Efficient and adapted estimation for semiparametric models. Johns Hopkins, Baltimore.

Cowell, R.G., Dawid, A.P., Lauritzen, S.L, and Spiegelhalter, D.J. (1999). Probabilistic networks in expert systems, New York: Springer-Verlag.

Donald, S.G. and Newey, W.K. (1994). Series estimation of the semilinear models. Journal of Multivariate Analysis, 5): 30-40.

Gill, R.D. and Robins, J.M. (2001). Causal inference for complex longitudinal data: the continuous case. *Annals of Statistics*, 29(6): 1785-1811

Hoffman, M. and Lepski, O. (2002). Random rates and anisotropic regression (with discussion and rejoinder). Annals of Statistics, 30: 325-396.

Li, KC. (1989). Honest Confidence Regions for Nonparametric Regression. The Annals of Statistics, 17(3):1001-1008.

Laurent, B. (1996). Efficient estimation of integral functionals of a density. Annals of Statistics, 24(2): 659 -681.

Laurent, B. and Massart, P. (2000). Adaptive estimation of a quadratic functional by model selection. *Annals of Statistics*, 28(5): 1302-1338.

Murphy, Susan. (2003). Optimal dynamic treatment regimes. *Journal of the Royal Statistical Society B*, 65(2):331-355.

Ritov, Y. and Bickel, P. (1990) Achieving information bounds in non- and semi- parametric models. Annals of Statistics, 18: 925-938.

Robins, J.M. (1986). A new approach to causal inference in mortality studies with sustained exposure periods - Application to control of the healthy worker survivor effect. *Mathematical Modelling*, 7:1393-1512

Robins, J.M. (1994). Correcting for non-compliance in randomized trials using structural nested mean models. *Communications in Statistics*, 23:2379-2412.

Robins, J.M. (1997). Causal Inference from Complex Longitudinal Data. Latent Variable Modeling and Applications to Causality. *Lecture Notes in Statistics* (120), M. Berkane, Editor. NY: Springer Verlag, pp. 69-117.

Robins, J.M. (1998a). Correction for non-compliance in equivalence trials. *Statistics in Medicine,* 17:269-302.

Robins, J.M., (1998b) Structural nested failure time models. **Survival Analysis,** P.K. Anderson and N. Keiding, Section Editors. *The Encyclopedia of Biostatistics.* P. Armitage and T. Colton, Editors. Chichester, UK: John Wiley & Sons. pp 4372-4389.

Robins, J.M. (1999). Marginal Structural Models versus Structural Nested Models as Tools for Causal Inference. *Statistical Models in Epidemiology: The Environment and Clinical Trials.* M.E. Halloran and D. Berry, Editors, IMA Volume 116, NY: Springer-Verlag, pp. 95-134.

Robins, J.M. (2000). Robust estimation in sequentially ignorable missing data and causal inference models. *Proceedings of the American Statistical Association Section on Bayesian Statistical Science* 1999, pp. 6-10.

Robins, J.M., Greenland, S. and Hu F-C. (1999). Rejoinder to Comments on "Estimation of the causal effect of a time-varying exposure on the marginal mean of a repeated binary outcome." *Journal of the American Statistical Association, Applications and Case Studies,* 94:708-712.

Robins, J.M. and Ritov, Y. (1997). Toward a curse of dimensionality appropriate (CODA) asymptotic theory for semi-parametric models. *Statistics in Medicine,* 16:285-319.

Robins J.M. and Rotnitzky A. (2001). Comment on the Bickel and Kwon article, "Inference for semiparametric models: Some questions and an answer" *Statistica Sinica*, 11(4):920-936. ["On Double Robustness."]

Robins, J.M. and Rotnitzky, A. (2003). Direct effects structural nested mean models. *Annals of Statistics*, (under review).

Robins, J.M., Rotnitzky, A. and Scharfstein, D. (1999a). Sensitivity Analysis for Selection Bias and Unmeasured Confounding in Missing Data and Causal Inference Models. In: *Statistical Models in Epidemiology: The Environment and Clinical Trials*. Halloran, E. and Berry, D., eds. IMA Volume 116, NY: Springer-Verlag, pp. 1-92.

Robins J.M., Rotnitzky A., van der Laan M. (2000). Comment on "On Profile Likelihood" by Murphy SA and van der Vaart AW. *Journal of the American Statistical Association – Theory and Methods*, 95(450):431-435.

Robins, J.M., Scheines, R., Spirtes, P., and Wasserman, L.(2003).Uniform consistency in causal inference. Biometrika, 90(3):491-515.

Robins, J.M. and Wasserman L. (1997). Estimation of Effects of Sequential Treatments by Reparameterizing Directed Acyclic Graphs. Proceedings of the Thirteenth Conference on Uncertainty in Artificial Intelligence, Providence Rhode Island, August 1-3, 1997. Dan Geiger and Prakash Shenoy (Eds.), Morgan Kaufmann, San Francisco, pp. 409-420.

Robins, J.M. and van der Vaart, A.W. (2003). Non parametric confidence sets by cross-validation. (Technical Report).

Robins, J.M. and van der Vaart, A.W. (2004). A unified approach to estimation in non-semiparametric models using higher order influence functions. (Technical Report)

Small, C.G. and McLeish, D. (1994). Hilbert space methods in probability and statistical inference. New York: Wiley.

Sutton, R.S. and Barto, A.G. (1998). Reinforcement learning: An introduction. Cambridge, MA: MIT Press.

van der Laan, M. and Dudoit (2003) Asymptotics of cross-validated risk estimation in model selection and performance assessment, revised for publication in Annals of Statistics.

van der Laan, M.J., Murphy, S., and Robins, J.M. (2003). Marginal structural nested models. (to be submitted).

van der Laan M.J., Robins JM (1998). Locally efficient estimation with current status data and time-dependent covariates. *Journal of the American Statistical Association*, 93:693-701.

van der Laan, M. and Robins, J.M. (2002). *Unified methods for censored longitudinal data and causality*. Springer-Verlag.

van der Vaart, A.W. (1991). On differentiable functionals. Annals of Statistics, 19:178-204.

Waterman, R.P. and Lindsay, B.G. (1996). Projected score methods for approximating conditional scores. *Biometrika*, 83(1): 1-13.

Wegkamp, M. (2003) Model selection in nonparametric regression. *Annals of Statistics*, 31(1):252-273.

Acknowledgements: I would like to thank Thomas Richardson for his very careful reading of the manuscript and many helpful suggestions, Andrea Rotnitzky for useful discussions, and Aad van der Vaart for his codevelopment of an important part of the statistical methodology used in this paper. This methodology is described in detail in our joint papers. This work was supported in part by NIH grant A1-32475.

Addresses for Contact Authors
(in the same order as the papers)

Norman Breslow
Department of Biostatistics
University of Washington
School of Public Health and Community Medicine
Box 357232
Seattle, WA 98195, U.S.A.
email: norm@u.washington.edu

Raymond J. Carroll
Department of Statistics
447 Blocker Building
Texas A&M University
College Station, TX 77843-3143, U.S.A.
email: carroll@stat.tamu.edu

Roderick J. A. Little
Department of Biostatistics
University of Michigan
1420 Washington Heights, M4045
Ann Arbor, MI 48109-2029, U.S.A.
email: rlittle@umich.edu

Lee-Jen Wei
Department of Biostatistics
Harvard School of Public Health
655 Huntington Avenue
Boston, MA 02115, U.S.A.
email: wei@hsph.harvard.edu

Ziding Feng
Fred Hutchinson Cancer Research Center
1100 Fairview Ave. N., MP 859
P. O. Box 19024
Seattle, WA 98109, U.S.A.
email: zfeng@fhcrc.org

Bruce W. Turnbull
School of Operations Research and Industrial Engineering
Cornell University
227 Rhodes Hall
Ithaca, NY 14853, U.S.A.
email: turnbull@orie.cornell.edu

David Oakes
Department of Biostatistics
University of Rochester Medical Center
601 Elmwood Avenue, Box 630
Rochester, NY 14642, U.S.A.
email: oakes@bst.rochester.edu

Ross L. Prentice
Program in Biostatistics
Division of Public Health Sciences
Fred Hutchinson Cancer Research Center
1100 Fairview Ave. N., M3-A410
PO Box 19024
Seattle, WA 98109, U.S.A.
email: rprentic@whi.org

Jon A. Wellner
Department of Statistics, Box 354322
University of Washington
Seattle, WA 98195, U.S.A.
email: jaw@stat.washington.edu

Mitchell H. Gail
Division of Cancer Epidemiology and Genetics
National Cancer Institute
Executive Plaza South, Room 8032
Bethesda, MD 20892, U. S. A.
email: gailm@mail.nih.gov

James Robins
Department of Epidemiology
Kresge Building, Room 823
677 Huntington Avenue
Boston, MA 02115, U. S. A.
email: robins@hsph.harvard.edu

List of Referees
(in alphabetical order)

Rebecca Betensky, *Harvard University*
Norman Breslow, *University of Washington*
Babette Brumback, *University of Washington*
Raymond Carroll, *Texas A&M University*
Scott Emerson, *University of Washington*
Ziding Feng, *Fred Hutchinson Cancer Research Center*
Mitchell Gail, *National Cancer Institute*
Patrick Heagerty, *University of Washington*
Li Hsu, *Fred Hutchinson Cancer Research Center*
Sin-Ho Jung, *Duke University*
Kathleen Kerr, *University of Washington*
Michal Kulich, *University of Washington*
Danyu Lin, *University of North Carolina*
Xihong Lin, *University of Michigan*
Roderick Little, *University of Michigan*
Thomas Lumley, *University of Washington*
Amita Manatunga, *Emory University*
Stephanie Monks, *University of Washington*
David Oakes, *University of Rochester*
Robert Platt, *McGill University*
Ross Prentice, *Fred Hutchinson Cancer Research Center*
James Robins, *Harvard University*
Jianguo Sun, *University of Missouri*
Bruce Turnbull, *Cornell University*
Ching-Yun Wang, *Fred Hutchinson Cancer Research Center*
Jonathan Wakefield, *University of Washington*
Jon Wellner, *University of Washington*

Lecture Notes in Statistics

For information about Volumes 1 to 126, please contact Springer-Verlag

155: Leon Willenborg and Ton de Waal, Elements of Statistical Disclosure Control. xvii, 289 pp., 2000.

156: Gordon Willmot and X. Sheldon Lin, Lundberg Approximations for Compound Distributions with Insurance Applications. xi, 272 pp., 2000.

157: Anne Boomsma, Marijtje A.J. van Duijn, and Tom A.B. Snijders (Editors), Essays on Item Response Theory. xv, 448 pp., 2000.

158: Dominique Ladiray and Benoît Quenneville, Seasonal Adjustment with the X-11 Method. xxii, 220 pp., 2001.

159: Marc Moore (Editor), Spatial Statistics: Methodological Aspects and Some Applications. xvi, 282 pp., 2001.

160: Tomasz Rychlik, Projecting Statistical Functionals. viii, 184 pp., 2001.

161: Maarten Jansen, Noise Reduction by Wavelet Thresholding. xxii, 224 pp., 2001.

162: Constantine Gatsonis, Bradley Carlin, Alicia Carriquiry, Andrew Gelman, Robert E. Kass Isabella Verdinelli, and Mike West (Editors), Case Studies in Bayesian Statistics, Volume V. xiv, 448 pp., 2001.

163: Erkki P. Liski, Nripes K. Mandal, Kirti R. Shah, and Bikas K. Sinha, Topics in Optimal Design. xii, 164 pp., 2002.

164: Peter Goos, The Optimal Design of Blocked and Split-Plot Experiments. xiv, 244 pp., 2002.

165: Karl Mosler, Multivariate Dispersion, Central Regions and Depth: The Lift Zonoid Approach. xii, 280 pp., 2002.

166: Hira L. Koul, Weighted Empirical Processes in Dynamic Nonlinear Models, Second Edition. xiii, 425 pp., 2002.

167: Constantine Gatsonis, Alicia Carriquiry, Andrew Gelman, David Higdon, Robert E. Kass, Donna Pauler, and Isabella Verdinelli (Editors), Case Studies in Bayesian Statistics, Volume VI. xiv, 376 pp., 2002.

168: Susanne Rässler, Statistical Matching: A Frequentist Theory, Practical Applications and Alternative Bayesian Approaches. xviii, 238 pp., 2002.

169: Yu. I. Ingster and Irina A. Suslina, Nonparametric Goodness-of-Fit Testing Under Gaussian Models. xiv, 453 pp., 2003.

170: Tadeusz Caliński and Sanpei Kageyama, Block Designs: A Randomization Approach, Volume II: Design. xii, 351 pp., 2003.

171: D.D. Denison, M.H. Hansen, C.C. Holmes, B. Mallick, B. Yu (Editors), Nonlinear Estimation and Classification. x, 474 pp., 2002.

172: Sneh Gulati, William J. Padgett, Parametric and Nonparametric Inference from Record-Breaking Data. ix, 112 pp., 2002.

173: Jesper Møller (Editor), Spatial Statistics and Computational Methods. xi, 214 pp., 2002.

174: Yasuko Chikuse, Statistics on Special Manifolds. xi, 418 pp., 2002.

175: Jürgen Gross, Linear Regression. xiv, 394 pp., 2003.

176: Zehua Chen, Zhidong Bai, Bimal K. Sinha, Ranked Set Sampling: Theory and Applications. xii, 224 pp., 2003

177: Caitlin Buck and Andrew Millard (Editors), Tools for Constructing Chronologies: Crossing Disciplinary Boundaries, xvi, 263 pp., 2004

178: Gauri Sankar Datta and Rahul Mukerjee , Probability Matching Priors: Higher Order Asymptotics, x, 144 pp., 2004

179: D.Y. Lin and P.J. Heagerty , Proceedings of the Second Seattle Symposium in Biostatistics: Analysis of Correlated Data, vii, 336 pp., 2004

180: Yanhong Wu, Inference for Change-Point and Post-Change Means After a CUSUM Test, xiv, 176 pp., 2004

181: Daniel Straumann, Estimation in Conditionally Heteroscedastic Time Series Models , x, 250 pp., 2004